The Antibody Molecule

IMMUNOLOGY

*An International Series of Monographs
and Treatises*

EDITED BY

F. J. DIXON, JR.
*Division of Experimental Pathology
Scripps Clinic and Research Foundation
La Jolla, California*

HENRY G. KUNKEL
*The Rockefeller University
New York, New York*

The Antibody Molecule

ALFRED NISONOFF

Department of Biological Chemistry
University of Illinois at the Medical Center
Chicago, Illinois

JOHN E. HOPPER

Department of Medicine
Pritzker School of Medicine
The University of Chicago
Chicago, Illinois

SUSAN B. SPRING

Laboratory of Infectious Diseases
National Institutes of Health
Bethesda, Maryland

Academic Press   New York   San Francisco   London   1975
A Subsidiary of Harcourt Brace Jovanovich, Publishers

ACADEMIC PRESS, INC.
111 Fifth Avenue, New York, New York 10003

United Kingdom Edition published by
ACADEMIC PRESS, INC. (LONDON) LTD.
24/28 Oval Road, London NW1

Library of Congress Cataloging in Publication Data

Nisonoff, Alfred.
        The antibody molecule.

        (Monographs in immunology)
        Includes bibliographical references and index.
        1.   Immunoglobulins.   I.   Hopper, John E. joint
author.   II.   Spring, Susan B., joint author.
III.   Title.   [DNLM: 1.   Antibodies.   2.   Immunoglobu-
lins.   QW570 N725a]
QR186.7.N57   599'.02'93   74-17989
ISBN 0–12–519950–3

Contents

3 HUMAN IMMUNOGLOBULINS

4 AMINO ACID SEQUENCES IN HUMAN IMMUNOGLOBULINS AND IN MOUSE LIGHT CHAINS

5 THE THREE-DIMENSIONAL STRUCTURE OF IMMUNOGLOBULINS

6 PROPERTIES AND INTERACTIONS OF THE LIGHT AND HEAVY CHAINS OF IMMUNOGLOBULINS

7 EVOLUTION OF THE IMMUNOGLOBULINS

8 IMMUNOGLOBULINS OF THE RABBIT, MOUSE, GUINEA PIG, AND HORSE

11 IDIOTYPIC SPECIFICITIES OF IMMUNOGLOBULINS

12 THEORIES OF THE GENETIC CONTROL OF DIVERSITY OF ANTIBODIES

Preface

Sixteen years ago little was known about the structure of an antibody molecule. Hydrodynamic measurements and electron microscopy had indicated that IgG is an elongated, flexible molecule, with antigen-binding sites located at its ends. Studies of amino acid sequences were hampered by the heterogeneity of an antibody population, by the (then unknown) multichain structure of the molecule, and by the fact that some immunoglobulin polypeptide chains do not possess a free terminal amino group. Starting in 1958 and 1959, parallel investigations initiated in the laboratories of Porter and Edelman elucidated the multichain structure of the molecule, the topological arrangement of the light and heavy chains in space, and the relationship of fragments released by proteolytic enzymes to the polypeptide chains. The demonstration by Edelman and Gally that Bence Jones proteins are light chains identical to those of the myeloma protein of the same patient plus Putnam's recognition of a relationship between the peptide maps of Bence Jones proteins and normal light chains set the stage for a thorough investigation of monoclonal proteins. This rapidly led to a delineation of classes and subclasses of immunoglobulins and of their genetic variants. A major contribution was made by Kunkel and his associates who utilized myeloma and other monoclonal proteins to study exhaustively the properties and genetic control of human immunoglobulins. This work was greatly facilitated by an awareness of allotypy discovered earlier by Oudin and by Grubb. The artificial induction of numerous plasmacytomas in mice, principally by Michael Potter, permitted parallel approaches to the study of immunoglobulins in that species. During this period the structural relationships among the immunoglobulins present in all vertebrates and the pattern of evolution of the immunoglobulin classes were extensively investigated.

The demonstration by Hilschmann and Craig in 1965 that there are contiguous variable and constant segments in a light chain clearly established the structural basis of antibody specificity, validated the use of monoclonal immunoglobulins associated with lymphoproliferative disease as a source of information on the patterns of sequences in normal immunoglobulins, and eventually led to the concept that separate genes encode the variable and constant portions of a heavy or light chain. The control of a single polypeptide chain by two structural genes is a phenomenon which is encountered very infrequently.

Crystallization of the Fab fragments of myeloma proteins and of Bence Jones proteins was followed by the detailed X-ray crystallographic analyses of Poljak, Davies, Edmundson, Huber, and their co-workers. This work yielded a three-dimensional outline of that segment of the molecule which contains the combining site, and crystallographic models of this region at the atomic level are now available. These provide intimate details of the folding of the polypeptide chains and the structure of the antibody-combining site and some information as to the nature of the antigen–antibody bond.

Fundamental questions remain unresolved. A wealth of data on amino acid sequences, acquired in the laboratories of Milstein, Hood, Hilschmann, and others, has failed to establish whether variability in sequence is solely a consequence of mutations occurring over evolutionary time, or whether somatic mutation takes place during the lifetime of the individual. A related, unanswered question is the basis of the hypervariability of certain segments of both heavy and light chains. The availability of homogeneous antibodies and myeloma proteins with antibody activity has made it possible to explore the relationship between the nature of the amino acid side chains in hypervariable regions and the chemical structure of the antigenic determinant. Important information on this subject should be forthcoming in the next few years.

We do not know, at the atomic level, the exact nature of the physical interactions between antigens of various structures and antibody nor the degree of variability in size and shape of the combining region. The intriguing possibility has been suggested that the antigen-binding site is larger than a typical antigenic determinant and that different regions of the same site can accommodate unrelated determinants. If correct, this would greatly reduce the number of different antibody molecules (and structural genes) required to provide an adequate system. The X-ray crystallographic analyses carried out so far do not exclude this possibility; in fact, the large size of the region containing hypervariable amino acid residues would favor it. Genetic material would also be conserved if unrelated, useful specificities could be generated by the interaction of a given heavy chain with different light chains or vice versa. While this seems rather likely, it remains to be proved.

There is strong evidence to indicate that a single gene controlling variable segments (V regions) of the heavy chain can act in concert with genes controlling the constant regions of the heavy chains of different immunoglobulin classes, thus yielding molecules with identical specificity but belonging to different classes. It seems probable that the interaction takes place at the DNA level and that the V_H gene is capable of translocation. While on a less firm basis, translocation of genes controlling the variable segments of light chains also seems likely. The physical chemical basis of this genetic mechanism is unknown.

Thus, there remain many areas of uncertainty with respect to the genetic control of antibody variability; but it would appear that knowledge of antibody structure is approaching a plateau in the sense that many of the underlying principles have been elucidated. While many details remain to be filled in, the general pattern of structure now seems to have a firm foundation. Although new and significant information appears regularly, and much more data on V region variability is needed, there is rarely any conflict with currently accepted views as to structural patterns in the immunoglobulins.

We have tried to present the important principles derived from research on antibody structure and to supply enough references so that the interested reader can trace the historical development of the field and locate the relevant experimental protocols. The bibliography is of necessity highly selective. When several or many investigations illustrate a point, the choice of one or a few for discussion was often arbitrary. In making such selections we have exercised the prerogatives of the writers of a text, but have tried to be inclusive in citing those investigations which represented important new advances.

Since the immunoglobulins of various species differ in their characteristics, a complete description was not feasible. Chapter 3 considers properties of human immunoglobulins in some detail, and many of the basic principles of structure common to all immunoglobulins are discussed in that chapter. Special properties of mouse, guinea pig, rabbit, and horse immunoglobulins are described in Chapter 8. The general pattern of evolution of the immunoglobulin classes, starting with the primitive vertebrates, is the subject of Chapter 7. Other topics covered include allotypy, idiotypy, homogeneous antibodies, and the properties of isolated heavy and light chains and their recombinants. The second chapter should serve as an introduction to the mechanism of action of antibodies, and deals with the fine specificity of the antibody-combining site as revealed by binding studies and affinity labeling and with rates and energetics of immune reactions.

The presentation of amino acid sequences in Chapter 4 is again selective, including mainly those of human, mouse, and rabbit immunoglobulins. Selected sequences are presented in other sections where relevant, in particular where they serve to define principles underlying the construction of the antibody molecule or to illuminate the genetic control of the immune response. The "Atlas of Protein Structure," published periodically, is a comprehensive source of amino acid sequences (Margaret O. Dayhoff, ed., The National Biomedical Research Foundation, Silver Spring, Maryland).

We were unable to avoid some redundancy. For example, it seemed necessary to consider allotypy, idiotypy, and amino acid sequences in separate chapters. Yet each subject is intimately related to the genetic control of the immune response. Therefore, similar generalizations are sometimes drawn from the data presented in the three sections. Chapter 12 on theories of the genetic basis of structural variability attempts to draw these discussions together.

The style of Chapter 11 on idiotypic specificity differs somewhat from that of the remainder of the book since it was prepared by updating a review article prepared by two of the authors. As a result, the topic is presented in somewhat greater detail than most other subjects.

The principal audience we address comprises immunologists who have not personally observed the development of this exciting period in the history of immunology. A perusal of the Contents will reveal that this is not an introductory or general textbook. It is hoped that it will provide useful supplemental reading for the serious student or investigator who wishes to become familiar with the nature of the antibody molecule, its genetic control, and mode of action. We have tried to present the material in a didactic style, and, whenever possible, have included current interpretations of experimental data.

The book owes a great deal to Dr. Lisa A. Steiner and Dr. Katherine L. Knight, and to Mr. Shyr-Te Ju, a graduate student at the University of Illinois, who read large segments of the manuscript critically and made numerous constructive suggestions. The authors are deeply indebted to them for this assistance. The valuable cooperation of Dr. Stephen K. Wilson is also gratefully acknowledged.

Alfred Nisonoff*
John E. Hopper
Susan B. Spring

* Present address: Rosenstiel Basic Medical Sciences Research Center, Brandeis University, Waltham, Massachusetts.

The Antibody Molecule

1

General Structural Features of Immunoglobulin Molecules; Myeloma Proteins

One purpose of this text is to review the literature leading to our current knowledge of the structure of immunoglobulins. In subsequent chapters, references are provided to much of the pertinent research. In this introductory section we will outline some of the basic structural characteristics of immunoglobulins without citing the references on which the information is based. The discussion will be brief and, at times, sketchy. Its purpose is to facilitate reading of the remainder of the book, and perhaps to permit the reading of other chapters without strict regard to their sequence.

Immunoglobulins are present throughout the vertebrate kingdom but have not been identified in invertebrates. A basic feature, maintained during evolution, is the four-chain structure, comprising two light (L) and two heavy (H) chains. Both the H and L chain contribute amino acid residues which form the antigen-binding site. Each H-L pair produces one binding site, and the four-chain structure thus yields two sites. An individual molecule normally contains one species of H chain and one species of L chain, so that the combining sites of a molecule are identical. This property has its origin in the expression of only one gene for an L chain (variable region) and of one gene for the H chain (variable region) in a lymphoid cell that is synthesizing antibody.

An immunoglobulin molecule may have more than four chains. Such molecules are polymers of the four-chain unit, which are held together by disulfide bonds. For example, molecules of the IgM class may have from 16 to 24 chains (4–6 four-chain units, or 8–12 potential binding sites), depending on the animal species. Serum IgA may also exist as a polymer, and secretory IgA, found in colostrum, tears, saliva, and other secretory fluids, generally occurs as a dimer of the four-chain unit.

Thus the minimum "valence" of an immunoglobulin is 2. The presence of more than one combining site on the antibody molecule is of biological importance because it permits aggregation of macromolecular or particulate antigens. Bivalence is essential for enhancement of phagocytosis by antibody and for fixation of complement in the presence of antigen. Also, bivalent or multivalent attachment of a single antibody molecule to a particle increases the energy of interaction or "avidity"; this is significant, for example, in the neutralization of viruses, particularly when the affinity of a single combining site is low, as is often the case early in the process of immunization.

It was demonstrated by R.R. Porter in 1958 that cleavage of rabbit IgG by papain at neutral pH gives rise to large fragments with distinctive properties. The nature of this cleavage, as it applies to rabbit IgG or human IgG1, is illustrated in Figs. 1.1 and 1.2. Papain selectively attacks each H chain at a site just N-terminal to the interheavy chain disulfide bonds. This liberates three large fragments. Two are called Fab fragments (ab for antigen-binding) and the other is fragment Fc (c for crystallizable). Each Fab fragment (mol. wt. $\sim 45,000$) has one antigen-binding site, i.e., is univalent. Fab fragments therefore cannot precipitate macromolecular antigens or agglutinate particulate antigens, but they can, when present in excess, block the precipitation or agglutination that would otherwise occur upon addition of untreated, bivalent antibody. The fragments do this by occupying antigenic determinants, thus denying access to bivalent antibodies. Each Fab fragment comprises a

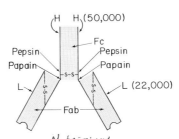

Fig. 1.1. Schematic diagram of the arrangement of polypeptide chains and interchain disulfide bonds in rabbit IgG [after Fleischman et al. (2)]. Reduction of the interchain disulfide bonds does not result in a decrease in molecular weight at neutral pH, owing to noncovalent interactions (shaded regions). A more accurate model would show the two L chains as being in very close proximity in the region of the interheavy chain disulfide bond, since in some immunoglobulins the L chains are disulfide bonded to one another. The molecule is flexible; the Fab fragments can rotate relative to one another around the "hinge region," which includes the sites of cleavage by papain and pepsin.

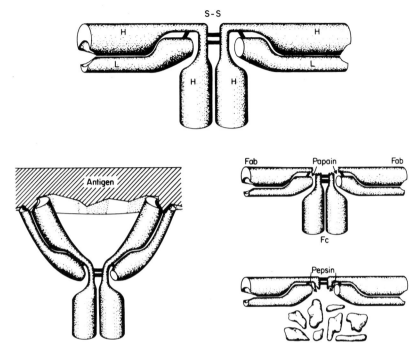

Fig. 1.2. Schematic diagram of the arrangement of polypeptide chains in human IgG1.

complete L chain and the N-terminal half of an H chain, designated fragment Fd. The L chain and fragment Fd are held together by noncovalent bonds and by a disulfide bond.

The third fragment, Fc (mol. wt. 50,000), crystallizes spontaneously in cold neutral buffer from a digest of rabbit IgG, which is heterogeneous. Crystallizability is generally associated with homogeneity and this was the first evidence for the presence of an invariant segment in the heterogeneous IgG molecules. We know now that fragment Fc consists of the C-terminal halves of two H chains, which are held together by noncovalent interactions.

Figures 1.1 and 1.2 also show the site of attack of rabbit or human IgG by pepsin at pH 4 to 4.5. Owing to the fact that its preferential site of cleavage is on the C-terminal, rather than the N-terminal side of the interheavy chain disulfide bond(s), a large bivalent fragment is liberated. Only the interheavy chain disulfide bond(s) join the two univalent fragments after peptic digestion; these bonds are very easily reduced, liberating two univalent fragments, designated Fab', which are slightly larger than fragment Fab. [The initial product of digestion is F(ab')$_2$.]

The Fab′ segments can be reunited, to form fragment F(ab′)$_2$, by reoxidation of the disulfide bond; this cannot, for obvious reasons, be accomplished with fragment Fab. Pepsin partially degrades fragment Fc, possibly owing to the low pH required for peptic activity.

Because of the susceptibility of a particular region in the middle of the H chain to attack by papain, pepsin, and other enzymes, it is generally thought that this region must be loosely folded. It has been designated the hinge region because the two univalent (Fab) fragments can move in space in relation to one another, and it is believed that the "swivel" is in this region of the chain.

This flexibility permits bivalent attachment of a single antibody to a particulate antigen (horseshoe configuration of the antibody) or, alternatively, the linking of two antigen particles with the antibody stretched out to its maximum length (about 140 Å for IgG). The combining sites are situated at the ends of the bivalent IgG molecule. A single, decavalent IgM molecule can attach itself to a particulate antigen through several combining sites. (Information of this kind is obtained by electron microscopy; the location of the combining site has been confirmed by X-ray crystallography, which also provides information as to the dimensions of the site.)

As indicated in Fig. 1.1, each H chain is joined to an L chain through a disulfide bond. In addition, strong noncovalent bonds serve to link the two chains. The latter can be disrupted by reagents such as 6 *M* guanidine hydrochloride, 8 *M* urea, or 1 *M* propionic acid. If the interchain disulfide bond joining the H to the L chain is first reduced, the chains can be separated on a preparative scale by gel filtration in the solvents mentioned. The chains reassociate as H-L pairs, in quite good yield, if the dissociating solvent is replaced by dialysis against neutral buffer. In the native molecule the H chains are joined to one another through disulfide and noncovalent bonds in the hinge and Fc regions. Under appropriate conditions it is possible to produce half-molecules, each consisting of a complete H chain and a complete L chain.

Besides L and H chains, secretory IgA contains a polypeptide called secretory component, or SC, which has a molecular weight of 65,000 − 70,000 and is bound to the H chains of the molecule. Another component, J chain (J for joining; mol. wt. 15,000), is found in the IgM of many primitive and advanced species, and in polymeric, but not monomeric (four-chain) IgA. J chain is linked to H chains through disulfide bonds. The amino acid sequences and antigenic properties of SC and J chain do not appear to be homologous to those of the immunoglobulin polypeptides; i.e., they do not seem to have a common evolutionary origin.

In humans and in many other species there are two "types" of L chain, κ and λ. The two types have sufficient homology of sequence to indicate a common evolutionary origin: phylogenetic evidence suggests that they both existed prior to the divergence of mammals and birds. It is possible that κ chains arose first in evolution since they appear, on the basis of limited data, to be the only type present in sharks. The two types of chain are approximately equal in length. Each chain has two (sometimes three) intrachain disulfide loops and a half-cystine through which the L chain is disulfide bonded to an H chain; this half-cystine is generally the C-terminal residue in a κ chain and the penultimate residue in a λ chain. The original discovery of κ and λ chains was made with human immunoglobulins, and the designation of a chain from another species as κ or λ is based on similarity of its amino acid sequence to the corresponding human protein. Even among mammalian species the percentages of κ and λ chains vary greatly—from 0 to 100% for each type. Humans have, on the average, 60% κ chains; rabbits, 70–90%; and mice, about 95%; the remainder are λ. When both types are present in a species, κ and λ chains are found in association with H chains of all classes and subclasses.

The size of an L chain is quite invariant (mol. wt. 22,000–23,000) in vertebrates throughout the phylogenetic scale. Also there are strong "homologies" among the amino acid sequences of L chains. (This applies to H chains as well.) In addition, definite homologies are observed when the sequences of H and L chains are compared with one another. This clearly suggests that there was a common ancestral gene for all the immunoglobulins.

The "primeval" polypeptide sequence probably had a molecular weight of 10,000 to 12,000 and comprised about 100–120 amino acid residues. Evidence for this can be seen, for example, in the structure of a typical human L chain, which contains about 214 amino acid residues. For a given type of L chain (κ or λ), the second half of the sequence, comprising about 107 residues at the C-terminal end of the chain, is invariant except for minor, inherited differences, or variants with nearly identical sequences found in all individuals. Wide variations of sequence are seen, however, in the first half (N-terminal 107 residues) of the chain. The sequence variations, in H as well as L chains, account for the differences in specificity among antibodies. It is clear that the L chain can be thought of as comprising two segments, about equal in size. In addition, there are resemblances in structure between the two halves. Principal among these is the intrachain disulfide loop, which is located nearly symmetrically in the two halves of the chain; this, again, is consistent with the concept that the primordial polypeptide chain comprises about 110 amino acids, and that the gene encoding this peptide underwent duplication and subsequent mutation.

The N-terminal half of the L chain is known as the variable, or V_L region; the C-terminal half is the C_L segment (C for constant). Terms used to designate the individual, 110- to 120-residue segments, are "domain" or "homology unit."

The H chain of human IgG consists of four domains (Fig. 1.3) including an N-terminal, V_H domain, with approximately 115 amino acid residues and three domains of invariant sequence (C_H1, C_H2, and C_H3; C for "constant"). All the domains are roughly equal in size, and each domain has the characteristic intrachain disulfide loop. It has been suggested that each domain may have one or more particular biological functions. For example, the V domain provides for antibody specificity, and the C_H2 domain is associated with complement fixation.

Figure 1.4 shows the amino acid sequence of the three C_H domains of human IgG1, worked out by Edelman and his collaborators for a myeloma protein (1). The three domains are aligned so as to exhibit maximum homology of sequences. The hyphens represent gaps artificially introduced into the sequence for this purpose. With the alignment shown any pair of domains exhibits about 30 to 33% homology, i.e., identities of amino acids. To maximize homology, positions 221 to 233 had to be omitted. These thirteen residues comprise the hinge region.

The term "invariant sequence" applies to members of the same class and subclass, for example the IgG1 subclass of IgG. Within a subclass there may be minor, genetically determined differences in the

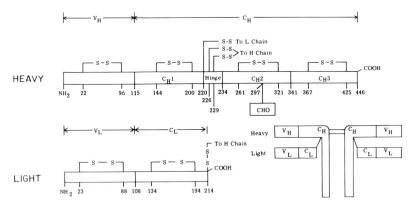

Fig. 1.3. Location of disulfide bonds in the sequence of the H chain of human IgG1 [protein Eu (1)] and of a human κ chain (3,4).

                    120   130

C_H1 (Residues 119–220) Ser Thr Lys Gly Pro Ser Val Phe Pro Leu Ala Pro Ser Ser Lys Ser - - Thr Ser Gly Gly Thr

C_H2 (Residues 234–341) Leu Leu Gly Gly Pro Ser Val Phe Leu Phe Pro Pro Lys Pro Lys Asp Thr Leu Met Ile Ser Arg Thr

C_H3 (Residues 342–446) Gln Pro Arg Glu Pro Gln Val Tyr Thr Leu Pro Pro Ser Arg Glu Glu - - Met Thr Lys Asn Gln

140   150   160

Ala Ala Leu Gly Cys Leu Val Lys Asp Tyr Phe Pro Glu Pro Val Thr Val Ser - Gly Ala Leu Thr Ser

Pro Glu Val Thr Cys Val Val Val Asp Val Ser His Glu Asp Pro Gln Val Lys Phe Asn Trp Tyr Val Asp Gly - Val Gln Val

Val Ser Leu Thr Cys Leu Val Lys Gly Phe Tyr Pro Ser Asp Ile Ala Val Glu - - Glu Trp Glu Ser Asn Asp - Gly Glu Pro

170   180   190

Gly - Val His Thr Phe Pro Ala Val Leu Gln Ser Ser Gly Leu Tyr Ser Leu Ser Ser Val Val Thr Val Pro Ser Ser Ser

His Asn Ala Lys Thr Lys Pro Arg Glu Glu Gln Tyr - Asp Ser Thr Tyr Arg Val Val Ser Val Leu Thr Val Leu His Gln Asn

Glu Asn Tyr Lys Thr Thr Pro Pro Val Leu Asp Ser - Asp Gly Ser Phe Phe Leu Tyr Ser Lys Leu Thr Val Asp Lys Ser Arg

200   210

Leu Gly Thr Gln - Thr Tyr Ile Cys Asn Val Asn His Lys Pro Ser Asn Thr Lys Val - Asp Lys Arg Val - - Glu Pro

Trp Leu Asp Gly Lys Glu Tyr Lys Cys Lys Val Ser Asn Lys Ala Leu Pro Ala Pro Ile - Glu Lys Thr Ile Ser Lys Ala Lys

Trp Gln Glu Gly Asn Val Phe Ser Cys Ser Val Met His Glu Ala Leu His Asn His Tyr Thr Gln Lys Ser Leu Ser Leu Ser Pro

220

Lys Ser Cys

Gly

Gly

Fig. 1.4. Amino acid sequences of the C_H1, C_H2, and C_H3 domains of a human IgG1 myeloma protein (Eu), aligned so as to maximize homologies (1).

C_H sequence, known as genetic or allotypic variants. Such variants are usually detected by means of naturally occurring or artificially induced antibodies which can discriminate among them. Genetic variants have so far been found mainly in C regions. An exception is the rabbit H chain in which allotypic variants are present in both the V_H and C_H segments of the chain. There are allotypes of L chains as well as H chains; most of the markers that have been localized so far appear to reside in the C_L region. Genes controlling allotypic markers have all proven to be codominant, autosomal, and inherited according to the simple Mendelian law of independent assortment.

The number of domains in the H chain is four in human IgG and IgA, four or five in IgD, and five in IgM and IgE. Thus the molecular weight of the H chain of IgM (the μ chain) is greater than that of the γ or α chain (since each chain has one V_H domain).[1] In the immunoglobulins of vertebrate species studied so far, the number of C_H domains appears to vary from two to four. There is no evidence for the presence of more than one V_H domain. There are significant homologies in sequence among the individual C_H domains of an H chain and, to a lesser extent, between a V_H and a C_H domain.

The class to which an immunoglobulin belongs is defined by the sequence of its C_H region. In many cases, the class (particularly IgG) is further divided into subclasses. For example, there are four subclasses of human IgG, IgG1, . . . , IgG4, each with a characteristic C_H sequence. The reason for designating these as subclasses rather than as four separate classes is the close relatedness of their amino acid sequences and antigenic structures. There is more than 90% homology of sequence between the C_H regions of any pair of subclasses of human IgG. By contrast, the degree of homology between the C_H region of human IgG and IgM is about 32%. This reflects a very early divergence of IgM and IgG during evolution, and a comparatively recent divergence of the subclasses.

The term "degree of homology" refers to the percentage of amino acids that are identical when the two chains are optimally aligned. In making such an alignment, it is often necessary to permit an occasional gap in the sequence in order to maximize homology. For example, if two chains containing 100 and 101 residues, respectively, were identical, except that the larger chain had an additional serine group in the middle of the chain, the degree of homology would not be much greater than 50% if the serine were retained in making the alignment, but would be 99% if

---

[1] The H chains of IgG, IgM, IgD, IgA, and IgE are designated γ, μ, δ, α, and ϵ, respectively.

a gap were inserted in the shorter chain sequence at a position corresponding to that of the serine.

Although the various classes and subclasses of immunoglobulin differ with respect to amino acid sequences of their C_H regions, one cannot in general differentiate among them on the basis of their L chains or V_H sequences. It is easy to understand how the various classes, defined on the basis of C_H region sequence, might share the same pool of L chains. The fact that they also share the same V_H sequences has led to the concept that two separate but linked genes, V_H and C_H, control the biosynthesis of a single H chain. There is strong evidence for this concept, which is widely accepted. In addition, there are considerable data to support the notion that a given cell line can switch from the biosynthesis of immunoglobulin of one class or subclass to another and that this switch involves only the gene controlling the C_H region; i.e., the L chain and V_H segment remain the same. This would imply that the combining site is unchanged, even though a different class of immunoglobulin is synthesized after the switch occurs. Although the genetic mechanism is obscure, some type of physical movement of the V_H gene, to make contact with one, then another C_H gene is implied. The existing data suggest that the joining of C_H and V_H takes place at the level of DNA, rather than RNA or polypeptide (Chapter 12).

Before discussing the nature of the sequence variability in V regions it is useful to define a V region subgroup. If one examines a large number of human V_κ sequences (variable halves of kappa chains), it becomes logical to divide them into three or four major subgroups. (Principles which apply to V_κ generally apply to V_λ and V_H as well.) Subgrouping is based on chain length and on linked substitutions within the chain. For example, proteins belonging to the $V_{\kappa I}$ subgroup usually have aspartic acid, alanine, lysine, and threonine, respectively, at positions 1, 13, 42, and 85 (counting from the N-terminus). At the same four positions, $V_{\kappa III}$ sequences typically have glutamic acid, leucine, glutamine, and valine. (Other positions, as well, could have been used in the example.) An occasional κ chain might have only three of the four amino acids specified; it would still in all probability be classified in the same subgroup. To permit alignment of the sequences of $V_{\kappa I}$ and $V_{\kappa III}$ it is necessary to introduce a single gap in the $V_{\kappa I}$ sequence after position 31. In comparing sequences of $V_{\kappa I}$ and $V_{\kappa II}$ a gap of six residues must be allowed in $V_{\kappa I}$ after position 31. It should be stressed that the number of V region subgroups varies markedly with the species. Thus, there are more V_κ subgroups in the mouse and rabbit than in man.

Within the V_κ region there are positions which are entirely invariant. Primary examples are the two half-cystines comprising the intrachain disulfide bond, which is a vital factor in maintaining the three-dimensional structure of the chain. When amino acid sequences of different L chains are compared the corresponding half-cystine groups are always aligned. The C-terminal half-cystine, which forms a disulfide bond with the H chain, is also invariant. Other examples of apparently invariant amino acids are interspersed along the length of the V_κ domain. It is possible that exceptions may be found as additional sequences are determined; this prediction is based on the fact that there are examples of positions in the V_κ sequence where all but one protein studied so far has the same amino acid. It is also probable that certain positions will be found to be completely invariant, owing to the requirement of a particular amino acid for structural integrity. In some positions substitutions occur but are conservative; i.e., a hydrophobic amino acid replaces another hydrophobic amino acid. A large preponderance of the data on which this discussion is based was obtained by sequencing L chains from myeloma proteins or urinary L chains (Bence Jones proteins) from patients with multiple myeloma. These proteins are discussed toward the end of this chapter.

Perhaps the most interesting segments of the V_L (or V_H) polypeptide chain are its hypervariable regions. There are three in $V_{\kappa I}$, starting at residues 30, 49, and 91 (counting from the N-terminus). Each spans 3 to 7 positions, but not all positions in each segment are equally variable. If two V_κ sequences, chosen at random, are compared, it is improbable that any of the three hypervariable segments will be identical. These regions are of great importance because, as shown by X-ray crystallography, the residues in the antibody molecule which comprise the antigen-binding site are mainly those of the hypervariable regions of L and H chains (Chapter 5). Thus, although hypervariable segments are widely separated in the V region sequence, they are brought into close proximity in the folded molecule.

Many positions in the V_κ regions are neither invariant nor hypervariable but, within a subgroup, show a moderate frequency of variation. The nature of this variability can best be understood by referring to amino acid sequences tabulated in Chapter 4. Usually, differences outside hypervariable regions, within a subgroup, are associated with a single base change in the DNA sequence.

A fundamental and still controversial question concerns the genetic basis of sequence variability in V regions. One school of thought maintains that there is a very large library of germ line *V* genes. An opposing view is that the number of germ line genes is very limited, perhaps to only one for each subgroup, and that additional *V* genes are generated by somatic mutation or recombination. A third suggestion is that the DNA encoding V regions is branched and that different sequences are generated by choosing different forks in the pathway. The theory of multiple germ line genes does not necessarily rule out the possibility of somatic processes, which would add to the library of genes. These questions are discussed in Chapter 12.

Of particular interest is the generation of diversity in hypervariable regions. If somatic mutation is responsible, the question remains as to whether these regions are "hot spots," or whether selection by antigen magnifies the pool of immunoglobulins in which mutations in hypervariable regions have occurred; i.e., a mutation in a hypervariable region could permit stimulation of the lymphocyte by a previously unrecognized antigen, whereas mutations outside hypervariable regions would ordinarily not generate new specificities.

Implicit in all of the above discussion is acceptance of Burnet's theory of clonal selection. There is general agreement that the formation of an antibody molecule initially takes place without informational input from, or the physical presence of the antigen. A decision is somehow made within a lymphocyte to synthesize a particular L and H chain pair. The antibody molecules take their place on the membrane of a B lymphocyte, where they act as receptors for antigen. Stimulation by antigen under appropriate conditions leads to differentiation — into cells such as plasma cells which can synthesize antibody at a higher rate — and to proliferation. All descendants of the lymphocyte are believed to synthesize the same antibody molecules, with the proviso of a possible switch in class (C_H region). The initial contact with antigen leads to aggregation and endocytosis of the immunoglobulin receptors. Little is known of the biochemical events which take place immediately after capture of the antigen and lead to differentiation and cell division.

The antibodies produced in response to antigenic challenge, even against a simple hapten, are ordinarily heterogeneous. However, it appears that there often are homogeneous subpopulations of significant size within a heterogeneous population of antibodies; for example, a rabbit might produce, say, 30 species of antibody molecule in significant quantity in response to challenge by a hapten, but one of these species might comprise 25% of the total weight of the antihapten antibody. Thus, it is sometimes possible to isolate homogeneous antibodies from a heterogeneous mixture. The outstanding current examples of useful homogeneous antibody populations are those directed to streptococcal or pneumococcal polysaccharides. These have been produced by immunization of various species, particularly rabbits and mice, with killed bacteria. Not only do homogeneous subpopulations appear quite frequently but the antibody titers are often very high (20 to 50 mg/ml is not uncommon), so that large quantities of homogeneous antibody can sometimes be isolated from an individual animal. Such preparations have been of great value in studies of the structure and genetic control of antibodies and are under intensive investigation.

MYELOMA AND BENCE JONES PROTEINS

A recurrent theme in this book is the use of myeloma or Bence Jones proteins in structural studies. Most of this work has been done with human and mouse myeloma proteins; some sequence studies have been carried out with myeloma proteins of the cat and the dog. Much of the recent progress in the field would have been difficult or impossible without these proteins, which are now accepted as being homogeneous but otherwise representative immunoglobulins. This concept has been reinforced by the failure to observe any basic differences in the structure of myeloma proteins and induced antibodies and by the discovery of myeloma proteins with antibody-like activity directed to a variety of antigens. Immunoglobulin fractions of serum and most populations of antibodies specific for a single antigen are, in contrast, very heterogeneous. The homogeneity of a myeloma protein reflects its biosynthesis by a malignant clone of cells, all producing molecules with essentially the same structure. The statement is qualified because electrophoretic microheterogeneity is frequently seen in myeloma proteins; this is generally attributed to postsynthetic hydrolysis of amide groups by serum enzymes, yielding negatively charged carboxylate groups, or to slight variations in the content of carbohydrate, including the negatively charged sialic acid.

All the known classes and subclasses of human immunoglobulin occur as monoclonal proteins. IgG, IgA, IgE, and, occasionally, IgM monoclonal proteins are found in patients with multiple myeloma. Homogeneous IgM occurs more often in the sera of patients with a form of malignant lymphoma referred to as Waldenström's macroglobulinemia. Multiple myeloma is a malignant disorder in which there is proliferation of plasma cells in the bone marrow, leading to marked anemia and destruction of bone. The proliferating cell type in Waldenström's macroglobulinemia is predominantly lymphocytic, with a wide distribution of cells in bone marrow, lymphoid organs, and peripheral blood. The disease is typically more benign than multiple myeloma; severe anemia and bone destruction are generally not observed, but the patient's immune system may be greatly impaired.

Monoclonal proteins of the IgD class usually occur in patients with a malignant lymphocytic lymphoma, not too dissimilar from Waldenström's macroglobulinemia. Patients with IgD monoclonal proteins tend to be considerably younger than those with Waldenström's disease, who are often over 65 years of age, and somewhat younger on the average than patients with myeloma proteins of the other classes.

In many instances, identification of a class or subclass either became possible or was greatly facilitated through the availability of the corresponding myeloma protein. To illustrate the point, IgD in normal human serum can be recognized with a specific antiserum. However, the isolation of IgD from normal serum is very difficult because of its low concentration (average 30 μg/ml). The preparation of a monospecific antiserum would therefore be quite impractical if it were not for the availability of IgD myeloma proteins. Similarly, delineation of the four subclasses of human IgG, or the two subclasses of IgA, would have been very difficult without the corresponding myeloma proteins. (The same considerations apply to mouse immunoglobulins.) Myeloma proteins have also been of great value in defining and localizing the allotypes, or genetic variants, of human and mouse immunoglobulins.

Bence Jones proteins are L chains (monomers or dimers; κ or λ) synthesized by patients with multiple myeloma or, infrequently, with Waldenström's disease. The L chains are present in the serum and urine. They are often easy to isolate from urine because of their relatively high concentration and the absence of other immunoglobulins. About 10–15% of patients with multiple myeloma produce only a Bence Jones protein, and about 40% synthesize a myeloma protein without significant amounts of a Bence Jones protein. When both types of protein are present in an individual the Bence Jones protein is generally identical in structure to the L chain of the serum myeloma protein; it therefore reflects the synthesis of excess L chains, as compared to H chains, by the malignant clone of cells.

The frequency of occurrence of human myeloma proteins of a particular class or subclass parallels rather closely the concentration of that class or subclass in normal human serum. It would appear that the events leading to malignant transformation occur with about the same probability, irrespective of the class of immunoglobulin synthesized by the lymphoid cell. Similar considerations apply to L chains of the κ and λ types; the number of myeloma proteins possessing each type of chain corresponds well with their proportions in normal human serum ($\kappa : \lambda = 6 : 4$). Myeloma proteins of the IgD class and IgG4 subclasses are exceptions to this general rule since a high proportion of IgD myeloma proteins are λ and the preponderance of IgG4 myeloma proteins are κ. Also about 75% of human myeloma proteins of the IgA class have V_H

regions belonging to the V_{HIII} subgroup, as compared to 20 to 25% of the total immunoglobulin population. A disproportionate number of IgA myeloma proteins appears in susceptible strains of mice after intraperitoneal irritation with mineral oil or certain plastics. This may be due to the large proportion of IgA-producing cells in the peritoneum.

Besides their essential role in the identification of classes, subclasses, and genetic variants (allotypes), monoclonal immunoglobulins have been invaluable in studies of amino acid sequences. They have been of particular importance in establishing V region sequences, since the V regions of normal immunoglobulins are too heterogeneous for detailed analysis. (Some data have, however, been obtained on V regions of homogeneous antibodies, particularly in the rabbit.) It is important in this regard that the variability seen in myeloma proteins is, in general, not inconsistent with that found in normal immunoglobulins. For example, κ chains of human myeloma proteins have methionine or leucine at position 4 (reading from the N-terminus); and only these two amino acids are found at position 4 of the κ chains of pooled normal human IgG. Although C region sequences can in principle be worked out with normal immunoglobulins, myeloma proteins, in species where they are available, have generally been used for this purpose as well because of the ease of obtaining them in a pure state and in large quantity.

X-Ray crystallographic studies have been carried out at high resolution with the Fab' fragments of a human and a mouse myeloma protein and with two human Bence Jones proteins. This work has resulted in the construction of crystallographic models which permit visualization of the three-dimensional structure including the region of the active site (Chapter 5).

The association of antibody activity with myeloma proteins has permitted the investigation, through chemical modifications including affinity labeling, of the nature of the amino acid side chains present in the active site. Also, many physicochemical investigations of immunoglobulins have utilized myeloma proteins because of their homogeneity; heterogeneous antibody populations may vary with respect to a parameter (e.g., circular dichroism) and the results may be difficult to interpret.

The association of a biological property (such as complement fixation) with a particular class or subclass has often been studied with the aid of myeloma proteins because of the difficulty of isolating the desired population from normal serum.

Malignant cell lines, maintained in culture, have been extensively used in studies of the biosynthesis of H and L chains and their assembly into complete immunoglobulin molecules. An important current area of research is the identification and characterization of mutants occurring in such cell lines. They are also employed for the isolation of mRNA specific for L or H chains, for use in studies of cell-free synthesis of immunoglobulin, and for hybridization with DNA. Hybridization studies may yield reliable values for the number of germ line structural genes encoding immunoglobulins.

NOMENCLATURE

The nomenclature of the immunoglobulins has evolved considerably over the years; the interested reader can consult references 5–7. The terminology used in this text is based on references 6 and 7.

REFERENCES

1. Edelman, G.M., Cunningham, B.A., Gall, W.E., Gottlieb, P.D., Rustishauser, U., and Waxdal, M.J. (1969). *Proc. Nat. Acad. Sci. U.S.* **63**, 78.
2. Fleischman, J.B., Pain, R.H., and Porter, R.R. (1962). *Arch. Biochem. Biophys. Suppl.* **1**, 174.
3. Hilschmann, N. and Craig, L.C. (1965). *Proc. Nat. Acad. Sci. U.S.* **53**, 1403.
4. Titani, K., Whitley, E., Jr., Avogardo, L., and Putnam, F.W. (1965). *Science* **149**, 1090.
5. *Bull. WHO* **30**, 447 (1964).
6. *Bull WHO* **41**, 975 (1969).
7. *J. Immunol.* **108**, 1733 (1972).

Nature of the Active Site of an Antibody Molecule and the Mechanism of Antibody–Hapten Interactions

This chapter will summarize information relating to the chemical nature of the active site of an antibody molecule and mechanisms of interaction with hapten. It will consider studies relating to the fine specificity of an antibody; the concept of an immunodominant antigenic grouping; forces involved in antibody–hapten interactions; the size and structure of the antibody combining site; kinetics and thermodynamics of antibody–hapten interactions; and affinity labeling of the active site as a probe for amino acid sequences in or near the site. Details of the structure of the combining regions of myeloma proteins, as ascertained by X-ray crystallography, are discussed in Chapter 5.

I. INHIBITION OF PRECIPITATION BY HAPTENS AND CHEMICAL MODIFICATION AS PROBES FOR ANTIBODY SPECIFICITY

A. Introduction

Much of our insight into the nature of antibody specificity has been acquired through experiments in which haptens were tested for their capacity to inhibit the precipitin reaction of antihapten antibody with a protein–hapten conjugate. The method was exploited for many years by K. Landsteiner and his collaborators, who combined ingenuity with enormous energy and established many of the basic principles of antibody specificity. Their work is summarized in a book published by Landsteiner in 1944 (1), near the end of his career. In the early 1940's this work was extended in a series of investigations by L. Pauling, D. Pressman, and their collaborators, who used quantitative methods for the determination of amounts of precipitate formed and brought sophistication in physical chemistry to the interpretation of data. Many other investigators have also contributed to this area of research. In this relatively brief discussion we will try to illustrate types of information that can be obtained by this method.

Suppose that antibody is elicited by immunization with a conjugate of a hapten of low molecular weight to a protein, which we can designate protein A. If protein A is not too heavily substituted by the hapten enough of its native structure will be retained so that antibodies will be elicited which react with the unconjugated protein. In addition, part of the induced antibody population will be specific for the hapten. This can be shown by allowing the antiserum to react with the homologous hapten conjugated to a protein (protein B) other than that used for immunization. The formation of a precipitate is evidence for antihapten specificity, since the animal had not been inoculated with protein B. Various haptens related in structure to that present on the immunogen will be found to inhibit this precipitin reaction. Figure 2.1 illustrates the mechanism of inhibition; free haptens of low molecular weight, if present in excess, will compete with the hapten groups attached to the carrier protein for the available antibody combining sites. The free hapten cannot form a precipitate with antibody since it only has a single site of attachment per molecule and precipitation requires the formation of a cross-linked network. It is evident that a variety of different haptens can

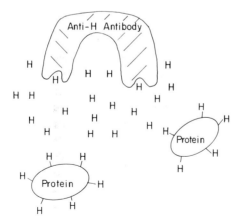

Fig. 2.1. Mechanism of inhibition by free hapten molecules of the precipitation of an antihapten antibody with a protein–hapten conjugate. Inhibition is attributable to the large excess of free molecules as compared to those bound to the carrier protein.

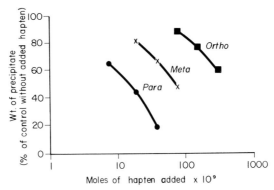

Fig. 2.2. Hapten inhibition of precipitation of rabbit antibodies to the *p*-azophenylar-sonate group. The precipitating antigen is ovalbumin-*p*-(*p'*-phenylazo)-phenylarsonate. Inhibiting haptens are ortho-, meta-, and para-nitro derivatives of phenylarsonate. Approximately 770 μg of precipitate formed in the absence of hapten. The data are from Pauling *et al.* (2).

rapidly be screened by this method for their capacity to bind specifically to the antibody.

One can also carry out a series of experiments in which the antibody and antigen concentrations are held constant and the concentration of free hapten is varied. Typical hapten inhibition curves are shown in Fig. 2.2. When a series of haptens is tested the relative inhibitory capacities will be dependent on binding affinities. The lower the association content the higher will be the concentration of hapten needed to cause 50% inhibition of precipitation. As shown by Pauling *et al.* (2) there should be an inverse proportionality between this concentration and the average binding affinity, K_0, of the hapten for antibody.[1] If one arbitrarily assigns to a particular hapten a K_0 value of 1.0, one can obtain the relative K_0 value for another, related hapten by determining the relative concentrations of the two haptens needed for 50% inhibition of precipitation. Thus, in Fig. 2.2, the K_0 values are in the order, *p*-nitrobenzoate > *m*-nitrobenzoate > *o*-nitrobenzoate. It should be noted that this method only gives comparative K_0 values. The actual K_0 must be obtained by a direct binding assay, such as equilibrium dialysis. Having obtained the K_0 for one hapten, however, the K_0 values for other haptens can then be calculated from data on inhibition of precipitation. Values thus obtained are not considered to be as precise as K_0 values measured directly for each hapten.

[1] This is based on the arbitrary assumption, discussed further below, that the distribution of combining energies (which are proportional to log K) in a normal antibody population obeys a Gauss error function. K_0, the "average" K value, is that represented by the peak of the distribution curve.

B. Specificity of Antibodies Directed to the Phenylazobenzoate Group

The nature of the specificity of antihapten antibodies can be demonstrated with a few examples of experimental results. Tables 2.1 and 2.2 present data on the specificity of rabbit antibody directed to the p,p'-azophenylazobenzoate hapten group (2a).[2] The immunizing antigen consisted of bovine serum proteins to which several hapten groups, per molecule of protein, had been conjugated by diazotization. (See Fig. 2.3.)

Relative K_0 values for various haptens were obtained by measuring their capacity to inhibit the precipitin reaction of the rabbit antiserum with a heterologous protein, ovalbumin, to which phenylazobenzoate groups had been coupled. In calculating relative K_0 values, that of unsubstituted benzoate was taken arbitrarily as 1.0.

The data in Table 2.1 indicate that the carboxylate group and the benzene ring of benzoate are both essential for effective interaction with the anti-p-p'-azophenylazobenzoate antibodies. Phenol and p-cresol, each of which has an uncharged hydroxyl group in place of the carboxylate, do not combine with the antibody. Similarly, acetate, which has a carboxyl group but not a benzene ring, failed to inhibit the precipitin reaction. Cyclohexane carboxylate, which has a saturated ring

TABLE 2.1

INTERACTION OF HAPTENS WITH RABBIT ANTIBODIES TO THE
p-PHENYLAZOBENZOATE GROUP[a,b]

Hapten	Relative K_0 value
Benzoate	1
Acetate	<0.01
Phenol	<0.01
p-Cresol	<0.01
Cyclohexane carboxylate	<0.01
p-Nitrophenol	0.23
Benzenesulfonate	<0.01
p-Arsanilate	<0.01
Benzenephosphonate	<0.01
Phenylacetate	<0.01

[a] From reference 2a.

[b] Data were obtained by measurement of the capacity of haptens to inhibit the precipitation of antibodies by ovalbumin to which p-azobenzoate groups were conjugated.

[2] These relatively recent data, obtained by using IgG fractions of antisera in precipitin tests, are selected for presentation since whole antiserum was used in most earlier investigations; the use of serum complicates the quantitative interpretation of results because albumin binds many anions.

TABLE 2.2

INTERACTION OF OTHER HAPTENS WITH RABBIT ANTIBODIES TO THE
p-PHENYLAZOBENZOATE GROUP

Hapten (benzoate derivative)	Relative K_0 value	Hapten (benzoate derivative)	Relative K_0 value	Hapten (benzoate derivative)	Relative K_0 value
Unsubstituted	1.0				
o-Chloro	0.11	*m*-Chloro	0.43	*p*-Chloro	5.3
o-Methyl	0.03	*m*-Methyl	0.21	*p*-Methyl	1.8
o-Iodo	0.013	*m*-Iodo	0.29	*p*-Iodo	9.0
o-Nitro	<0.01	*m*-Nitro	0.12	*p*-Nitro	1.8
o-Carboxy	<0.01	*m*-Carboxy	0.90	*p*-Carboxy	5.3
o-Acetamino	0.13	*m*-Acetamino	1.3	*p*-Acetamino	1.6
				p-Phenylazo	67
				p-(*p'*-Methyl- phenylazo)	65
				p-(*p'*-Hydroxyl- phenylazo)	111
				p-(*o'*-Methyl-*p'*-hy- droxyphenylazo)	81
				p-(*m'*-Methyl-*p'*-hy- droxyphenylazo)	125
				H-acid-*p*-azobenzoate	89
				H-acid-*p*-azo- nitrobenzene	<0.01

structure, also was ineffective as an inhibitor. This indicates great specificity for the benzene ring since the cyclohexane group is also hydrophobic but is somewhat larger and different in shape than the benzene ring.

The data in Table 2.1 also demonstrate a close fit of the antibody around the carboxylate group. Benzene sulfonate (ϕSO_3^-), benzene phosphonate ($\phi PO_3 H_2^-$), and *p*-arsanilate ($NH_2—\phi—AsO_3 H_2^-$) did not interact with the antibody, although the requirements of a benzene ring and a negative charge are fulfilled. The failure to combine is probably attributable to the larger size of the charged groups, as compared to carboxylate, and resulting steric interference. Similarly, phenylacetate had no measurable affinity, indicating that the extra $—CH_2—$ group, between the benzene ring and carboxyl group, could not be accommodated by the antibody. It is evident that errors of even 1 or 2 Å in spatial relationships between the hapten and antibody cannot be tolerated, at least in this region of the hapten molecule.

As indicated above, phenol, which is uncharged, did not interact with the antibody. In contrast, *p*-nitrophenol, for example, which is partly ionized at neutral pH,

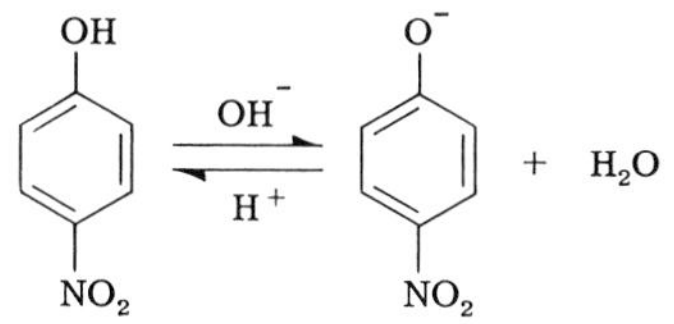

interacted quite effectively. The fact that an ionized phenol but not, for example, benzenesulfonate, can combine with the antibody is probably attributable to steric factors; the $-O^-$ group but not the larger $-SO_3^-$ can be accommodated in the active site.

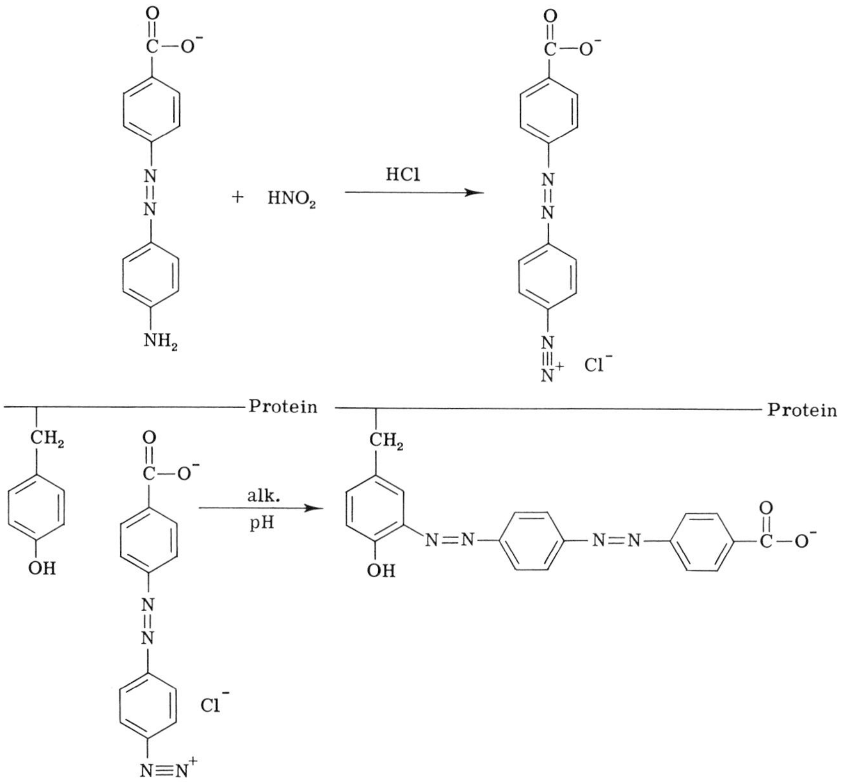

Fig. 2.3. Conjugation of a hapten to a protein carrier by diazotization. This method of conjugation has been used in many investigations (e.g., 1,2) and is applicable to a wide variety of aniline derivatives.

The closeness of fit of the antibody site around the hapten is also illustrated by the effect of ortho substitution in the benzoate group, which, in nearly all instances, resulted in a large decrease in combining affinity (Table 2.2). Ortho substitutents may interfere sterically and also tilt the carboxylate group out of the plane of the benzene ring; this slight displacement is sufficient to hinder the specific combination markedly.

Similarly, meta substitution tends to reduce the combining affinity, suggesting that there is a close fit of antibody around the meta as well as the ortho position. However, the reductions in K_0 are much less striking than in the case of ortho substitution, indicating a somewhat less critical fit of the antibody around the meta position (Table 2.2). Two exceptions are *m*-acetaminobenzoate and *m*-phthalate (*m*-carboxybenzoate). The *m*-acetamino group also occupies space around the para position and para substitution is associated with increased affinity (see below); two opposing tendencies may therefore be involved. In the case of *m*-phthalate, steric interference associated with meta substitution may be overcome by interaction of the second negatively charged group with a positively charged side chain in the active site. The possibility of the presence of such a positive charge is considered more fully below.

For para substitution the results are strikingly different. All such substituents tested caused an increase in the K_0 value relative to that of unsubstituted benzoate (Table 2.2). The highest values of K_0 are associated with the presence of a *p*-azo group and a second benzene ring.

One can readily understand how para substituents can be accommodated without steric interference, since the antibody was prepared against a *p*-phenylazobenzoate group. The reason for the increase in K_0 associated with every para substituent tested is less clear. Pressman *et al.* (3) ascribed such increases in similar systems to nonspecific dispersion forces that act between any two atoms in close proximity; in this case the atoms would belong to the hapten and antibody, respectively. It is not certain whether apolar (hydrophobic) forces may also play a role in the interactions taking place in the para region.

The very high values of K_0 associated with the presence of a *p*-azo group and a second benzene ring are attributable to the close structural relationship of these compounds to the immunogen. The data thus show that the antibody combining site encompasses the second benzene ring. The large relative increase in K_0 associated with the second ring and the azo group does not prove that this region of the hapten molecule contributes more to the energy of interaction than the first benzene ring and its associated carboxylate group. From the relationship

$$\Delta G^0 = -RT \ln K_0$$

one calculates that a factor of 100 in K_0 is roughly equivalent to a change in the free energy of interaction of 2.5 kcal/mole. Benzoate itself, which interacts with a K_0 value of about 10^4 to 10^5 M^{-1}, would contribute roughly 5–6 kcal/mole to the free energy of interaction, or more than two-thirds of the energy of a compound which also contains a second ring.

On this basis one might predict that the fit around the benzoate group might be closer than that around the second benzene ring. This is borne out by the effects of substitution in the second ring, which are much less important than those in the first benzene ring; the presence of a methyl group in the ortho or meta positions of the second ring had very little effect on K_0 (Table 2.2). The picture that emerges is one of a close fit of antibody around the first benzene ring. There is considerable energy of interaction with the second ring and the *p*-azo group; this is based, however, on a relatively loose fit.

C. Evidence for the Presence of a Positively Charged Group in the Active Site of Antibodies Directed to Certain Negatively Charged Haptens

The data we have just cited strongly suggests that a positively charged side chain may be present in the active site of anti-*p*,*p'*-azophenylazobenzoate antibodies; they showed that only benzoate derivatives or a negatively charged phenol have appreciable affinity for the antibody. The simplest explanation would be the presence of an oppositely charged lysine or arginine side chain as a contact residue in the active site of the antibody.

Further evidence in support of this possibility was obtained by comparing, as inhibitors in the same system, "H-Acid" *p*-azobenzoate with "H-Acid" *p*-azonitrobenzene.[3] (The H-acid component was needed to solubilize the *p*-azonitrobenzene.) (See Table 2.2.) It was found that "H-acid" *p*-azobenzoate is a highly effective competitor ($K_0 = 89$) whereas "H-acid" *p*-azonitrobenzene has no detectable affinity for the antibody, despite the fact that the nitro group has virtually the same size and structure as carboxylate, and that both the nitro and carboxylate groups are coplanar with the benzene ring. The presence of the negative charge appears essential.

Through chemical modifications of antibodies, Pressman, Grossberg, and collaborators (4,5) have obtained direct evidence for the presence of positively charged amino acid side chains in the active sites of rabbit antibodies directed to the following negatively charged haptens: *p*-

---

[3] H-Acid is 8-amino-1-naphthol-3,6-disulfonic acid.

azobenzoate, *p*-azobenzenearsonate, and *p*-azobenzenephosphonate. In each case the presence of a positively charged group could be demonstrated in a substantial fraction, but not all of the antibody population. In principle, their method consists of selective chemical modification of lysine or arginine side chains, each of which is positively charged. Loss of activity upon modification is not, however, taken as proof of the presence of the amino acid in the active site unless protection against loss of activity is conferred by the hapten, present in excess in the reaction mixture. (The hapten can fill the active site and sterically prevent access of the reagent used for chemical modification.)

Modification by 2,3-butanedione of 54% of the 44–46 arginine groups in a molecule of specifically purified rabbit anti-*p*-azobenzoate antibody resulted in a loss of 0.6 binding sites per molecule of bivalent antibody. When chemical modification was carried out in the presence of 0.1 *M* hapten, *p*-nitrobenzoate, no combining sites were lost when the same fraction, 54%, of the arginine groups had been modified. This result is interpretable on the basis that the hapten, when bound to antibody, sterically protects an arginine group in the active site from modification by 2,3-butanedione.

Similar experiments demonstrated the presence of arginine side chains in the active sites of at least one-third of rabbit antibody molecules specific for the *p*-azobenzenearsonate group. The fact that complete inactivation by 2,3-butanedione was not attained can be understood on the basis that an antibody population is heterogeneous with respect to the presence or absence of an arginine side chain in the active site.

Evidence was obtained for the presence of lysine side chains in active sites of rabbit antibodies directed to the *p*-azobenzoate, *p*-azobenzenearsonate, and *p*-azobenzenephosphonate groups (5). The minimum fractions of active sites containing lysine, in the three antibody populations, were 15, 45, and 25%, respectively. Maleic anhydride was used for the chemical modification. Conditions were chosen so as to minimize reactions with tyrosine, serine, and threonine. The values cited for percentages of active sites specifically modified were obtained from data on maximum hapten-binding capacity per molecule of antibody before and after treatment. Specific modification was taken as the difference between the numbers of sites inactivated in the presence of absence of a protective hapten.

Freedman *et al.* (6) were also able to show that anti-*p*-azobenzenearsonate antibodies can be fractionated into two separate populations having arginine or lysine side chains, respectively, in their active sites. Lysine residues were first reacted with maleic anhydride without protecting hapten present; this allowed modification of lysine groups in the active site. About one-half of the hapten-binding capacity was lost as a result of this treatment. The modified population was applied to an immunoadsorbent column containing covalently bound benzenearsonate groups. Approximately one-half of the antibodies now failed to become attached to the column. As might be expected, the unbound population possessed very few hapten-binding sites, and presumably comprised those molecules whose active sites had been modified by maleic anhydride. Proof for this supposition was obtained by removal of the attached maleyl groups by hydrolysis at pH 3.5. This treatment restored the hapten-binding capacity to a value of approximately 2 molecules of hapten per molecule of antibody; also, the K_0 value was approximately the same as that of untreated antibody. This restored population was then treated with glyoxal, a reagent which specifically modifies the guanidinium group of arginine side chains. Sufficient reagent was used to modify 77% of the arginine groups in the antibody. Despite the fact that no protective hapten was present no loss of hapten-binding activity occurred. The authors concluded that those antihapten antibodies which have a lysine group in the active site do not also have arginine.

Other experiments demonstrated, however, that arginine side chains are present in the active sites of another subpopulation of antibenzenearsonate antibodies of the same pool. The subpopulation which adhered to the immunoadsorbent after maleylation (presumably lacking a lysine group in the active site), was eluted at low pH, neutralized, and subjected to glyoxylation to modify arginine. This resulted in a loss of 75% of the hapten-binding sites (as compared to zero loss in the nonadherent population). The loss of activity was prevented when glyoxylation was carried out in the presence of a protective hapten. Thus, a substantial fraction of the population has either lysine or arginine in the active site, but these subpopulations do not overlap. A mixture of the two reagents, glyoxal and maleic anhydride, inactivated about 90% of the hapten-binding sites; only 10% were lost when chemical modification was done in the presence of the hapten, *p*-nitrobenzenearsonate.

Chemical modifications with 2,3-butanedione, glyoxal, and maleic anhydride, were also carried out with specifically purified rabbit antibodies directed toward a positively charged and a neutral hapten group (*p*-azophenyltrimethylammonium and 3-azopyridine, respectively) (6). Even after extensive modification of arginine, or virtually complete modification of lysine side chains, there was no significant loss of hapten-binding sites. These experiments provided excellent controls for the studies with antibodies to negatively charged haptens. Related experiments with antibodies to negatively charged hapten groups are reported in references 7–9.

Another type of evidence for the presence of positively charged side chains in the active sites of antibodies directed to negatively charged hapten groups was reported by Koshland and Englberger (10). Very careful analyses of amino acid composition demonstrated a higher arginine content in specifically purified rabbit antibodies directed to the *p*-azobenzenearsonate group, as compared to those antibodies against the positively charged *p*-azobenzenetrimethylammonium group ($—N\!=\!N—\emptyset—N(CH_3)_3{}^+$). The difference amounted to 2 to 4 arginine groups per molecule of antibody. Similar results were obtained when pools of serum from several rabbits were compared or when an individual rabbit was immunized with both antigens and the two antibodies were subsequently purified and analyzed. Conversely, they found that rabbit antibodies to the positively charged anti-*p*-azobenzenetrimethylammonium group are richer in negatively charged aspartic side chains. These results provide supportive evidence for the presence of oppositely charged side chains in antibodies directed to charged hapten groups.

D. Active Site of Antibody Directed to a Positively Charged Hapten Group

Several types of evidence suggest the presence of a complementary, negatively charged side chain in the active sites of rabbit antibodies directed to the positively charged *p*-azotrimethylammonium group: (a) Substitution of the uncharged tertiary butyl group, $—C(CH_3)_3$, for trimethylammonium, $—N(CH_3)_3{}^+$, results in approximately an eightfold decrease in K_0, despite the fact that the two groups are otherwise almost identical in structure (11); (b) as already indicated, M.E. Koshland found a consistently greater aspartic acid content in rabbit antibodies directed to the *p*-azotrimethylammonium group, as compared with antibodies directed to a negatively charged hapten; (c) chemical modification studies suggest the presence of a carboxylate group in the active sites of a substantial proportion of rabbit antibodies directed to the same hapten. The reagent used was diazoacetamide

$$N_2—CH_2—\overset{\overset{\displaystyle O}{\|}}{C}—NH_2$$

which esterifies carboxylate groups in aspartic acid or glutamic acid side chains, as well as terminal carboxylate groups. Forty percent of the hapten-binding sites were inactivated by treatment with the reagent, but the presence of a protective hapten of high affinity almost completely prevented the loss of activity (12). In contrast, esterification of carboxylate groups in rabbit antibody specific for the negatively charged *p*-azobenzoate group causes virtually no loss of activity.

E. Specificity of Antibodies to the 2,4-Dinitrophenyl (Dnp) Hapten Group

Throughout the 1960's antibodies to the Dnp hapten were studied intensively in a number of laboratories, in particular that of H.N. Eisen. Dnp groups are readily coupled to a carrier protein with the reagent, 2,4-dinitrophenylsulfonate (Dnp-sulfonate) (13):

At pH 10 the reagent is conjugated, through a substitution reaction, mainly to the ϵ-amino groups of lysyl side chains and to amino-terminal groups. The sulfonate group is split off during the process. Anti-Dnp antibodies are of particular interest because the Dnp group, when attached to protein, is uncharged; many of the earlier studies of specificity had involved antibodies to charged hapten groups.

Antibodies of very high affinity ($K_0 \geqslant 10^8 \ M^{-1}$) can be elicited by prolonged immunization with Dnp–protein conjugates (14). These antibody populations are highly heterogeneous, showing a broad spectrum of combining affinities. Data illustrating the specificity of rabbit anti-Dnp antibodies are presented in Table 2.3. The results were obtained by measurements of fluorescence quenching (Section VI,D) or, in the case of one hapten of low affinity, by equilibrium dialysis using radiolabeled hapten.

The contribution of the lysine group to the interaction may be seen by comparing ϵ-Dnp-L-lysine and *m*-dinitrobenzene; the K_0 value for the former compound is approximately 40 times greater. There is not a strict requirement for an L-lysine group, since the enantimorph, ϵ-Dnp-D-lysine, combines almost as well. The 6-carbon chain of lysine is also not essential; γ-Dnp-aminobutyrate interacts with an affinity nearly as great as that of ϵ-Dnp-L-lysine. There is a decrease in affinity, however, associated with substitution of L-phenylalanine or L-norleucine for the lysine in ϵ-Dnp-L-lysine. This decrease is probably due to the presence of the negatively charged carboxylate group, close to the Dnp group in the phenylalanyl or norleucyl derivatives. The anti-Dnp antibody com-

TABLE 2.3

BINDING OF SOME 2,4-DINITROPHENYL (DNP) DERIVATIVES BY
RABBIT ANTI-DNP ANTIBODIES[a,b]

Hapten	K_0 $(M^{-1} \times 10^{-7})$	$-\Delta G^0$ (kcal mole^{-1})
ϵ-Dnp-L-lysine	2.30	10.30
ϵ-Dnp-D-lysine	1.20	9.82
α-Dnp-L-alanine	0.88	9.63
α-Dnp-L-norleucine	0.54	9.33
α-Dnp-L-phenylalanine	0.31	8.99
ϵ-Dnp-aminocaproate	2.85	10.37
γ-Dnp-aminobutyrate	2.00	10.12
Dnp-glycine	0.46	9.27
2,4-Dinitrophenol	0.027	7.52
m-Dinitrobenzene	0.06	8.02
2,4-Dinitroaniline	0.22	8.86
p-Mononitroaniline	0.00075	5.47
o-Mononitroaniline	(0.00060)	(5.2)

[a] Data from Eisen and Siskind (14).
[b] Data were obtained by the method of fluorescence quenching for all compounds except p-mononitroaniline, for which equilibrium dialysis was used.

bining site is probably hydrophobic and would therefore not readily accommodate a charged group. The fact that various nonpolar substituents increase the affinity of Dnp groups for antibody indicates specificity for a hydrophobic portion of the protein carrier as well as for Dnp itself. This is consistent with the fact that most Dnp groups are attached to apolar lysyl side chains in the antigen used for immunization. (The lysine side chain loses its positive charge when Dnp is attached.)

The disadvantageous effect of a negatively charged substituent is also indicated by a comparison of the binding affinities of 2,4-dinitroaniline and 2,4-dinitrophenol. The latter compound, which exists to a large extent as the negatively charged phenolate at neutral pH, has a K_0 value 8 times lower than that of the closely related 2,4-dinitroaniline.

Of much greater importance are substitutions on the benzene ring. Elimination of the 2-nitro group, as in p-nitroaniline, is associated with a very large diminution in K_0. A similar decrease occurs if the 4-nitro group is absent (as in o-nitroaniline).

In some respects the results are reminiscent of those obtained with anti-p-p'-phenylazobenzoate antibodies. First, the energy of interaction is very sensitive to alterations in the first benzene ring. Second, appropriate substitutions in the 1 position (the point of attachment to the carrier protein) are associated with very significant increases in K_0, but the exact chemical configuration of the substituent seems relatively unimportant. The data are suggestive of close complementarity with the first ring and less stringent structural requirements for the more distal groups. The great importance to specificity of groups which are exposed, or protrude the most from the carrier protein, is a general phenomenon. Such protruding groups, referred to generically as "immunodominant" groups, are considered in greater length later in this chapter.

F. Size of the Combining Region of Antidextran Antibodies

Extensive studies of antibodies to dextran, a polymer of glucose of high molecular weight, and of mouse myeloma proteins with antidextran activity, have been carried out in the laboratory of E.A. Kabat. An early investigation was done with human immune serum containing substantial amounts of precipitating antibody (15). Oligosaccharides of increasing length, comprising glucose residues in $\alpha(1 \rightarrow 6)$ linkage, were tested for their capacity to inhibit the precipitin reaction. In a typical experiment the dimer of glucose, isomaltose, was ineffective; the inhibitory capacity per molecule increased with size from the tri- to the hexasaccharide, but no further increase in inhibitory capacity was observed with additional increase in the size of the glucose polymer. The pentamer was only slightly less effective than the hexamer. From these data, Kabat concluded that the size of the combining site in many antibody molecules is large enough to accommodate five or six linked glucose residues.

Some heterogeneity in size of the active site was also noted. The relative effectiveness of the glucose trimer, as compared to the hexamer, varied among the antisera tested; with one antiserum the trimer was nearly as effective as the hexamer. This was interpreted as reflecting a larger percentage of relatively small combining sites in the antibodies of that serum.

Additional evidence for heterogeneity was obtained by fractionating the antidextran antibody population (16). The antibodies were bound to an immunosorbent and eluted successively with the dimer, isomaltose, or the trimer, followed by the hexamer. Precipitin reactions of antibodies eluted by the hexamer were not at all inhibitable by the dimer, whereas reactions of antibodies eluted with the dimer or trimer could be inhibited to some extent by the glucose dimer. Antibodies eluted by the trimer reacted equally well with the pentamer and the hexamer. These results were taken to indicate that antibodies eluted by the smaller glucose polymers had, on the average, smaller combining sites than the antibodies in the total population.[4]

G. Size of Combining Region of Antibodies to Blood Group A Substance

In a more recent investigation, Moreno and Kabat (17) studied human antibodies to hog blood group A substance, which are reactive with haptens containing N-acetylgalactosamine as an end group. The antibodies were purified specifically by immunoadsorption onto an insoluble polymer containing blood group A substance and subsequent elution with hapten. Haptens used for elution of different subpopulations of the antibody included N-acetylgalactosamine and a pentasaccharide containing a terminal α-D-N-acetylgalactosamine residue. The polysaccharides were prepared from hog blood group A substance. Sizes of combining sites were estimated by comparing the capacity of N-acetylgalactosamine, the pentasaccharide and a trisaccharide containing N-acetylgalactosamine to inhibit specific precipitin reactions of the human anti-A antibodies. With each of the two eluted antibody preparations, the pentasaccharide was much more effective on a molar basis than N-acetylgalactosamine and somewhat more effective than the specific trisaccharide.

When tested against antibodies eluted from the column by N-acetylgalactosamine, the N-acetylgalactosamine inhibited the specific precipitin reaction with A substance, whereas there was no appreciable inhibition by N-acetylgalactosamine of antibodies eluted with the pentasaccharide. The results were interpreted on the basis that the sizes of the combining sites of anti-A substance vary markedly in the human antibody population.

Investigations of a similar nature were subsequently carried out with myeloma proteins having antibody activity against $\alpha(1\rightarrow3)$dextran and levan (18). Oligosaccharides comprising glucose residues in $\alpha(1\rightarrow3)$ linkage were tested for their capacity to inhibit the precipitin reaction of the appropriate myeloma protein with $\alpha(1\rightarrow3)$dextran of high molecular weight. The inhibitory capacity per mole of glucose polymer increased with increasing size to the glucose pentamer. The hexamer and heptamer were no more effective than the pentamer, suggesting that the size of the

---

[4] Perhaps a more precise way of phrasing this would be to say that the area of contact with antigen is smaller in the population eluted with dimer or trimer. Eventually we may define the size of the combining site, on the basis of X-ray crystallography, as comprising that portion of the surface of the molecule which is made up of amino acids in the hypervariable regions of the polypeptide chains (Chapter 5). The antigen may not make contact with the entire region.

active site of the myeloma protein corresponded approximately to that of the pentamer. These results were strikingly similar to those obtained with induced antibodies.

The effective size of the active site of the myeloma protein with anti-levan activity appeared to be somewhat smaller. A trimer of the basic subunit of levan, fructose, showed maximum inhibitory capacity on a molar basis. The similarity in the type of specificity noted in myeloma proteins and in induced antibody provides one type of evidence for the concept that myeloma proteins have all the properties of induced antibodies.

H. Immunodominant Region in the Glucose Molecule

Evidence for the primary importance or immunodominance, of the protruding portion of a hapten determinant was obtained by Torii *et al.*, who worked with human antibodies to $\alpha(1 \to 6)$ dextran (19). An $\alpha(1 \to 6)$ linked pentamer or hexamer of glucose was a potent inhibitor of the specific precipitin reaction. Glucose itself was inhibitory at high concentrations. Substitution of a methyl group in the 2 or 3 position of glucose greatly diminished the inhibitory capacity, whereas substitution in the 6 position had little effect and actually somewhat enhanced the binding to antibody. The data thus indicated that the antibody fits most closely around the protruding end of the antigen molecule.

II. SPECIFICITY OF ANTIBODIES TO SYNTHETIC POLYPEPTIDES

In this section we will summarize a few of a very large number of investigations carried out in several laboratories, particularly those of M. Sela, P. Maurer, and T.J. Gill. Investigations selected for discussion are those which illustrate certain characteristics of antibody combining sites. The relationship of structure to the immunogenicity of various types of synthetic polypeptides will not be considered (see 20,21 for discussions of this question). Methods used for the preparation of synthetic polymers are described in the references cited below.

A. Size and Specificity of Active Sites of Antibodies to Polyalanyl Peptides

Studies of the specificity of antibodies directed to poly-D- or poly-L-alanyl groups were reported by Schechter *et al.* (22,23). (See also 23a.) Rabbit antibodies were elicited by immunization with a protein carrier, ribonuclease, to which polyalanyl side chains were attached by reaction of the protein with the *N*-carboxy anhydride of alanine. Attachment occurs principally to the ε-amino groups of lysine side chains. The size of the polyalanyl groups attached varied from about 6 to 10 amino acid residues. Specificity of the antibodies was investigated by measuring the capacity of various haptens (small polyalanyl peptides) to inhibit precipitation with an unrelated carrier protein, rabbit serum albumin, to which polyalanyl groups were conjugated.

It was found that antibodies specific for poly-L-alanyl side chains were nonreactive with D-alanyl peptides, and vice versa. Results of measurements of inhibition of precipitation with alanine polymers of increasing length are indicated in Fig. 2.4. The alanine monomer had no significant activity in either system. Increasing values of K_0 were observed with the dimer, trimer, and tetramer, respectively, but further increases in length were not associated with greater inhibitory capacity. The authors tentatively concluded that the size of most of the antibody combining sites (or more precisely, contact regions) corresponds to that of the alanine tetramer. However, a subsequent investigation, discussed below, suggested that the size actually resembles more closely that of the trimer. This is somewhat smaller than the size of a typical contact region postulated by Kabat on the basis of his studies with dextran as antigen.[4]

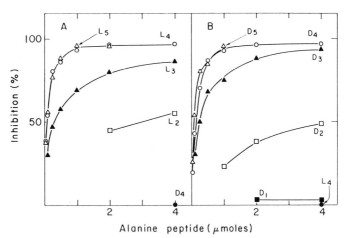

Fig. 2.4. Inhibition by alanine peptides of the precipitates obtained by reacting: (A) IgG obtained from anti-poly-L-alanyl–human serum albumin with poly-L-alanyl–rabbit serum albumin; (B) IgG obtained from anti-poly-D-alanyl–HSA with poly-D-alanyl–RSA. L, L-alanine; D, D-alanine; L2 is the polymer containing two L-alanine groups, etc. Reprinted by permission from Schechter *et al.* (22).

Antibodies to poly-L-alanyl side chains, which show greatest affinity for oligopolymers containing three or more L-alanine groups, exhibit heterogeneity with respect to their affinity for the dimer (24). When antipolyalanyl antibodies were bound to a specific immunosorbent and eluted with the alanine dimer, the antibodies purified in this way showed significant affinity for the dimer, although not nearly as great as their affinity for the trimer or tetramer. The unfractionated antibody population, however, had very little affinity for the dimer; the results are therefore indicative of heterogeneity in the total population. In contrast to the conclusions derived from studies with antidextran antibodies (Section I,F) these results suggested that the effective size of all the antibody combining sites was approximately the same, but that there is heterogeneity with respect to the "fit" around the alanine dimer. It is evident that the size distribution of the contact regions can vary with the antigen and/or species.

An innovative approach to the question of the size of the antibody combining site was made by Schechter *et al.*, who prepared rabbit antibodies against proteins conjugated to peptides of increasing length (25). The structure of these peptides is (D-alanyl)$_n$-glycyl–ribonuclease. The peptide is attached almost exclusively to lysine side chains in the protein molecule. To estimate the contribution of the lysine side chain to specificity, affinities of peptides with the structure (D-alanyl)$_n$-glycyl-ϵ-aminocaproate were compared with the corresponding peptides lacking the ϵ-aminocaproate group, When $n = 1$ or 2, the presence of the ϵ-aminocaproate group caused a large increase in affinity, indicating that the antibody combining site recognized the lysine side chain in the carrier protein. (Lysine and ϵ-aminocaproate are very similar in structure.) When $n = 3$, the presence of the ϵ-aminocaproate had no enhancing effect on affinity; i.e., (D-alanyl)$_3$-glycine had an affinity similar to that of (D-alanyl)$_3$-glycyl-ϵ-aminocaproate. One can interpret these results on the basis that the antibody combining site can accommodate a polypeptide approximately the size of (D-alanyl)$_3$-glycine; the side chain of the carrier protein plays a role in determining specificity only when the hapten group is smaller than this. From these results one would conclude that the antibody combining site accommodates a polypeptide with a backbone consisting of 10 to 12 carbon atoms. This corresponds quite closely to the depth of certain antibody combining sites estimated by studies of spin-labeled haptens (Section VI,D), or by electron microscopic investigation of interactions of antibodies with haptens of increasing size (Chapter 5).

Studies with rabbit anti-polyalanyl antibodies also provided support for the concept of an "immunodominant" group; i.e., the region farthest

TABLE 2.4

THE EFFECT OF SIDE CHAIN SUBSTITUTION ON THE CAPACITY OF
TETRAPEPTIDES TO INHIBIT THE PRECIPITATION OF
RABBIT ANTIPOLYALANYL ANTIBODIES[a]

Peptide	C (mM)	Peptide	C (mM)[b]	Peptide	C (mM)[b]
Ala Ala Ala Ala	0.09				
Ala Ala Ala *Phe*	0.10			Ala Ala Ala *Gly*	0.09
Ala Ala *Phe* Ala	0.18			Ala Ala *Gly* Ala	0.18
Ala *Phe* Ala Ala	2.1	Ala *Val* Ala Ala	>3 (32%)	Ala *Gly* Ala Ala	0.70
Phe Ala Ala Ala	>3 (24%)	*Val* Ala Ala Ala	>3 (24%)	*Gly* Ala Ala Ala	2.9

[a] Reprinted by permission from Schechter (23).

[b] The symbol C represents the concentration of peptide required for 50% inhibition of precipitation. When 50% inhibition was not achieved the percentage inhibition at maximal peptide concentration tested is given in parentheses. All amino acids are L. The N-terminus is at the left.

removed from the protein carrier appears to be of prime importance in determining specificity (23). This point is illustrated by the data in Table 2.4, obtained with antibody directed to poly-L-alanyl side chains. Substitution of phenylalanine, valine, or glycine for one L-alanine in the tetramer decreased its capacity to combine with the antibody. This decrease was greatest when the substitution was at the N-terminal end (i.e., most distal from the protein carrier). The next most sensitive position was that adjacent to the N-terminus. Substitution in the third and fourth positions had much less of an adverse effect on the interaction with antibody. Again we are led to the conclusion that the "fit" is most critical around the protruding, or distal portion of the hapten.

In a related investigation (26) it was noted that the specificity and apparent size of the antibody combining site, as determined with poly-D-alanyl hapten groups, are essentially identical for antibodies of the IgG and IgM classes. This work was done with goat, as well as rabbit antibodies.

A more detailed investigation of antibodies specific for poly-L-alanyl determinants was reported by Schechter (23), who utilized specifically purified rabbit antibodies directed to polyalanyl side chains. He found that the trimer was actually as effective as the tetramer, provided that the terminal carboxylate group of the trimer was amidated

$$(-\overset{\overset{\text{O}}{\|}}{\text{C}}-\text{NH}_2).$$

It was concluded that the negative charge of the terminal carboxylate group is disadvantageous to binding; in the case of the trimer this can be overcome either by amidation or by adding a fourth alanyl group, either of which reacts with the carboxylate of the third alanyl group. When amide derivatives were compared, the trimer, tetramer, and pentamer showed about equal affinity for anti-polyalanyl antibodies. The increase in affinity resulting from amidation of the terminal carboxylate in the trimer also suggested that the complementary region of the antibody combining site is hydrophobic and can therefore not tolerate a negative charge in the hapten.

Using the alanine tetramer, Schechter (23) also quantified the contribution of the methyl group side chain of each alanine to the free energy of interaction $(\Delta G^0)^5$ by substitution for alanine of glycine, which lacks the methyl group (Table 2.4). The change in free energy associated with substitution of glycine for alanine in the N-terminal position was 2.1 kcal/mole; in the second position the change was 1.25 kcal/mole and in the third position, 0.42 kcal/mole. When glycine was substituted in both the first and second positions the change in ΔG^0 was 3.38 kcal/mole, which agrees closely with the summation of effects due to the single replacements $(2.1 + 1.25 = 3.35$ kcal/mole). Effects on ΔG^0 of substitution at the second and third positions were also found to be additive.

It was concluded that the contributions of the methyl group of alanine to binding energy at each position are additive and thus essentially independent of one another. As already indicated, the importance of the methyl group decreases with increasing distance from the N-terminal end of the chain; this is in accord with the concept that the grouping which protrudes most from the carrier molecule tends to be immunodominant.

B. Evidence for Immunodominant Groups in Synthetic Polypeptides with Branched Chains (Multichain Copolymers)

Early investigations supporting the concept that exposed haptenic determinants are immunodominant were carried out by Sela and his collaborators, who prepared antibodies against a number of synthetic polypeptides of high molecular weight with the general structure illustrated in Fig. 2.5. The backbone of the polymer consists of poly-L-lysine. The

---

[5] Changes in free energy of interaction were calculated from relative binding affinities by using the expression, $\Delta G^0 = -RT \ln K_0$ (A change in K_0 by a factor of 10 corresponds to a change in ΔG^0 of about 1.3 kcal/mole at 25°.)

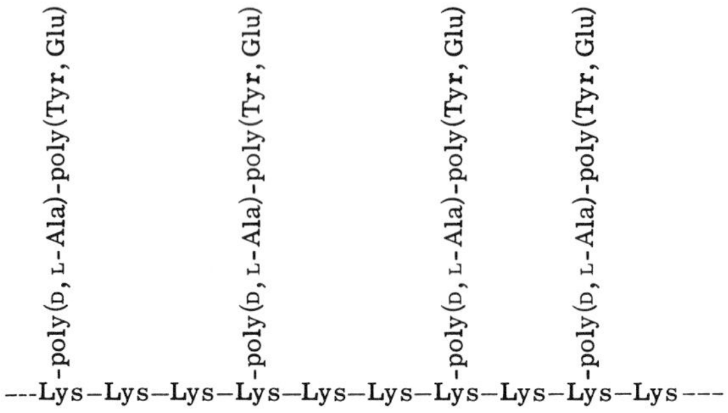
-poly(D, L-Ala)-poly(Tyr, Glu)
-poly(D, L-Ala)-poly(Tyr, Glu)
-poly(D, L-Ala)-poly(Tyr, Glu)
-poly(D, L-Ala)-poly(Tyr, Glu)
---Lys–Lys–Lys–Lys–Lys–Lys–Lys–Lys–Lys–Lys---

Fig. 2.5. Structure of a multichain polymer containing a backbone of polylysine and an external random copolymer of tyrosine and glutamic acid (molar ratio, Lys:Tyr:Glu:D,L-Ala = 1:1.8:3.7:24). The average molecular weight of the polymer used as antigen in the experiments discussed in the text is 35,000. From Fuchs and Sela (27,28).

ϵ-amino side chains of lysine residues are used as points of initiation for attachment of either an oligopolymer (polyalanine in the illustration) or a random copolymer. Still a third polypeptide chain [poly(Tyr,Glu) in the illustration] is then attached to the amino terminus of the second chain (i.e., to the polyalanine). The number of ϵ-amino groups of the polylysine which are modified, and the lengths of the attached chains can vary markedly depending on conditions used for coupling and the molar ratios of the reagents. *N*-Carboxy anhydrides of amino acids are used to prepare the polymers (27,28).

In one set of experiments (27) a copolymer with the general structure shown in Fig. 2.5 was used to immunize rabbits. Antiserum was eventually obtained which precipitated the immunogen specifically. Precipitation could be inhibited by the random copolymer poly(Tyr,Glu). Maximum inhibition was obtained when the ratio of tyrosine to glutamic acid in the copolymer was 1.0:1.1. When the ratio in the copolymer was 1:4, only partial inhibition was possible, even with very high concentrations of the inhibitor, and no inhibition of precipitation was obtained when the ratio was 1:9 [a ratio widely different from that in the immunogen (Fig. 2.5, legend)].

The same antibodies were not at all inhibited by polylysine or by polyalanine, i.e., by the backbone polypeptide or by the first chain attached. These results again provide strong evidence that the most exposed portion of the molecule, in this case poly(Tyr,Glu), is also the most immunogenic.

C. Suggestive Evidence for the Presence of Two Negative Charges in an Antibody Combining Site

Using random copolymers, such as $Glu_{56}Lys_{38}Tyr_6$,[6] of high molecular weight as antigens, Gill was able to elicit precipitating antibodies in rabbits (29). Inhibition of precipitation was obtained with certain diamines, NH_3^+—$(CH_2)_n$—NH_3^+. When $n = 2$, inhibition was very weak; inhibitory capacity increased with increasing values of n, reaching a maximum in 1,5-pentanediamine ($n = 5$). The corresponding uncharged dialcohol, 1,5-pentanediol, was ineffective. These results were interpreted on the basis that the combining site of this antibody contains two negative charges (presumably complementary to positive charges in lysine side chains in the copolymer) and that the spacing between the two negatively charged groups corresponds in length to that of pentanediamine.

D. Size of the Combining Region of Antibodies to α-Dnp-Polylysine

Schlossman and Levine (30) prepared antibodies in guinea pigs against poly-L-lysine to which Dnp (2,4-dinitrophenyl) groups were coupled at the α-amino position:

$$O_2N-\overset{\displaystyle NO_2}{\underset{\displaystyle }{\bigcirc}}-NH-Lys-Lys-Lys---Lys-Lys-Lys-COOH$$

To prepare such antibodies, an α-Dnp-substituted polymer, which had an average chain length of 11 lysine groups, was conjugated to bovine serum albumin for use as the immunogen. Synthetic poly-L-lysine preparations of increasing length, with Dnp groups attached at the α-NH_2-terminal position, were tested as inhibitors of the precipitin reaction of the immunogen with its rabbit antibodies. (Polylysines without an attached Dnp group were noninhibitory.) On a molar basis the Dnp-substituted peptides increased in effectiveness as inhibitors with increasing length up to the pentamer; thereafter increases in length had relatively little effect, although the heptamer was slightly more effective than the pentamer. The apparent size of the combining region deduced from these investigations would appear somewhat larger than that derived from

---

[6] The subscripts represent the percent of each amino acid in the random copolymer. Each amino acid is of the L series.

studies with polyalanine as the antigenic group, but roughly comparable to sites on antibodies specific for dextran.

In an earlier study with rabbit antibodies to poly-L-lysine, Arnon *et al.* had deduced that the antibody combining site was complementary to an area encompassing 5 to 6 lysine residues (31). Stollar *et al.* (32) studying naturally occurring anti-DNA antibodies in two patients with systemic lupus erythematosus concluded that the antibody combining site could accommodate an oligonucleotide polymer comprising 4 or 5 thymidylate groups.

III. STABILIZATION OF THE ANTIBODY MOLECULE BY INTERACTION WITH HAPTEN

Evidence for stabilization by hapten was reported by Metzger and Singer (33), who showed that it is more difficult to dissociate H and L chains of anti-Dnp antibody in the presence of hapten than in its absence. Subsequently, Cathou and Haber (34) studied the effect of guanidine hydrochloride on the optical rotatory dispersion of rabbit anti-Dnp antibody and concluded that the hapten, ϵ-Dnp-L-lysine, stabilizes the molecule against denaturation by 4 M guanidine hydrochloride. Very similar findings were reported by Cathou and Warner (35) who investigated rabbit anti-Dnp antibodies, but measured circular dichroism rather than optical rotatory dispersion. On the basis of the strong protection afforded against unfolding by a small hapten molecule the authors correctly predicted that the active site must involve amino acid residues located at positions widely separated in the linear sequence, but brought into proximity in the folded molecule, and that both the L chain and the Fd segment are involved.

IV. INDUCTION OF OPTICAL ACTIVITY IN HAPTEN BOUND TO ANTIBODY

Two groups of investigators (36–38) have demonstrated the induction of optical activity in Dnp and Tnp (2,4,6-trinitrophenyl) derivatives upon interaction with the corresponding antihapten antibody or with a myeloma protein having the appropriate antihapten antibody activity; in the absence of antibody the haptens are optically inactive. Nonspecific immunoglobulins are without effect. Glazer and Singer refer to this phenomenon as an extrinsic Cotton effect. Since the optical activity is maximal at a wavelength corresponding to an absorption peak of the hapten, it must be attributed to the hapten and not to the protein molecule. The effect is ascribed to the interaction of the asymmetric environment of the antibody binding site with the inherently symmetrical chromophore of the hapten.

The circular dichroic spectra vary with the Dnp derivatives tested (37,38). Spectra of ϵ-Dnp-lysine and ϵ-Dnp-aminocaproate, interacting with anti-Dnp antibody, are quite similar, reflecting the similarity in structure of the haptens, but they differ markedly from the spectra of Dnp-glycine or ϵ-Tnp-lysine.

The method is also capable of differentiating among different antibody populations with the same specificity. Mouse anti-Dnp antibodies elicited by immunization with Dnp derivatives induce circular dichroic patterns, upon interaction with ϵ-Dnp-lysine, that are strikingly different from those induced by MOPC 315, a mouse IgA myeloma protein with anti-Dnp activity (38). It was concluded that the combining site of protein 315 must differ in its fine structure from that of the majority of induced mouse anti-Dnp antibodies.

V. THE QUESTION OF CONFORMATIONAL CHANGES INDUCED IN ANTIBODIES UPON INTERACTION WITH ANTIGEN OR HAPTEN

It is attractive, as an explanation for certain properties of antibodies, to assume that conformational changes may occur within the antibody molecule as a consequence of combination with antigen. For example, the Fc region of the antibody molecule has been implicated in complement fixation, which occurs after combination with antigen; the latter reaction takes place in the Fab segment. This could conceivably be explained by an antigen-induced conformational change extending to the Fc segment; i.e., by a mechanism analogous to an allosteric effect. It should be pointed out, however, that there is no strong evidence for this and that alternative explanations are conceivable.

Conformational changes in antibody have been suggested to explain the triggering of immunocompetent cells as a result of the interaction of membrane-bound receptors (immunoglobulins) with antigen. Again, there is no direct proof that a conformational change is involved. Recent demonstrations of surface migration of cell-bound receptors, after interaction with an antiglobulin reagent or with antigen (39–41), suggest the possibility of a triggering mechanism based on such massive migration rather than on a conformational change in antibody. Again, this is conjectural, but it illustrates the fact that alternative hypotheses exist.

There is one type of conformational change in antibodies whose existence is generally accepted. This involves the potential for movement of the two Fab segments in relation to one another. The evidence, discussed in greater detail in Chapter 5, was obtained by electron microscopy. IgG antibody molecules have been seen in an extended form, attached to two virus particles, or in a horseshoe or Y-shaped configuration with both combining sites apparently linked to the same particle (42,43). Additional evidence that the angle between two Fab fragments of IgG can vary was obtained by Feinstein and Rowe (44) and by Valentine and Green (45), who examined by electron microscopy both free antibody molecules and antibody with its combining sites attached to an antigen (ferritin, Dnp-ferritin, or small bivalent Dnp compounds). Angles of extension between the two Fab fragments varied from 10° to 180° with no suggestion of a preferred angle.[7] Molecules were seen in a Y-configuration in the absence as well as the presence of antigen. This freedom of rotation is generally attributed to flexibility in the hinge region of the chain. It obviously imparts great versatility to the antibody in combining with two receptors on the same or on different particles.[8] Physicochemical studies relating to the flexibility of the antibody molecule are discussed in Chapter 5.

This type of conformational change, involving the flexible movements of large segments of the molecule, is not necessarily germane to the related question whether alterations of internal structure occur upon interaction with antigen. Several early studies failed to reveal significant changes in optical rotation of antihapten antibodies, resulting from combination with hapten (46–48). Ishizaka and Campbell (46) observed changes in optical rotation upon interaction of antibodies with multivalent antigens. Metzger points out that these changes may have involved the antigen exclusively, since the effects were greatest in the presence of excess antibody (49).

The possibility of a conformational change is suggested by the work of Holowka *et al.* (50), who found significant changes in the circular dichroic spectra of three homogeneous preparations of rabbit anti-type

---

[7] The possibility has not been ruled out that differences in angle reflect heterogeneity of antibody structure rather than flexibility; however, this seems rather unlikely.

[8] There is no clear evidence as to whether the IgG molecule interacts more effectively with the first component of complement when a wide angle separates the two Fab segments. An alternative possibility to account for the enhanced ability of antibody to interact with C1q after forming a complex with antigen is that C1q can combine more effectively with two adjacent antibody molecules than with a single molecule, owing to the energetic advantages of multivalent attachment. Support for this view comes from the capacity of aggregated IgG to fix complement in the absence of antigen.

III pneumococcal polysaccharides in the presence of a complementary hexasaccharide. The spectral changes (in the ultraviolet) were attributed to changes in the optical activity of the antibodies, since the hapten alone showed no absorbance at the same wavelengths. These effects were interpreted as indicating either a conformational change in the antibody, occurring as a result of the interaction with hapten, or changes in the asymmetric environments of tyrosine or tryptophan side chains in the presence of hapten.

Data interpreted as suggestive of a conformational change were obtained by Warner *et al.* (51). They observed a decrease of about 1% in the sedimentation coefficient of rabbit antibody to the azophenyl-β-lactoside group upon interaction with free hapten. The investigators concluded that the hapten induces a structural change, resulting in a more compact configuration of the antibody molecule. The degree of structural change necessary for this very small effect cannot be readily estimated. No such increase in sedimentation rate was noted, however, with antibody to a different hapten, the Dnp group, as a result of specific interaction of the antibody with monovalent hapten.

Attempts to demonstrate conformational changes in a monoclonal human IgM protein with anti-Dnp activity were made by Ashman and Metzger (52). They noted no changes in circular dichroic spectra, even when more than 90% of the hapten-binding sites were occupied. Hydrogen-exchange studies, carried out with tritiated water, indicated that some hydrogen atoms of the myeloma protein were trapped (i.e., were no longer free to exchange), in the presence of hapten. The number of hydrogen atoms involved corresponded to about 10 amino acid residues per active site. Trapping was confined to atoms in the Fab fragment, indicating the absence of long-range effects. Alternative explanations for the results, suggested by the authors, were (a) that hapten stabilizes thermal motions in certain amino acid side chains, greatly retarding the release of hydrogen atoms or (b) that a small conformational change occurs as a consequence of binding of hapten.

A change in conformation upon interaction with a hapten is indicated by the study of Pilz *et al.* (52a), who investigated the interaction of rabbit anti-poly-D-alanyl antibodies with tetra-D-alanine by the method of small-angle X-ray scattering. The interaction was associated with a significant contraction in volume (3–10%) and a small decrease in the radius of gyration of the antibody. The volume contraction was attributed to a conformational change.

Tumerman *et al.* (52b) observed an increase in rotational relaxation time, associated with an antibody–hapten interaction, which they thought might reflect decreased flexibility.

Studies of diffraction patterns of crystallized immunoglobulins, in the presence or absence of ligands of low molecular weight bound in the active site, have so far not revealed any significant conformational changes (Chapter 5).

A. Resistance of Antibody to Proteolysis in the Presence of Hapten

Two investigations, one with conventionally induced antibody and the other with a myeloma protein having known hapten-binding activity, have indicated that the presence of hapten affords some protection to the antibody against the action of proteolytic enzymes. There are at least two possible interpretations of these results. One is that hapten induces a conformational change which results in a more compact, enzyme-resistant structure. A second interpretation postulates that the hapten sterically protects susceptible bonds in the binding site against attack by an enzyme. It is relevant that cleavage of a single peptide bond can result in partial unfolding, making other bonds susceptible to enzymatic attack (zipper effect). Therefore, steric protection of even a small region of the molecule by hapten could be significant.

Grossberg et al. worked with specifically purified antibodies directed to the p-azobenzenearsonate and the p-azobenzenetrimethylammonium hapten groups (53). Antibodies were radiolabeled with iodine and the degree of proteolysis by chymotrypsin was assayed by measuring the amount of radioactivity that remained in solution after precipitation of the protein with sulfosalicylic acid. The experiments were carefully controlled by labeling one of the antibodies with ^{131}I and the other with ^{125}I and treating the mixture with chymotrypsin in the presence of a hapten reactive with one or the other antibody. The amounts of each isotope that became nonprecipitable after proteolysis were measured. The presence of specific hapten caused a decrease in the amount of radioactivity released after a given period of digestion. In a typical experiment, 10% of the radioactivity became nonprecipitable after 5 hours of digestion in the absence of hapten, whereas only 7% failed to precipitate when digestion was carried out in the presence of hapten. Antibody, present in the same reaction mixture, that was nonreactive with the hapten was digested to the same extent in the presence or absence of hapten. The protective action of hapten was confined to the Fab fragment of the molecule. Two possible interpretations of these results, one of which does not require a conformational change, were discussed above.

Effects of binding of hapten on the resistance of an immunoglobulin to proteolysis were also investigated by Ashman and Metzger (54), who utilized a Waldenström macroglobulin (IgM) having anti-Dnp activity. They found that the presence of hapten retarded the rate of proteolysis, when the IgM protein was exposed to subtilisin or to chymotrypsin. The retardation was confined to the Fab fragment of the molecule. The results were interpreted as indicative of a small conformational change or of steric protection by hapten of certain enzyme-sensitive peptide bonds.

B. Absence of Major Interactions between the Two Combining Sites of a Bivalent Antibody Molecule

If hapten caused a major conformational change in an antibody molecule, one manifestation might be an allosteric alteration of the binding properties of one combining site upon interaction of the other site with hapten. The experimental data indicate that such an effect, if it occurs at all, must be small. Thus, Nisonoff *et al.* (55) measured the binding of hapten to specifically purified rabbit anti-*p*-azobenzoate antibody (IgG) and to its Fab fragments. The average binding affinity, K_0, and the index of heterogeneity agreed within experimental error for the two preparations; i.e., the binding curves were virtually superimposable. This observation indicated that combination of hapten with one combining site did not influence the affinity of the other site. It should be noted that these results may not necessarily apply to all classes of immunoglobulin.

Similar results were obtained by Velick *et al.* (56), using rabbit anti-Dnp antibody, and by Ashman and Metzger (57), who studied a human monoclonal IgM protein with anti-Dnp activity.

VI. RATES AND ENERGETIC ASPECTS OF ANTIGEN–ANTIBODY REACTIONS

A. Kinetic Measurements

This discussion of reaction rates will be concerned principally with antibody–hapten interactions. While much valuable information has been obtained with protein antigens (58–63), the data are more difficult to analyze because of the possibility of multivalent attachment of a single antibody molecule to the same antigen particle and the effect of the growth of a lattice on the rates and affinities of attachment of subsequent antibody molecules. Very rapid measurements of initial rates of reactions of antibodies with protein antigens, such as those of Dandliker and his colleagues (62,63), overcame many of these problems but will be omitted because of space limitation. We should mention one important conclusion derived from that work, namely, that the initial rate of reaction of antibody with a protein antigen appears to be at least 100 times slower than a typical antibody-hapten reaction. This is attributable to the more rapid diffusion rates of small ligands.

With the exception of a myeloma protein with anti-Dnp activity, preparations used for these studies have been specifically purified anti-hapten antibodies, which are heterogeneous. The velocity constants reported, as well as equilibrium constants, are therefore average values.

To study rates of antibody–hapten reactions the principal methods employed have involved stopped flow or temperature jump techniques. The former was first used by Sturtevant *et al.* (64) and Day *et al.* (65). The temperature jump method has been employed by Froese, Sehon, and their collaborators (66–68) and more recently by Pecht *et al.* (69). Both methods are utilized in conjunction with very rapid optical measurements (in the millisecond range). For example, Sturtevant *et al.* took advantage of a spectral shift which occurs upon combination of anti-Dnp antibody with the dye, 2-(Dnp-azo)-1-naphthol-3,6-disulfonic acid (64). With the same hapten, and with ϵ-Dnp-L-lysine and ϵ-Dnp-6-aminocaproate, Day *et al.* (65) used the method of fluorescence quenching (Section VI,D) with a stopped flow apparatus. In the temperature jump technique the components are first equilibrated, a temperature increment is rapidly induced (up to 10°C in 0.1 μsecond), and the rate of reequilibration at the new temperature is measured. Velocity constants can be estimated from the data; the mathematical approaches required are described in the references cited.

Table 2.5 summarizes data obtained with a number of haptens and their corresponding antibodies. Except for protein 315, a mouse myeloma protein with anti-Dnp activity, specifically purified rabbit antibodies were used. The data on reaction rates are expressed in terms of a second-order velocity constant, k_{12}, where the forward reaction velocity is $v = k_{12}(A)\,(L)$; v is in mole/liter/second; (A) and (L) are the molar concentrations of free (unoccupied) antibody combining sites and of ligand, respectively. The units of k_{12} are 1/mole/second ($M^{-1}\mathrm{sec}^{-1}$). In measuring rates it is essential to have a method for detection of the product at a low concentration, since the concentrations of reactants must be sufficiently small so that the velocity of the reaction is not too rapid to measure.

The rate of the reverse reaction is k_{21} (AL), where (AL) is the concentration of the antibody–hapten complex. The units of k_{21} are reciprocal seconds. If initial forward rates are measured with sufficient rapidity

TABLE 2.5

FORWARD AND REVERSE RATE CONSTANTS FOR SOME ANTIBODY–HAPTEN INTERACTIONS

Antibody preparation[a]	Hapten	Average association constant (K_0) (M^{-1})	t (°C)	k_{12} ($M^{-1} sec^{-1}$)	k_{21} (sec^{-1})	Method[b]	Calculated $K_0 (k_{12}/k_{21})$ (M^{-1})	Reference
Anti-p-azophenyl-arsonate	N-R'-arsonate[c]	—	31	2×10^7	50	A	4×10^5	66
Anti-Dnp	ε-Dnp-lysine	9×10^7	25	8×10^7	1.1^f	B	—	65
Anti-Dnp	ε-Dnp-aminocaproate	9×10^7	25	1×10^8	4.1^f	B	—	65
Anti-Dnp	1 N-2,5S-4Dnp[d]	2.4×10^5	29	1.7×10^7	70	A	2.4×10^5	67
Anti-Dnp	1 N-2,5S-4-np[e]	$\sim 1 \times 10^4$	29	1.4×10^7	410	A	3.4×10^4	67
Anti-Dnp	ε-Dnp-lysine	2.2×10^7	25	1.1×10^7	0.5^f	B	—	68
Anti-Dnp (Fab)	ε-Dnp-lysine	2.5×10^7	25	1.8×10^7	0.8^f	B	—	68
Protein 315 (monomer)	ε-Dnp-lysine	2.0×10^6	25	1.3×10^8	53	A	2.5×10^6	69
Protein 315	Dnp-glycine	Not done	25	1.9×10^8	1300	A	1.5×10^5	69
Protein 315 (Fab')	Dnp-lysine	2.0×10^6	25	1.5×10^8	68	A	2.2×10^6	69

[a] All preparations are specifically purified rabbit antibodies except for protein 315, which is a mouse myeloma protein with anti-Dnp activity.

[b] Method used for rate measurements: A, Temp. jump; B, fluorescence quenching, stopped flow.

[c] 1-Napthol-4[4(4'-azobenzeneazo)]-phenylarsonate.

[d] 1-Hydroxy-4-(2,4-dinitrophenylazo)-2,5-naphthalene disulfonate.

[e] 1-Hydroxy-4-(4-nitrophenylazo)-2,5-naphthalene disulfonate.

[f] Obtained from the relationship $k_{21} = k_{12}/K_0$; k_{21} not determined directly.

the effect of reversibility on the measurement is negligible. The temperature jump method has the unique advantage of permitting the simultaneous estimation of both k_{12} and k_{21}, since the rate of reequilibration is dependent on both the forward and reverse reaction rates. When initial rates are measured by stopped flow techniques, k_{21} can still be estimated from the relationship $K = k_{12}/k_{21}$, if the equilibrium constant, K, has been determined independently. Conversely, the equilibrium constant can be calculated from values of k_{12} and k_{21} obtainable by the temperature jump technique. Agreement of this calculated value with one obtained by independent means helps to establish the validity of the data. Such calculations are necessarily greatly oversimplified since antihapten antibodies of a single specificity are heterogeneous with respect to rate and equilibrium constants. By the same token, the data in Table 2.5, with the exception of those for the myeloma protein, represent average values.

One striking feature of the data in Table 2.5 is the small range of values of k_{12}. The second-order rate constants for these interactions are among the highest seen in biochemical reactions. It is estimated that they approximate the value for a diffusion controlled reaction involving a macromolecule, i.e., that the limiting factor is the frequency of collision of hapten with the antibody combining region. There is little difference in this respect between the myeloma protein (MOPC 315) with anti-Dnp activity and induced anti-Dnp antibody.

Since the forward rate constants do not vary greatly it is apparent that the equilibrium constant must reflect the rate constant of the reverse reaction, k_{21}. Thus, an antibody combining site with a binding affinity, K, of $10^5\ M^{-1}$ might have a dissociation rate constant about 10^3 times as great as that of an antibody with $K = 10^8\ M^{-1}$. As indicated in Table 2.5 there are marked variations in the dissociation rate constants.

It has been suggested that the very high forward velocity constant, which is indicative of a low energy of activation, precludes the occurrence of a major conformational change during the antibody–hapten interaction. A minor, rapidly occurring change in antibody structure is not ruled out, however, or is a conformational change which might occur after the changes in optical properties are registered.

The value of k_{21} is directly related to the half-life of a hapten group within the combining site (half-life $= 0.693/k_{21}$). Thus, for a reaction with $k_{21} = 1\ \text{sec}^{-1}$ the half-life is 0.69 sec. For an antibody with a binding affinity of $10^9\ M^{-1}$ and a typical forward velocity constant of $2 \times 10^9\ M^{-1}\ \text{sec}^{-1}$ the half-life in the active site would be about 30 sec. As a consequence it is difficult to remove hapten from an antibody of very high affinity by dialysis or gel filtration.

For a univalent fragment of antihapten antibody the forward velocity constant, k_{12}, is about the same as that of the whole antibody. In one careful investigation directed to this question [Table 2.5 (68)] the value for the fragment was greater by about a factor of 2; this could be explained by the smaller size and hence greater diffusion constant of the fragment. That the equilibrium constants for the association of antibody or its univalent fragments with hapten are approximately the same had been reported earlier (55).

B. Thermodynamics of Antigen–Antibody Reactions

In recent years many investigations in cellular immunology as well as immunochemistry have made use of thermodynamic concepts. For example, it has been shown that there is frequently a gradual increase in the affinity of circulating antibody with time after initial immunization, with IgG more likely to increase in affinity than IgM; that a low dose of antigen favors the production of antibody of high affinity; and that the affinity of a receptor on a B cell reflects that of the antibody that will be produced by the cell and its descendants. These findings had their inception in the investigations of Jerne (70) and of Eisen and Siskind (12).

Quantitative experiments require the measurement of binding affinities, which are determined by thermodynamic properties. Thermodynamic parameters (ΔG^0, ΔH^0, and ΔS^0) have also been investigated in efforts to analyze the mechanisms of antigen–antibody reactions. For example, a high affinity could be attributable to a large negative value for the standard enthalpy change, ΔH^0, or heat of the reaction, or to a large increase in entropy (ΔS^0) resulting from the antigen–antibody reaction, or to both. A knowledge of these parameters can in theory contribute to an understanding of the mechanism of antigen–antibody reactions. In fact, however, numerous investigations of this type, carried out over a period of many years, have failed to reveal intimate details of the reaction mechanism. Possible reasons for this are suggested below. We will therefore summarize only briefly work directed toward the determination of ΔH^0 and ΔS^0 and will concentrate on methods for determining equilibrium constants, which have proved very useful.

We will consider first some of the relationships that are most relevant to this type of analysis of antibody–hapten reactions. The basic equation is:

$$Ab + H \rightleftharpoons (AbH); \qquad K = b/cA_f \qquad (2.1)$$

where K is the equilibrium constant, or association constant, for the reaction; b and c are the molar concentrations of hapten bound and free, respectively, when equilibrium is attained, and A_f is the molar concentration of antibody combining sites remaining unoccupied at equilibrium. In a typical set of experiments the total concentration of antibody is held constant while the hapten concentration is increased. Under these conditions b will increase, and A_f will decrease until saturation of the antibody combining sites is approached. Equation (2.1) is not directly applicable, in general, to actual antibody–hapten interactions, since normal antibody populations are heterogeneous with respect to K. Its application to heterogeneous antibodies is discussed later.

The equilibrium constant, K, is related to the standard free energy change, ΔG^0, of the reaction by the expression, $\Delta G^0 = -RT \ln K$, where is the gas constant and T the absolute temperature. Thus, if K is known, ΔG^0 can be calculated.

The value of the enthalpy change, ΔH^0, can be calculated from the van't Hoff equation.

$$(d\ln K)/dT = \Delta H^0/RT^2 \quad \text{or} \quad \ln K_2/K_1 = (\Delta H^0/R)(1/T_1 - 1/T_2) \quad (2.2)$$

where K_1 and K_2 are the equilibrium constants at two temperatures T_1 and T_2. Thus, ΔH^0 can be calculated if the value of K is known for at least two temperatures. (A larger number is preferable.) A linear relationship should exist between $\ln K$ and $1/T$; the slope of the line is $-\Delta H^0/R$. Again this would apply to a homogeneous antibody population.

Finally, the expression

$$\Delta G^0 = \Delta H^0 - T\Delta S^0 \quad (2.3)$$

permits calculation of the standard entropy change, ΔS^0, when ΔH^0 and ΔG^0 have been determined. Thus, an evaluation of K at different temperatures permits the calculation of the three basic thermodynamic parameters, and the value of K at a single temperature allows computation of the standard free energy change, ΔG^0, at that temperature.

There are major difficulties in using this approach for estimating ΔH^0 and ΔS^0 of immune reactions. These derive from the heterogeneity of antibodies. The value of K that one calculates is necessarily some type of average value for that population of antibodies, and one cannot predict how temperature changes will affect the average. For example, two different groups of antibody molecules in the same population might combine with the same hapten by making preferential use of different types of noncovalent forces (e.g., hydrogen bonding versus van der

Waal's interactions). The relative contributions of ΔH^0 and ΔS^0 to the interaction might be quite different for the two sets of molecules; the effect on K of an increase in temperature might conceivably be positive for one antibody and negative for the other. It therefore involves unproved assumptions to make a direct calculation of ΔH^0 from average values of K at two temperatures.

Secondly, calculation of an average K value necessarily requires an *ad hoc* assumption as to the nature of the distribution of heterogeneous antibody molecules with respect to their binding affinities. A commonly used approximation is that values of ΔG^0 (or ln K) follow a Gauss error function (see below). On the basis of this assumption one can calculate an average value of K through measurement of binding with varying concentrations of hapten. However, recent work on the actual distribution of antibody molecules has demonstrated that a few homogeneous subpopulations may account for the bulk of the antibodies of a given specificity in many antisera. In the Gaussian distribution all values of K are represented, and the "average K," or K_0, is that corresponding to the peak of the distribution curve. Using this assumption for estimation of K_0 values at different temperatures could lead to indeterminate errors in the calculated values of ΔH^0 and ΔS^0.

Perhaps the most reliable data for ΔH^0 have been obtained by direct measurements, using microcalorimetry (71,72). The measurements were carried out initially with specifically purified anti-2,4-dinitrophenyl (anti-Dnp) antibodies from hyperimmune rabbits and the hapten, ϵ-Dnp-lysine. That fraction (30%) of the population which had the highest affinity exhibited an enthalpy change on binding hapten of -23 kcal/mole. Assuming a maximum standard free energy change of -12 kcal/mole this would correspond to a decrease in entropy of at least 35 cal/deg/mole. In other words, the entropy change strongly opposes the binding reaction but is overcompensated by the large decrease in enthalpy. The average value of ΔH^0 for the total population was estimated as -17.5 kcal/mole. The authors did not propose a molecular mechanism to account for this surprisingly large value.

It was also observed that the experimental value of $-\Delta H^0$ was about 50% greater (more negative) than that obtained by the use of Eq. (2.5), the van't Hoff expression; the latter value was determined by measuring K_0 at three temperatures. The difference in the two sets of results was attributed to a lack of knowledge as to which subpopulation of the heterogeneous antibody contributes most significantly to the changes in K observed with changing temperature. These careful experiments cast serious doubt on the validity of earlier evaluations of ΔH^0 and ΔS^0 of antibody–hapten reactions, based on the variation of K_0 with temperature.

In a subsequent investigation, it was shown that there is agreement between values of ΔH^0, estimated by microcalorimetry or from the van't Hoff equation, when myeloma proteins with antihapten activity rather than induced antibodies are studied (72); this finding is consistent with the homogeneity of myeloma proteins. The mouse myeloma proteins studied, MOPC 315 and MOPC 460, both have specificity for Dnp derivatives. The driving force for the interaction of either protein with polynitro derivatives of aromatic compounds is enthalpy (-12 to -20 kcal/mole). The interaction with the naphthaquinone derivative, menadione, is, in contrast, dependent on an increase in entropy. The authors suggest that the data are consistent with charge transfer, involving tryptophan in the active site, as a mechanism for the interaction of the polynitro compounds with the myeloma proteins. The possibility of charge transfer had been suggested earlier on the basis of other data (Section VI,D).

C. Direct Measurement of Antibody–Hapten Interactions; General Considerations

Equation (2.1) above is arithmetically equivalent to the following:

$$K = b/(nA_t - b)c \qquad (2.4)$$

where A_t is the total (rather than free) concentration of antibody molecules and n is the number of binding sites per molecule of antibody (the valence). This is readily transformed into[9]

$$r/c = nK - rK \qquad (2.5)$$

where r is the number of moles of hapten bound per mole of antibody. This equation predicts, for homogeneous antibody, a linear relationship between r/c and r, with a slope of $-K$, an intercept on the abscissa of n, and an intercept on the ordinate of nK. Thus, the intercept on the abscissa is the valence of the antibody.

Figure 2.6 illustrates a typical curve for the binding of hapten by a purified rabbit antihapten antibody (73). The binding curves for a homogeneous Waldenström macroglobulin with specific activity toward the 2,4-dinitrophenyl (Dnp) group, and for some of the substructures of the macroglobulin, are shown in Fig. 2.7 (57).

---

[9] The molar concentration of antibody, needed to obtain r, is calculated from its molecular weight, by use of the assumption that the antibody is pure.

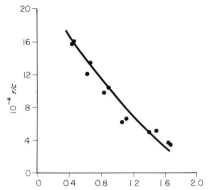

Fig. 2.6. Data on the binding of ^{125}I-*p*-iodobenzoate to specifically purified rabbit anti-*p*-azobenzoate antibody. Based on the assumption of a molecular weight of 145,000, the concentration of antibody was 7.0×10^{-6} *M*. Data are from reference 73. The curve drawn through the points is theoretical, based on the values of the index of heterogeneity *a*, obtained as described in the text (see Fig. 2.8). K_0, equal to $1/c$ when $r = 1$ [log $r/(2-r) = 0$], is 9.8×10^4 M^{-1}. The curve is theoretical and is based on the straight line Sips plot shown in Fig. 2.8.

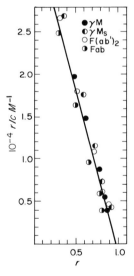

Fig. 2.7. Results of equilibrium dialysis of a homogeneous IgM preparation, its IgMs (cysteine-produced) subunit and its F(ab')$_{2\mu}$, and Fab$_\mu$ fragments, with ^{3}H-Dnp-ε-aminocaproate. The data are expressed as moles of hapten bound per mole of heavy-light chain pair (*r*) in each molecular species at varying concentrations of free hapten (*c*). The line was drawn by the method of least squares, using all the data. The IgM used is a human Waldenström macroglobulin which happened to have anti-Dnp activity. Reprinted by permission from Ashman and Metzger (57).

The macroglobulin, its 4-chain subunit, IgMs, or the univalent Fab fragment derived from the macroglobulin, give the predicted linear relationship, indicating both homogeneity with respect to binding sites and an absence of significant interactions between the sites; i.e., combination of one site with hapten does not alter the combining affinity of the other site. The fact that different sites do not interact had been indicated in the case of induced antibodies by the identity of binding curves for intact antibody and its Fab fragments (55). There are two binding sites per 4-chain subunit.

The binding curve for the specifically purified antibenzoate antibody (Fig. 2.6) similarly extrapolates to an r value close to 2. However, the relationship between r/c and r is obviously not linear but rather is convex toward the ordinate. This is typical of induced antibody populations and reflects heterogeneity of binding sites with respect to K. Thus, from binding measurements with heterogeneous, purified antibodies one can estimate the valence directly by extrapolation. The visual extrapolation is subject to error if there are substantial amounts of antibody of very low affinity present (discussed below). Since the r/c versus r relationship is not linear, assumptions must be made in order to calculate an average value of K.

One approach is to assume that there is a continuous distribution of antibody populations with respect to the free energy of interaction with hapten, or with respect to $\ln K$, which is proportional to ΔG^0. One can assume a Gauss error distribution (74), or the Sips relationship (75,76), which closely approximates a Gaussian type of distribution curve. On the basis of the latter assumption one obtains the following relationship:

$$1/b = 1/A_t{}' (K_0 c)^a + 1/A_t{}' \qquad (2.6)$$

This is arithmetically equivalent to the expression (74):

$$\log r/(n-r) = a \log K_0 + a \log c \qquad (2.7)$$

$A_t{}'$ represents the total concentration of antibody combining sites; the term A_t is reserved to indicate the total concentration of antibody molecules. The symbols r, n, and c have their usual significance, and K_0 is the equilibrium constant corresponding to the peak of the distribution curve; i.e., the "most frequently occurring" K. The assumed distribution of K values ranges from $-\infty + \infty$ but the number of molecules associated with a given K value decreases on either side of K_0.

The term, a, in the above equations is the Sips index of heterogeneity, which is a measure of the broadness of the distribution curve.[10]

TABLE 2.6

DISTRIBUTION OF COMBINING AFFINITIES CORRESPONDING TO SEVERAL
VALUES OF THE HETEROGENEITY INDEXES a AND $\sigma^{a,b}$

a (Sips equation)	Corresponding σ value (Gauss distribution)	Range containing 75% of sites
0.5	4.3	0.025 to 40 K_0
0.7	2.4	0.16 to 6 K_0
0.8	1.8	0.27 to 3.7 K_0

[a] From Nisonoff and Pressman (76).

[b] The range of K's corresponding to a given value of a was obtained by plotting theoretical curves of relative number of sites versus log K, as calculated from the Sips distribution function, and measuring appropriate areas under the curves. The corresponding σ values were calculated as described by Pauling *et al.* (2).

This is illustrated by the data in Table 2.6. Thus, when $a = 0.7$, a typical value, 25% of the combining sites have K values greater than 6 K_0 and less than $K_0/6$; the other 75% of the sites fall within the range, $K_0/6$ to $6K_0$. For a homogeneous population of combining sites, such as may be associated with a myeloma protein having antibody activity, $a = 1$ and the equation becomes

$$\log r/(n{-}r) = \log K_0 + \log c \qquad (2.8)$$

$$r/(n{-}r) = Kc \quad \text{or} \quad r/c = nK{-}rK \qquad (2.9)$$

This is identical to Eq. (2.5), which relates r to c for a homogeneous population of combining sites.

On the assumption of the Sips distribution curve, which leads to Eq. (2.7), K_0 can be evaluated experimentally, since it equals the reciprocal of the free hapten concentration ($1/c$) when $r = 1$, i.e., when one-half the combining sites are occupied (76). This is independent of a knowledge of the index of heterogeneity, a. Thus, for bivalent antibody, when $r = 1$ Eq. (2.7) becomes

$$\log 1/(2{-}1) = a \log K_0 + a \log c$$

$$0 = a \log K_0 + a \log c \quad \text{or} \quad K_0 = 1/c$$

From an experimental plot of r/c versus r, one obtains the value of $1/c$ when $r = 1$; this value equals K_0, the average association constant.

[10] The derivation of the Sips equation, which is mathematically complex, is given in (75).

The value of a, the index of heterogeneity, can be estimated by plotting log $[r/(n-r)]$ versus log c; the slope is a [Eq. (2.7)]. Alternatively, a can be determined (76) by plotting $1/b$ versus $(1/c)^a$ [Eq. (2.6)] for various assumed values of a to determine that value of a which gives the best straight line. This approach has the important advantage that it is not necessary to assume that the antibody is pure, whereas an equation containing the term r requires a knowledge of the total concentration of antibody molecules.[11]

In Fig. 2.8 the data of Fig. 2.6 are replotted according to Eq. 2.7, and a least squares straight line is fitted to the data. The slope, a, or index of heterogeneity is 0.92.

Tables 2.5 and 2.7 present a few of the many experimental values of

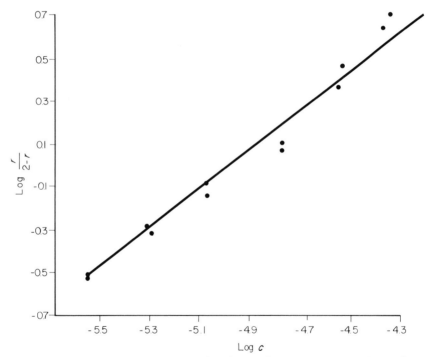

Fig. 2.8. The data of Fig. 2.6 are replotted according to Eq. (7), which is based on a Sips distribution function for binding energies. A straight line is fitted by the method of least squares. The index of heterogeneity, a, calculated from the slope of the line is 0.92.

[11] One can alternatively estimate the concentration of antibody by assuming bivalence and extrapolating the binding curve (r/c versus r) to the abscissa to estimate the total concentration of combining sites. This extrapolation requires the assumption that no disproportionate amount of low affinity antibody is present.

TABLE 2.7

A Few Examples of Equilibrium Constants and Indexes of Heterogeneity[a]

Ligand	$K_0 \ (M^{-1})$	a^b	Antibody specificity	Reference
p-(p′-Hydroxyphenylazo)-phenylarsonate	3.5×10^5	—	p-Azophenylarsonate	81[c]
p-Iodobenzoate	2.5 to 7×10^4	0.65–1	p-Azobenzoate (several preps.)	76
p-(p′-Dimethylaminobenzeneazo)-phenyl-β-lactoside	1.6×10^5	—	p-Azophenyl-β-lactoside	99
3-Nitro-4-hydroxyphenyl acetate	2.0 to 5.4×10^6	0.9–1.0	3-Nitro-4-hydroxy-5-iodophenylacetyl (several preps.)	100
ε-Dnp-L-lysine	6×10^5 to 2.5×10^8	0.3–0.9	2,4-Dinitrophenyl (Dnp) (several preps.)	14[d]
ε-Dnp-L-lysine	1.0×10^7	~1.0	MOPC 315 (mouse myeloma protein)	101
ε-Dnp-6-aminocaproate	3.8×10^4	~1.0	IgM (Waldenström macroglobulin)	57

[a] See also Table 2.4 and reference 74. This represents only a small fraction of a voluminous literature. Except for the last two proteins listed the preparations used are specifically purified rabbit antibodies.

[b] Sips index of heterogeneity.

[c] This investigation first established the bivalence of IgG antibodies.

[d] This study is discussed in some detail in the text.

K_0 that have been reported in the literature. Table 2.6 includes some values of a as well. An example of a binding curve for a homogeneous immunoglobulin was presented above (Fig. 2.7). A list of K_0 values compiled earlier by Karush (74) may also be consulted. One can generalize that rabbit antibodies to charged or polar hapten groups, such as azobenzoate, azophenylarsonate, or derivatives of phenyl-β-lactoside usually have K_0 values between 10^4 and 10^6 M^{-1}. Much higher association constants have been observed with antibodies to dinitrophenyl or trinitrophenyl derivatives, when animals were hyperimmunized using small dosages of antigen, preferably over a long period of time (14,77). As would be predicted, monoclonal proteins (Table 2.7) generally give a values approximating 1.0. Many studies have not been capable of detecting antibodies with average $K_0 < 10^4$ M^{-1} because of practical limitations on the concentration of antibody used.

The reader is referred to a paper by Pinckard and Weir (78) for a careful and detailed examination of approaches to the estimation of K_0 and a.

It should be emphasized that the ability of a set of assumptions, regarding the distribution of K values, to generate a binding curve that agrees with the experimental curve does not indicate that the assumptions are correct. Data matching the experimental set within experimental error can ordinarily be generated by assuming a variety of values for the numbers of homogeneous subpopulations and the K values assigned to each. The usefulness of an arbitrary assumption as to the nature of the distribution (which gives a reasonable fit to the actual data) is that comparisons among different antibody populations can then be made on an objective, i.e., consistent, basis. Classic examples are the change in affinity of antibody with time after immunization or with dosage of antigen or the use of the Gauss error function to compare K_0 values of different, related haptens.

Studies described in detail in Chapter 10 have indicated that many, if not most, specifically purified antibody populations contain significant amounts of homogeneous subpopulations. It is therefore evident that the Gauss error function must provide an inaccurate picture of the actual distribution of K values. Attempts have therefore been made to analyze experimental data in terms of the real distributions (79,80).

The approach of Werblin and Siskind (80) involves an effort to approximate the actual distribution curve of K values by assuming a discrete number (say 10) of homogeneous subpopulations with assigned K values (e.g., 1×10^5, 7×10^5, . . . , 1×10^{11}). As a first approximation, each of the ten populations is assumed to be equal in size and a theoretical binding curve is generated by a computer. This, of course, will represent a poor match to the actual, experimental set of data at hand. Next, the assumed sizes of each of the ten subpopulations are varied upward or downward in a systematic fashion until the best fit of the calculated and experimental binding curves is obtained.

The method is of particular value for demonstrating the presence of a bimodal distribution, with peaks of concentrations of molecules of high and low affinity. (The Gauss error function assumes a single peak with decreasing concentration of molecules on each side.) Werblin and Siskind used their computational techniques to demonstrate the continued presence of low affinity antibody, up to one year after initial immunization, coexisting with antibody of high affinity present after the first few weeks. As with other techniques, the lower limit of affinity detectable is dependent on the antibody concentration.

D. Methods of Measuring the Binding of Haptens by Antibodies

1. Equilibrium Dialysis

If a solution of hapten in buffer is placed inside a small dialysis bag, which is then immersed in a small quantity of buffer, hapten will diffuse out until the concentrations inside and outside of the bag are equal. If, however, antibody is present inside the dialysis sac, some of the hapten will be bound to antibody and therefore unable to participate in the diffusion equilibrium. When equilibrium is attained the concentration of free hapten will be the same in the two compartments but the total hapten concentration inside the bag will be greater, with the difference between the concentrations of hapten in the two compartments representing the concentration bound to antibody.[12] The molar concentration in the outer compartment is c in Eq. (2.1) or (2.5); r is the bound concentration, b, divided by the concentration of antibody. If r and c are determined for a set of increasing values of c, with the antibody concentration held constant, the data can be plotted according to Eq. (2.7) for the evaluation of the index of heterogeneity, a, and of K_0.

In practice, it is necessary to work with very low concentrations of hapten because the molar concentration of antibody is small. For example, with a concentration of specifically purified antibody (IgG) of 1 mg/ml, the antibody concentration is approximately 7×10^{-6} M. If the free hapten concentration greatly exceeds this value, the concentration of hapten bound will necessarily be low in relation to the total hapten concentration and the difference in concentrations inside and outside the bag will be too small to measure accurately. Thus, the concentration of

---

[12] The Donnan effect is negligible with the isotonic solutions normally employed in handling antibodies.

hapten must be of the same order of magnitude or lower than the antibody concentration. For this reason, radioactive hapten or a hapten that absorbs light strongly in the visible region is generally used for equilibrium dialysis. Tables 2.5 and 2.7 present values of K_0 determined in a few systems.

In setting up binding experiments it is also necessary to consider the binding affinity of the antibody. With an antibody of low affinity, relatively high concentrations of antibody must be used. This can be seen from the basic relationship (Eq. 2.1),

$$K = b/A_f c \qquad \text{or} \qquad KA_f = b/c$$

Let us assume that $K = 10^5 \ M^{-1}$, and that the total concentration of antibody combining sites is $10^{-8} \ M$. Then the value of b/c cannot exceed $10^5 \times 10^{-8}$ or 10^{-3}.[13] In other words, a maximum of only 1 part in 1000 of hapten can be bound; this cannot be measured by equilibrium dialysis. For convenient measurements, it is necessary that the antibody concentration approximate or exceed the reciprocal of the average binding affinity. From similar considerations it can be shown that antibodies of very high affinity must be used at very low antibody concentrations. If, for example, the average $K = 10^8$, the antibody concentration should be of the order of $10^{-8} \ M$.[14] This, in turn, necessitates the use of correspondingly low concentrations of hapten; with relatively high concentrations of hapten the percentage that can be bound by a low concentration of antibody becomes too small to measure accurately.

Any extrapolation to the r axis to obtain the valence requires either a visual approximation or an *ad hoc* assumption as to the nature of the distribution of K values. In particular, the presence of a substantial concentration of antibodies of low affinity would not be experimentally detectable unless very high antibody concentrations were employed. In the case of IgG antibodies, the extrapolation, either visual or through the Sips approximation, has generally yielded a valence close to 2 for specifically purified IgG antibodies. This was first shown by Eisen and Karush in a classic investigation (81). (The number of molecules of antibody present is calculated by assuming that the preparation is uncontaminated.) Since a value of 2 is in accord with our present understanding of IgG structure (two H–L pairs), the validity of the extrapolation is generally accepted. In contrast, when certain early studies gave a

---

[13] This is a maximum value, based on a very low hapten concentration. With increasing concentration of hapten, b/c will decrease because A_f decreases.

[14] With high antibody concentrations nearly all of the hapten is bound at low hapten concentrations and K_0 is difficult to evaluate.

value of 5 for the valence of IgM, which has 10 H–L pairs, the extrapolation to obtain the valence was questioned, and subsequent work suggested the presence of additional combining sites of low affinity. It is evident that antibody concentrations should be as high as possible in experiments designed to determine the valence.

2. THE METHOD OF FLUORESCENCE QUENCHING

If a protein molecule which contains tryptophan is exposed to ultraviolet radiation of appropriate wavelength, it will fluoresce, emitting light at a longer wavelength. This can be measured in a spectrofluorometer, which is frequently used so as to detect radiation emitted at an angle of 90° to the incident light. For antibodies, optimal wavelengths for the incident and emitted radiations are 280 nm and 330–360 nm, respectively (56,82). Nearly all of the fluorescence measured at 330–360 nm is attributable to tryptophan. If the combining site of an antibody is occupied by a hapten capable of absorbing the emitted radiation, it will decrease or "quench" the fluorescence of the antibody. One can increase the hapten concentration so as to saturate the active sites and determine the maximal percentage of quenching attainable. If the maximal quenching is, say, 70% of the total fluorescence, one can make the assumption that the degree of quenching will be 35% when one-half of the sites are occupied; i.e., that the degree of quenching is directly proportional to the fraction of combining sites occupied. This, then, provides an alternative method for measuring hapten binding as a function of hapten concentration. The free hapten concentration is calculated as the difference between the total concentration present and the concentration bound. The algebraic analyses already described can then be applied for evaluation of K_0 and the index of heterogeneity, a.

This method was first applied to antibodies by Velick *et al.* (56) and has since found widespread application, particularly in studies of antibodies directed to the dinitrophenyl and trinitrophenyl groups. Its major advantages are rapidity of measurement, which is essentially limited only by the rate of temperature equilibration, and a requirement for small amounts of antibody. (A typical concentration of antibody is 50 μg/ml.) A disadvantage is that the method is essentially restricted to purified antibody. If, for example, an IgG fraction containing 10% of specific antibody is used, not more than 10% of the total fluorescence can be quenched by hapten. This would greatly decrease the accuracy of the measurements.

It seems likely that quenching may occur even when the bound hapten is spatially quite distant from the fluorescing group; thus, more than 90% of the fluorescence of an Fab fragment of high-affinity anti-

Dnp antibody can be quenched in the presence of the hapten, ϵ-Dnp-L-lysine (83). The fact that only about 70% of the fluorescence is quenched in the intact antibody is consistent with the possibility that the fluorescence of fragment Fc is not quenched by the hapten. This is attributable to the distance between the hapten-binding site and the Fc fragment. In addition, the loosely folded hinge region connecting the Fab and Fc fragment may not efficiently transmit the excitation energy from fragment Fc to fragment Fab (84).

Effective quenching of fluorescence seems to require that the antibody have a compact conformation. Affinity labeling, with a Dnp derivative, of a myeloma protein possessing anti-Dnp activity caused marked quenching of the fluorescence of the protein. However, quenching by the bound hapten was greatly diminished in the presence of 7 M guanidine (85). This reagent causes unfolding of the protein molecule but does not cause dissociation of the covalently bound hapten.

There appears to be a greater degree of fluorescence quenching associated with high-affinity antibodies than with antibodies of lower affinity (83). Also, the amount of fluorescent radiation emitted by high-affinity anti-Dnp antibody is somewhat greater than that of a low-affinity antibody; in addition, the extinction coefficient at 278 nm of high-affinity antibodies is somewhat higher (83,86). The latter two properties of high-affinity antibodies are attributable to a higher tryptophan content, which has been localized to the Fd segment and which in all probability resides in the V_H region; it may well be part of the active site. The tryptophan content of L chains, or of the Fc fragments, of antibodies of high and low affinity are approximately the same. The difference in tryptophan content between high- and low-affinity anti-Dnp antibodies is about 4 moles per mole of IgG antibody, or approximately 2 residues per H chain (86).

The relatively high tryptophan content of high-affinity antibody leads to an apparent anomaly in fluorescence quenching measurements with low concentrations of hapten. In a heterogeneous antibody population the higher-affinity antibodies preferentially bind the hapten and, because of their relatively high tryptophan content, the degree of quenching appears to be disproportionately large. This may introduce an error into the calculated value of an average equilibrium constant for antibody populations containing molecules with a spectrum of affinities, since binding curves are interpreted on the assumption that the degree of quenching is directly proportional to the number of sites occupied.

a. Variations in Affinity of Antibodies during the Immune Response. Using the method of fluorescence quenching, Eisen and

Siskind carried out extensive investigations of changes in affinity of anti-Dnp antibody populations during the immune response (14). Some of their conclusions may be summarized as follows: (1) When a rabbit is inoculated with a small amount of antigen (bovine γ-globulin–Dnp conjugate), in incomplete Freund's adjuvant, followed 3 weeks later by 1 mg of the antigen injected intravenously, the average affinity (K_0) of the circulating anti-Dnp antibody increases with time from $\sim 10^6\ M^{-1}$, 2 weeks after the second inoculation, to about 10^8 to $10^9\ M^{-1}$ 6 weeks later. The average affinity of the early antibodies, and the change in affinity with time were decreased when large doses of antigen (50–250 mg) were used in the initial inoculations. These findings have since been amply confirmed. The data may be interpreted on the basis that low concentrations of antigen are captured preferentially by B cells having receptors (antibodies) of high affinity. The cells are stimulated by the antigen to differentiate and divide and their progeny produce antibodies identical to the receptors. This would explain the higher average affinity of antibodies produced in response to low doses of antigen and also the increase in average affinity with time, since the concentration of available antigen would be expected to diminish. A possible alternative explanation was considered, namely, that residual antigen might preferentially react with and cause the removal of antibodies of high affinity. A high concentration of antigen might in this way lower the average affinity of circulating antibody. This appears to be ruled out by the experiments of Steiner and Eisen, who found that lymph node cells from animals immunized with low doses of antigen produce antibodies of relatively high affinity (87). They incubated antibody-producing cells with radiolabeled amino acid and measured relative affinities of the antibodies synthesized through their capacity to be coprecipitated with unlabeled antibody in the presence of increasing concentrations of antigen. (Antibodies of higher affinity are precipitated with lower concentrations of antigen.)

Another striking observation made by Eisen and Siskind in their original investigations concerned the degree of heterogeneity of anti-Dnp antibodies. Rabbit anti-Dnp antiserum was fractionated by successive precipitations with small increments of a Dnp-protein conjugate. The antibody was purified from each precipitate and its affinity for ϵ-Dnp-L-lysine was determined by the method of fluorescence quenching. As would be predicted, K_0 values were highest for the antibodies initially precipitated and gradually diminished in successive fractions. In one antiserum K_0 values ranged from 10^4 to $10^7\ M^{-1}$; in another the range was 10^5 to $10^9\ M^{-1}$. These results vividly illustrate the versatility of the immune capability against a single hapten group.

b. Evidence that Tryptophan is a "Contact Residue" in the Active Site of Anti-Dnp Antibody. Although the evidence is not conclusive there are strong indications, based on the work of Little, Eisen, and their associates, that Dnp or Tnp haptens make direct contact with one or more tryptophan residues in the active site of their corresponding antibody molecules; this appears to be true for a number of species.

First, upon combination with their specific antibodies, Dnp and Tnp derivatives undergo a characteristic spectral shift (red shift)[15] which is quantitatively and qualitatively similar to a spectral shift which occurs when such haptens are mixed with free tryptophan in solution (88). This spectral shift is believed to result from the transfer of an electron from the indole ring of tryptophan to the highly electropositive dinitrophenyl or trinitrophenyl group. Electrostatic attraction between the oppositely charged groups may then account for part of the energy of interaction. The tryptophan side chain has the greatest ability to act as an electron donor; also none of the other common amino acids gives a comparable spectral shift. It does not occur when Dnp or Tnp haptens are added to nonspecific immunoglobulins, nor when anti-Dnp antibodies are mixed with unrelated haptens (88). The possibility of charge transfer had been postulated earlier on theoretical grounds and on the basis of the strong quenching of tryptophan fluorescence in anti-Dnp antibodies by Dnp derivatives (12).

Second, as indicated above, the tryptophan content is relatively high in rabbit anti-Dnp and anti-Tnp antibodies of high affinity. These additional tryptophan groups are in the Fd segment; it will be of great interest to establish whether they are in hypervariable regions.

Although the direct interaction with tryptophan may well account for part of the energy of interaction of Dnp or Tnp haptens with antibody, other forces are undoubtedly operative as well. The energy of interaction of haptens with free tryptophan is only a fraction ($\sim 10\%$) of the energy of interaction with antibody (88).

This capacity to interact with tryptophan side chains is apparently not restricted to polynitrobenzene determinants. Antibodies specific for folate, which includes an electron-accepting pteridine group, show similar spectral shifts and fluorescence quenching upon combination with the homologous hapten. Furthermore, in the presence of folate, 2 tryptophan side chains of antifolate antibody were protected against oxidation by N-bromosuccinimide, a finding consistent with the presence of tryptophan in the active site. A spectral shift at 390 nm similar to that

---

[15] For anti-Dnp antibodies, the maximum changes in absorbance take place at 390 and 470 nm; for anti-Tnp, maximum changes occur at 380 and 470 nm. Similar values are obtained with antibodies of a number of different species (88).

observed with antibody was seen upon mixing folate with free tryptophan (89).

3. STUDIES WITH SPIN-LABELED HAPTENS

An interesting series of investigations has been based on the electron spin resonance of certain chemical groups, which can be part of a hapten. Such groups are free radicals containing an unpaired electron. The group which has been employed most extensively is the nitroxide radical (see below). The free radical has a characteristic paramagnetic resonance spectrum which depends on adjacent groups and on their rotational freedom. Details of the chemistry may be found in reference (90). The technique was first applied to antibodies by Stryer and Griffith (91).

When the rotational freedom of the nitroxide group is restricted, owing to an interaction with an antibody combining site, changes in the paramagnetic resonance spectrum take place. The specific interaction which is measured is that which occurs between the unpaired electron and the nitrogen atom of the nitroxide radical. One such molecule, which contains both a nitroxide radical and a Dnp group, has the following structure.

This compound will combine with anti-Dnp antibodies (91).

The very marked changes which occur upon interaction of another nitroxide derivative with anti-Tnp antibody are illustrated in Fig. 2.9 (92). When all the hapten is combined with antibody, peaks a, b, and c are absent. When only a fraction of the hapten molecules is combined the peaks corresponding to unbound hapten are present but are diminished in size. The areas under the peaks can be compared with those corresponding to unbound hapten to calculate the percentage of hapten bound.

Using the Dnp derivative illustrated above, Stryer and Griffith showed that the K_0 value for its interaction with anti-Dnp antibody is similar to that of ϵ-Dnp-L-lysine. By measurements of electron spin resonance they found an inverse stoichiometric relationship between the amount of antibody present and the percentage of hapten which exhibited the characteristic spectrum of unbound spin-labeled material.

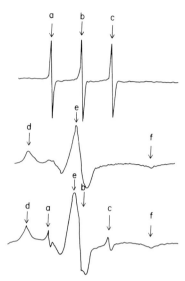

Fig. 2.9. Electron spin resonance spectra of N-(1-oxyl-2,2,5,5-tetramethyl-3-aminopyrrolidinyl)-2,4,6-trinitrobenzene, i.e., TNP-SL(5). Top, Free TNP-SL(5) (1×10^{-5} M) spectrum in the presence of 1×10^{-5} M normal RIgG. Middle, Pure immobilized spectrum of TNP-SL(5), 1.5×10^{-5} M, with anti-TNP-antibody (5×10^{-5} M) from a secondary response. Bottom, Mixture of free and immobilized TNP-SL(5) and antibody. Concentrations 4×10^{-5} M, and 5×10^{-5} M, respectively. Peaks a,b,c and d,e,f are explained in the text. All spectra were recorded at $22° \pm 2°C$ in 0.15 M NaCl-0.02 M phosphate buffer at pH 7.4. Reprinted by permission from Hsia and Little (92).

When the molar ratio of hapten to antibody exceeded 2 to 1 some unbound hapten appeared.[16]

Perhaps the most important and unique application of the method is in ascertaining when the nitroxide radical is actually present within the active site of the antibody. For example, one can synthesize haptens in which the nitroxide radical is spatially separated from the dinitrophenyl group by the insertion of chemical groups, e.g. $(—CH_2—)_n$. If the radical is sufficiently far removed from the dinitrophenyl group it will not be located within the antibody combining site when the hapten is combined with antibody. Under these circumstances the paramagnetic resonance spectrum corresponds to that of the unbound free radical.

Thus, two types of information can be obtained: (a) the fraction of hapten bound (when the free radical is located within the active site); (b) the apparent depth of the antibody combining site. The latter is es-

[16] These measurements were done at relatively high antibody concentrations so that nearly all of the hapten was bound when the concentration of antibody combining sites exceeded the hapten concentration.

timated by increasing the distance between the dinitrophenyl group and the nitroxide radical until the paramagnetic resonance spectrum indicates unrestricted rotational freedom.

An experiment to estimate the depth of the antibody combining site was carried out by Hsia and Piette (93). They synthesized compounds with the general structure; $H-d-SL$ where H represents the 2,4-dinitrophenyl hapten, d is a spacer which can be varied in size, and SL is the spin-labeled group,

The chemical groups comprising d were methyl, glycyl, β-alanyl, γ-butyryl, and ϵ-caproyl. The length, $H + d$, for this series of compounds varies from 8 to 17 Å. When $H + d$ was 10 Å or less the spin-labeled group showed marked rotational restriction in the presence of anti-Dnp antibody, indicating an interaction with the antibody combining site. When $H + d$ was 12 Å or more, the rotational restriction was greatly reduced, as evidenced by the paramagnetic spin resonance spectrum. From these results the authors concluded that the depth of the antibody combining site is 10-12 Å.

In the same investigation confirmatory evidence concerning the depth of the site was obtained through another approach. It was found that bifunctional Dnp derivatives, $Dnp-d-Dnp$ are capable of forming dimers with anti-Dnp antibody only when the total length of the compound exceeds 21 Å. Dimer formation was demonstrated by ultracentrifugation and gel filtration. It was once more concluded that the effective depth of the site is 10 to 11 Å; when the length of the bifunctional hapten is less than twice this value steric interference prevents combination with two antibody molecules. A similar value (12 to 13 Å) had been estimated by Valentine and Green (45) who used electron microscopy (Chapter 5). Recent X-ray crystallographic data confirm the hypothesis that the active site contains a cavity, although the depth in the monoclonal proteins studied so far varies markedly.

The method was extended to rabbit anti-*p*-azobenzoate and anti-*p*-azophenyltrimethyammonium antibodies by Piette *et al.* (94). Both antibodies were shown to immobilize their corresponding spin-labeled haptens. Variations in the degree of immobilization of bound hapten were indicated by the amount of separation of the first and third spin-resonance peaks. In the case of anti-*p*-azobenzoate antibodies, antibodies of higher affinity appeared to cause a greater degree of immobilization of the spin-labeled group, when the hapten was bound to the active site.

4. THE METHOD OF FLUORESCENCE ENHANCEMENT

As first shown by Winkler (95) the fluorescence of certain dyes, generally polycyclic aromatic compounds, is enhanced upon interaction with specific antibody. An example is 4-anilinonaphthalene-1-sulfonate (ANS).

Antibodies are prepared by diazotizing the corresponding 4-amino derivative (lacking the third benzene ring) and coupling it to a protein carrier for immunization. Compound 4,1-ANS is virtually nonfluorescent in aqueous solution but fluoresces in a hydrophobic solvent or when it interacts with specific (anti-ANS) antibody in aqueous solution.

This property gives the method of fluorescence enhancement a unique advantage over other techniques for studying the binding of hapten to antibody, since it permits the measurements of interactions involving very low binding affinities. Suppose that the binding affinity of an antibody, K_0, is 10^3 M^{-1}. Then at antibody concentrations normally employed ($\sim 10^{-5}$ M or less) a large excess of hapten is needed for appreciable binding to occur. Under these circumstances the fraction of hapten bound is small and not accurately measurable by equilibrium dialysis. Fluorescence quenching also is not generally applicable because high concentrations of hapten cause nonspecific quenching. In contrast, 4,1-ANS, even at high concentration, shows little fluorescence when present in aqueous solution, so that the increase in fluorescence is measurable even when a very small fraction of the dye is bound. The method has therefore found its major application in the accurate measurement of low binding affinities. It can also be used when the antibody is impure; it must then be proved that the antibody is responsible for the enhancement observed.

The technique was used by Yoo *et al.* to demonstrate binding by L chains isolated from specifically purified rabbit antibody reactive with 4,1-ANS (96). The average binding constant determined by this method was approximately 10^2 M^{-1}. L chains from nonspecific rabbit IgG or from antibodies reactive with unrelated haptens showed much weaker interaction with 4,1-ANS. Several controls suggested that the binding by specific L chains was not due to slight contamination by undissociated antibody.

Parker and Osterland demonstrated that rabbit antibodies of several different specificities, nonspecific rabbit or human IgG, and several human myeloma proteins are capable of binding 8,1-ANS with low to moderate affinity (97). Equilibrium dialysis measurements yielded values for K_0 of 8×10^2 to 2×10^4 M^{-1}. All of these preparations enhanced the fluorescence of 8,1-ANS, and most of the enhancing activity was associated with the Fab fragment. In the case of anti-Dnp antibody, the degree of enhancement, per molecule of 8,1-ANS bound, showed direct correlation with the binding affinity for ϵ-Dnp-L-lysine. Dinitrophenyl derivatives, which appear structurally quite different from 8,1-ANS, were able to displace the compound from anti-Dnp antibody. This suggests that 8,1-ANS interacts with the specific combining site of anti-Dnp antibody, although the affinity is relatively low (e.g., 2×10^4 M^{-1} for one preparation). This conclusion was supported by the finding that a maximum of approximately 2 molecules of 8,1-ANS could be bound per molecule of antibody. Light chains of rabbit anti-Dnp antibody and, to a lesser extent, nonspecific L chains also interacted weakly with 8,1-ANS.

The fact that anti-ANS and anti-Dnp antibodies, like hydrophobic solvents, cause fluorescence enhancement, suggests that the combining site of either antibody is a hydrophobic region. This is in accord with the nonpolar nature of the hapten. The direct correlation of binding affinity of anti-Dnp antibodies (for Dnp derivatives) with the degree of fluorescence upon interaction with 8,1-ANS might be interpreted on the basis that higher affinity is associated with increased hydrophobicity of the antibody combining site.

Binding of 8,1-ANS, with low affinity, was also observed with a number of myeloma proteins (97). For two such proteins with relatively high K_0 values ($\sim 10^3$ M^{-1}), the binding curves were indicative of a homogeneous population of combining sites. In only one instance, however, were Dnp derivatives able to displace 8,1-ANS from the myeloma protein.

The possibility was considered that the cross-reactions between Dnp-containing haptens and 8,1-ANS might be attributable to the fact that both possess aromatic rings, i.e., that these are typical but weak immunological cross-reactions. It was found, however, that octanoate (an aliphatic hydrocarbon derivative) was as effective an inhibitor as 8,1-ANS of the interaction of Dnp-valine with anti-Dnp antibody. It would appear then that these weak cross-reactions are based largely upon hydrophobic interactions rather than precise structural relationships. This may well account for the frequency of occurrence of myeloma proteins with weak anti-Dnp activity (Chapter 10).

Analogous findings, with enzymes rather than antibodies, were reported by Glazer (98) who showed that a number of different enzymes have appreciable binding affinity for a variety of hydrophobic compounds, apparently unrelated in structure to the substrate of the enzyme. As shown by competition with substrate, these compounds combined only with the active site of the enzyme. The hydrophobic substances tested comprised a number of aromatic dyes containing 2–4 benzene rings. To account for his results, Glazer postulated that the active sites of the enzymes studied are hydrophobic regions which can interact with nonpolar compounds, even if the "fit" is not exact. He pointed out that the active regions of several enzymes have been shown, by X-ray crystallography, to resemble a cleft, which might provide a number of possible modes of binding to a rigid molecule. Further accommodation may be possible if the active site has a certain amount of flexibility; such flexibility has indeed been demonstrated for lysozyme, one of the enzymes used in Glazer's study.

E. Enhancement of the Energy of Interaction of Antibodies through Multivalent Binding

It was first noted by Greenbury *et al.* that bivalent antibodies exhibit a higher effective energy of interaction ("avidity") in their reaction with red blood cells than the corresponding univalent (Fab') fragments; the ratio of effective combining affinities was 150:1 to 450:1 (102). This was attributed by the authors to bivalent attachment of a single antibody molecule to antigenic determinants on the same erythrocyte. This would lead to a very large decrease in the rate of dissociation and hence to a large increase in the effective binding affinity. Mathematical treatments are given by Greenbury *et al.*, by Crothers and Metzger (103), and by Bell (104).

Onoue *et al.* (105) showed that IgM antihapten antibodies, with approximately the same hapten-binding affinity as IgG antibodies of the same specificity, are much more effective per unit weight in agglutinating red blood cells coated with the hapten. These studies have been extended to a number of other systems, including viral neutralization, by Karush and his collaborators. Their work is reviewed in references 106 and 107, which also cite relevant studies of other investigators. It is now generally accepted that multivalent attachment is an important biological feature of antibody molecules, and that multivalence is significant because of the increased avidity that it confers, as well as its role in linking antigen molecules or particles. IgM, which appears to be present in almost all vertebrates, may be particularly effective because of its multivalence, and the multivalence of sIgA may similarly be of biological significance.

VII. AFFINITY LABELING OF ANTIBODY MOLECULES OR MYELOMA PROTEINS WITH ANTIBODY ACTIVITY

A. Affinity Labeling with Diazonium Derivatives

Starting in 1962, S.J. Singer and his associates, in particular L. Wofsy and H. Metzger, developed a very useful technique for covalent attachment of a small molecule to an amino acid side chain in the active site of an antibody molecule (108–112). The method, designated affinity labeling, is in principle applicable to antihapten antibodies with a wide range of specificities. Covalent attachment of a marker to a side chain in the active site permits identification of amino acid sequences in or near the site. To be most efffective the affinity labeling reagent should be radioactive so that its location in the amino acid sequence can subsequently be traced. One antibody studied extensively by Singer's group is rabbit anti-Dnp. The immunogen used to elicit the antibody comprises a protein with a number of 2,4-dinitrophenyl groups attached, principally to lysyl and tyrosyl side chains. An effective affinity labeling reagent is *m*-nitrobenzenediazonium fluoroborate (MNBDF).

The *m*-nitrobenzene group cross-reacts with Dnp, and the diazonium group is capable of forming covalent bonds with tyrosyl, histidyl, or lysyl side chains. Fluoroborate is simply an anion which forms a stable salt with the positively charged diazonium group but plays no part in the reaction. By virtue of the nitrobenzene hapten group the molecule rapidly becomes attached noncovalently to the active site of anti-Dnp antibodies; the diazonium group then reacts to form a covalent bond

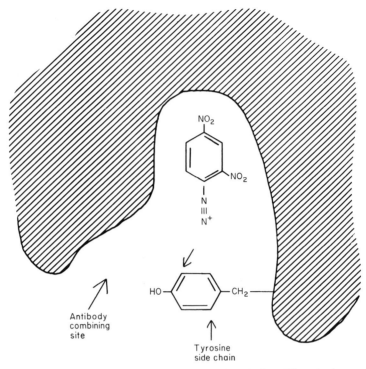

Fig. 2.10. Illustration of the mechanism of affinity labeling. When the hapten is in its most favored position in the active site the reactive diazonium group is in close proximity to a side chain (tyrosine in the figure) with which it is capable of forming a covalent bond.

with a side chain in the active site. For example, the reaction with a tyrosine side chain leads to the following product (see Fig. 2.10).

A remarkable and essential feature of the reaction is its very high velocity constant, relative to the rate of reaction of the affinity labeling reagent with side chains outside the active site. For example, the rate of reaction of MNBDF with a tyrosine in the active site of rabbit anti-Dnp is several hundred times as great as its total rate of reaction with all tyrosine side chains outside the active site, despite the fact that there are about 50 tyrosine groups in the molecule. The very high relative rate of affinity labeling must be attributed to favorable steric factors resulting from the noncovalent binding of the hapten to the active site of the antibody (108).

Singer and his collaborators introduced several lines of evidence to demonstrate that the covalent binding of the affinity labeling reagent takes place primarily within the active site of anti-Dnp antibody. (a) The very rapid initial reaction rate is not observed with nonspecific IgG; (b) the rapid reaction with antibody is prevented by the presence of an excess of specific hapten, such as ε-Dnp-L-lysine, which is capable of forming a noncovalent bond to the antibody; the hapten occupies the active site and denies access to the affinity labeling reagent; (c) affinity labeling results in a loss of hapten binding capacity. At low levels of labeling there is nearly a one-to-one relationship between the number of molecules of affinity label taken up by the antibody and the loss of binding sites. (As the concentration of affinity label is increased, some labeling of residues outside the active site begins to take place.) (d) The absorption spectrum, in the visible region, of MNBDF bound to rabbit anti-Dnp antibody indicates that tyrosine groups are predominantly labeled. In contrast, when nonspecific IgG or specific antibody protected by hapten is treated with the affinity labeling reagent the spectral characteristics indicate labeling of both tyrosine and histidine side chains. This result is interpretable on the basis that active sites contain a tyrosine, but not a histidine group, in a sterically favorable position.

In a typical rabbit anti-Dnp population, about 30% of the active sites can be affinity labeled. It is not certain whether the remaining sites lack tyrosine or whether tyrosine (or histidine) may be present but sterically inaccessible or unfavorably located with respect to the reactive group of the labeling reagent. Table 2.8 shows a typical set of data.

If rabbit anti-Dnp antibody is affinity labeled with MNBDF and its H and L chains are then separated, about two-thirds of the label is found in the H chains (113). In a number of antibodies of different specificities and from different species, a greater percentage of the affinity labeling compound has most frequently been found in the H chain, although the L chain contains appreciable amounts (112). One interpretation is that the H chain may play a predominant role in the formation of the active site. [Stronger support for this conjecture is the fact that H chains, but rarely L chains, generally possess appreciable specific antibody activity (Chapter 6).] Alternatively, the greater degree of affinity labeling of H chains may be attributable to the fact that many of the studies have used reagents which attack tyrosine side chains (112) and that H chains may be more likely to possess strategically located tyrosine groups in the region of the active site.

TABLE 2.8

AFFINITY LABELING OF RABBIT ANTI-DNP ANTIBODY[a]

Reaction condition	Whole antibody		Heavy chains ^{3}H	Light chains ^{3}H	2 Heavy + 2 light ^{3}H
	^{3}H[b]	Antibody binding sites lost			
Experiment 1					
Unprotected	0.68		0.215	0.117	0.66
Protected[c]	0.059		0.013	0.007	0.04
Experiment 2					
Unprotected	0.51	0.50	0.136	0.072	0.42

[a] From Singer and Doolittle (110).

[b] Results obtained by labeling specifically purified anti-Dnp antibody with tritiated *m*-nitrobenzenediazonium fluoroborate. Data are given in moles per mole of antibody or polypeptide chain. These experiments were terminated at a level of labeling of about 0.6 mole per mole of antibody in order to maintain a high specificity of labeling.

[c] Affinity labeling reaction carried out in the presence of the hapten, ε-Dnp-6-aminocaproate.

The same methods were applied to specifically purified anti-Dnp antibodies of the sheep, guinea pig (IgG1 and IgG2), and mouse (114). The results were remarkably similar to those observed with rabbit antibodies with respect to preferential labeling of tyrosine, ratio of H to L chains labeled, and percentage of active sites capable of accepting the label (see Table 2.9). These data suggest some structural homology among the antibodies of the various species.

Efforts to determine the site of attachment of MNBDF to rabbit and mouse anti-Dnp antibodies were made by Thorpe and Singer (115). As in previous studies the affinity label was predominantly attached to tyrosine. After separating H and L chains from the labeled antibody, the polypeptide chains were digested with the enzymes Nagarse or pronase to obtain small peptides. Most of the label was present on fragments having an average molecular weight of about 400, a value consistent with that of a dipeptide containing tyrosyl-azo-mononitrobenzene as one of its components. The authors made use of purified anti-Dnp antibody and affinity chromatography to recover the labeled dipeptide from the digest, then subjected it to an Edman degradation. The labeled tyrosine constituted the C-terminus of each dipeptide. In each polypeptide chain examined there was considerable heterogeneity with respect to the nearest neighbor of the labeled tyrosine. However, 50% of the dipeptides isolated from rabbit H chains had the structure Thr-Tyr and 52%

TABLE 2.9

AFFINITY LABELING OF ANTI-DNP ANTIBODIES FROM
VARIOUS SPECIES BY MNBDF[a,b]

Species	Reaction condition	Whole antibody	H chains	L chains	R[e]	2 H + 2 L
Rabbit	Unprotected	0.66[d]	0.23	0.113	2.0	0.69
	Protected[c]	0.057	0.013	0.007		0.04
Guinea pig IgG1	Unprotected	0.670	0.222	0.059	2.5	0.562
	Protected	0.365	0.117	0.020		0.274
Guinea pig IgG2	Unprotected	0.638	0.214	0.065	3.7	0.558
	Protected	0.171	0.044	0.019		0.126
Sheep	Unprotected	0.832	0.261	0.050	4.8	0.622
	Protected	0.199	0.033	0.003		0.072
Mouse	Unprotected	0.49	0.159	0.087	1.8	0.49
	Protected	0.18	—	—	—	—

[a] Reprinted by permission from Good *et al.* (114).

[b] *m*-Nitrobenzenediazonium fluoroborate.

[c] Reaction carried out in the presence of an excess of a Dnp hapten incapable of forming a covalent bond.

[d] Values in the table are given in moles of attached affinity label per mole of protein.

[e] Ratio of above values for the H and L chains of the antibody.

of the dipeptides from mouse L chains were Asp-Tyr. By analogy with known amino acid sequences in mouse and human myeloma proteins, the authors tentatively concluded that the labeled tyrosine in the mouse L chain is at position 86, and in the rabbit H chain is at a position homologous to residue 86 of the mouse L chain (112). (More recent sequence data suggest that this would be residue 95 in the rabbit H chain.) This would place each tyrosine close to a hypervariable region. Later in this section we will describe data indicating that hypervariable regions in monoclonal proteins possessing antibody activity are frequently the site of attachment of affinity labeling reagents. However, X-ray crystallographic analyses suggest that in the human λ or γ_1 chain the residues corresponding to Tyr 86 of the mouse κ chain or Tyr 95 of the rabbit γ chain are actually in the interior of the molecule and not part of the active site (116,117). This, however, is an exception. Most residues that have been affinity labeled are in hypervariable regions and, according to X-ray crystallographic studies, are exposed to solvent and are an integral part of the active site.

Rabbit anti-*p*-azobenzenearsonate antibodies have also been the subject of extensive affinity labeling investigations (108,109,118), which utilized specifically purified antibody and, as affinity labeling reagent, p-(arsonic acid)-benzenediazonium fluoroborate.

$$AsO_3H_2^-$$

$$N$$
$$\underset{N^+BF_4^-}{\overset{|||}{}}$$

The evidence for successful affinity labeling was essentially the same as that summarized in discussing anti-Dnp antibodies. When antibodies purified from the pooled sera of several rabbits were used, tyrosine was found to be the principal residue labeled. However, sera from individual rabbits have revealed marked differences, with one antibody preparation having a substantial proportion of labeled histidine and another failing to accept an appreciable amount of the label (108,118).

The experiments of Wofsy and Parker indicated that one cannot generalize concerning the presence of tyrosine, capable of being affinity labeled, in the active sites of antibodies (119). Horse antibodies specific for haptens containing carbohydrate (a β-lactoside or a β-galactoside derivative) were affinity labeled with an appropriate diazonium reagent. The affinity label was found principally in association with histidine in both the H and the L chains. Some tyrosine groups were labeled, however, in rabbit H chains in antibody of the same specificity; L chains were also affinity labeled, but the amino acid side chain involved was not established.

Cebra and his co-workers have affinity labeled specifically purified antibodies from inbred (strain 13) guinea pigs. In contrast, for example, to rabbit antibodies, certain antihapten antibodies from these inbred animals exhibit restricted heterogeneity. Ray and Cebra (120) used radiolabeled m-nitrobenzenediazonium fluoroborate to label anti-Dnp antibodies. The label was essentially confined to tyrosine residues in V regions; the ratio of labeled residues in H(γ_2) and L chains was approximately 8 to 1. Most of the label in the γ_2 chains was attached to tyrosines at positions 32/33 or 60, in the first and second hypervariable regions, respectively. In another investigation (121), anti-p-azobenzenearsonate antibodies from guinea pigs of the same strain were affinity labeled with radiolabeled bromoacetylmono-(p-azobenzenearsonic acid)-L-tyrosine; the bromoacetyl derivative is capable of reacting with lysyl as well as tyrosyl side chains. Much of the label was attached to lysine 59, in the second hypervariable region. Since the lysine side chain is positively charged, the suggestion was made that it may make contact with the negatively charged phenylarsonate derivative when the latter is bound in the antibody combining site.

Another example of affinity labeling within hypervariable regions is afforded by the work of Franek with porcine anti-Dnp antibodies; the reagent he used was *m*-nitrobenzenediazonium fluoroborate. Tyrosyl side chains were labeled at positions 33 and 93 in the λ chain and between positions 22 and 36 in the H chain (122,123).

B. Bromoacetyl Derivatives

An interesting approach to affinity labeling of anti-Dnp antibodies was developed by Strausbach *et al.* (124). They synthesized a series of four reagents, each containing the hapten moiety (Dnp), and a chemically reactive bromoacetyl group; however, the spacing between the Dnp and bromoacetyl varied. The smallest and largest of the four reagents are bromoacetyl-*N*-Dnp ethylenediamine (BADE) and a lysine derivative (BADL):

BADE $\quad O_2N-\underset{NO_2}{C_6H_3}-NH-CH_2-CH_2-NH-\overset{O}{\overset{\|}{C}}-CH_2-Br$

BADL $\quad O_2N-\underset{NO_2}{C_6H_3}-NH-CH_2-CH_2-CH_2-CH_2-\underset{COOH}{CH}-NH-\overset{O}{\overset{\|}{C}}-CH_2-Br$

Each reagent was prepared with a ^{14}C label. In goat anti-Dnp antibody from three immunized animals, 30 to 90% of the active sites were affinity labeled. With each reagent a somewhat larger proportion of the label appeared on the H chain than on the L chain. In both chains attachment occurred to lysyl and tyrosyl side chains, but the ratios were different in individual goats. For an individual animal the characteristic labeling pattern was invariant during the course of prolonged immunization. The very interesting results obtained when these reagents were applied to myeloma proteins with anti-Dnp activity will be discussed below.

C. Photoactivated Reagents

Another class of affinity labeling reagents, which are photoactivated, was adapted to immunoglobulins by Fleet *et al.* (125–127) and by Converse and Richards (128). To illustrate, we may designate an immunogen as follows:

Protein

The azide group is inert in the dark but becomes highly chemically reactive when exposed to light. Since the azide, because of its exposed location, is part of an immunodominant group and is capable when activated of displacing hydrogen atoms from carbon to form a covalent bond, it can react with almost any side chain with which it may be in contact when the hapten is bound to antibody. In the conventional type of affinity labeling reagent, contact of the functional reactive group with an appropriate protein side chain is dependent on the precise geometry of the binding situation; also, most reagents are highly restricted with respect to the type of side chain that will react. By comparison, photoactivated reagents are extremely versatile.

An example of such a reagent is ε-(4-azido-2-nitrophenyl)-L-lysine (NAP-lysine) (126).

A useful feature of this reagent is that it cross-reacts antigenically with conventional anti-Dnp antibody and thus can be used as an affinity label for anti-Dnp as well as for its homologous antibody. Rabbit anti-NAP antibodies had a relatively high average binding affinity ($7 \times 10^6 \ M^{-1}$), and were readily affinity labeled upon exposure to tritiated NAP-lysine in the dark, followed by photoactivation. There is considerable variation in different preparations with respect to the number of combining sites that can be labeled (126,127). Typically, 70 to 80% of the label was found in the H chain and the remainder in the L chain. This ratio is quite similar to that observed in other systems already discussed and adds support to the view, based on antibody activity in isolated chains, that the H chain may contribute more directly to the binding site of many antibodies. Although the heterogeneity of rabbit antibodies complicated the precise localization of the affinity label, part of it was found to be attached to half-cystine 97 and part to alanine 98 in the H chain, both located near the major hypervariable region starting at position 100 (126).

Rabbit anti-Dnp antibodies ($K = 1 \times 10^6\ M^{-1}$) also were labeled by NAP-lysine, but not as efficiently as anti-NAP antibodies (126). About 40 to 54% of the active sites were affinity labeled, again with the bulk of the label bound to the H chain. Precise localization of the bound labeling reagent has not yet been reported in this system. In all instances, sites that were affinity labeled lost the capacity to bind hapten.It is of interest that even this type of reagent does not label the entire population of antibody molecules; evidently geometric considerations are still of significance.

An important sidelight was the finding that within an individual antibody molecule both sites were either affinity labeled or both were unlabeled (126). Those molecules capable of being bound to a hapten-specific immunoadsorbent after the labeling procedure were essentially free of the label, indicating that few if any molecules were labeled only in one site. Furthermore, antibody molecules absorbed to and eluted from the immunoadsorbent after the initial treatment were resistant to affinity labeling. Thus, antibody molecules appear symmetrical with respect to the capacity of their two active sites to be affinity labeled.

In a subsequent study, Fisher and Press localized the ϵ-(4-azido-2-nitrophenyl)-L-lysine group, after affinity labeling, within two distinct hypervariable regions (positions 29–34 and 95–114) of the H chain of the homologous rabbit antibody (129). The exact identities of the labeled side chains were not determined, possibly owing to a reaction with more than one side chain in each hypervariable segment. About 20 to 25% of the affinity label was bound to L chains.

Photoaffinity labeling of myeloma proteins is discussed in the next section.

D. Affinity Labeling of Myeloma Proteins with Antibody Activity

Potentially, there are many significant advantages associated with affinity labeling of myeloma proteins, as compared to conventional antibodies. (The myeloma proteins must, of course, have antihapten activity.) The homogeneity of the protein permits detailed sequence analysis and thus a precise localization of the affinity label. In addition, one might expect that in theory all of the sites of the myeloma protein population could be labeled. In the case of conventional antibodies this has generally not been possible because of heterogeneity of active sites; evidently not all sites contain an appropriate side chain, or some side chains subject to attack by the affinity label are not sterically available.

Experiments with myeloma proteins have so far largely been confined to mouse proteins (designated 315 and 460) with anti-Dnp activity. Each protein binds ϵ-Dnp-L-lysine with a rather high affinity (10^6 to 10^7 M^{-1}); a high affinity appears to facilitate affinity labeling. Two classes of reagent have been successfully employed in addition to the photoactivated diazo compounds already discussed. In one, the functional group is a diazonium salt, in the other, a bromoacetyl group. The reagents have in common a mononitrophenyl or a dinitrophenyl group (the hapten).

Using a *m*-diazonium derivative of nitrobenzene, Goetzl and Metzger were able to affinity label most of the hapten-binding sites in protein 315 (130,131). The net result, however, was a 50-fold decrease in binding affinity, rather than the complete loss of activity generally observed. The isolated L chain contained all the affinity label, which was bound to tyrosine at position 34. Since this is in a hypervariable region of the polypeptide chain, the result strongly supports the inference that the labeled tyrosine is in the active site.

An interesting chemical experiment was carried out by Hadler and Metzger (132). After affinity labeling protein 315 with the *m*-nitrobenzene diazonium salt, the azotyrosine group formed in the process of affinity labeling was reduced with dithionite to form 3-aminotyrosine.

Subsequently they allowed the derivatized protein to react with the bifunctional reagent, 1,5-difluoro-2,4-dinitrobenzene. Cross-links were formed between L and H chains, as shown by the failure of the two chains to separate under the usual conditions. The chemical reaction presumably proceeds in the following schematic manner.

Cross-linking did not occur if the protein was not affinity labeled. This experiment indicated that portions of the H and L chains are in close proximity in or very near the hapten-binding site of the myeloma protein. The side chain involved on the H chain was not identified.

Another very useful set of affinity labeling reagents was devised by

Weinstein *et al.* (133), and applied to protein 315 (314–136). Bromo-acetyl-*N*-Dnp-ethylenediamine (BADE) was found to be capable of affinity labeling at least 70% of the active sites of protein 315 with little modification of side chains outside the site. Ninety-six percent of the radioactive affinity label was found in the L chain, where it was localized to tyrosine 34 — the same residue that was labeled with Metzger's diazonium reagent. The evidence is thus convincing that this tyrosine, located in a hypervariable region, is intimately associated with the Dnp-binding site.

Another set of experiments utilized a reagent with somewhat greater separation between the Dnp and the functional bromacetyl group (BADL). (Section VII,B). This also proved very effective as an affinity labeling reagent but, in contrast to BADE, labeled H chains almost exclusively (95%). Again the affinity label was attached to a side chain (lysine 54) which is in or very close to a hypervariable region. The simplest explanation for the result obtained with the two bromoacetyl derivatives is that the exact site of labeling is controlled by steric factors. With the Dnp group in its favored position in the active site, the bromoacetyl group in compound BADE is in close proximity to tyrosine 34 in the L chain; in compound BADL, which is 5 Å longer, the bromoacetyl group is evidently near lysine 54 of the H chain.

Direct proof of the importance of steric factors was obtained with a bifunctional reagent containing two bromoacetyl groups, one located in the same position as in compound BADE and the other corresponding closely in its position to that of the bromoacetyl group in compound BADL (135).

$$\text{Dnp}-\text{NH}-\text{CH}_2-\underset{\underset{\underset{\underset{\text{CH}_2-\text{Br}}{|}}{\overset{\text{C}=\text{O}}{|}}}{\overset{\text{NH}}{|}}}{\text{CH}}-\overset{\overset{\text{O}}{\|}}{\text{C}}-\text{NH}-\text{NH}-\overset{\overset{\text{O}}{\|}}{\text{C}}-\text{CH}_2-\text{Br}$$

When protein 315 was treated with this compound the active sites were affinity labeled according to all the usual criteria. However, in addition, the H and L chains were covalently cross-linked, as evidenced by their failure to separate under the usual dissociating conditions. This experiment, together with those of Goetzl and Metzger, firmly established the participation of both the H and L chain in the formation of an active site, a conclusion subsequently confirmed by X-ray crystallography.

Results of considerable interest were obtained with related reagents, varying in the amount of spatial separation between the Dnp and bromoacetyl groups (135). Reagents larger than compound BADL (which labels H chains), or smaller than compound BADE (which labels L chains), failed to affinity label protein 315. Reagents intermediate in size between the two compounds were quite effective as affinity labeling reagents but labeled both chains.

Protein 460, another mouse myeloma protein with anti-Dnp activity, was also affinity labeled by compound BADE (136). The label was found on the L chain, as in protein 315, but attached to a lysyl rather than a tyrosyl side chain. The locus of attachment was in a hypervariable region, at position 54.

The fact that the spacing between the Dnp and the functional bromoacetyl group is critical for affinity labeling suggests that covalent attachment takes place, at least in protein 315, without much movement of the hapten from its favored noncovalently bound position, i.e., that after noncovalent binding of the hapten group the bromoacetyl is very close to the side chain which it will attack.

More direct evidence for this postulate was secured by Givol *et al.* (135), who took advantage of a small spectral shift at 460 to 470 nm, which occurs in certain Dnp derivatives when bound to protein 315. They were able to compare the spectral shifts for covalently and noncovalently bound affinity labeling reagents because covalent attachment occurs very slowly at 4°C. Both for compounds BADE and BADL the spectral shift was virtually the same whether the binding was covalent or noncovalent. This was interpreted as indicating that the covalent bond could form with little if any displacement of hapten from its normal position in the binding site of the protein.

A photoactivated molecule was exploited for affinity labeling of myeloma proteins by Rosenstein and Richards (137). The molecule, 1-methyl-2,4-naphthaquinone-^{3}H-3-thioglycollyl diazoketone, abbreviated ^{3}H-menadione diazoketone or ^{3}H-MenDK, has the following structure.

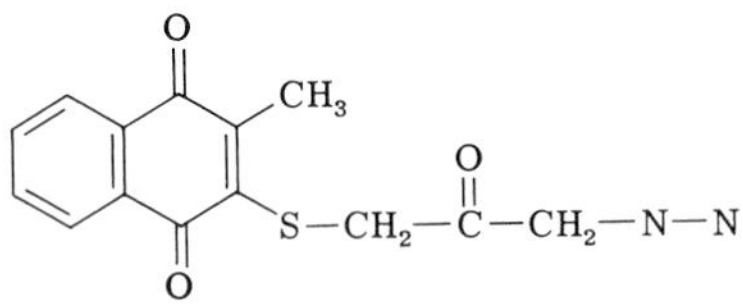

The diazo group becomes activated in the presence of light. The usefulness of this reagent is based, in part, on the fact that certain mouse myeloma proteins (MOPC 315 and 460) with anti-Dnp activity also react with menadione.

This immunologic cross-reaction, whose chemical basis is not readily apparent, is also observed with rabbit anti-Dnp antibodies. In any event, it has been possible to affinity label myeloma protein 460, which has anti-Dnp activity, with ^{3}H-MenDK. Approximately two-thirds of the active sites of the myeloma protein were covalently labeled; about 85% of the label was present in the H chain (130).

Yoshioka *et al.* (138,139) allowed two different photoaffinity labeling reagents to react with protein 460. Each reagent, Dnp-alanyl diazoketone and Dnp-1-azide, competed for binding to the active site with other Dnp derivatives in the dark and formed covalent bonds to the protein when exposed to light. The number of combining sites inactivated was equivalent to the number of molecules of labeling reagent that were covalently bound. The ketone derivative predominantly labeled lysine 54, in the second hypervariable region of the L chains; the azide derivative reacted mainly with the H chain at a site or sites not yet identified.

REFERENCES

1. Landsteiner, K. (1944). "The Specificity of Serological Reactions." (revised edition), Harvard Univ. Press, Cambridge, Massachusetts.
2. Pauling, L., Pressman, D., and Grossberg, A.L. (1944). *J. Amer. Soc.* **66**, 784.
2a. Nisonoff, A. and Pressman, D. (1957). *J. Amer. Chem. Soc.* **79**, 1616.
3. Pressman, D., Swingle, S.M., Grossberg, A.L., and Pauling, L. (1944). *J. Amer. Chem. Soc.* **66**, 1731.
4. Grossberg, A.L. and Pressman, D. (1968). *Biochemistry* **7**, 272.
5. Freedman, M.H., Grossberg, A.L., and Pressman, D. (1968). *Biochemistry* **7**, 1941.
6. Freedman, M.H., Grossberg, A.L., and Pressman, D. (1968). *J. Biol. Chem.* **243**, 6186.
7. Joniau, M., Grossberg, A.L., and Pressman, D. (1970). *Immunochemistry* **7**, 755.
8. Joniau, M., Grossberg, A.L., and Pressman, D. (1971). *Immunochemistry* **8**, 457.
9. Mayers, G.L., Grossberg, A.L., and Pressman, D. (1972). *Immunochemistry* **9**, 169.
10. Koshland, M.E. and Englberger, F.M. (1963). *Proc. Nat. Acad. Sci. U.S.* **50**, 61.
11. Pressman, D. and Siegel, M. (1953). *J. Amer. Chem. Soc.* **75**, 686.
12. Grossberg, A.L. and Pressman, D. (1960). *J. Amer. Chem. Soc.* **82**, 5478.
13. Eisen, H.N. (1964). *Methods Med. Res.* **10**, 94.
14. Eisen, H.N. and Siskind, G.W. (1964). *Biochemistry* **3**, 996.

15. Kabat, E.A. (1960). *J. Immunol.* **84**, 82.
16. Schlossman, S.F. and Kabat, E.A. (1962). *J. Exp. Med.* **116**, 535.
17. Moreno, C. and Kabat, E.A. (1969). *J. Exp. Med.* **129**, 871.
18. Lundblad, A., Steller, R., Kabat, E.A., Hirst, J.W., Weigert, M.G., and Cohn, M. (1972). *Immunochemistry* **9**, 535.
19. Torii, M., Kabat, E.A. and Weigel, H. (1966). *J. Immunol.* **96**, 797.
20. Sela, M. (1969). *Science* **166**, 1365.
21. Pinchuck, P. and Maurer, P.H. (1968). *In* "The Regulation of the Antibody Response" (B. Cinader, ed.), p. 97. Thomas, Springfield, Illinois.
22. Schechter, I., Schechter, B., and Sela, M. (1966). *Biochim. Biophys. Acta* **127**, 438.
23. Schechter, I. (1970). *Nature (London)* **228**, 639.
23a. Sage, H.J., Deutsch, G.F., Fasman, G.D., and Levine, L. (1964). *Immunochemistry* **1**, 133.
24. Schechter, B., Schechter, I., and Sela, M. (1970). *Immunochemistry* **7**, 587.
25. Schechter, B., Schechter, I., and Sela, M. (1970). *J. Biol. Chem.* **245**, 1438.
26. Haimovich, J., Schechter, I., and Sela, M. (1969). *Eur. J. Biochem.* **7**, 537.
27. Fuchs, S. and Sela, M. (1963). *Biochem. J.* **87**, 70.
28. Fuchs, S. and Sela, M. (1962). *Biochem. J.* **85**, 223.
29. Gill, T.J. (1963). *J. Biol. Chem.* **238**, 108.
30. Schlossman, S.F. and Levine, H. (1967). *J. Immunol.* **98**, 211.
31. Arnon, R., Sela, M., Yaron, D., and Sober, H.A. (1965). *Biochemistry* **4**, 948.
32. Stollar, D., Levine, L., Lehrer, H.I., and van Vunakis, H. (1962). *Proc. Nat. Acad. Sci. U.S.* **48**, 874.
33. Metzger, H. and Singer, S.J. (1963). *Science* **142**, 674.
34. Cathou, R.E. and Haber, E. (1967). *Biochemistry* **6**, 513.
35. Cathou, R.E. and Warner, T.C. (1970). *Biochemistry* **9**, 3149.
36. Rockey, J.H., Dorrington, K.J., and Montgomery, P.C. (1971). *Nature (London)* **232**, 192.
37. Rockey, J.H., Dorrington, K.J., and Montgomery, P.C. (1971). *J. Immunol. Methods*, **1**, 67.
38. Glazer, M. and Singer, S.J. (1971). *Proc. Nat. Acad. Sci. U.S.* **68**, 2477.
39. Taylor, R.B., Duffus, W.P.H., Raff, M.C., and dePetris, S. (1971). *Nature New Biol.* **233**, 225.
40. Dunham, E.K., Unanue, E.R., and Benacerraf, B. (1972). *J. Exp. Med.* **136**, 403.
41. Loor, F., Forni, L., and Pernis, B. (1972). *Eur. J. Immunol.* **2**, 203.
42. Almeida, J.D., Cinader, B., and Howatson, A. (1963). *J. Exp. Med.* **118**, 327.
43. Lafferty, K.J. and Oertelis, S. (1963). *Virology* **21**, 91.
44. Feinstein, A. and Rowe, A.J. (1965). *Nature (London)* **205**, 147.
45. Valentine, R.C. and Green, N.M. (1967). *J. Mol. Biol.* **27**, 615.
46. Ishizaka, K. and Campbell, D.H. (1959). *J. Immunol.* **83**, 318.
47. Steiner, L. and Lowey, S. (1966). *J. Biol. Chem.* **241**, 231.
48. Cathou, R.E., Kulczycki, A., and Haber, E. (1969). *Biochemistry* **7**, 3958.
49. Metzger, H. (1970). *Annu. Rev. Biochem.* **39**, 889.
50. Holowka, D.A., Strosberg, A.D., Kimball, J.W., Haber, E., and Cathou, R.E. (1972). *Proc. Nat. Acad. Sci. U.S.* **69**, 3399.
51. Warner, C., Schumacher, V., and Karush, F. (1970). *Biochem. Biophys. Res. Commun.* **38**, 125.
52. Ashman, R.F. and Metzger, H. (1971). *Immunochemistry* **8**, 627.
52a. Pilz, I., Kratky, O., Licht, A., and Sela, M. (1973). *Biochemistry* **12**, 4998.

52b. Tummerman, L.A., Nezlin, R.S., and Zagyansky, Y.A. (1972) *FEBS Lett.* **19**, 290.
53. Grossberg, A.L., Markus, G., and Pressman, D. (1965). *Proc. Nat. Acad. Sci. U.S.* **54**, 942.
54. Ashman, R.F. and Metzger, H. (1971). *Immunochemistry* **8**, 643.
55. Nisonoff, A., Wissler, F.C., and Woernley, D.L. (1960). *Arch. Biochem. Biophys.* **88**, 241.
56. Velick, S.F., Parker, C.W., and Eisen, H.N. (1963). *Proc. Nat. Acad. Sci. U.S.* **46**, 1470.
57. Ashman, R.F. and Metzger, H. (1969). *J. Biol. Chem.* **244**, 3405.
58. Farr, R.S. (1958). *J. Infect. Dis.* **103**, 239.
59. Berson, S.A. and Yalow, R.S. (1959). *J. Clin. Invest.* **38**, 1996.
60. Talmage, D.W. (1960). *J. Infect. Dis.* **107**, 115.
61. Samuels, A. (1960). *Biophys. J.* **1**, 437.
62. Dandliker, W.B. and Levison, S.A. (1968). *Immunochemistry* **5**, 171.
63. Levison, S.A., Portmann, A.J., Kierazenbaum, F., and Dandliker, W.B. (1971). *Biochem. Biophys. Res. Commun.* **43**, 258.
64. Sturtevant, J.M., Wofsy, L., and Singer, S.J. (1961). *Science* **134**, 1434.
65. Day, L.A., Sturtevant, J.M., and Singer, S.J. (1963). *Ann. N.Y. Acad. Sci.* **103**. 611.
66. Froese, A., Sehon, A.H., and Eigen, M. (1962). *Can. J. Chem.* **40**, 1786.
67. Froese, A. (1968). *Immunochemistry* **5**, 253.
68. Kelly, K.A., Sehon, A.H., and Froese, A. (1971). *Immunochemistry* **8**, 613.
69. Pecht, J., Givol, D., and Sela, M. (1972). *J. Mol. Biol.* **68**, 241.
70. Jerne, N.A. (1951). *Acta Pathol. Microbiol. Scand. Suppl.* **87**, 99.
71. Barisas, B.G., Sturtevant, J.M., and Singer, S.J. (1971). *Biochemistry* **10**, 2816.
72. Johnston, M.F.M., Barisas, B.G., and Sturtevant, J.M. (1974). *Biochemistry* **13**, 390.
73. Nisonoff, A. and Pressman, D. (1959). *J. Immunol.* **83**, 138.
74. Karush, F. (1962). *Advan. Immunol.* **2**, 1.
75. Sips, R. (1948). *J. Chem. Phys.* **16**, 490.
76. Nisonoff, A. and Pressman, D. (1958). *J. Immunol.* **80**, 417.
77. Siskind, G.W. and Benacerraf, B. (1969). *Advan. Immunol.* **10**, 1.
78. Pinckard, B.N. and Weir, D.M. (1973). *In* "Handbook of Experimental Immunology" (D.M. Weir, ed.), 2nd ed., p. 16. F.A. Davis, Philadelphia, Pennsylvania.
79. Medof, M.E. and Aladjem, F. (1971). *Fed. Proc. Fed. Amer. Soc. Exp. Biol.* **30**, 657.
80. Werblin, T.P. and Siskind, G.W. (1972). *Immunochemistry* **9**, 987.
81. Eisen, H.N. and Karush, F. (1949). *J. Amer. Chem. Soc.* **71**, 363.
82. Eisen, H.N. (1964). *Methods Med. Res.* **10**, 115.
83. McGuigan, J.E. and Eisen, H.N. (1968). *Biochemistry* **7**, 1919.
84. Noelken, M.E., Nelson, C.A., Buckley, C.E., and Tanford, C. (1966). *J. Biol. Chem.* **240**, 218.
85. Haimovich, J., Eisen, H.N., and Givol, D. (1971). *Ann. N.Y. Acad. Sci.* **190**, 352.
86. Little, J.R. and Eisen, H.N. (1968). *Biochemistry* **7**, 711.
87. Steiner, L. and Eisen, H.N. (1967). *J. Exp. Med.* **126**, 1161.
88. Little, J.R. and Eisen, H.N. (1967). *Biochemistry* **6**, 3119.
89. Rubenstein, W.A. and Little, J.R. (1970). *Biochemistry* **9**, 2106.
90. Hamilton, C. and McConnell, H. (1968). "Structural Chemistry and Molecular Biology," p. 115. Freeman, San Francisco, California.
91. Stryer, L. and Griffith, O.H. (1965). *Proc. Nat. Acad. Sci. U.S.* **54**, 1785.
92. Hsia, J.C. and Little, J.R. (1971). *Biochemistry* **10**, 3742.
93. Hsia, J.C. and Piette, L.H. (1969). *Arch. Biochem. Biophys.* **129**, 296.

94. Piette, L.H., Kiefer, E.F., Grossberg, A.L., and Pressman, D. (1972). *Immunochemistry* **9**, 17.
95. Winkler, M.H. (1962). *J. Mol. Biol.* **4**, 118.
96. Yoo, T.J., Roholt, O.A., and Pressman, D. (1967). *Science* **157**, 707.
97. Parker, C.W. and Osterland, C.K. (1970). *Biochemistry* **9**, 1074.
98. Glazer, A.N. (1970). *Proc. Nat. Acad. Sci. U.S.* **65**, 1057.
99. Karush, F. (1957). *J. Amer. Chem. Soc.* **79**, 3380.
100. Hoffman, D.R., Grossberg, A.L., and Pressman, D. (1971). *Immunochemistry* **8**, 769.
101. Underdown, B.J., Simms, E.S., and Eisen, H.N. (1971). *Biochemistry* **10**, 4359.
102. Greenbury, C.L., Moore, D.H., and Nunn, L.A.C. (1965). *Immunology* **8**, 420.
103. Crothers, D.M. and Metzger, H. (1972). *Immunochemistry* **9**, 341.
104. Bell, G.I. (1974). *Nature (London)* **248**, 430.
105. Onoue, K., Tanigaki, N., Yagi, and Pressman, D. (1965). *Proc. Soc. Exp. Biol. Med.* **120**, 340.
106. Karush, F. (1970). *Ann. N.Y. Acad. Sci.* **169**, 56.
107. Hornick, C.L. and Karush, F. (1972). *Immunochemistry* **9**, 325.
108. Wofsy, L., Metzger, H., and Singer, S.J. (1962). *Biochemistry* **1**, 1031.
109. Metzger, H., Wofsy, L., and Singer, S.J. (1964). *Proc. Nat. Acad. Sci. U.S.* **51**, 612.
110. Singer, S.J. and Doolittle, R.F. (1966). *Science* **153**, 13.
111. Singer, S.J., Slobin, L.I., Thorpe, N.O., and Fenton, J.W. (1967). *Cold Spring Harbor Symp. Quant. Biol.* **32**, 99.
112. Singer, S.J., Martin, N., and Thorpe, N.O. (1971). *Ann. N.Y. Acad. Sci.* **190**, 342.
113. Good, A.H., Traylor, P.S., and Singer, S.J. (1967). *Biochemistry* **6**, 873.
114. Good, A.H., Ovary, Z., and Singer, S.J. (1968). *Biochemistry* **7**, 1304.
115. Thorpe, N.O. and Singer, S.J. (1969). *Biochemistry* **8**, 4523.
116. Schiffer, M., Girling, R.L., Ely, K.R., and Edmundson, A.B. (1973). *Biochemistry* **12**, 4620.
117. Poljak, R.J., Amzel, L.M., Avey, H.P., Chen, B.L., Phizackerley, R.P., and Saul, F. (1973). *Proc. Nat. Acad. Sci. U.S.* **70**, 3305.
118. Koyama, J., Grossberg, A., and Pressman, D. (1968). *Biochemistry* **7**, 1935.
119. Wofsy, L. and Parker, D.A. (1967). *Cold Spring Harbor Symp. Quant. Biol.* **32**, 111.
120. Ray, A. and Cebra, J.J. (1972). *Biochemistry* **11**, 3647.
121. Koo, P.H. and Cebra, J.J. (1974). *Biochemistry* **13**, 184.
122. Franek, F. (1971). *Eur. J. Biochem.* **19**, 176.
123. Franek, F. (1973). *Eur. J. Biochem.* **33**, 59.
124. Strausbach, P.H., Weinstein, Y., Wilchek, M., Shaltiel, S., and Givol, D. (1971). *Biochemistry* **10**, 4342.
125. Fleet, G.W.J., Porter, R.R., and Knowles, J.R. (1969). *Nature (London)* **224**, 511.
126. Press, E.M., Fleet, G.W.J., and Fisher, C.E. (1971). "Progress in Immunology" (B. Amos, ed.), Vol. 1, p. 233. Academic Press, New York.
127. Fleet, G.W.J., Knowles, J.R., and Porter, R.R. (1972). *Biochem. J.* **128**, 499.
128. Converse, C.A. and Richards, F.F. (1969). *Biochemistry* **8**, 4431.
129. Fisher, C.E. and Press, E.M. (1974). *Biochem. J.* **139**, 135.
130. Goetzl, E.J. and Metzger, H. (1970). *Biochemistry* **9**, 1267.
131. Goetzl, E.J. and Metzger, H. (1970). *Biochemistry* **9**, 3862.
132. Hadler, N.M. and Metzger, H. (1971). *Proc. Nat. Acad. Sci. U.S.* **68**, 1421.
133. Weinstein, Y., Wilchek, M., and Givol, D. (1969). *Biochem. Biophys. Res. Commun.* **35**, 694.

134. Haimovich, J., Givol, D., and Eisen, H.N. (1970). *Proc. Nat. Acad. Sci. U.S.* **67,** 1656.
135. Givol, D., Strausbach, P.H., Hurwitz, E., Wilchek, M., Haimovich, J., and Eisen, H.N. (1971). *Biochemistry* **10,** 3461.
136. Haimovich, J., Eisen, H.N., Hurwitz, E., and Givol, D. (1972). *Biochemistry* **11,** 2389.
137. Rosenstein, R.W. and Richards, F.F. (1972). *J. Immunol.* **108,** 1467.
138. Yoshioka, M., Lifter, J., Hew, C-L., Converse, G.A., Armstrong, M.Y.K., Konigsberg, W.H., and Richards, F.F. (1973). *Biochemistry* **12,** 4679.
139. Hew, C-L., Lifter, J., Yoshioka, M., Richards, F.F., and Konigsberg, W.H. (1973). *Biochemistry* **12,** 4685.

3

Human Immunoglobulins

Because the immunoglobulins of all species have important structural features in common, many of the principles underlying antibody structure can be presented through reference to one species. Human immunoglobulins were selected because of the general interest in human proteins and because more detailed information is available on human immunoglobulins than on those of any other species. This is due in part to the existence of myeloma and Bence Jones proteins, which lend themselves to sequence analysis and X-ray crystallography. Although many studies have been carried out with mouse myeloma proteins, more sequences of human H and L chains — particularly complete sequences — have been published. X-Ray crystallographic analyses have been carried out on both human and mouse immunoglobulins (Chapter 5).

We will describe some of the general structural features and properties of the various classes of human immunoglobulin. The chapters on amino acid sequences, X-ray crystallography, interactions of H and L chains, allotypy, and idiotypy deal in part with human immunoglobulins.

I. GENERAL STRUCTURAL PROPERTIES

Table 3.1 lists the classes and subclasses of human immunoglobulins and presents some of their properties. No subclasses of IgM are indicated in the table since reports of the presence of two subclasses have not been well substantiated. We will consider first some of the properties common to all the classes and make some comparisons among them.

TABLE 3.1 PROPERTIES OF HUMAN IMMUNOGLOBULINS

Ig	H chain designation	Chain structure	Mol. wt. ($\times 10^{-3}$)	No. of domains in H chain	Mol. wt. of H chain ($\times 10^{-3}$)	Percentage of CHO	Normal serum conc. (mg/ml)	Half-life (days)	Fixation of guinea pig complement	Attachment to monocytes
IgG1	γ_1		146	4	51	2–3	9	21 ± 5	+	+
IgG2	γ_2		146	4	51	2–3	3	20 ± 2	±	−
IgG3	γ_3	a	165	4	60	2–3	1	7 ± 1	+	+
IgG4	γ_4	b	146	4	51	2–3	0.5	21 ± 2.5	−[d]	−
IgM	μ	5 + J	970	5	72	9–12	1.5	5	+	−
IgA1	α_1	b	160	4	52–56	7–11	3	6	−[d]	−
IgA2 A2m(1)	α_2	b								
A2m(2)	α_2	b	160	4	55–58	7–11	0.5	6	−[d]	
sIgA	α_1 or α_2	2 + J + SC	380–390	4	52–58	7–11	0–0.05	6	−	
IgD	δ	b	172–200	4 or 5	60–69	9–11	0.03	3	−	
IgE	ϵ	c	188–196	5	72–76	12	0.0003	2.3–4	−[d]	−

[a] The number of interheavy chain disulfide bonds may be as high as 15 (53).   [b] The number of interheavy chain disulfide bonds is uncertain.
The number of interheavy chain disulfide bonds is uncertain (probably 3 to 5).   [c] Complement can be activated by aggregated molecules via an alternate pathway.

87

Nature of the Forces Joining Polypeptide Chains and Subunits in Immunoglobulins

As shown by the structures depicted in Table 3.1, interchain disulfide bonds play a major role in maintaining the structural integrity of the immunoglobulins. In general, however, H and L chains do not separate upon cleavage of these bonds, which indicates that noncovalent interactions are also important. Elucidation of the multichain nature of immunoglobulins and the forces joining the chains began with the work of Edelman in 1959 (1,2). He showed initially that the average molecular weight of human IgG is reduced to 48,000 by reduction with mercaptoethylamine in the presence of urea; sulfhydryl groups formed as a result of the reduction were alkylated with iodoacetate to prevent reoxidation during subsequent handling of the protein (1). Edelman and Poulik found that rabbit IgG is dissociated under similar conditions to products having an average molecular weight of 42,000 (2). The immunoglobulins of various species have since been dissociated into smaller products by similar methods. This work demonstrated that the polypeptide chains are held together by strong noncovalent bonds as well as by interchain disulfide bonds. Some information as to the nature of the noncovalent bonds has come from X-ray crystallographic analyses and from physicochemical measurements (Chapter 5).

Edelman and Poulik further characterized the polypeptide structure of human IgG by separating subunits of the reduced, alkylated protein in 6 or 8 M urea, electrophoretically on starch gel at low pH, or by chromatography on carboxymethylcellulose. They were able to determine the approximate molecular weight of the L chain and to identify H chains. The degree of aggregation of the latter precluded an accurate determination of the molecular weight. Subsequent studies by R.R. Porter, J.B. Fleischman, R.H. Pain, and E.M. Press led to the determination of the molecular weight of the H chain, the elucidation of the topological arrangement of the H and L chains, and the relationship of fragments Fab and Fc to the two types of chain (3–5) (See Figs. 1.1 and 1.2). One key feature of their studies was the use of mild conditions for reduction of interchain disulfide bonds (i.e., neutral buffer, in the absence of any protein dissociating agent). Reduction in the presence of concentrated urea, guanidine, or dilute detergent results in the cleavage of intrachain, as well as interchain disulfide bonds, and in extensive denaturation of the polypeptide chains. After selective reduction of interchain disulfide bonds, H and L chains could be separated by gel filtration in 1 M propionic or acetic acid. The L chains obtained in this way are quite soluble; the H chains tend to aggregate but remain in solution at pH 5 and below. Subsequent studies have shown that the H and L chains of all immunoglobulins can be separated by reduction, usually under mild conditions, followed by exposure to an agent that dissociates noncovalent bonds in proteins. In a few immunoglobulins that have been studied, the L and H chains are linked only by noncovalent interactions and not by disulfide bonds. The yield of L chains from the IgG of mammalian species is approximately 30% by weight. Thus, the weight ratio of L to H chains in human IgG (3:7) is the same as the molecular weight ratio (22,000:50,000), indicating the presence of an equal number of L and H chains in a molecule. A 1:1 ratio of L to H chains is a constant feature of all immunoglobulins, with the possible exception of those of the hagfish and lamprey.

A major advance was made by Edelman and Gally (6) who showed that Bence Jones proteins are L chains, identical in structure to L chains of the serum myeloma protein of the same patient (in those patients who manifest both types of protein). The presence of a urinary protein in association with multiple myeloma had been reported by Henry Bence Jones in 1847 (7). Such proteins have the interesting property of precipitating when the urine is heated to 50°–60°C, redissolving at 100°, and reprecipitating upon cooling. The criteria used by Gally and Edelman to relate the Bence Jones protein and myeloma L chain included the amino acid composition and the mobility of the protein bands upon electrophoresis in starch gel.

Bence Jones proteins occur as monomers or, more frequently, as dimers of L chains. In dimers the L chains are joined by noncovalent interactions and, in general, by an interchain S–S bond, which involves the same half-cystine that normally joins the L chain to an H chain in an immunoglobulin molecule (8). This half-cystine is the C-terminal residue in a κ chain and the penultimate residue in a λ chain. In a κ Bence Jones monomer the half-cystine is disulfide bonded to another, otherwise unattached half-cystine group (8).

$$\text{Protein-N} \underset{\underset{\displaystyle CH_2 - S - S - CH_2}{|}}{\overset{\overset{\displaystyle H \quad H}{|\ \ \ |}}{-C-COO^-}} \ ^+H_3N - \overset{\overset{\displaystyle H}{|}}{C} - COO^-$$

As indicated in Fig. 3.1, human IgM is a pentamer of 4-chain units, linked by disulfide bonds. These bonds are readily cleaved by reduction at neutral pH, liberating five 4-chain subunits, designated IgMs (9,10). Thus, the IgMs subunits are not held together by strong noncovalent interactions. IgMs has a sedimentation coefficient of about 7 S as compared to 19 S for the intact IgM molecule. IgA in serum occurs principally as the 4-chain monomer; also generally present in low concentration are IgA polymers, in which the monomers are held together by disulfide bonds (11). These bonds are readily reduced, yielding

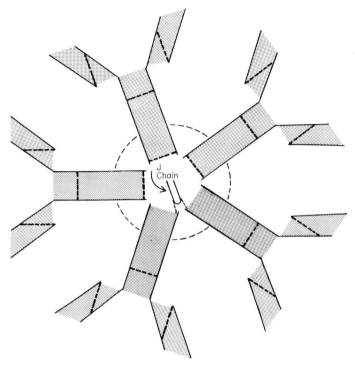

Fig. 3.1. Structural model of human IgM. There is some uncertainty as to whether J chain is linked to one or two μ chains, and as to whether or not it joins two IgMs subunits. The dashed lines represent interchain disulfide bonds.

4-chain molecules. Secretory IgA, which normally contains two 4-chain units, is more difficult to dissociate, owing to the presence of secretory component (SC); it can, however, be separated into 4-chain components and free SC, or into H and L chains, under appropriate conditions (see Section V). IgM, polymeric IgA, and secretory IgA (sIgA) also contain a J chain (see Sections IV and V) which is disulfide bonded to H chains, but is not bound through noncovalent interactions.

II. KAPPA AND LAMBDA CHAINS

All classes or subclasses, defined on the basis of the amino acid sequence of the C_H region, appear to share the same repertoires of L chains and of V_H regions although, as will be seen, there is some selectivity. Korngold and Lipari first showed that Bence Jones proteins fall into two groups, distinguishable on the basis of antigenic determinants

(12). Subsequently, it was demonstrated that all normal human immunoglobulins and myeloma proteins can be divided into the same two antigenic groups, which are now designated κ and λ (for Korngold and Lipari) (13–20). The ratio of κ to λ myeloma proteins, Bence Jones proteins, or Waldenström's macroglobulins is about 6 to 4 (16). The same ratio is found in normal human immunoglobulins (17). There is, however, a high proportion of IgD(λ) (21–23) and IgG4(κ) (24) myeloma proteins. The reason for this is unknown.[1] Kappa and lambda chains both have a molecular weight of 22,000 to 23,000. Some of their general structural features were described in the preceding chapter. The two types of chain are readily distinguishable by sequences in either the variable or constant half of the chain; i.e., an L chain does not have a V_κ and a C_λ sequence, or vice versa. The degree of homology between the human C_κ and C_λ sequences is about 40%, which indicates a common evolutionary origin. There is, however, little if any antigenic cross-reactivity.

In man, there are no known genetic markers for λ chains; in the rabbit, where markers exist for both κ and λ chains, the corresponding genes are unlinked, suggesting a probable absence of linkage in man as well. The C_κ sequence exists in three known polymorphic forms or allotypes, designated Inv groups, which are under control of allelic genes. These genetic markers are associated with a leucine–valine interchange at position 191 and an alanine–valine interchange at position 153 (Chapter 9). Although the C_λ region also exhibits polymorphism, this is evidently based on the presence of more than one, nonidentical C_λ gene in each individual, so that certain polymorphic forms, sometimes referred to as subtypes, have been found in all normal sera tested. The following substitutions are observed in λ chains (26–28): Oz(+), Lys 190; Oz(−), Arg 190; Kern(+), Gly 152; Kern (−), Ser 152. The presence of each subtype in all normal sera examined has been demonstrated for the Kern subtype with anti-subtype antiserum (29) and for both Oz and Kern subtypes by the isolation and characterization of the relevant peptides from normal sera (30,31). Other amino acid substitutions in the C_λ region have occasionally been observed in myeloma proteins.

Cohen and Gordon (32) found that the pH required for dissociation of IgA(λ) and IgG(λ) proteins into H and L chains is, on the average, shifted to higher values than that observed for type κ proteins. (There is heterogeneity with respect to the required pH for either type of immunoglobulin.) Thus, a large fraction of reduced IgG(λ) protein dissociates at pH 3.3, whereas only a small percentage of reduced IgG(κ) is

---

[1] Another example of nonrandom distribution is the high percentage of IgA molecules associated with the V_{HIII} subgroup [about 75% as compared with 25% for the average of all human immunoglobulins (25)].

dissociated at the same pH; both types dissociate almost completely at pH 2.4 (in 1 N acetic acid). This property can be utilized to effect a partial separation of κ and λ chains from a mixture of normal immunoglobulins.

Since the various classes of immunoglobulin possess the same spectrum of L chains they also cross-react antigenically; e.g., an antiserum prepared against an IgG(λ) protein will cross-react with IgA(λ). (Some cross-reactivity may also result if the antiserum recognizes determinants in V_H regions.) To render the antiserum specific for IgG it must be absorbed with a type λ immunoglobulin of a class other than IgG. Fab fragments of the IgG(λ) protein would also be effective. Absorption with free λ chains may not always be successful since some antigenic determinants are altered upon isolation of L chains; i.e., they are dependent on the L chain conformation in the native molecule.

Despite the presence of significant amounts of sequence homology, the C_H regions of the five classes of human immunoglobulin do not in general cross-react antigenically; an exception is IgD versus IgM; C_δ and C_μ are cross-reactive but not antigenically identical. There are, however, strong cross-reactions among the four subclasses of IgG and between the two subclasses of IgA, reflecting a more recent evolutionary divergence.

III. IgG AND ITS SUBCLASSES

IgG constitutes about 75% of the immunoglobulin in normal human serum. The percentage composition with respect to subclasses is IgG1, 66 ± 8, IgG2, 23 ± 8; IgG3, 7 ± 4; and IgG4, 4 ± 2.5 (33). The values given are ± 1 standard deviation for 145 Caucasian children. For each subclass the incidence among myeloma proteins falls within the ranges given; thus, about 4% of myeloma proteins are IgG4 and 70% are IgG1 (24,34). The four subclasses were initially defined by immunological methods (35,36). Despite strong antigenic cross-reactivity each subclass has at least two unique antigenic determinants, localized in two or three of the C_H domains (37,38). Certain subclass-specific determinants are also found in the Fab fragment (C_H1 domain) and other determinants are shared by two or three subclasses but not by all four (24,39,40); antisera to such shared determinants are, of course, less useful for subclass typing, although they may provide supplementary information.

Antiserum specific for a subclass is generally obtained by immunization with a myeloma protein or its Fc fragment and absorption of the antiserum with myeloma proteins of the other subclasses. Primates are often used for the production of anti-IgG2, while rabbits are used for the other subclasses. Natvig and Kunkel (24) stress the difficulty of preparing antiserum specific for IgG1 and the problems arising from the presence in antisera of antibodies specific for κ chains in association with the particular class of H chain present in the immunogen; i.e., the determinant expressed by a κ chain can be influenced by the class of H chain to which it is joined. Thus, an antiserum that appears to be recognizing H chains of a particular subclass may sometimes be reacting with κ chains associated with such H chains and fail to react with λ proteins of the same subclass. As a result of these problems, antisera specific for subclasses have not, unfortunately, become commercially available although a number of laboratories have prepared them.

A chemical method for determining the subclass of an IgG myeloma protein was described by Frangione *et al.* (41). It is based on differences in the number and location of the interchain disulfide bonds (principally the interheavy chain bonds) in the four subclasses. The protein is first reduced under mild conditions, so that all interchain but few intrachain disulfide bonds are cleaved. The reduced protein is alkylated with ^{14}C-iodoacetate, converting cysteine to radiolabeled carboxymethylcysteine. The protein is digested with pepsin, then with trypsin, and subjected to zone electrophoresis in one dimension. Peptides containing carboxymethylcysteine can be detected by autoradiography. Bands appear in a pattern characteristic of the class and subclass of the myeloma protein. The L chain type is identified at the same time from the bands formed by its carboxymethylcysteine-containing peptides.

A. Interchain Disulfide Bonds in the IgG Subclasses

Sketches of the interchain disulfide bonds in molecules of the four IgG subclasses are shown in Table 3.1. [The number of interheavy chain bonds in IgG3 is not indicated since it may be as high as 15 (see below).] In each subclass one disulfide bond joins the H chain to an L chain (to the C-terminal half-cystine of a κ chain or the penultimate half-cystine residue of a λ chain) (42). In the H chain, the H–L disulfide bond originates at a different position in IgG1 than in the other subclasses (43–47). In the γ_1 chain the half-cystine involved is in the hinge region (position 220). In γ_2, γ_3, and $\gamma4$ chains the half-cystine corresponds to position 131 (Eu numbering system); the H–L bond originates at a corresponding position in the H chains of several other classes of human immunoglobulin (Table 3.1) and in the rabbit γ chain (47–49), as well as in immunoglobulins of certain other species.

All interheavy chain disulfide bonds localized so far originate in the hinge region. There is marked variability, however, among the sub-classes with respect to the number of such bonds (43–47,49–52). There are two H–H disulfide bonds in IgG1 and IgG4 and four in IgG2. Early evidence suggested the presence of five H–H bonds in IgG3 (51). This figure has been challenged by Michaelsen (53) who reports a value of 15 S–S bridges, all located in or near the hinge region of IgG3. The result was supported by amino acid analysis and by quantitative determinations of radioactive carboxymethylcysteine after reduction and alkylation with ^{14}C-iodoacetate. Especially convincing is Michaelsen's finding of a total of 58 half-cystine groups per molecule of IgG3, as compared to 33 in IgG1 and 38 in IgG2; his values for IgG1 and IgG2 are in accord with earlier reports. Localization of S–S bonds to the hinge region was based on the difference in the number of half-cystine groups in an Fab' (pepsin) fragment versus an Fab (papain) fragment (25 versus 10). The data also suggest that the hinge region may contain an extra intrachain disulfide bond.

The molecular weight of the H chain of IgG3 is about 60,000 (54,55). This is approximately 10,000 daltons higher than the weight of a γ_1 chain, which contains about 450 residues, and would indicate the presence of approximately 95 additional amino acid residues in the γ_3 chain, since there is no major difference in carbohydrate content. From a comparison of the molecular sizes of the papain and pepsin cleavage products of IgG1 and IgG3, Damacco *et al.* (55) suggested that the additional residues in IgG3 are present in the form of an extended hinge region. This might explain the relatively great susceptibility of this subclass to proteolysis and thus its rapid catabolism (Table 3.1). (The latter property may also be attributable in part to the tendency of IgG3 to aggregate.)

B. Limited Proteolysis of IgG of Different Subclasses

The enzymes papain and pepsin have been used most extensively in studies of the proteolysis of human IgG. When normal IgG, comprising all of the subclasses, is treated with papain, Fab and Fc fragments are liberated (56). Papain cleaves molecules of each subclass in the hinge region, on the N-terminal side of the interheavy chain disulfide bonds; e.g., in IgG1 the principal site of attack is between positions 225 and 226. Fc fragments can be crystallized only with difficulty from a digest of whole IgG (57) but more readily from a digest of certain myeloma proteins (58). Pepsin, at pH 4–4.5, cleaves the H chain on the C-terminal side of the interheavy chain disulfide bonds, yielding bivalent $F(ab')_2$ fragments. The C_H2 domain is degraded but a dimer of the C_H3 domain can be recovered from molecules of each subclass of IgG.

There are marked differences among subclasses with respect to their rate of proteolysis by papain or pepsin. As a consequence, measurements of such rates can help in identifying the subclass to which a myeloma protein belongs (59–64). Myeloma proteins of the IgG3 subclass and most IgG1 myeloma proteins are very susceptible to digestion with papain, even in the absence of cysteine; some IgG1 proteins, however, require 0.01 M cysteine. IgG2 myeloma proteins are resistant to digestion in the absence of cysteine and, in many instances, in the presence of 0.01 M cysteine as well; higher concentrations of the reducing agent are required for such proteins. There is considerable variation among individual IgG4 proteins, most but not all of which require 0.01 M cysteine for cleavage by papain. Thus, the order of decreasing susceptibility to papain is IgG3 > IgG1 > IgG4 > IgG2; because of individual variability this precise order does not apply to all myeloma proteins.

After short-term digestion of normal IgG with papain, crystals were found which proved to consist of the Fc fragment of IgG1 (65). This is in accord with the facts that IgG1 is readily digested and is present at the highest concentration in normal serum.

IgG2 proteins are initially hydrolyzed by papain on the C-terminal side of the interheavy chain disulfide bonds, yielding F(ab)₂ fragments which are subsequently digested further to Fab (63,64). Significant yields of F(ab)₂ fragments can also be obtained from IgG1 and IgG4 myeloma proteins if conditions are carefully selected (66). Short-term digestion of normal IgG without cysteine yielded an interesting product, comprising one Fab fragment joined to the Fc fragment; this is produced by the cleavage of one, rather than both H chains (67). The fragment was mainly derived from IgG1. A similar product has been obtained by careful digestion of rabbit IgG with papain (68,69).

Relative rates of digestion of the various subclasses by pepsin and papain are quite different (61,70). IgG1, which is very susceptible to papain, is the most resistant of the subclasses to peptic digestion; IgG3 and IgG4 are very sensitive, whereas IgG2 is quite resistant to pepsin. Molecules of each subclass yield F(ab')₂ fragments if the conditions of digestion are appropriate (61).

C. The pFc' and Fc' Fragments

Although peptic digestion does not produce an intact Fc fragment, owing to degradation of the C_H2 domain, a useful subfragment of Fc, designated pFc' (2.4 S; mol. wt. 25,000) can be recovered (71,72). The pFc' fragment, which corresponds closely to a dimer of the C_H3 domain, can be produced from each of the four subclasses (61,70). In IgG1 each segment of the dimer comprises residues 335 or 336 to the C-terminus (position 446) (73). The ability to prepare pFc' fragments has aided in the localization of isotypic and allotypic (Gm) markers (Chapter 9). The pFc' fragment has its counterpart in rabbit IgG; a large C-terminal segment, designated Pep III', is liberated from the Fc region by peptic digestion (74).

In addition to fragment Fc, a papain digest of human IgG contains a lower concentration of subfragments designated Fc' (72,75–80). Such a fragment can also be prepared by further digestion with papain of fragment Fc or the pepsin fragment, pFc', of any of the subclasses (76,78). Thus, Fc' is smaller than pFc'. In IgG1 it is a dimer of residues extending from positions 342 to 432 (14 residues short of the C-terminus) (73). It thus comprises a large segment of the two C_H3 domains. The dimers comprising pFc' and Fc' are held together by noncovalent bonds but not by interchain disulfide bonds.

A fragment, designated stFc by Utsumi (81), is obtained by digestion of rabbit IgG with papain at pH 4.5. It has a molecular weight of 25,000 and contains only the C-terminal antigenic determinants of the molecule. The fragment, therefore, resembles human Fc' or pFc'.

D. Biological Properties Associated with Subclasses of IgG

1. INTERACTION WITH COMPLEMENT

Of the four subclasses of human IgG only IgG4 is unable to fix guinea pig or human complement. Among the other subclasses the order of effectiveness is IgG3 > IgG1 > IgG2. This was shown by experiments in which myeloma proteins of the four subclasses were aggregated with a bifunctional chemical reagent, bisdiazotized benzidine; each of the aggregated proteins except IgG4 fixed guinea pig complement. The activity was independent of L chain type or Gm type of the γ chain (82). Complement-fixing activity had previously been localized to the Fc fragment of normal IgG, which comprises a mixture of the four subclasses. These conclusions were confirmed by direct binding experiments in which it was shown that monomeric myeloma proteins of each subclass except IgG4 are capable of binding human or guinea pig $C\overline{1}$, the activated form of C1. Except for IgG4, binding was considerably enhanced when the immunoglobulins were aggregated. The Fc fragment of IgG1 was as effective as the intact molecule (83).

2. BINDING TO MONOCYTES OR MACROPHAGES

Sorkin (84) first showed that certain immunoglobulins have the capacity to bind to macrophages. In the human this cytophilic capability is most pronounced in IgG1 and IgG3. Thus, only IgG1 and IgG3 can inhibit phagocytosis by human macrophages of particles coated with immunoglobulin (85–87). In addition, only IgG1 and IgG3 combine strongly with human monocytes, as shown by direct binding measurements using radiolabeled myeloma proteins and radioautography (88). When guinea pig macrophages were tested, only IgG1 was bound (89). Binding to human monocytes requires the presence of the Fc fragment (90). A rabbit or human macrophage typically possesses 1 to 2×10^6 receptors for IgG; the number tends to increase after stimulation by Freund's adjuvant.

3. LYMPHOCYTE-MEDIATED CYTOTOXICITY

^{51}Cr-Labeled chicken erythrocytes coated with rabbit antierythrocyte antibody are lysed by unsensitized human lymphocytes. This lysis is inhibited by human IgG1, IgG3, or by aggregated IgG2, but not by IgG4. The inhibitory activity is localized in the Fc fragment (91). These experiments suggest that IgG4, and possibly IgG2, may prove to be incapable of sensitizing target cells for lymphocyte-mediated, antibody requiring cytotoxicity.

4. PROPERTIES OF INDIVIDUAL DOMAINS

Crystallographic models of an Fab fragment and of an L chain suggest that each domain of an immunoglobulin has a discrete, self-contained tertiary structure, stabilized by the intrachain disulfide loop, by hydrophobic interactions, and by a substantial amount of β-pleated sheet structure (Chapter 5). There is a close resemblance among the three-dimensional structures of the polypeptide chains in each domain. The V_L and V_H domains are in intimate contact as are the V_L and C_H1 domains. The term "module" will be used to describe such a pair of domains. Edelman and Gall proposed that each domain has its own particular biological function (92,93). The major function of the pair of V domains, or V module, is apparent since it provides for antibody specificity. It was suggested that the module comprising the C_L and C_H1 domains might add stability to the combining site (92). While this is quite likely, it appears that the V module is, in some immunoglobulins, sufficiently stable that it can be isolated and retain antibody activity (the Fv fragment).

There is evidence that the module comprising a pair of C_H2 domain of IgG (the N-terminal half of the Fc fragment) is involved in complement (C) fixation. Thus, Fab or F(ab')$_2$ fragments do not fix C through the conventional pathway, whereas aggregated fragment Fc has this capability; however, a fragment of rabbit IgG (Facb) lacking only the

C_H3 domains is capable of C fixation (93a). This would appear to localize the property to the C_H2 module. Kehoe and Fougereau found that a fragment from the C_H2 domain of a mouse IgG2 myeloma protein, prepared with cyanogen bromide and comprising about 60 amino acids, is capable of fixing guinea pig C when adsorbed to polystyrene latex particles (94). Other large fragments released by cyanogen bromide cleavage failed to fix C. By similar methods, a fragment approximating a dimer of the C_H2 domain, isolated from human IgG myeloma protein, was found to fix C (95). Cleavage between the C_H2 and C_H3 regions was accomplished by exposing Fc fragments to pH 2.5, then digesting for less than a minute with trypsin at neutral pH. The C_H3 fragment failed to fix complement. The properties of these fragments also suggested that the C_H3 domain may be responsible for the cytophilic activity of human IgG toward macrophages (96); the C_H3 dimer, but not the C_H2 dimer, inhibited the binding of sheep erythrocytes, coated with a human IgG1 myeloma protein, to guinea pig macrophages. Fc fragments and whole IgG, but not Fab fragments, were also inhibitory.

Effector functions that have been localized to the Fc fragment but not definitely to one domain include the capacity for transplacental transfer (IgG); fixation to guinea pig skin for mediation of "reverse" passive cutaneous anaphylaxis (IgG); control of catabolic rate of the immunoglobulin; binding to mast cells or basophilic leukocytes (IgE). Allotypic determinants of IgG have been localized in each of the C region domains. Also, an important isoantigen, termed the Ga antigen, reactive with many different preparations of rheumatoid factor, is present in the C_H2 domain of IgG1, IgG2, and IgG4 (97).

Failure to demonstrate a particular biological activity in a fragment does not prove that the activity is not associated with that segment of the molecule. The fragment may be altered during isolation or require cooperation from another portion of the molecule.

5. OTHER PROPERTIES

Half-lives of IgG molecules of the various subclasses in normal individuals are shown in Table 3.1 (98). These are mean values based on rates of clearance of several ^{125}I-labeled myeloma proteins. The rate of catabolism does not correlate with L chain type, Gm type, carbohydrate content, or net charge (99). The relatively short half-life of IgG3 may be related to its tendency to form aggregates (100) or to its large hinge region, which is a principal site of attack by proteolytic enzymes.

Studies of the nature of immunoglobulins on the surface of human B lymphocytes indicate that IgG2 is the dominant subclass present; it was found on 3 to 5% of the peripheral lymphocyte population (101). It is of interest in this context that the IgG2 subclass may have been the first to evolve (Chapter 7).

IV. STRUCTURE AND PROPERTIES OF HUMAN IgM

Representations of the structure of IgM and the μ chain are shown in Figs. 3.1 and 3.2. The molecule is a pentamer of 4-chain subunits, containing ten L chains, ten H chains, and one J chain (mol. wt. 15,000), and has ten combining sites which are probably identical (10,102–106). The pentameric structure is also shown by electron micrographs of human IgM (e.g., reference 106a) which closely resemble those of the mouse IgM depicted in Fig. 8.1.

Figure 3.2 is based to a considerable extent on the complete amino acid sequences of μ chains from two Waldenström macroglobulins, which were recently reported from the laboratories of N. Hilschmann (107) and F.W. Putnam (108,109). The two proteins investigated had different V_H sequences, as expected, but very similar C_H sequences. In addition to a few individual substitutions there is disagreement with respect to a stretch of 8 or 9 residues around position 267 (Ou numbering system); in view of very large size of the μ chain the differences may well be attributable to experimental error. (There is no conclusive evidence for the existence of subclasses of human IgM, although allotypic markers have been identified (Chapter 9). Proteins Ou and Gal both have κ chains belonging to the $V_{\kappa I}$ subgroup. The V_H regions of the two proteins are in the V_{HII} and V_{HIII} subgroups, respectively.

The sequences of the μ chains of proteins Gal and Ou comprise 571 and 588 amino acid residues, respectively, and include five domains (1

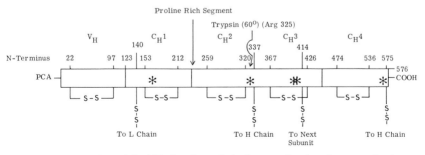

Fig. 3.2. Location of disulfide bonds, carbohydrate, and point of enzymatic cleavage of the human μ chain (107,108,110). Asterisks, carbohydrate at positions 170,332, 395,402, and 563. Trypsin at 60°C degrades the C_H2 segment from residue 213 to 325.

V_H, 4 C_H). Individual domains of the μ chain are roughly as large as those of the γ chain, as are the five intrachain disulfide loops, which enclose 59 to 72 residues (Ou) or 58 to 63 residues (Gal). Carbohydrate, which represents about 10% by weight of the molecule, is attached at five positions in the C_μ region (Fig. 3.2) (107,108,110). Each of the five oligosaccharides, in the IgM protein, Dau, studied by Hurst *et al.* (110) contained 5–12 sugar residues. Two consisted only of mannose and *N*-acetylglucosamine. These sugars, and also galactose and fucose, were found in other glycopeptides. Sialic acid was present in the H chain but was not localized.

A segment rich in proline, around residue 230, may possibly be homologous with the hinge region of IgG, but it lacks the interchain disulfide bonds characteristic of that region and shows no extra length of polypeptide in alignment with the other domains (Fig. 3.2). It is, however, one site of attack by trypsin (109). The complete sequence of the μ chain of protein Ou is presented in Chapter 4 (Fig. 4.10).

The single J chain in IgM (106) is disulfide bonded to the penultimate half-cystine residue of one, or possibly two μ chains (111,112). This would suggest an asymmetry in the IgM molecule, since a half-cystine linked to a J chain cannot also be part of an intrasubunit disulfide bond, and it is believed that most of the penultimate half-cystines do form such bonds; this question requires further clarification. The L–H disulfide bonds in IgM involve half-cystine 140 in the H chain; in this respect IgM is similar to molecules of the various subclasses of IgG, except for IgG1 in which the L–H disulfide bond utilizes a half-cystine in the hinge region of the γ chain.

The molecular weight of protein Ou, calculated from the known amino acid sequence and estimated carbohydrate content, is 956,000, or 971,000 including the J chain (109). This agrees fairly well with earlier data on molecular weight of human IgM based on sedimentation analysis (104). Kabat, in 1939, obtained molecular weights averaging 1,000,000 for the IgM of the cow, horse, and pig (113). The molecular weight of the μ chain of protein Ou is 72,000 daltons.

IgM can be separated into its H and L chains by the usual methods of reduction in neutral buffer, alkylation of sulfhydryl groups, and gel filtration in dilute acetic or propionic acid (114,115). The L chain peak contains J chains, which can be separated from L chains by virtue of their high anodal electrophoretic mobility.

A. Reduction of IgM to IgMs

The 19 S IgM molecule is readily broken down into 7 S subunits by mild reduction at neutral pH (9). J chain is released at the same time and is easily separated; it represents such a small fraction (about 2%) of the protein mass that until 1971 it was overlooked. The 7 S subunit contains two H and two L chains and is designated IgMs (s for subunit). A careful investigation (116) showed that IgMs can be produced quantitatively, without disrupting H–L or H–H intrasubunit disulfide bonds, by using 0.015 M 2-mercaptoethylamine for the reduction. Only two carboxymethylcysteine groups were present on each reduced, alkylated IgMs subunit, indicating that the intersubunit disulfide bonds were the only ones cleaved. The great lability of such bonds is ascribable to their accessibility and to the increase in entropy accompanying the liberation of subunits.

When rabbit or human IgM is reduced to IgMs with 0.1 to 0.2 M 2-mercaptoethanol it dissociates further, upon dilution in neutral buffer, into half-molecules (5 S) containing one H and one L chain. At higher concentration the half-molecules reassociate and it is possible in this way to prepare hybrid IgMs from two different IgM preparations (117,118).

Miller and Metzger found that 25 disulfide bonds in human IgM (a Waldenström macroglobulin) are readily reducible in neutral buffer (10). Ten of these (one per L chain) were H–L disulfide bonds. They detected a total of about 95 disulfide bonds in the molecule, a value in close accord with present information on the amino acid sequence. The value of 25 bonds was obtained by determining the number of —SH groups released as a function of time in the presence of 0.001 M dithiothreitol; it attained a plateau of 50 groups. Interchain disulfide bonds are characteristically more labile than intrachain bonds. In one of the models they proposed, the IgMs subunits are arranged as a circular pentamer, linked by intersubunit S–S bonds (Fig. 3.1). Such a model would be in accord with electron micrographs. Our current concept is in agreement with that of Miller and Metzger, except for the presence of two interheavy chain bonds and one intersubunit bond per IgMs subunit, rather than the reverse. A total of 25 interchain bonds is still appropriate (Fig. 3.1); there may, however, be an additional contribution by the J chain. On the basis of these studies one can arrange the disulfide bonds of IgM in order of decreasing lability as follows: intersubunit; interchain intrasubunit; intrachain.

More recently, Tomasi showed that after very mild reduction, in which less than half the IgM is transformed to IgMs, the remaining 19 S IgM is stabilized only by noncovalent bonds and breaks down to IgMs in the presence of guanidine hydrochloride; i.e., the partially reduced molecule is stabilized somehow by noncovalent interactions after cleavage of disulfide bonds (119). The mechanism of this stabilization is unclear since the slightly more severe reduction that liberates IgMs from all the molecules would not seem likely to disrupt noncovalent bonds. One possibility is that the partially reduced J chain holds the molecule together through noncovalent interactions.

B. Reassociation of IgMs Subunits and J Chain

If IgM is reduced to IgMs without subsequent alkylation, and the reducing agent is removed by dialysis or gel filtration, reassembly occurs to varying degrees and polymers with sedimentation coefficients of 10 to 19 S as well as larger aggregates have been reported. After reduction to produce IgMs under minimal conditions [0.02 M mercaptoethylamine (120)] a substantial amount of IgM of the original size was recovered upon reoxidation, and few products of intermediate size were formed. Similar results were obtained by Parkhouse *et al.* upon careful reduction and reoxidation of mouse IgM (121). More recently, Ricardo and Inman showed that IgM, reconstituted from IgMs, contained approximately as much J chain, covalently bound, as native human IgM (122); i.e., J chain was reincorporated during reoxidation. Again, no reoxidation products intermediate in size between IgMs and IgM were observed. Della Corte and Parkhouse observed that complete reassembly of both IgA and IgM is greatly facilitated if a disulfide-interchange enzyme, obtained from bovine liver, is present in the mixture together with J chain (123). Monomeric IgA and IgMs subunits, isolated from plasma cell tumors, failed to polymerize unless both J chain and the enzyme were present. Despite the obviously important role of J chain, IgM reconstituted in its absence (from IgMs prepared by reduction of IgM, as contrasted with naturally occurring IgMs) can still fix complement and may retain full antibody activity (124). Hybrid IgM molecules were formed by reoxidizing a mixture of rabbit and human IgMs (125); certain practical applications of the method are described by the authors.

C. Proteolysis of IgM

IgM can be cleaved into large fragments by a variety of enzymes, including trypsin, papain, pepsin, and chymotrypsin. Many of these procedures have been reviewed by Metzger (104). A few of the more widely used methods will be outlined.

Miller and Metzger (126) treated the IgMs subunit of a human macroglobulin with trypsin at 25°C and recovered a major 3.6 S product (mol. wt. 47,000) with properties characteristic of fragment Fab; it comprises an L chain and the N-terminal segment of an H chain. When intact IgM is treated with trypsin an early product [F(ab')$_2$] has a molecular weight of 114,000 and consists of two Fab-like fragments, linked only by one disulfide bond. Stone and Metzger showed that the Fab fragments in a tryptic digest of monoclonal IgM retain full antigen-binding activity; each of the Fab fragments of the IgM molecule appeared equivalent in its binding properties (127). Fab fragments of approximate molecular weight 50,000 can also be produced by digestion of human IgM (128,129) or IgMs (130) with papain.

In contrast to the ease of preparation of Fab fragments it has proved relatively difficult to obtain Fc fragments of IgM. Onoue *et al.* (129) found that treatment of a macroglobulin with papain in the absence of cysteine yields Fab fragments and a polymer, apparently consisting of five Fc fragments linked by disulfide bonds [(Fc)$_{5\mu}$]. This 10.6 S polymer has a molecular weight of 320,000; upon reduction 3.2 S fragments (Fc) are formed. A very similar product is produced by tryptic digestion of IgM at 56°C for 30 min, or at 65°C for 8 min (131). The yield of (Fc)$_{5\mu}$ obtained by this method exceeds 70% of the theoretical value. The product has a molecular weight of 340,000, which decreases to 67,000 upon mild reduction, indicating that the five Fc fragments are joined by disulfide bonds. The Fab$_\mu$ fragment produced by tryptic digestion at high temperature has a molecular weight of 40,000 to 48,000. This procedure appears to be the method of choice for preparing Fc fragments. It is stated that optimal conditions for the digestion are 20 min at 60°C (132).

According to Putnam *et al.* (109) (see Fig. 3.2) the sequence of the Fc fragment produced by trypsin at 60°C begins adjacent to arginine 325 and continues to the C-terminus. Fragment (Fc)$_{5\mu}$ contains five dimers of such segments. Each chain segment comprises the C_H4 and C_H5 domains of the μ chain. The Fab$_\mu$ fragment contains the L chain and a segment of the μ chain from the N-terminus to position 213. The C_H3 domain is degraded. (The points of cleavage do not correspond precisely to the beginning or end of a domain.)

D. Naturally Occurring Human IgM of Low Molecular Weight (7 S IgM)

Many species of fish synthesize IgM of both high (14–19 S) and low (7 S) molecular weight, which are antigenically very similar or identical (Chapter 7), and are believed to have similar or identical H chains, i.e., belonging to a single class. IgM of low molecular weight ($\sim$ 7 S) can also be detected at a low concentration in certain normal human sera (133–135). It is present at higher concentration in some, but not all, patients with immunological disorders such as systemic lupus erythematosus (SLE), ataxia telangiectasia, rheumatoid arthritis, Waldenström's macroglobulinemia, multiple myeloma, and lymphoma (136,137). Among patients with SLE the incidence is about 15 to 20%; in Waldenström's macroglobulinemia it is roughly 30–50%. The concentration of 7 S IgM is most likely to be substantial (>1 mg/ml) in the presence of a high concentration of 19 S IgM, although the concentrations are not directly correlated. There is evidence that 7 S IgM can be synthesized independently and is not necessarily a breakdown product of IgM (136,138). IgM of low molecular weight has been shown to have antibody activity, for example, against red blood cell antigens, casein, or cell nuclei. Since intracellular IgM is mainly in the forms of IgMs, the appearance of 7 S IgM in serum could result from a defect in the assembly process, conceivably as a result of a deficiency of J chain within the cell; this is, however, speculative.

E. Valence of IgM

There has been some disagreement as to the number of antigen binding sites per molecule, or valence, of IgM; values reported in the literature are either 5 or 10. (It is still not clear why intermediate values have not been obtained with antihapten antibodies.) It now appears that, at least in rabbit and human IgM, there are 10 combining sites per molecule, as would be predicted from the presence of ten H–L pairs (139–142). With large antigens the apparent valence may be less than 10 because of steric interference; i.e., a large molecule of antigen bound in one combining site can block access of antigen to another combining site. This is shown clearly by the investigation of Edberg et al. (143), who found that the apparent valence of rabbit antidextran antibody decreases from 10 with isomaltose (mol. wt. 342) as ligand to 2.3 for dextran of mol. wt. 1.8×10^6. For dextrans of molecular weight 7000–237,000 the apparent valence was 5; the constant valence over such a wide range of molecular weight of antigen suggests that pairs of combining sites are in close proximity, so that occupancy of one of them by a fairly large molecule blocks the other. Reports of a valence of 5 for certain IgM antihapten antibodies might be explained on the basis that part of the isolated antibody population has such a low K value ($<1 \times 10^4$ M^{-1}) so as to be difficult to detect by the methods used for measuring binding of hapten.

F. Interaction with Complement

Human IgM is capable of binding the activated first component of human or guinea pig complement, $C\bar{1}$ (83). When the purified components were mixed and analyzed in the ultracentrifuge, the relative binding capacity increased with increasing state of aggregation of IgM; the 19 S molecule was 15 times as effective, per unit weight, as the IgMs, 4-chain subunit. A 35 S aggregate of IgM had approximately four times as much binding capacity per unit weight as 19 S IgM. It is of interest that the IgMs subunit was about as effective as IgG1. The greater capacity of IgM, as compared to IgG, for binding $C\bar{1}$ may therefore be due to the close proximity of multiple Fc units in the IgM pentamer.

V. STRUCTURE AND PROPERTIES OF HUMAN IgA

A. Physical and Chemical Properties[2]

IgA was first identified in human serum by Grabar and Williams (146), who used their newly developed technique of immunoelectrophoresis. It was related to myeloma proteins of the same class by the antigenic analyses of Slater *et al.* (147). The electrophoretic mobility of IgA at slightly alkaline pH (in the slow β region) is on the average faster than that of IgG although there is overlap owing to the charge heterogeneity of both classes. IgA was isolated from a globulin fraction of normal human serum by Heremans *et al.* (148), who exploited the observation that IgG, but not IgA is precipitated by 0.1 M zinc sulfate at neutral pH. IgA is much easier to isolate in good yield when it occurs as a myeloma protein. Specific antiserum to IgA (directed to the C_α region) is readily prepared with a myeloma protein as immunogen; the antiserum is absorbed with immunoglobulin of one or more classes other than IgA to render it specific.

Although IgA constitutes about 20% of normal serum immunoglobulins, serum IgA does not have any obvious special properties, as compared to IgG, that are known to be essential in host defense. IgA does play a unique role in secretory fluids surrounding mucous membranes, where it occurs in a different form and generally constitutes the major immunoglobulin class. In human serum it exists primarily as a

---

[2] The properties of IgA are reviewed in references 144 and 145.

4-chain monomer (7 S) but also, in varying amounts, as disulfide bonded polymers of the 4-chain unit (10–18 S) (11). IgA myeloma proteins are similarly heterogeneous in size, owing to the presence of disulfide bonded polymers. The polymers are readily broken down to 4-chain (7 S) units by mild reduction. Monomeric IgA has a molecular weight of about 160,000 and a relatively high carbohydrate content (Table 3.1). (The nature of the carbohydrate is discussed in Chapter 4.) Partial amino acid sequence analyses of the α chain (Chapter 7) indicate a closer evolutionary relationship between IgM and IgA than between IgM and IgG; it has been suggested that both the α and γ chain evolved from the μ chain and that divergence of the α chain took place more recently.

Two subclasses of IgA, IgA1 and IgA2, have been identified in normal human serum by antisera prepared in goats, monkeys, or rabbits (149–151). IgA2 myeloma proteins occur less frequently than IgA1, in accord with the relatively low concentration of IgA2 (about 10 to 20% of total IgA) in normal serum (152,153). In exocrine secretions, secretory IgA (sIgA) contains roughly equal concentrations of α_1 and α_2 chains (152). The α_2 chain appears, on the basis of the higher average anodal mobility of IgA2 myeloma proteins, to be more negatively charged than the α_1 chain. The molecular weights of the α_1 and α_2 chains were reported as 52,000 and 58,000, respectively (154,155); this suggests the presence of four domains in each subclass. Where the extra amino acids in IgA2 are located is uncertain. The α_1 and α_2 chains differ somewhat with respect to carbohydrate content. For example, one or two galactosamine-containing carbohydrate moieties are present in the hinge region of α_1 but not α_2 chains (156). The Fc regions of the α_1 and α_2 chains yielded two glucosamine-containing glycopeptides in which the peptide appeared identical in the two subclasses; an additional glycopeptide was isolated from an α_1 chain (157). The deficiency of carbohydrate in the hinge region of the α_2 chain is associated with a deletion of 12 amino acids as compared to the α_1 chain (158); the hinge region of the α_1 chain contains a duplicated stretch of seven amino acids which is not present in α_2.

There are two known genetic markers of IgA2, designated $A_2m(1)$ and $A_2m(2)$ (Chapter 9). Molecules of allotype $A_2m(1)$ have an unusual chain structure with the L chains disulfide bonded to one another but not to H chains (152) (Table 3.1). Perhaps to compensate for the absence of L–H disulfide bonds, the noncovalent forces linking L to H chains are stronger in IgA2 than in IgA1 (159). This type of chain structure is also seen in the IgA myeloma proteins of BALB/c mice.

B. Proteolysis of IgA

It has proved difficult to obtain Fc fragments of human IgA; however, there is evidence for the production of 3.5 S Fab-like fragments after digestion with papain (160). Peptic digestion of an IgA(κ) 10 S serum myeloma protein yielded a fragment with a sedimentation coefficient of 4.8 S which was reduced to 3.4 S by treatment with mercaptoethanol (161). This fragment did not react with antibodies specific for the Fc portion but did react with anti-κ chain antibody. It would appear that the 4.8 and 3.4 S molecules correspond to F(ab')$_2$ and Fab', respectively.

C. Secretory IgA

In 1963, Chodirker and Tomasi made the important discovery that IgA is the predominant class of immunoglobulin in human saliva, colostrum, and tears (162). This was subsequently extended to include nasal, bronchial, and other fluids bathing the mucous membranes of the respiratory and digestive systems. Its presence is associated with plasma cells containing IgA, which are very numerous in the lamina propria of these tracts. Although 7 S IgA is found in secretory fluids the predominant form has a sedimentation coefficient of 11 S (163) and a molecular weight of 380,000 to 390,000 (164–166). A molecular weight of 370,000 was reported for rabbit sIgA (167). These values agree well with that

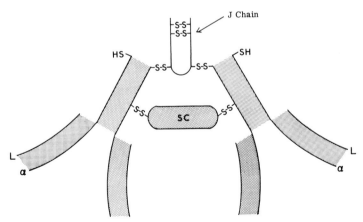

Fig. 3.3. Hypothetical structural model of secretory IgA. It is uncertain whether the J chain is linked to one or two α chains.

calculated from the sum of the molecular weights of its components (about 400,000). A molecule of sIgA is made up of two molecules of IgA, one of secretory component (SC) (65,000–70,000) and one J chain (15,000). A hypothetical model of the arrangement of polypeptide chains in sIgA is shown in Fig. 3.3. The J chain is linked to the Fc region of α chains through disulfide bonds; the penultimate half-cystine of one or two α chains is joined to the single J chain (168). It is uncertain whether the J chain links two IgA monomers, as shown in the figure, joins two α chains in one monomer, or is linked to only a single α chain. Secretory component is joined to α chains through strong noncovalent interactions; it is bound, in addition, through disulfide bonds in at least 80% of the sIgA molecules in human colostrum (165). Separation of SC from IgA thus requires reduction and exposure to a reagent, such as urea, guanidine, or detergent, which will disrupt noncovalent interactions. Small amounts of sIgA (average concentration, 0.03 mg/ml) were found in the sera of about 50% of normal individuals (169–171).

D. Secretory Component

Tomasi *et al.* (163) showed in 1965 that the IgA of secretions contains a component which is antigenically unrelated to monomeric IgA. The finding was confirmed by South *et al.* (172), who also demonstrated that the immunologically distinct component is present in unbound form in the saliva of persons lacking IgA; these include patients with agammaglobulinemia or ataxia telangiectasia and newborns (172). The protein, now referred to as secretory component (SC), can be separated from secretory IgA by reduction and gel filtration in the presence of a dissociating agent (164,173). It consists of a single polypeptide chain and contains about 9% carbohydrate (165,174), and is also found in unbound form in colostrum and milk (164,175). The molecular weight of SC has been variously reported as 54,000 to 80,000, with values for free SC component tending to be higher than those obtained with SC isolated from sIgA (144); a molecular weight of about 70,000 is now generally accepted. There is one molecule of SC per molecule of sIgA. Secretory component is antigenically unrelated to IgA, to J chain, or to other immunoglobulins, and there is no evidence for an evolutionary origin in common with the immunoglobulins. Partial amino acid sequence analysis and peptide mapping revealed no differences between SC occurring in free form in human mucous secretions or bound to IgA (176).

An extensive investigation of the interaction of SC with serum IgA was reported by Mach (175), who isolated free SC from human and bovine milk. The SC was labeled with ^{125}I and tested for its capacity to bind to the IgA of various species by a method involving autoradiography after immunoelectrophoresis; the presence of radioactivity in a specific precipitin band containing IgA was taken as evidence for binding of SC. Human and bovine SC were found to bind to serum IgA of the nine different mammalian species tested. Binding occurred to lesser extent to IgM but not at all to IgG or to monomeric IgA. The binding to IgM is of interest since the IgM of patients with IgA deficiency was reported to contain antigenic determinants of SC (177). The biological significance of this is not known, and, in general, SC is not found in association with immunoglobulins other than IgA. Secretory component can be synthesized by patients who do not produce IgA; the concentration of free SC in secretory fluids is often increased in such cases (172). The IgA1 and IgA2 subclasses are both capable of binding SC. When SC was allowed to combine with a IgGA2 myeloma protein of allotype $A_2m(1)$, which lacks L–H disulfide bridges, the stability of the molecule in the presence of denaturing agents was greatly increased (178). Bienenstock *et al.* have shown that human SC is bound by a chicken secretory immunoglobulin, which appears to be the counterpart of mammalian IgA (179).

E. J Chain

Our understanding of the structure of polymeric immunoglobulins was advanced by Halpern and Koshland, when they demonstrated the presence of J chain in human and rabbit sIgA (180). Its detection had been complicated by its similarity in size to L chain. J chain was discovered by virtue of its relatively high negative charge at alkaline pH, which causes it to move more rapidly than L chain toward the anode during electrophoresis of reduced and alkylated IgA. A J chain, which is apparently identical to that in sIgA, was subsequently shown to be present in IgM and in polymers of IgA (lacking secretory component) (105,181). J chain is not found in monomeric serum IgA or in IgMs. It has been detected in the polymeric immunoglobulins of a wide variety of vertebrates (Chapter 7), including a primitive species, the shark (182).

J chain has a molecular weight of 15,000 to 15,500 and is rich in half-cystine groups (7–8 residues per molecule) (122,183–185). This, its presence only in polymeric immunoglobulins, and the fact that it is disulfide bonded to the Fc region of an α or μ chain (112,186,187), suggest a role as a "joining" (J) protein, responsible for the polymerization of 4-chain monomers through disulfide bonding (180). More recently it was found that, in human IgM, the single J chain is disulfide bonded to the penultimate half-cystine of the μ chain (111). Since there is evidence that the intersubunit bonds in IgM are initiated much closer to the N-terminus, at position 424 (protein Ou), it would appear that the J chain is not required to join two IgMs subunits. It may, however, help in some manner to initiate polymerization.

As in the μ chain, J chain is attached to the half-cystine which is next to the C-terminus of the α chain (168). Only 2 out of a total of 7 to 8 half-cystines in the J chain are involved in linking the chain to a μ chain (106), and 1 or 2 half-cystines join the J chain to an α chain (168). It is uncertain whether the J chain is linked to two 4-chain subunits, or to two H chains within a subunit, of IgM or IgA; the former would seem to represent a more useful function.

J chain is synthesized by the same cells that produce the immunoglobulin to which it is attached (188,189). It is linked to IgM or to polymeric IgA shortly before secretion from a lymphoid cell. In the case of a myeloma tumor secreting both monomeric and dimeric IgA, the amount of dimer produced appears to be a function of the quantity of J chain available (189,190).

By carefully determining the amino acid composition of a mixture of L and J chains from human sIgA, Halpern and Koshland obtained a value of 1.02 moles J chain per mole of sIgA dimer and 1.3 moles per mole of an sIgA tetramer (8 H and 8 L chains); both proteins were isolated from human colostrum (191). A value of 1 mole per mole of IgM was obtained in experiments in which all the half-cystines in the J chain and IgM were reduced and carboxymethylated with labeled iodoacetate, and the ratios of radioactivities in isolated J, μ, and L chains were determined (106).

As already indicated, J chain moves more rapidly than L chain to the anode during electrophoresis. This, or ion-exchange chromatography, provides a means of purification on a preparative scale. Alternatively, one can take advantage of the greater lability of L–α disulfide bonds, as compared to J–α disulfide bonds, to selectively cleave the former, separate L chains by gel filtration, then cleave the J–α bonds, and repeat the gel filtration to separate J from α chains. Residual α or L chains can be removed with an immunoadsorbent containing bound anti-α and anti-L chain antibodies (184). The low solubility of J chain in salt-free water has also been used to effect a partial separation from L chains (192). Isolated J chain appears homogeneous, although the possibility of minor polymorphism has not been ruled out. The chain is highly elongated, with an axial ratio (assuming a prolate ellipsoid shape) of about 18:1 (184). J chain is quite hydrophilic; it is rich in arginine, isoleucine, and aspartic acid as well as cysteine, and has a low content of phenylalanine, serine, and glycine.

Antiserum against isolated J chain reacts well with IgM or polymeric IgA only after the immunoglobulin has been reduced and alkylated; thus, the J chain is either not exposed or is in an unreactive conformation in the native molecule (181). The J chain has similar antigenic properties whether or not its four disulfide bonds have been reduced; this suggests that its conformation is not greatly affected by the status of those bonds (M.E. Koshland, personal communication).

There is no evidence for a common evolutionary origin of J chain and the immunoglobulins. Their peptide maps, antigenic determinants, and partial sequences have shown no similarities (105,181). A minor resemblance to H chains is the presence in J chains of a blocked N-terminus (pyrrolidonecarboxylic acid) (193).

F. Assembly of the sIgA Molecule

Studies of the products secreted by mouse plasma cell tumors *in vitro* indicate that the J chain is synthesized by the same plasma cells that synthesize IgA (or IgM) (123,188–190). In each investigation the cells were exposed to tritiated leucine to label the immunoglobulin being actively synthesized. J chain was identified and its radioactivity determined through its characteristic rapid mobility toward the anode in polyacrylamide gel. Polymeric IgA and IgM were found to contain J chain, linked through disulfide bonds, in roughly the expected proportions, thus establishing the plasma cell as its site of synthesis; monomeric IgA lacks J chain. Since intracellular IgA and IgM are largely monomeric (4-chain units) it would appear that the J chain is added shortly before secretion. It is present, however, within that fraction of the intracellular IgA which is polymeric (188).

In contrast to J chain, secretory component (SC) is not synthesized by the plasma cell. Tourville *et al.* used fluoresceinated antisera to localize IgA and SC; the latter was found within epithelial cells of the mucosa of all tissues studied; these included parotid and submaxillary glands, bronchi, pancreas, gastrointestinal tract, and other tissues (194). No SC was identified within plasma cells. It is uncertain where IgA and SC are joined. The authors inability to visualize IgA within epithelial cells suggested that the combination takes place in spaces between those cells. They did not rule out an alternative possibility (195) that IgA passes through epithelial cells, where joining occurs, but is present in very low concentration and is, therefore, not detectable. The latter possibility is supported by the study of Roger and Lamm (196), who concluded that assembly of SC and IgA probably occurs in the Golgi zone or in the adjacent apical cytoplasm of the epithelial cell. Heremans and

Vaerman (195) have proposed that secretion through epithelial cells is restricted to IgA dimers, which constitute a large proportion of the IgA synthesized by plasma cells located below the epithelium. That SC and IgA are synthesized in separate cells is also indicated by the studies of Lawton et al. (197) who found that IgA, treated so as to remove SC, will compete with newly synthesized IgA for combination with SC. Since the IgA added presumably cannot enter the plasma cell, this would indicate that joining occurs elsewhere. The authors made the additional interesting observation that IgA lacking SC, but not intact IgA, stimulates the biosynthesis of SC.

G. Biological Role of sIgA

The importance of the secretory immune system as a first line of defense, present at external surfaces, is apparent, and IgA antibodies against a large variety of pathogens have been demonstrated (174). Although IgA does not fix complement by the conventional pathway it may nevertheless enhance phagocytosis, and neutralize viruses. The multivalence of sIgA may be of considerable significance in viral neutralization since it can confer greater avidity on the antibody molecule. Secretory IgA may also combine with and prevent the absorption of various antigens, such as those present in food (144). This could have the effect of reducing the incidence of allergic reactions and the presence of harmful immune complexes in body fluids. IgA antibodies in colostrum may be significant in limiting infections in newborns.

It has been suggested (174) that sIgA may possess a significant biological advantage over IgG by virtue of its increased resistance to proteolysis; this could be of particular importance in external secretions, particularly those of the gastrointestinal tract, which contain potent proteolytic enzymes. Brown et al. (198) compared the susceptibility of human exocrine and serum immunoglobulins to trypsin, chymotrypsin, and enzymes in duodenal fluid; changes in molecular size and antibody activity were monitored. Secretory IgA proved to be considerably more resistant to digestion than either IgG or serum IgA. In other investigations it was found that a proportion of sIgA is more resistant to pepsin than serum IgA (199,200). The IgA2 fraction of serum IgA was found to be somewhat more resistant to pepsin than IgA1. Underdown and Dorrington (201) showed that sIgA is considerably more resistant than IgG1 and somewhat more resistant than monomeric IgA to papain or to pronase.

These investigations indicate that IgA is more resistant to pro-teolysis than IgG and that the presence of SC and/or J chain confers ad-ditional protection against the action of a variety of proteolytic enzymes.

VI. IgE

A. General Considerations

This class of immunoglobulin, which is present at very low concen-trations in serum, has assumed great importance since its discovery in 1966 and the demonstration that antibodies of the IgE class mediate reactions of immediate hypersensitivity. In humans, IgE is probably the only class having skin-sensitizing activity, and the Prausnitz–Küstner (P–K) test for sensitivity is thus a test for the presence of IgE antibodies against the antigen in question.[3] Levels of IgE are frequently elevated in atopic conditions or as a consequence of parasitic infections. IgE is found in the circulation of nonallergic, as well as allergic individuals, and normal individuals can respond to challenges by antigen with the pro-duction of reaginic antibodies, which are undoubtedly IgE (202,203). IgE appears to have antigen-binding characteristics similar to those of other immunoglobulins; thus reaginic activity can be removed with an insoluble adsorbent containing the specific antigen (204), and IgE an-tibodies are capable of agglutinating erythrocytes coated with the corre-sponding allergen (205). This is consistent with the bivalence predicted on the basis of the chain structure of the molecule (two H and two L chains).

What particular beneficial effects IgE antibodies have is uncertain. On the basis of the high levels of IgE often observed in patients with parasitic infections it has been proposed that a principal function may in-volve combating parasitic organisms. The increases in vascular perme-ability associated with the reaction of IgE with antigen may confer pro-tection against bacterial infections as well (206).

The discovery by K. Ishizaka and T. Ishizaka of the IgE class of immunoglobulin was a major accomplishment of immunochemical re-search. Its presence had escaped many investigators, owing mainly to its

---

[3] In the Prausnitz-Küstner test a dilution of serum to be tested for the presence of reagin is introduced into the skin of a nonallergic individual. After 1 or 2 days this is followed by the allergen. A wheal and erythema reaction indicates the presence of reagin in the donor's serum.

very low serum concentration. The Ishizakas fractionated reagin-containing sera from atopic patients by chromatography on DEAE-cellulose and gel filtration through Sephadex G-200 (207). The skin-sensitizing activity did not run parallel with the concentration of either IgA or IgG and, further, was not precipitated by anti-IgG or anti-IgA. It was coprecipitated by IgG reacting with antibodies to L chains, indicating that reaginic activity is mediated by an immunoglobulin. As little as 1 ng of an impure preparation served to sensitize human skin for the P–K reaction. This work contradicted earlier investigations which suggested that P–K activity is a property of IgA; it succeeded because of the absence of anti-IgE in the absorbed antiserum used. In a related study it was demonstrated by similar methods that reaginic activity is not associated with IgD or IgM; this indicated the existence of a fifth class of immunoglobulin, now designated IgE (208).

The next step was to prepare an antiserum specific for this class of immunoglobulin (209). This was done by immunization of a rabbit with Cohn fraction III from a normal individual. The resulting antiserum, after absorption with an IgA myeloma protein, would no longer react with IgA, IgG, or L chains, but did form a precipitin band when tested against a reagin-rich fraction of the serum of a patient allergic to ragweed pollen. Also, a component of the precipitin band was shown by radioimmunoelectrophoresis to bind ^{125}I-labeled antigen E, an important allergen in ragweed. Finally, the absorbed antiserum was capable of removing, by precipitation, reaginic activity from the patient's serum. This work clearly established the existence of the new class of immunoglobulin.

The concentration of IgE in normal serum is so low (mean value, about 0.3 μg/ml) that it is virtually impossible to isolate the protein by chemical techniques. A major advance was the discovery of a patient with multiple myeloma whose myeloma protein proved to be of the IgE class (210,211). The antigenic and structural identity of the myeloma protein with the IgE class discovered by Ishizaka was established through a collaborative effort of the two laboratories (212). The myeloma protein (type λ) was present at a concentration of about 40 mg/ml. Thus, 1 ml of the patient's serum contained as much IgE as 130 liters of normal serum. The unique antigenic determinants on the protein were localized to H chains and eventually to the Fc fragment. Since this initial discovery, at least 3 other patients with IgE myeloma proteins have been identified (213–215) and the myeloma protein from the patient of Ogawa *et al.* (213) has been studied extensively.

A radioimmunoassay was used to quantitate IgE in normal sera (211); the technique involves competition of unlabeled IgE in the unknown sample with ^{125}I-labeled, myeloma IgE for combination with anti-IgE; the latter is bound to an insoluble matrix. IgE was found in all normal sera tested; in more than 90% of the samples the range of concentrations was 0.1 to 0.7 μg/ml.

The discovery of an IgE myeloma protein facilitated many avenues of research: (a) It permitted detailed studies of the structure of IgE, including amino acid sequence analysis. (b) It became possible to investigate the biological properties of IgE and its Fab and Fc fragments, in studies requiring substantial amounts of the purified protein. Among these properties are fixation to various cell types and the consequent liberation of vasoactive substances, biological half-life, fixation of complement by aggregated IgE, etc. (c) The production of large amounts of specific antiserum was made possible; only a few milligrams are needed, for example, to produce liter quantities of a potent goat antiserum. Anti-IgE is now available commercially and is being used to determine IgE levels in the sera of a wide variety of patients in efforts to establish correlations with disease states. One also can assay for the level of IgE antibody of a particular specificity if the antigen is available in a pure form; a radioimmunoassay is generally employed. One type of assay for total IgE in serum requires purified, labeled IgE (nanogram quantities) in addition to anti-IgE.

B. Physical and Chemical Properties of IgE

Following their isolation of the myeloma protein, Johansson and Bennich investigated a number of its properties. This work was reviewed in 1971 (216). The protein migrates in the fast γ region and has a carbohydrate content of about 11.5%, localized in the ϵ chains. Upon reduction, exposure to acid, and gel filtration about 20% of the protein was recovered as λ chains, the remainder as ϵ chains. The sedimentation coefficient is 8.0 ± 0.1 S and the molecular weight is 188,000–196,000, which is close to that of IgD. This would indicate a molecular weight for the ϵ chain of 72,000 to 76,000, or 61,000 to 65,000 without the carbohydrate, a range consistent with the presence of five domains. Direct determination of the molecular weight of the ϵ chain gave a value of 61,000 with the carbohydrate subtracted. This is 3000 daltons higher than the similarly corrected value for a μ chain. The molecular weight determined for a second IgE myeloma protein is 185,000 and that of its ϵ chain is 69,700, or 58,500 with the carbohydrate content subtracted (217). The latter value is consistent with the presence of about 540 amino acid residues per chain. The difference between the two proteins is probably within the range of experimental error.

One disulfide bond joins each L chain to an H chain. The number of interheavy chain disulfide bonds is uncertain, but the number of half-cystines in the ϵ chain (about 15) suggests that there are approximately 4 (217,218).

Digestion of an IgE myeloma protein with papain liberates an Fc fragment with a sedimentation coefficient of 5 S and a molecular weight of about 98,000; it contains nearly all of the carbohydrate and the antigenic determinants characteristic of IgE, but lacks L chain determinants (216,219). Fragment Fc exhibits microheterogeneity and is gradually degraded into smaller fragments. An Fab fragment can also be isolated after short-term digestion, but it is quite labile to papain and difficult to prepare in good yield. An F(ab')$_2$ fragment is produced by digestion with pepsin. It comprises about 75% of the molecule and contains all but the C-terminal portions of the two ϵ chains. Pepsin thus cleaves the ϵ chains at a position farther from the N-terminus than does papain. The F(ab')$_2$ fragment is split, apparently in half, by reduction of interheavy chain disulfide bonds. Papain fragment Fc and pepsin fragment F(ab')$_2$ share antigenic determinants, present in the N-terminal portion of the Fc fragment; IgE differs from other human immunoglobulins in this respect.

C. Amino Acid Sequence Analysis and Composition

The amino acid sequence of the C-terminal domain of IgE, worked out by Bennich *et al.* (220) is shown in Fig. 4.13. With optimal alignment of the 118 C-terminal residues there are 40 positions of identity with respect to the $\gamma 1$ chain and 32 with respect to the μ chain. The number of positions of identity in this segment of the γ and μ chains is 45.[4] On the basis of the greater difference between ϵ and μ, the authors suggest that the genes controlling these chains diverged earlier in evolution than those controlling γ and μ chains. The overall amino acid composition of IgE is quite similar to that of IgM. Significant differences are the presence of a higher content of cysteine (40 versus 26 residues per 4-chain monomer) and methionine (20 versus 14) (217).

D. Levels of IgE in Human Sera

IgE is present at a very low concentration in the cord serum of the newborn (mean concentration $\sim$ 40 ng/ml) (221,222) where IgG is the

[4] At the end of the μ chain there is an additional tail of 19 residues, not included in these comparisons. An extra sequence of 19 residues is also present in IgA (Table 7.5).

major immunoglobulin component. The average IgE concentration rises gradually during childhood to a mean value in adults of 250 to 300 ng/ml. In colostrum, the average concentration is several times greater than that of serum; relatively high concentrations are also found in urine (223) but not in most other secretions.

Concentrations of IgE are often elevated in adult patients with hay fever or asthma; average serum concentrations are several times greater than normal and are particularly high in patients with positive skin or bronchial provocation tests (224,225). No such elevated concentrations of IgG, IgA, IgM, or IgD were observed. Most children with asthma, but only about one-third of those with hay fever, have significantly elevated levels of IgE. Levels tend to be higher during the pollination season and to increase during hyposensitization procedures (225). Administration of disodium cromoglycate, sometimes used in the treatment of asthma, did not affect levels of serum IgE (226).

Among a group of children sampled in Addis Ababa, the mean level of IgE was about 3000 ng/ml, as compared to an average of 160 ng/ml among Swedish children of the same age. This was attributed to parasitic infestation, since the highest levels were seen in children with stools positive for *Ascaris lumbricoides* (227). Other investigations, some of which are reviewed by Bennich and Johansson (216), have also demonstrated an association between parasitic diseases and high levels of IgE. One individual, with ankylostomiasis, had a serum IgE concentration of 140,000 ng/ml (cited in reference 216).

Raised levels of IgE were found among groups of patients with various helminth infections, including schistosomiasis and hookworm (228). Depending on the disease, the average values ranged from 2 to 20 times the average normal level of 0.3 μg/ml. Elevated IgE concentrations (average values, 2–3 times normal) were present in patients with certain types of dermatosis, including eczema; an occasional patient had more than 3000 ng/ml (229). Numerous other reports correlating elevated IgE levels with atopic conditions have appeared.

Correlations with atopic disease states are in general better if measurements are made of the concentration of serum IgE antibodies specific for the allergen in question, rather than total IgE; the correlations are never perfect but are often high enough to have useful predictive value. One frequently encountered difficulty is the unavailability of a pure allergen. When a reasonably homogeneous preparation is at hand, measurement of IgE antibody levels can generally be made by radioimmunoassay. An example is the radioallergosorbent test or RAST (230). The allergen is first linked to an insoluble adsorbent. Next, the patient's serum is added; any antibodies to the allergen, including antibodies of the IgE class, are bound. The latter can then be quantitated by adding radiolabeled anti-IgE; the uptake of radioactivity is a measure of the concentration in the patient's serum of IgE antibodies directed to the allergen.

A few examples of atopic states in which correlations have been found between levels of specific IgE antibodies and the presence of clinical symptoms are: allergy to horse dandruff or timothy pollen (231), cod extract, bird pollen, house dust (232), animal danders, and various pollens (233). Zeiss *et al.* (234) observed a highly significant correlation between levels of IgE antibody specific for ragweed antigen E and the sensitivity of the patients leukocytes to the antigen, as evidenced by histamine release.

We have discussed the initial evidence identifying IgE as the reaginic antibody. In further comfirmatory work Ishizaka and collaborators showed that the skin-sensitizing activity of a patient's sera, as indicated by the highest dilution still capable of giving a P–K reaction, closely paralleled the concentration of IgE antibody specific for the allergen (ragweed extract) (235). By making the assumption that the antigen-binding capacities, per molecule, of IgE and IgG antibodies are comparable, Ishizaka *et al.* calculated the concentration of IgE antibody present and concluded that about 0.2 ng/ml suffices to give a positive P–K reaction.

Results of "reverse" P–K tests were also informative. Here, a wheal and erythema reaction was caused simply by the intracutaneous injection of anti-IgE but not by antibody against other classes of human immunoglobulin. Evidently the anti-IgE reacts with cell-bound normal IgE to give the reaction (236) (See Fig. 3.4.) Experiments with monkey or human lung tissue indicated that the vasoactive substances released are histamine and slow-reacting substance (SRS-A) (237,238). Human lung fragments also release a chemical mediator which is chemotactic for eosinophils (239). Each of these three substances plays a role in allergic reactions.

Autoradiographic studies with ^{125}I-labeled anti-IgE and electron microscopic investigations using anti-IgE with an electron-dense marker have shown that the site of fixation of IgE is the basophilic leukocyte in blood and the mast cell in skin; IgE is attached to membrane receptors through its Fc region (240–244). The latter is shown by the capacity of fragment Fc, but not Fab, when present in excess to block the P–K reaction or the passive sensitization of cells by IgE (using specific antigen for the test), and by the capacity of fragment Fc to combine with cells and give a "reverse-type" reaction upon addition of anti-IgE (Fig. 3.4) (240–242).

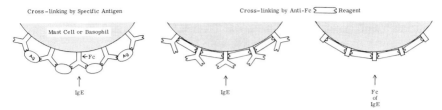

Fig. 3.4. Alternative mechanisms for IgE-mediated release of histamine or SRS-A from mast cells or basophils. This occurs as a consequence of cross-linking which can be caused by antigen or by an antiglobulin reagent.

The reverse reaction (IgE or its Fc fragment on the cell, followed by anti-IgE) can be brought about by bivalent F(ab')$_2$ fragments of anti-IgE but not by monovalent Fab' (237,245). This indicates that aggregation of IgE on the cell surface is required for a reaction of immediate hypersensitivity. The criteria for such a reaction include the P–K test and the release of histamine from leukocytes or from monkey lung tissues (245). This result implies that antigen may act in a similar way, by aggregating *specific* IgE molecules on the cell surface. Aggregation need not, however, be induced by antigen or by anti-IgE; simply injecting aggregated IgE myeloma protein, or its aggregated Fc fragment, results in a wheal and erythema reaction (242–246).

E. Complement Fixation

IgE fails to fix complement through the normal pathway when allowed to react with antigen, and aggregated IgE is similarly inactive [in contrast to aggregated IgG or IgM (246)]. Studies (247) carried out in the light of the discovery of the alternate pathway of complement fixation (248,249) showed that aggregated IgE, or its aggregated Fc fragment, can fix complement through this alternate mechanism, which bypasses C1,4,2.

VII. IgD

A. General Considerations

The IgD class of immunoglobulin was discovered in 1965 by Rowe and Fahey (250,251), who identified it in the serum of a patient with multiple myeloma. The isolated protein was found to have fast γ mobility and Fc fragments with unusually high anodal mobility; it possessed antigenic determinants not present in IgG, IgA, or IgM. The myeloma protein was used to produce antiserum specific for IgD. Using such antisera, a number of studies of the incidence of IgD myeloma proteins were carried out; it was found in 1–3% of cases of multiple myeloma (21–23,252). A high proportion (~80%) of IgD myeloma proteins have λ chains; the reason for this selectivity is not known (21–23). IgD myeloma proteins are present, on the average, at lower concentration than myeloma proteins of the IgG and IgA classes. Typically, the concentration of the monoclonal IgD is less than 15 mg/ml; it can therefore be missed in certain types of routine screening procedure. The average age of patients with IgD myeloma proteins is lower than that of patients with other classes of myeloma protein and the tumor is often located in tissues other than bone; it is, however, sometimes present in the immediate vicinity of bone tissue (22). The monoclonal protein has its counterpart in normal human serum, where its concentration is quite variable but averages about 30 μg/ml (251), a value less than 1% of that of IgG. Its concentration is somewhat higher in the serum of pregnant women near term (253,254). Although IgD has been detected in the cord serum of a small percentage of newborns (255), its concentration generally becomes appreciable only at the age of about 6 months and gradually increases during childhood (256). Normal IgD has been reported to have antibody activity, but the significance of these results has been questioned (257). A review of the properties of IgD was written by Spiegelberg in 1972 (257a).

B. Physical and Biological Properties

IgD has a sedimentation coefficient of about 6.5 S. Its molecular weight has been variously reported as 172,000 to 200,000 (258–261). The value of 172,000 was supported by molecular weights of the separated chains (H = 60,000; L = 23,000), which would give a total for two H and two L chains of 166,000 (260). In another study of three IgD myeloma proteins, however, the average molecular weight of the δ chain was found to be 69,700 daltons; this would correspond to a molecular weight for IgD of approximately 184,000 (262). If the latter value is correct there may be five domains in the δ chain; this question should eventually be settled by amino acid sequence analysis.

The molecule has the usual single disulfide bond joining each H and L chain pair, and a single bond between the H chains (260). In the latter respect it differs from other human immunoglobulins but resembles rabbit IgG (263). IgD has a carbohydrate content of 11%, which is restricted to the δ chain in the majority of proteins.

The contents of *N*-acetylglucosamine and of sialic acid are high as compared to levels in other classes of immunoglobulin (259,260,264). IgD is heat labile, losing much of its antigenic structure after 1 hour at 56°C (265).

The location of interchain disulfide bridges in constant regions permits "chemical typing" of IgD myeloma proteins by reduction, alkylation with ^{14}C-iodoacetic acid, and enzymatic degradation. After electrophoresis of the peptides, those containing carboxymethylcysteine are identified by autoradiography. Peptides containing half-cystine groups involved in H–H and H–L linkage migrate in a pattern uniquely characteristic of IgD [All the classes and subclasses of human immunoglobulins can be identified in this way (218,264)]. These and other studies (260) indicated, as noted above, that one disulfide bond joins each H–L pair and one links the H chains.

The amino acid composition of the δ chain is quite similar to that of human γ chains. Carbohydrate is present in at least three separate positions on the δ chain (260).

IgD of normal serum has proved difficult to isolate because of its low concentration and because of sensitivity to proteolysis. On standing for a few days, even in the cold, IgD in serum may be broken down into Fab and Fc fragments (21,266,267). A systematic study of the cleavage of IgD myeloma proteins by papain, trypsin, and plasmin was carried out by Griffiths and Gleich (261), who compared the rates of digestion of IgD, IgG1, IgG2, IgA, and IgM monoclonal proteins. IgD was the most rapidly degraded and IgG1 the next most susceptible. IgG2 and IgM were quite resistant and IgA was not fragmented under the conditions employed. No IgD remained intact after only 5 minutes exposure to trypsin (30 μg/ml) at 24°C, and it was also cleaved rapidly by papain. The degradation of IgD in serum has been attributed to the action of plasmin since it is retarded by the addition of a plasmin inhibitor, ε-aminocaproate. Spiegelberg *et al.* (260) found that papain and trypsin both cleave IgD on the N-terminal side of the single interheavy chain disulfide bond but that trypsin cleaves about 15 amino acid residues closer to the bond, thus liberating a somewhat larger Fab fragment.

IgD myeloma proteins fail to elicit reverse passive cutaneous anaphylactic reactions in guinea pigs and aggregated IgD (in contrast to IgG) does not fix guinea pig complement (268,269). IgD normally does not cross the human placental barrier (255,256); or does IgD interact with human neutrophils (270) or mast cells (206).

C. IgD on Lymphocyte Membranes

Although the particular biological functions of IgD remain obscure, its presence on lymphocyte membranes has led to some provocative speculation. The presence of IgD on adult lymphocytes was observed by Van Boxel *et al.* (271), who used a fluorescent anti-IgD reagent. Rowe *et al.* showed that the percentage of lymphocytes bearing IgD is, on the average, more than twice as large in the cord blood of the newborn child as in the adult; the average value in newborns is about 14%, a figure that is very high in relation to the amount of IgD in normal serum (about 0.2% of total immunoglobulins) (257,272). Of considerable interest was the finding (272) that about 75% of lymphocytes, from newborns or adults, having surface IgD also stain for IgM, and vice versa. The intensity of staining with anti-IgD and anti-IgM indicated considerable variability in the relative proportions of IgD and IgM on an individual cell. Two factors appear to rule out the possibility that the IgD is passively absorbed from serum. When IgD was removed from cells by exposure to anti-IgD, followed by capping, the IgD reappeared on the surface in an IgD-free medium; second, lymphocytes carried only one type of L chain, κ or λ, and IgM thus had the same L chain type as the IgD on the same cell. This is difficult to explain on the basis of passive absorption.

Of the IgD positive cells, about 55 and 41% had κ or λ chains, respectively; this remains to be reconciled with the fact that about 80% of IgD myeloma proteins are λ. IgM and IgD form caps independently on the same cell, indicating that they are not linked (272,273).

The presence of IgD and IgM on the same cell is striking since only one class had been considered to be present on the surface of a normal lymphocyte. Rowe *et al.* (272) suggest that the IgD and IgM may have identical V_H regions and L chains and are related through a switch in the C_H regions (Chapter 11). They further propose that IgD is the antigen receptor initially present and that IgM is synthesized and appears on the cell membrane as a first step toward differentiation into a plasma cell. This seems to imply that IgM appears after stimulation by antigen; if so, one would have to make the rather difficult assumption that most circulating small lymphocytes have made contact with their specific antigens.

D. IgD on Lymphocytes in Lymphoproliferative Diseases

IgD has been identified, with fluorescent antibodies, on the surface of neoplastic lymphocytes in certain types of malignant lymphoma and in chronic lymphocytic leukemia (CLL) (274–277); the latter represents a leukemic phase of well-differentiated lymphocytic lymphoma and thus may be considered in this context as a form of malignant lymphoma. Earlier studies indicated that IgM is the major Ig class detectable on the surface of CLL lymphocytes, usually in a monoclonal distribution (274,276,278–281). Except for IgE, the other immunoglobulin classes, alone or coexistent with IgM, have frequently been demonstrated as well. More recent investigations have shown that IgD is often present together with IgM on the membrane of CLL lymphocytes (274–276). Fu *et al.* (276) investigated 15 patients with CLL. In ten instances the CLL lymphocyte population exhibited a high percentage of IgD positive cells. Surface IgM was concomitantly present with IgD in the majority of these cases; in three cell populations, however, IgD was present alone, and in four others, IgM was expressed without IgD.

Immunofluorescent analyses of surface Ig determinants have also been carried out on malignant lymphocytes obtained from patients with poorly differentiated lymphocytic lymphoma (PDL), which is often designated as lymphosarcoma (274,275,277). The PDL lymphocytes frequently exhibit surface Ig of multiple heavy-chain classes, including IgD, IgM, IgG, and IgA. Generally, the surface Ig is restricted to a single L chain type, although in several instances both L chain types, together with all four H chain classes have been represented on the majority of cells. Independent capping of IgD and IgM is observed when antibody preparations with two different fluorescent labels are used.

Increased percentages of IgD staining cells were present in 5 of 7 patients with Sjogren's syndrome (282); the data also suggested the presence of multiple Ig classes on individual lymphocytes from all five cell populations exhibiting increased IgD positivity. It should be noted that there is a marked increase in the occurrence of malignant lymphoma among patients with Sjogren's syndrome although none of these patients showed evidence of overt or occult lymphoma (283,284).

The interpretation of these results remains speculative. CLL and PDL lymphocytes are somewhat analogous to fetal lymphocytes in their surface Ig characteristics. It is therefore conceivable that the neoplastic transformation of these cells results in an induced oncofetal state of immune differentiation of the malignant lymphocytic clone (277). Further, the marked increase in frequency of appearance of IgD on poorly differentiated neoplastic lymphocytes suggests that IgD may indeed represent the first Ig produced by the lymphocyte and that this Ig class may play a key role in the ontogenetic development of the lymphoid clone. The association of IgD with IgM on individual lymphocytes has led to speculation that IgD, rather than IgM, might represent the earliest Ig class in the phylogenetic development of the immunoglobulin proteins. The role of the IgD class in both the ontogeny and phylogeny of immunoglobulins should be further defined in the near future.

VIII. β_2-MICROGLOBULIN (β_2m)

A. General Properties

This is a protein of molecular weight 11,600, which is related structurally to the immunoglobulins but whose biological function is still unknown. It was discovered in 1968 by Berggard and Bearn who isolated it from the urine of patients with kidney disorders (285). It is found in the serum, urine, cerebrospinal fluid, saliva, and colostrum of normal individuals. Its concentration is increased in the urine of persons with disorders of the renal tubules, associated with a reduced glomerular filtration rate; this greatly facilitates its isolation. Patients with renal disorders studied by Berggard and Bearn had 3–89 mg in a 24-hour urine sample. Some individuals with cancer or autoimmune diseases have elevated levels of β_2m (286).

The protein was found on the outer membranes of circulating leukocytes (287–290). It can be solubilized from cells by sonication, acidification, or treatment with sodium deoxycholate. Platelets, mononuclear cells, and polymorphonuclear cells were reported to contain, on the average, about 0.5×10^5, 18×10^5, and 7×10^5 molecules per cell, respectively (291). None was found in erythrocytes. A substantial fraction of the total β_2m of lymphocytes or platelets is present on cell membranes (289,291).

Bernier and Fanger observed that β_2m is synthesized by lymphocytes in culture, particularly when stimulated by phytohemagglutinin or by Concanavalin A. The absence of stimulation by pokeweed mitogen suggested that the T cell might be the major lymphocyte source. This conjecture was supported by the observation that cells with surface immunoglobulin (B cells) absorb less fluorescent anti-β_2m than those without surface immunoglobulin (T cells) (290,292). Nevertheless, β_2m is present on B as well as T lymphocytes (293), including B cells in established cultures, and on platelets and polymorphonuclear cells as well (291–294). The protein is also synthesized by cultures of nonlymphoid cells, including glial fibroblasts, gliomas, adult skin fibroblasts, kidney epithelium, and various carcinomas and sarcomas (287,295,296). The observation that nonlymphoid cells synthesize β_2m suggests that the protein may have functions unrelated to those of the immunoglobulins.

Although $\beta_2 m$ and immunoglobulin coexist on the B cell membrane they are independent of one another. Anti-immunoglobulin antibodies cause the "modulation"[5] of immunoglobulin surface antigens but not of $\beta_2 m$; conversely, antibodies to $\beta_2 m$ did not affect the expression of immunoglobulin antigens on the cell surface (295).

$\beta_2 m$ is about the size of a typical immunoglobulin domain, has the characteristic intrachain disulfide loop (encompassing 57 residues), and shows substantial homology of sequence with individual domains of human L and H chains. The closest homology (about 28%) is with the $C_H 3$ domain of the γ chain. No antigenic cross-reactivity has, however, been detected between $\beta_2 m$ and immunoglobulins. The complete sequence of human $\beta_2 m$ is shown in Fig. 4.17. The protein comprises 100 amino acid residues and is devoid of carbohydrate.

A homologous protein has been isolated from the urine of dogs used in kidney transplantation experiments (297). The sequence of the N-terminal 42 residues was determined and found to be identical to that of the human protein at 35 or 36 positions. Nevertheless, antigenic cross-reactivity was not observed. Rabbit antibodies were used; antibodies from a nonmammalian species are generally more discriminatory in this type of comparison. Since $\beta_2 m$ was also detected in chimpanzee serum (297), it may be anticipated that the homolog of $\beta_2 m$ will be found in many mammalian species.

B. Association of $\beta_2 m$ with Other Components of the Lymphocyte Surface

Although the biological role of $\beta_2 m$ is still unclear, there is evidence suggesting that it may somehow be involved in the recognition processes of lymphocytes. This possibility is especially provocative in view of the structural relationship of $\beta_2 m$ to the immunoglobulins. (There is no suggestion that $\beta_2 m$ itself is a primary recognition unit since its structure seems to be invariant.) Bach *et al.* showed that two T cell functions are blocked by antibodies to $\beta_2 m$: the mixed lymphocyte reaction of human lymphocytes to allogenic, mitomycin-treated lymphocytes and the proliferative response to phytohemagglutinin (298). Both responses were quantitated by measuring uptake of tritiated thymidine in cell cultures. Treatment of one cell population with mitomycin ensures that the other is the responding population. The anti-$\beta_2 m$ necessarily acted on the responding cells in the case of PHA stimulation and presumably did so in

---

[5] Disappearance of antigen from the surface, generally because of aggregation, followed by endocytosis.

the mixed lymphocyte reaction. The authors proposed that β_2m is a component of a recognition unit on the cell surface.

There is evidence for a close molecular association between β_2m and HL-A antigens on the lymphocyte membrane. Studies using immunofluorescence showed that anti-β_2m induces aggregation of β_2m molecules on the cell surface, producing a cap. HL-A antigens were found in the same cap, suggesting that the β_2m and HL-A antigens are joined to one another (299). After the loss of both antigens from the cell surface which follows capping with anti-β_2m, HL-A and β_2m reappeared on the surface at about the same rate. Poulik et al. suggest that the binding of β_2m to HL-A antigens may tend, somehow, to stabilize the association of HL-A antigens with the cell surface. Antibodies to HL-A antigen cause capping of some but not all of the β_2m on the cell surface (300).

When HL-A antigens are isolated from lymphocytes they are found to comprise one unit of molecular weight 30,000–33,000 and another of molecular weight 11,000–12,000 (301–303). Nakamura et al. first proposed, on the basis of amino acid composition, size, and distribution in tissues, that the smaller subunit is β_2m (302). This was confirmed by the antigenic analyses of Peterson et al. (303) who showed also that free HL-A antigens are capable of binding β_2m isolated from urine.

High salt concentration, low pH, or the presence of detergent or concentrated urea suffices to separate HL-A from β_2m. There is no apparent antigenic relationship between the two proteins. The precise role of the invariant β_2m subunit, in its association with the variety of HL-A antigens, remains to be elucidated.

IX. RHEUMATOID FACTORS[6]

The sera of most patients with rheumatoid arthritis contain an IgM antibody (19 or 7 S) reactive with the IgG of the patient and of other individuals. Such antiglobulins are found also in other chronic inflammatory disorders and in the sera of certain normal individuals; the incidence in normal persons increases with age. They frequently are found in the sera of normal relatives of rheumatoid patients. These antiglobulins, termed rheumatoid factors (RF), may also be of the IgG or IgA class. RF of the IgM class frequently circulates in the patient's serum in the form of a 22 S complex made up of the RF and several

[6] For discussions of monoclonal rheumatoid factors, cryoglobulins, and cold agglutinins, see Chapter 11.

bound molecules of IgG (304); complexes are also found in synovial fluid and may be responsible entirely or in part for the synovitis associated with rhematoid arthritis. The complexes dissociate in acid solution, permitting isolation of the RF by gel filtration. Most RF's are capable of cross-reacting with IgG of various other mammalian species. Actually, the presence of RF in the sera of rheumatoid patients was first recognized by Waaler (305) on the basis of the capacity of the serum to agglutinate sheep red blood cells sensitized with rabbit antibody.

Possible beneficial effects of RF are conjectural. Goldberg and Fudenberg (306) speculate that RF may play a role in clearing immune complexes from the serum. There are conflicting data on this point since RF can inhibit phagocytosis of certain antibody–bacterial complexes, presumably by combining with opsonic IgG and preventing its attachment to phagocytes (307). RF does, however, have the capacity to bind to certain soluble antigen–antibody complexes and to cause their precipitation (308). It can also combine with infectious complexes of herpes simplex virus with its human antibodies; subsequent treatment of the RF–antibody–virus complex with complement or with anti-IgM results in loss of infectivity of the virus (309). It is nevertheless possible that RF's, which are products of an autoimmune process, are of little beneficial value to the host.

Very often, RF precipitates more strongly with denatured or aggregated IgG than with native IgG. Normansell and Stanworth (310,311) have found, however, that the affinity of a rheumatoid factor for aggregated IgG is no greater than its affinity for the IgG monomer. The enhanced precipitability, then, is probably attributable to the increased antigenic valence of the aggregated IgG. An alternative possibility, that has frequently been advanced but not proved, is that new antigenic determinants, reactive with RF, are exposed upon denaturation or aggregation of IgG (312). Actually, the two alternative explanations could be applicable to different RF-containing sera.

Monomeric IgG is frequently a poor inhibitor of the aggregation by RF of red cells coated with aggregated IgG. This again, could be due either to the exposure of new determinants, reactive with RF, upon aggregation of IgG or to multivalent attachment of single IgM molecules to aggregates of IgG on the red cell surface; multivalent attachment is associated with high avidity.

There exist both heterogeneous and monoclonal rheumatoid factors. Most patients with rheumatoid arthritis possess heterogeneous antiglobulins, although monoclonal factors sometimes appear after prolonged illness. A substantial number of monoclonal proteins with anti-IgG activity have, however, been found in the sera of patients with

Waldenström's disease; these are often referred to as rheumatoid factors despite the absence of symptoms of rheumatoid arthritis.

RF generally, although not always, reacts with the Fc portion of IgG. A given RF may react with from one to four of the human IgG subclasses (313); however, certain patterns of specificity may recur. For example, a number of RF's have been found to react with IgG1, IgG2, and IgG4, but not with IgG3 (24). The isotypic antigenic determinant, designated Ga, present in the C_H2 domain of IgG1, IgG2, and IgG4 accounts, in many instances, for such specificity (24,39,314). An RF may also react with L chains, for example, with an Inv allotypic determinant (315), with allotypic determinants on the Fc or Fd portion of the H chain, or with "nonmarkers," which are allotypic markers in one subclass of human IgG and isotypic determinants in other subclasses (24,316). Many sera used for identification of human Gm allotypes are from patients with rheumatoid arthritis. An occasional RF may react more strongly with IgG from a nonhuman species, such as the rabbit, than with human IgG. This is particularly apt to be true of monoclonal rheumatoid factors (313,317).

One standard test for RF uses polystyrene latex particles coated with human IgG. The relative concentration of RF in an unknown serum is estimated from the maximum dilution at which it is still capable of aggregating the coated particles. Alternatively, rheumatoid factor can be estimated through its ability to agglutinate sheep erythrocytes sensitized with a subagglutinating dose of rabbit antisheep erythrocyte antibody. A variety of related procedures has been utilized in various laboratories.

REFERENCES

1. Edelman, G.M. (1959). *J. Amer. Chem. Soc.* **81**, 3155.
2. Edelman, G.M. and Poulik, M.D. (1961). *J. Exp. Med.* **113**, 861.
3. Fleischman, J.B., Pain, R.H., and Porter, R.R. (1962). *Arch. Biochem. Biophys. Suppl.* **1**, 174.
4. Fleischman, J.B., Porter, R.R., and Press, E.M. (1963). *Biochem. J.* **88**, 220.
5. Pain, R.H. (1963). *Biochem. J.* **88**, 234.
6. Edelman, G.M. and Gally, J.A. (1962). *J. Exp. Med.* **116**, 207.
7. Bence Jones, H. (1847). *Phil. Trans. Roy. Soc. London* **138**, 55.
8. Milstein, C. (1966). *Biochem. J.* **101**, 338.
9. Deutsch, H. and Morton, J.I. (1958). *J. Biol. Chem.* **231**, 1107.
10. Miller, F. and Metzger, H. (1965). *J. Biol. Chem.* **240**, 4740.
11. Vaerman, J.P., Fudenberg, H.H., Vaerman, C., and Mandy, W.J. (1965). *Immunochemistry* **2**, 263.

12. Korngold, L. and Lipari, R. (1956). *Cancer* **9,** 262.
13. Mannik, M. and Kunkel, H.G. (1962). *J. Exp. Med.* **116,** 859.
14. Franklin, E.C. (1962). *Nature (London)* **195,** 393.
15. Migita, S. and Putnam, F.W. (1963). *J. Exp. Med.* **117,** 81.
16. Fahey, J.L. and Solomon, A. (1963). *J. Clin. Invest.* **42,** 811.
17. Mannik, M. and Kunkel, H.G. (1963). *J. Exp. Med.* **117,** 213.
18. Korngold, L. (1963). *Int. Arch. Allergy Appl. Immunol.* **23,** 9.
19. Fahey, J.L. (1963). *J. Immunol.* **91,** 438.
20. Fahey, J.L. (1963). *J. Immunol.* **91,** 448.
21. Fahey, J.L., Carbone, P.P., Rowe, D.S., and Bachmann, R. (1968). *Amer. J. Med.* **45,** 373.
22. Hobbs, J.R. and Corbett, A.A. (1969). *Brit. Med. J.* **1,** 412.
23. Fishkin, B.G., Glassy, F.J., Hattersley, P.G., Hirose, F.M., and Spiegelberg, H.L. (1970). *Amer. J. Clin. Pathol.* **53,** 209.
24. Natvig, J.B. and Kunkel, H.G. (1973). *Advan. Immunol.* **16,** 1.
25. Capra, J.D. (1974). Personal communication.
26. Ein, D. and Fahey, J.L. (1967). *Science* **156,** 947.
27. Appella, E. and Ein, D. (1967). *Proc. Nat. Acad. Sci. U.S.* **57,** 1449.
28. Ponstingl, H., Hess, M., Langer, B., Steinmetz-Kayne, M., and Hilschmann, N. (1967). *Hoppe Seyler's Z. Physiol. Chem.* **348,** 1213.
29. Hess, M., Hilschmann, N., Rivat, L., Rivat, C., and Ropartz, C. (1971). *Nature New Biol.* **234,** 58.
30. Ein, D. (1968). *Proc. Nat. Acad. Sci. U.S.* **60,** 982.
31. Gibson, D., Levanson, M., and Smithies, O. (1971). *Biochemistry* **10,** 3114.
32. Cohen, S. and Gordon, S. (1965). *Biochem. J.* **97,** 460.
33. Yount, W.J., Hong, R., Seligmann, M., Good, R., and Kunkel, H.G. (1970). *J. Clin. Invest.* **49,** 1957.
34. Schur, P.H. (1972). *In* "Progress in Clinical Immunology" (R. Schwartz, ed.), Vol. I. Grune & Stratton, New York.
35. Grey, H.M. and Kunkel, H.G. (1964). *J. Exp. Med.* **120,** 253.
36. Terry, W.D. and Fahey, J.L. (1964). *Science* **146,** 400.
37. Ballieux, R.E., Bernier, G.N., Tominaga, K., and Putnam, F.W. (1964). *Science* **145,** 168.
38. Franklin, E.C. and Frangione, B. (1969). *Annu. Rev. Med.* **20,** 155.
39. Allen, J.C. and Kunkel, H.G. (1966). *Arthritis Rheum.* **9,** 758.
40. Gaarder, P.I. and Natvig, J.B. (1970). *J. Immunol.* **105,** 928.
41. Frangione, B., Milstein, C., and Franklin, E.C. (1969). *Nature (London)* **221,** 149.
42. Milstein, C. (1965). *Nature (London)* **205,** 1171.
43. Steiner, L.A. and Porter, R.R. (1967). *Biochemistry* **6,** 3957.
44. Edelman, G.M., Cunningham, B.A., Gall, E.W., Gottlieb, P.D., Rutishauser, U., and Waxdal, M. (1969). *Proc. Nat. Acad. Sci. U.S.* **63,** 78.
45. Frangione, B. and Milstein, C. (1967). *Nature (London)* **216,** 939.
46. Milstein, C. (1969). *Nature (London)* **221,** 145.
47. Milstein, C. and Pink, J.R.L. (1970). *Progr. Biophys. Mol. Biol.* **21,** 209.
48. Smyth, D.S. and Utsumi, S. (1967). *Nature (London)* **216,** 332.
49. Pink, R., Wang, A-C., and Fudenberg, H.H. (1971). *Annu. Rev. Med.* **22,** 145.
50. Pink, J.R.L. and Milstein, C. (1967). *Nature (London)* **216,** 941.
51. Frangione, B. and Milstein, C. (1968). *J. Mol. Biol.* **33,** 893.
52. Milstein, C. and Frangione, B. (1971). *Biochem. J.* **121,** 217.
53. Michaelsen, T.E. (1973). *Scand. J. Immunol.* **2,** 523.

54. Saluk, P.H. and Clem, L.W. (1971). *J. Immunol.* **107**, 298.
55. Damacco, F., Michaelsen, T.E., and Natvig, J.B. (1972). *FEBS Lett.* **28**, 121.
56. Edelman, G.M., Heremans, J.F., Heremans, M.-Th., and Kunkel, H.G. (1960). *J. Exp. Med.* **112**, 203.
57. Hershgold, E.J., Cordoba, F., Charache, P., and Gitlin, D. (1963). *Nature (London)* **199**, 284.
58. Humphrey, R.L. (1967). *J. Mol. Biol.* **29**, 525.
59. Gergely, J., Medgyesi, G.A., and Stanworth, D.R. (1967). *Immunochemistry* **4**, 365.
60. Kunkel, H.G. and Grey, H.M. (1967). *Biochemistry* **6**, 2326.
61. Turner, M.W., Bennich, H.H., and Natvig, J.B. (1970). *Clin. Exp. Immunol.* **7**, 603.
62. Jeffries, R., Weston, P.D., Stanworth, D.R., and Clamp, T.R. (1968). *Nature (London)* **219**, 646.
63. Gergely, J., Fudenberg, H.H., and von Loghem, E. (1970). *Immunochemistry* **7**, 1.
64. Wang, A-C. and Fudenberg, H.H. (1972). *Nature New Biol.* **240**, 24.
65. Virella, G. and Parkhouse, R.M.E. (1971). *Immunochemistry* **8**, 251.
66. Michaelsen, T.E. and Natvig, J.B. (1973). *Scand. J. Immunol.* **2**, 299.
67. Michaelsen, T.E. and Natvig, J.B. (1972). *Scand. J. Immunol.* **1**, 255.
68. Nelson, C.A. (1964). *J. Biol. Chem.* **239**, 3727.
69. Goodman, J.W. (1965). *Biochemistry* **4**, 2350.
70. Turner, M.W., Bennich, H.H., and Natvig, J.B. (1970). *Clin. Exp. Immunol.* **7**, 627.
71. Heimer, R., Schnoll, S.S., and Primack, A. (1967). *Biochemistry* **6**, 127.
72. Turner, M.W. and Bennich, H. (1968). *Biochem. J.* **107**, 71.
73. Turner, M.W., Komvopoulos, A., Bennich, H., and Natvig, J.B. (1972). *Scand. J. Immunol.* **1**, 53.
74. Utsumi, S. and Karush, F. (1965). *Biochemistry* **4**, 1766.
75. Poulik, M.D. (1966). *Nature (London)* **210**, 133.
76. Grey, H.M. and Abel, C.A. (1967). *Immunochemistry* **4**, 315.
77. Frangione, B., Milstein, C., and Franklin, E.C. (1968). *Biochem. J.* **106**, 15.
78. Iramajiri, S., Franklin, E.C., and Frangione, B. (1968). *Immunochemistry* **5**, 383.
79. Iramajiri, S., Franklin, E.C., and Woods, K.R. (1968). *Nature (London)* **220**, 612.
80. Natvig, J.B. and Turner, M.W. (1971). *Clin. Exp. Immunol.* **8**, 685.
81. Utsumi, S. (1969). *Biochem. J.* **112**, 343.
82. Ishizaka, T., Ishizaka, K., Salmon, S., and Fudenberg, H.H. (1967). *J. Immunol.* **99**, 82.
83. Augener, W., Grey, H.M., Cooper, N.R., and Müller-Eberhard, H.J. (1971). *Immunochemistry* **8**, 1011.
84. Sorkin, E. (1964). *Int. Arch. Allergy Appl. Immunol.* **25**, 129.
85. Huber, H. and Fudenberg, H.H. (1968). *Int. Arch. Allergy Appl. Immunol.* **34**, 18.
86. Abramson, N., Gelfand, E.W., Jandl, J.H., and Rosen, F.S. (1970). *J. Exp. Med.* **132**, 1207.
87. Huber, H., Douglas, S.O., Nubacher, J., Kochwa, S., and Rosenfeld, R.E. (1971). *Nature (London)* **229**, 419.
88. Hay, F.C., Torrigiani, G., and Roitt, I.M. (1972). *Eur. J. Immunol.* **2**, 257.
89. Inchley, E., Grey, H.M., and Uhr, J.W. (1970). *J. Immunol.* **105**, 362.
90. LoBuglio, A.F., Cotran, R.S., and Jandl, J.H. (1967). *Science* **158**, 1582.
91. Wistoff, F., Michaelsen, T.E., and Froland, S.S. (1974). *Scand. J. Immunol.* **3**, 29.
92. Edelman, G.M. and Gall, W.E. (1969). *Annu. Rev. Biochem.* **38**, 415.
93. Edelman, G.M. (1970). *Biochemistry* **9**, 3197.
93a. Connell, G.E. and Porter, R.R. (1971). *Biochem J.* **124**, 53P.
94. Kehoe, J.M. and Fougerau, M. (1969). *Nature (London)* **224**, 1212.

95. Ellerson, J.R., Yasmeen, D., Painter, R.H., and Dorrington, K.J. (1972). *FEBS Lett.* **24**, 318.
96. Yasmeen, D., Ellerson, J.R., Dorrington, K.J., and Painter, R.H. (1973). *J. Immunol.* **110**, 1706.
97. Natvig, J.B., Munthe, E., and Gaarder, P.C. (1971). *In* "Rheumatoid Arthritis" (W. Muller, H.G. Haerwerth, and K. Fehr, eds.), p. 343. Academic Press, New York.
98. Morell, A., Terry, W.D., and Waldmann, T.A. (1970). *J. Clin. Invest.* **49**, 673.
99. Spiegelberg, H.L., Fishkin, B.G., and Grey, H.M. (1968). *J. Clin. Invest.* **47**, 2323.
100. Capra, J.D. and Kunkel, H.G. (1970). *J. Clin. Invest.* **49**, 610.
101. Froland, S.S. and Natvig, J.B. (1972). *Scand. J. Immunol.* **1**, 1.
102. Miller, F. and Metzger, H. (1965). *J. Biol. Chem.* **240**, 3325.
103. Lamm, M. and Small, P.A., Jr. (1966). *Biochemistry* **5**, 287.
104. Metzger, H. (1970). *Advan. Immunol.* **12**, 57.
105. Mestecky, J., Zikan, J., and Butler, W.T. (1971). *Science* **171**, 1163.
106. Chapuis, R.M. and Koshland, M.E. (1974). *Proc. Nat. Acad. Sci. U.S.* **71**, 657.
106a. Feinstein, A., Munn, E.A., and Richardson, N.E. (1971). *Ann. N.Y. Acad. Sci.* **190**, 104.
107. Watanabe, S., Barnikol, H.U., Horn, J., Bertram, J., and Hilschmann, N. (1973). *Hoppe Seyler's Z. Physiol. Chem.* **354**, 1505.
108. Putnam, F.W., Florent, G., Paul, C., Shinoda, T., and Shimizu, A. (1973). *Science* **182**, 287.
109. Putnam, F.W., Shinoda, T., Shimizu, A., Paul, C., Florent, G., and Raff, E. (1973). *Specific Receptors of Antibodies and Antigens, 3rd Int. Convoc. Immunol.*, p. 40. Karger, Basel.
110. Hurst, M.M., Niedermeier, W., Zikan, J., and Bennett, J.C. (1973). *J. Immunol.* **110**, 840.
111. Mestecky, J., Schrohenloher, R.E., and Kulhavy, R. (1974). *Fed. Proc. Fed. Amer. Soc. Exp. Biol.* **33**, 747.
112. Inman, F.P. and Ricardo, M.J. (1974). *J. Immunol.* **112**, 229.
113. Kabat, E.A. (1939). *J. Exp. Med.* **69**, 103.
114. Carbonara, A.D. and Heremans, J.F. (1963). *Arch. Biochem. Biophys.* **102**, 137.
115. Cohen, S. (1963). *Biochem. J.* **89**, 334.
116. Morris, J.E. and Inman, F.P. (1968). *Biochemistry* **7**, 2851.
117. Frank, M.M. and Humphrey, J.H. (1969). *Immunology* **17**, 237.
118. Solheim, B.G. and Harboe, M. (1972). *Immunochemistry* **9**, 623.
119. Tomasi, T.B., Jr. (1973). *Proc. Nat. Acad. Sci. U.S.* **70**, 3410.
120. Mukkur, T.K.S. and Inman, F.P. (1971). *J. Immunol.* **107**, 705.
121. Parkhouse, R.M.E., Askonas, B.A., and Dourmashkin, R.R. (1970). *Immunology* **18**, 575.
122. Ricardo, M.J., Jr., and Inman, F.P. (1974). *Biochem. J.* **137**, 79.
123. Della Corte, E. and Parkhouse, R.M.E. (1973). *Biochem. J.* **136**, 597.
124. Kownatski, E. and Drescher, M. (1973). *Clin. Exp. Immunol.* **15**, 557.
125. Harboe, M. and Solheim, B.O. (1972). *Scand. J. Immunol.* **1**, 62.
126. Miller, F. and Metzger, H. (1966). *J. Biol. Chem.* **241**, 1732.
127. Stone, M.J. and Metzger, H. (1968). *J. Biol. Chem.* **243**, 5977.
128. Mihaesco, C. and Seligmann, M. (1968). *J. Exp. Med.* **127**, 431.
129. Onoue, K., Kishimoto, T., and Yamamura, Y. (1968). *J. Immunol.* **100**, 238.
130. Onoue, K., Kishimoto, T., and Yamamura, Y. (1967). *J. Immunol.* **98**, 303.
131. Plaut, A.G. and Tomasi, T.B., Jr. (1970). *Proc. Nat. Acad. Sci. U.S.* **65**, 318.
132. Zikan, J. and Bennett, J.C. (1973). *Eur. J. Immunol.* **3**, 415.

133. Killander, J. (1963). *Acta Soc. Med. Upsal.* **68**, 230.
134. Hunter, A., Feinstein, A., and Coombs, R.R.A. (1968). *Immunology* **15**, 381.
135. Solomon, A. (1969). *J. Immunol.* **102**, 496.
136. Rothfield, N.E., Frangione, B., Franklin, E.C., Stobo, J.P., and Tomasi, T.B., Jr. (1967). *J. Clin. Invest.* **46**, 1329.
137. Solomon, A. and Kunkel, H.G. (1967). *Amer. J. Med.* **42**, 958.
138. Solomon, A. (1967). *Fed. Proc. Fed. Amer. Soc. Exp. Biol.* **26**, 529.
139. Onoue, K., Grossberg, A.L., Yagi, Y., and Pressman, D. (1968). *Science* **162**, 574.
140. Stone, M.J. and Metzger, H. (1968). *J. Biol. Chem.* **243**, 5049.
141. Merler, E., Karlin, L., and Matsumoto, S. (1968). *J. Biol. Chem.* **243**, 386.
142. Makela, O., Ruoslahti, E., and Seppälä, I. (1970). *Immunochemistry* **7**, 917.
143. Edberg, S.C., Bronson, P.M., and Van Oss, C.J. (1972). *Immunochemistry* **9**, 273.
144. Tomasi, T.B., Jr., and Grey, H.M. (1972). *Progr. Allergy* **16**, 81.
145. Vaerman, J.P. (1973). *In* "Research in Immunochemistry and Immunobiology" (J.B.G. Kwapinski and E.D. Day, eds.), Vol. 3, p. 91. Univ. Park Press, Baltimore, Maryland.
146. Grabar, P. and Williams, C.A., Jr. (1953). *Biochem. Biophys. Acta* **10**, 193.
147. Slater, R.S., Ward, S.M., and Kunkel, H.G. (1955). *J. Exp. Med.* **85**, 101.
148. Heremans, J.F., Heremans, M.-Th., and Schultze, H.E. (1959). *Clin. Chem. Acta* **4**, 96.
149. Kunkel, H.G. and Prendergast, R.A. (1966). *Proc. Soc. Exp. Biol. Med.* **122**, 910.
150. Feinstein, D. and Franklin, E.C. (1966). *Nature (London)* **212**, 1496.
151. Vaerman, J.P. and Heremans, J.F. (1966). *Science* **153**, 647.
152. Grey, H.M., Abel, C.A., Yount, W.J., and Kunkel, H.G. (1968). *J. Exp. Med.* **128**, 1223.
153. Vaerman, J.P., Heremans, J.F., and Laurell, C.B. (1968). *Immunology* **14**, 425.
154. Montgomery, P.C., Dorrington, K.J., and Rockey, J.H. (1969). *Biochemistry* **8**, 1427.
155. Dorrington, K.J. and Rockey, J.H. (1970). *Biochim. Biophys. Acta* **200**, 584.
156. Abel, C.A. and Grey, H.M. (1971). *Nature New Biol.* **233**, 29.
157. Despont, J-P.J. and Abel, C.A. (1974). *J. Immunol.* **112**, 1623.
158. Frangione, B. and Wolfenstein-Todel, C. (1972). *Proc. Nat. Acad. Sci. U.S.* **12**, 3673.
159. Zimmerman, B. and Grey, H.M. (1971). *Fed. Proc. Fed. Amer. Soc. Exp. Biol.* **30**, 594.
160. Bernier, G.M., Tominaga, K., Easley, C.W., and Putnam, F.W. (1965). *Biochemistry* **4**, 2072.
161. Ballieux, R.E., Stoop, J.W., and Zegers, B.J.M. (1968). *Scand. J. Hematol.* **5**, 179.
162. Chodirker, W.B. and Tomasi, T.B., Jr. (1963). *Science* **142**, 1080.
163. Tomasi, T.B., Jr., Tan, E.M., Solomon, A., and Prendergast, R.A. (1965). *J. Exp. Med.* **121**, 101.
164. Newcomb, R.W., Normansell, D., and Stanworth, D.R. (1968). *J. Immunol.* **101**, 905.
165. Tomasi, T.B., Jr. and Calvanico, N. (1968). *Fed. Proc. Fed. Amer. Soc. Exp. Biol.* **27**, 617.
166. Hurlimann, T., Waldesbuhl, M., and Zuber, C. (1969). *Biochim. Biophys. Acta* **181**, 393.
167. Cebra, J.J. and Small, P.A. (1967). *Biochemistry* **6**, 503.
168. Mestecky, J., Schrohenloher, R.E., Kulhavy, R., Wright, G.P., and Tomana, M. (1974). *Proc. Nat. Acad. Sci. U.S.* **71**, 544.
169. Brandtzaeg, P. (1971). *J. Immunol.* **106**, 318.

170. Thompson, R.A. and Asquith, P. (1970). *Clin. Exp. Immunol.* **7**, 419.
171. Waldman, R.H., Mach, J.-P., Stella, M.M., and Rowe, D.S. (1970). *J. Immunol.* **105**, 43.
172. South, M.A., Cooper, M.D., Wolheim, F.A., Hong, R., and Good, R.A. (1966). *J. Exp. Med.* **123**, 615.
173. Hong, R., Pollara, B., and Good, R.A. (1966). *Proc. Nat. Acad. Sci. U.S.* **56**, 602.
174. Tomasi, T.B., Jr., and Bienenstock, J. (1968). *Advan. Immunol.* **9**, 1.
175. Mach, J.-P. (1970). *Nature (London)* **228**, 1278.
176. Cunningham-Rundles, C., Lamm, M.E., and Franklin, E.C. (1974). *Fed. Proc. Fed. Amer. Soc. Exp. Biol.* **33**, 747.
177. Thompson, R.A. (1970). *Nature (London)* **226**, 946.
178. Jerry, L.M., Kunkel, H.G., and Adams, L. (1972). *J. Immunol.* **109**, 275.
179. Bienenstock, J., Percy, B.Y.E., Gauldie, J., and Underdown, B.J. (1972). *J. Immunol.* **109**, 403.
180. Halpern, M.S. and Koshland, M.E. (1970). *Nature (London)* **228**, 1276.
181. Morrison, S.L. and Koshland, M.E. (1972). *Proc. Nat. Acad. Sci. U.S.* **69**, 124.
182. Klaus, G.B., Halpern, M.S., Koshland, M.E., and Goodman, J.W. (1971). *J. Immunol.* **107**, 1785.
183. O'Daly, J.A. and Cebra, J.J. (1971). *Biochemistry* **10**, 3843.
184. Wilde, C.E., III and Koshland, M.E. (1973). *Biochemistry* **12**, 3218.
185. Schrohenloher, R.E., Mestecky, J., and Stanton, T.H. (1973). *Biochim. Biophys. Acta* **295**, 576.
186. Meinke, G. and Spiegelberg, H.L. (1971). *Fed. Proc. Fed. Amer. Soc. Exp. Biol.* **30**, 468.
187. Mestecky, J., Kulhavy, R., and Kraus, F.W. (1971). *Fed. Proc. Fed. Amer. Soc. Exp. Biol.* **30**, 468.
188. Halpern, M.S. and Coffman, R.L. (1972). *J. Immunol.* **109**, 674.
189. Parkhouse, R.M.E. (1972). *Nature New Biol.* **236**, 9.
190. Della Corte, E. and Parkhouse, R.M.E. (1973). *Biochem. J.* **136**, 589.
191. Halpern, M.S. and Koshland, M.E. (1973). *J. Immunol.* **111**, 1653.
192. Kang, Y.S., Calvanico, N.J., and Tomasi, T.B., Jr. (1974). *J. Immunol.* **112**, 162.
193. Meinke, G. and Spiegelberg, H.L. (1972). *J. Immunol.* **109**, 903.
194. Tourville, D., Adler, R., Bienenstock, J., and Tomasi, T.B., Jr. (1969). *J. Exp. Med.* **129**, 411.
195. Heremans, J.F. and Vaerman, J.P. (1971). *Progr. Immunol. Proc. 1st Int. Congr. Immunol.*, p. 695. Academic Press, New York.
196. Roger, M.E. and Lamm, M.E. (1974). *J. Exp. Med.* **139**, 629.
197. Lawton, A.R., Asofsky, R., and Mage, R.G. (1970). *J. Immunol.* **104**, 397.
198. Brown, W.R., Newcomb, R.W., and Ishizaka, K. (1970). *J. Clin. Invest.* **49**, 1374.
199. Wilson, I.D. and Williams, R.C. (1969). *J. Clin. Invest.* **45**, 321.
200. Shuster, J. (1971). *Immunochemistry* **8**, 405.
201. Underdown, B.J. and Dorrington, K.J. (1974). *J. Immunol.* **112**, 949.
202. Zohn, B. (1939). *Amer. J. Dis. Child.* **57**, 1067.
203. Davidson, A.G., Baron, B., and Walzer, M. (1947). *J. Allergy* **18**, 359.
204. Gyenes, L. and Sehon, A. (1960). *Can. J. Biochem. Physiol.* **38**, 1249.
205. Ishizaka, K. and Ishizaka, T. (1973). *Specific Receptors of Antibodies, Antigens, and Cells, 3rd Int. Convoc. Immunol.*, p. 69. Karger, Basel.
206. Ishizaka, K. (1973). *In* "The Antigens" (M. Sela, ed.), p. 479. Academic Press, New York.
207. Ishizaka, K. and Ishizaka, T. (1966). *J. Allergy* **37**, 169.

208. Ishizaka, K., Ishizaka, T., and Lee, E. (1966). *J. Allergy* **37**, 336.
209. Ishizaka, K., Ishizaka, T., and Hornbrook, M.M. (1966). *J. Immunol.* **97**, 75.
210. Johansson, S.G.O. and Bennich, H. (1967). *Immunology* **13**, 381.
211. Johansson, S.G.O., Bennich, H., and Wide, L. (1968). *Immunology* **14**, 265.
212. Bennich, H., Ishizaka, K., Ishizaka, T., and Johansson, S.G.O. (1969). *J. Immunol.* **102**, 826.
213. Ogawa, M., Kochwa, S., Smith, C., Ishizaka, K., and McIntyre, O.R. (1969). *New Engl. J. Med.* **281**, 1217.
214. Fishkin, B.G., Orloff, N., Scaduto, L.E., Borucki, D., and Spiegelberg, H.L. (1972). *Blood* **39**, 361.
215. Stefani, D.V. and Mokeeva, R.A. (1972). *Probl. Hematol. Blood Transfus. (USSR)* **6**, 44.
216. Bennich, H. and Johansson, S.G.O. (1971). *Advan. Immunol.* **13**, 1.
217. Kochwa, S., Terry, W.D., Capra, J.D., and Yang, N.L. (1971). *Ann. N.Y. Acad. Sci.* **190**, 49.
218. Mendez, E., Frangione, B., and Kochwa, S. (1973). *FEBS Lett.* **33**, 4.
219. Bennich, H. and Johansson, S.G.O. (1967). *In* "Gamma Globulins" (J. Killander, ed.), p. 199. Wiley (Interscience) New York.
220. Bennich, H., Milstein, C., and Secher, D.C. (1973). *FEBS Lett.* **33**, 49.
221. Johansson, S.G.O. and Bennich, H. (1967). *In* "Gamma Globulins" (J. Killander, ed.), p. 193. Wiley (Interscience), New York.
222. Johansson, S.G.O. (1968). *Int. Arch. Allergy Appl. Immunol.* **34**, 1.
223. Turner, M.W., Johansson, S.G.O., Barrat, T.M., and Bennich, H. (1970). *Int. Arch. Allergy Appl. Immunol.* **37**, 409.
224. Johansson, S.G.O. (1967). *Lancet* **ii**, 951.
225. Berg, T. and Johansson, S.G.O. (1969). *Int. Arch. Allergy Appl. Immunol.* **36**, 219.
226. Arner, B., Berg, B., Bertler, Å., and Johansson, S.G.O. (1971). *Acta Allergol.* **26**, 383.
227. Johansson, S.G.O., Mellbin, T., and Vahlqvist, B. (1968). *Lancet* **i**, 1118.
228. Kojima, S., Yokogawa, M., and Tado, T. (1972). *Amer. J. Trop. Hyg.* **21**, 913.
229. Gurevitch, A.W., Heiner, D.C., and Reisner, R.M. (1973). *Arch. Dermatol.* **107**, 712.
230. Wide, L., Bennich, H., and Johansson, S.G.O. (1967). *Lancet* **ii**, 1105.
231. Foucard, T. (1972). *Int. Arch. Allergy Appl. Immunol.* **42**, 711.
232. Aas, K. and Johansson, S.G.O. (1971). *J. Allergy Clin. Immunol.* **48**, 134.
233. Berg, T., Bennich, H., and Johansson, S.G.O. (1971). *Int. Arch. Allergy Appl. Immunol.* **40**, 770.
234. Zeiss, C.R., Pruzansky, J.J., Paterson, R., and Roberts, M. (1973). *J. Immunol.* **110**, 414.
235. Ishizaka, K., Ishizaka, T., and Hornbrook, M.M. (1967). *J. Immunol.* **98**, 490.
236. Ishizaka, K. and Ishizaka, T. (1968). *J. Immunol.* **100**, 554.
237. Ishizaka, T., Ishizaka, K., Orange, R.P., and Austen, K.F. (1970). *J. Immunol.* **104**, 335.
238. Orange, R.P., Kaliner, M.A., and Austen, K.F. (1971). *In* "Biochemistry of the Acute Allergic Reactions" (K.F. Austen and E. Becker, eds.), p. 189. Blackwell, Oxford.
239. Kay, A.B. and Austen, K.F. (1971). *J. Immunol.* **107**, 899.
240. Stanworth, D.R., Humphrey, J.H., Bennich, H., and Johansson, S.G.O. (1968). *Lancet* **ii**, 17.
241. Ishizaka, K., Tomioka, H., and Ishizaka, T. (1970). *J. Immunol.* **105**, 1459.
242. Ishizaka, K., Ishizaka, T., and Lee, E.H. (1970). *Immunochemistry* **7**, 687.

243. Ishizaka, K., Tomioka, H., and Ishizaka, T. (1971). *J. Immunol.* **106,** 705.
244. Sullivan, A.L., Grimley, P.L., and Metzger, H. (1971). *J. Exp. Med.* **134,** 1403.
245. Ishizaka, K. and Ishizaka, T. (1969). *J. Immunol.* **103,** 588.
246. Ishizaka, T., Ishizaka, K., Bennich, H., and Johansson, S.G.O. (1970). *J. Immunol.* **104,** 854.
247. Ishizaka, T., Sian, C.M., and Ishizaka, K. (1972). *J. Immunol.* **108,** 848.
248. Osler, A.G., Oliveira, B., Shin, H.S., and Sandberg, A.L. (1969). *J. Immunol.* **102,** 269.
249. Sandberg, A.L., Osler, A.G., Shin, H.S., and Oliveira, B. (1970). *J. Immunol.* **104,** 329.
250. Rowe, D.S. and Fahey, J.L. (1965). *J. Exp. Med.* **121,** 171.
251. Rowe, D.S. and Fahey, J.L. (1965). *J. Exp. Med.* **121,** 185.
252. Zawadski, Z.A. and Edwards, G.A. (1967). *Amer. J. Clin. Pathol.* **48,** 418.
253. Klapper, D.G. and Mendenhall, H.W. (1971). *J. Immunol.* **107,** 912.
254. Leslie, G.A. (1973). *Proc. Soc. Exp. Biol. Med.* **144,** 741.
255. Leslie, G.A. and Swate, T.E. (1972). *J. Immunol.* **109,** 47.
256. Rowe, D.S., Crabbe, P.A., and Turner, M.W. (1968). *Clin. Exp. Immunol.* **3,** 477.
257. Rowe, D.S., Hug, K., Faulk, W.P., McCormick, J.N., and Gerber, H. (1973). *Nature New Biol.* **242,** 155.
257a. Spiegelberg, H.L. (1972). *In* "Contemporary Topics in Immunochemistry," (F.P. Inman, ed.), Vol. 1, p. 165. Plenum, New York.
258. Rowe, D.S., Dolder, F., and Weischer, H.D. (1969). *Immunochemistry* **6,** 437.
259. Saha, H., Chowdhury, P., Sambury, S., Behelak, Y., Heiner, D.C., and Rose, B. (1970). *J. Immunol.* **105,** 238.
260. Spiegelberg, H.L., Prahl, J.W., and Grey, H.M. (1970). *Biochemistry* **9,** 2115.
261. Griffiths, R.W. and Gleich, G.J. (1972). *J. Biol. Chem.* **247,** 4543.
262. Leslie, G.A., Clem, L.W., and Rowe, D. (1971). *Immunochemistry* **8,** 565.
263. Palmer, J.L. and Nisonoff, A. (1964). *Biochemistry* **3,** 863.
264. Perry, M.B. and Milstein, C. (1970). *Nature (London)* **228,** 934.
265. Heiner, D.C., Saha, A., and Rose, B. (1968). *Fed. Proc. Fed. Amer. Soc. Exp. Biol.* **27,** 489.
266. Skvaril, F. and Rádl, J. (1967). *Clin. Chim. Acta* **15,** 544.
267. Spengler, G.A., Butler, R., Pflugshaupt, R., Lopez, V., and Barundun, S. (1967). *Schweiz. Med. Wochenschr.* **97,** 170.
268. Henney, C.S., Welscher, H.D., Terry, W.D., and Rowe, D.S. (1969). *Immunochemistry* **6,** 445.
269. Ovary, Z. (1969). *J. Immunol.* **102,** 790.
270. Lawrence, D.A., Spiegelberg, H.L., and Weigle, W.O. (1974). *Fed. Proc. Fed. Amer. Soc. Exp. Biol.* **33,** 801.
271. Van Boxel, J.A., Paul, W.E., Terry, W.D., and Green, I. (1972). *J. Immunol.* **109,** 648.
272. Rowe, D.A., Hug, K., Forni, L., and Pernis, B. (1973). *J. Exp. Med.* **138,** 965.
273. Knapp, W., Bolhuis, R.L.H., Radl, J., and Hijmans, W. (1973). *J. Immunol.* **111,** 1295.
274. Aisenberg, A.C. and Bloch, K.J. (1972). *New Engl. J. Med.* **287,** 272.
275. Piessens, W.F., Schur, P.H., Moloney, W.C., and Churchill, W.H. (1973). *New Engl. J. Med.* **228,** 176.
276. Fu, S.M., Winchester, R.J., and Kunkel, H.G. (1974). *J. Exp. Med.* **139,** 451.
277. Hopper, J.E. (1974). *Clin. Res.* **22,** 394.
278. Papamichail, M., Brown, J.C., and Holbarow, E.J. (1971). *Lancet* **ii,** 850.

279. Grey, H.M., Rabellino, E., and Pirofsky, B. (1971). *J. Clin. Invest.* **50**, 2368.
280. Froland, S.S., Natvig, J.B., and Staven, P. (1972). *Scand. J. Immunol.* **1**, 351.
281. Preud'homme, J.L. and Seligimann, M. (1972). *Blood*, **40**, 777.
282. Van Boxel, J.A., Hardin, J.A., Green, I., and Paul, W.E. (1973). *New Engl. J. Med.* **289**, 823.
283. Anderson, L.G. and Talal, N. (1972). *Clin. Exp. Immunol.* **10**, 199.
284. Cummings, N.A., Schall, G.L., Asofsky, R., Anderson, L.G., and Talal, N. (1971). *Ann. Int. Med.* **75**, 937.
285. Berggard, I. and Bearn, A.G. (1968). *J. Biol. Chem.* **243**, 4095.
286. Evrin, P.E. and Wibell, L. (1973). *Clin. Chim. Acta* **43**, 183.
287. Nilsson, K., Evrin, P.E., Berggard, I., and Ponten, J. (1973). *Nature New Biol.* **244**, 44.
288. Poulik, M.D. and Motwani, N. (1972). *Clin. Res.* **20**, 795.
289. Peterson, A., Cunningham, B.A., Berggard, I., and Edelman, G.M. (1972). *Proc. Nat. Acad. Sci. U.S.* **69**, 1697.
290. Bernier, G.M. and Fanger, M.W. (1972). *J. Immunol.* **109**, 407.
291. Evrin, P.E. and Pertoft, H. (1973). *J. Immunol.* **111**, 1147.
292. Fanger, M.W. and Bernier, G.M. (1973). *J. Immunol.* **111**, 609.
293. Poulik, M.D., Motwani, N., Nakamura, F., and Bloom, A.D. (1973). *Fed. Proc. Fed. Amer. Soc. Exp. Biol.* **32**, 983.
294. Poulik, M.D. and Bloom, A.D. (1973). *J. Immunol.* **110**, 1430.
295. Hutteroth, T.H., Cleve, H., Litwin, S.D., and Poulik, M.D. (1973). *J. Exp. Med.* **137**, 838.
296. Evrin, P.E. and Nilsson, K. (1974). *J. Immunol.* **112**, 137.
297. Smithies, O. and Poulik, M.D. (1972). *Proc. Nat. Acad. Sci. U.S.* **69**, 2914.
298. Bach, M.L., Huang, S.W., Hong, R., and Poulik, M.D. (1973). *Science* **182**, 1350.
299. Poulik, M.D., Bernocca, M., Bernocca, D., and Ceppellini, R. (1973). *Science* **182**, 1352.
300. Neauport-Sautes, C., Bismuth, A., Kourilsky, F.M., and Manuel, Y. (1974). *J. Exp. Med.* **139**, 957.
301. Creswell, P., Turner, M.J., and Strominger, J.L. (1973). *Proc. Nat. Acad. Sci. U.S.* **70**, 1603.
302. Nakamura, N., Tanigaki, N., and Pressman, D. (1973). *Proc. Nat. Acad. Sci. U.S.* **70**, 2863.
303. Peterson, P.A., Rask, L., and Lindblom, J.B. (1974). *Proc. Nat. Acad. Sci. U.S.* **71**, 35.
304. Franklin, E.C., Müller-Eberhard, H.J., Holman, H., and Kunkel, H.G. (1957). *J. Exp. Med.* **105**, 425.
305. Waaler, E. (1940) *Acta Pathol. Microbiol. Scand.* **17**, 172.
306. Goldberg, L.S. and Fudenberg, H.H. (1971). *Vox. Sang.* **20**, 1.
307. Messner, R.P., Caperton, E.M., Jr., King, R.A., and Williams, R.C., Jr. (1969). *Ann. N.Y. Acad. Sci.* **168**, 93.
308. Edelman, G.M., Kunkel, H.G., and Franklin, E.C. (1958). *J. Exp. Med.* **108**, 105.
309. Ashe, W.K., Daniels, C.A., Scott, G.S., and Notkins, A.L. (1971). *Science* **172**, 176.
310. Normansell, D.E. and Stanworth, D.R. (1968). *Immunology* **15**, 549.
311. Normansell, D.E. (1971). *Immunochemistry* **8**, 593.
312. Kunkel, H.G. and Tan, E.M. (1964). *Advan. Immunol.* **4**, 351.
313. Mackenzie, M.R., Goldberg, L.S., Barnett, E.V., and Fudenberg, H.H. (1968). *Clin. Exp. Immunol.* **3**, 931.

314. Natvig, J.B., Gaarder, P.I., and Turner, M.W. (1972). *Clin. Exp. Immunol.* **12,** 177.
315. Ropartz, C., Rivat, R., and Rousseau, P.Y. (1964). *Proc. 5th Congr. Nat. Transfusion Sanguine,* Montpelier, p. 313.
316. Grubb, R. (1970). "The Genetic Markers of Human Immunoglobulins." Springer-Verlag, New York.
317. Stone, M.J. and Metzger, H. (1969). *J. Immunol.* **102,** 222.

4

Amino Acid Sequences in Human Immunoglobulins and in Mouse Light Chains[1]

I. INTRODUCTION

A large proportion of the available data on amino acid sequences of immunoglobulins relates to human and mouse proteins. This is attributable to the availability of myeloma proteins in both species and to the intrinsic interest in human proteins. Multiple myeloma, which is a relatively rare disease in humans, can be induced in BALB/c or NZB mice by prolonged treatment with mineral oil, certain other hydrocarbons, plastics, or immunological adjuvants. Tumors can be maintained by transplantation into mice of the same inbred strain; this makes it possible to accumulate large amounts of serum or ascites fluid containing a homogeneous myeloma protein. A thorough review of this topic has been written by Potter (1).

Multiple myeloma is frequently accompanied by the presence of a high concentration of homogeneous, urinary L chains (Bence Jones proteins) which correspond in structure to the L chains of the individual's serum myeloma protein. Owing to their high concentration, myeloma or Bence Jones proteins can generally be isolated in reasonably pure form.

[1] In the figures showing amino acid sequences the following conventions are used. A solid line indicates identity of sequence with the prototype (the first sequence listed in the group). A short dash (hyphen) indicates a gap, artificially inserted for the purpose of maximizing homologies in a group of sequences. Empty parentheses indicate that amino acids are present but not determined. Filled parentheses indicate that the composition of the peptide shown within parentheses is known but that its sequence has not been established. Frequently, parentheses are omitted on the basis of a comparison with known sequences in related immunoglobulins.

This, together with their homogeneous character, makes such proteins eminently suitable for physicochemical studies, amino acid sequence analyses, and X-ray crystallography.

In this chapter we will discuss amino acid sequences of human and mouse L chains and of human and rabbit H chains. A few sequences of rabbit L chains are also tabulated. Other partial amino acid sequences are presented in connection with the phylogeny of immunoglobulins (Chapter 7), and allotype-related sequences are discussed in Chapter 9. The amino acid sequences to be discussed here represent only a small fraction of the existing literature but should serve to illustrate principles of immunoglobulin structure.

All the known classes and subclasses of human and mouse immunoglobulins occur as myeloma proteins. In addition, studies are being extended to strains other than BALB/c and NZB through the use of congenic mice, in which the genetic locus controlling C_H regions of another strain is introgressively backcrossed onto a BALB/c background (1). Such congenic mice have most characteristics of the BALB/c strain, and are therefore subject to artificial induction of multiple myeloma, but they synthesize immunoglobulins characteristic of the second strain.

Myeloma proteins are ordinarily isolated by salt fractionation, gel filtration, and either ion-exchange chromatography or zone electrophoresis. H and L chains are obtained from the purified proteins by reduction of interchain disulfide bonds, followed by gel filtration in a solvent which disrupts noncovalent interactions between the chains. Bence Jones proteins are another major source of L chains.

Homogeneous H chain segments can be isolated from the C_H regions of normal immunoglobulins as well as from myeloma proteins; nevertheless most studies of human and mouse H chain sequences have utilized myeloma proteins because of the ease with which they may be obtained in large quantity, and the difficulty of isolating certain classes or subclasses of immunoglobulin from normal serum. Known sequences of rabbit H chains are those of nonspecific immunoglobulins and homogeneous antibody preparations, since multiple myeloma does not occur in that species. Rabbit L chain sequences are based almost entirely on homogeneous antibody preparations.

II. NUMBERING SYSTEM

No general agreement has yet been reached as to the numbering system to be used for immunoglobulin polypeptide chains. Standardization with respect to V region sequences is particularly difficult, because of variations in length among V region subgroups, even for a particular type of polypeptide chain in a single species. We have selected the following proteins as a basis for alignment and numbering: Protein Eu (IgG1; ref. 2)[2] for C_H regions of human IgG and its subclasses and for the C_H region of rabbit IgG. The numbering system used for V_H sequences corresponds to that of protein He (3), except for the insertion of three gaps at positions 86–88 of protein He to permit alignment with other V_H sequences. Proteins Roy (4) and New (5) are used for alignment of human V_κ and V_λ, respectively. No separate system is used for mouse L chains; when they are compared with human L chains the human numbering system is employed.

Having selected a particular numbering system, insertions or deletions are then made in other related sequences in order to maximize homologies. This is done either by placing a gap in the listing of the sequence or, if necessary, by using numbers such as 31a, 31b, etc., in order to permit the best alignment with the prototype sequence (in this case at position 32).[1]

III. AMINO ACID SEQUENCES IN HUMAN L CHAINS

A. General Considerations

In Chapter 3, evidence was cited which indicated that a Bence Jones protein is a homogeneous representative of the heterogeneous normal L chain population (6,7). Because of their homogeneity these proteins are suitable for amino acid sequence analyses; the latter have conclusively shown that Bence Jones proteins are typical, although homogeneous, L chains.

The first detailed studies of amino acid sequences were reported by Hilschmann and Craig (8). These investigators had spent considerable effort in learning how to purify Bence Jones proteins by countercurrent distribution. This, however, proved to be unnecessary. An ammonium sulfate fraction of urine, which contains the Bence Jones protein, finally was used. Although such preparations are not completely pure, methods of peptide analysis can often be successfully applied in the presence of small amounts of contaminants.

An important series of findings was reported by Hilschmann and

[2] Protein Eu was the first immunoglobulin whose complete amino acid sequence was determined.

Craig in their first publication. Studying two Bence Jones proteins of the κ type, they were able to isolate all the peptides of one of these proteins (protein Roy) and to arrange them in their correct order in the sequence. They established the precise location within the sequence of 96 of the total of 212 amino acid residues.

Working with a second Bence Jones protein (designated Cum) they succeeded in isolating 18 of the 21 tryptic peptides expected on the basis of arginine and lysine content. Ten of these peptides had their counterpart in protein Roy; nine were identical and one had a single amino acid replacement. By analyzing a chymotryptic digest they showed that the ten tryptic peptides were in the same order as in protein Roy and occupied the entire sequence from positions 106 to 212, i.e., the C-terminal half of the chain. None of the remaining peptides isolated from protein Cum (N-terminal half) was identical to peptides in Roy, although certain similarities were noted. These findings led them to the conclusion that the N-terminal half of an L chain is variable whereas the C-terminal half, for a given type of L chain, is essentially invariant in sequence. That Bence Jones proteins of the same type (κ or λ) have regions of sequence in common as well as other, nonidentical sequences had been demonstrated earlier by the peptide mapping studies of Putman and Easley (9).

The single amino acid substitution observed at position 191 was shown by this and subsequent work (10–12) to correspond to a difference in allotype between the two κ chains; κ chains of allotype Inv(1) have leucine at position 191 whereas Inv(3) proteins have valine. (See also Chapter 9.)

The concept that the N-terminal half of the protein is variable whereas the C-terminal half is invariant was supported by the studies of Milstein, and of Baglioni *et al.*, who isolated cysteine-containing peptides from a large number of different Bence Jones proteins. All peptides isolated from the C-terminal half were invariant in structure, except for the single substitution noted above. Peptides from the N-terminal portion showed variability of sequence (10–12).

A significant contribution was made by Putnam and collaborators (13,14) who determined the complete amino acid sequence of a third protein of the κ type (protein Ag). Their data conclusively established the presence of variable and invariant linear segments in the chain.

The work of Hilschmann and Craig, together with studies of Milstein (15), also demonstrated that the half-cystine residues at positions 134 and 194 form an intrachain disulfide loop. A second loop is formed by half-cystines at positions 23 and 88. The half-cystine at the C-terminus of the κ chain forms a disulfide bond with an adjoining H chain.

```
                                             VARIABLE REGIONS

L Chain                                                                                  To Cys 88
                                  10                                      20             ↑                        27a  b   c          30
Human κ  Roy    Asp Ile Gln Met Thr Gln Ser Pro Ser Ser Leu Ser Ala Ser Val Gly Asp Arg Val Thr Ile Thr Cys Gln Ala Ser Gln  –   –   –  Asp (Ile Ser) Ile Phe Leu Asn Trp
Mouse κ  M-41   ——————————————————————————————————————————————————————— Leu —— Glu ———— Ser Leu ———— Arg ——————————          Asx —— Gly Ser Leu Ser Asx ——
Human λ  Bo     Glp Ser Ala Leu ———— Pro ——— – ——— Ala ——— Gly ——— Pro ——— Gln Ser ———————— Ser ——— Thr Gly Thr Ser Ser Asp Val Gly Asp Asn Lys Tyr Val Ser ——
Mouse λ  M104E  Glx Ala Val Val ———— Gln Ser  –  Ala ——— Thr Thr ——— Pro ——— Glu Thr Thr Val Leu ———— Arg Ser ——— Thr Gly Ala Val Thr Thr ——— Asn Tyr Ala ————

                         40                                        50                                      60                                    70
Human κ  Roy    Tyr Gln Gln Lys Pro Gly Lys Ala Pro Lys Leu Leu Ile Tyr Asp Ala Ser Lys Leu Glu Ala Gly Val Pro Ser Arg Phe Ser Gly Thr Gly Ser Gly Thr Asp Phe Thr Phe
Mouse κ  M-41   Leu Glx Glx (Asx ———— Glx Thr) Ile ——— Arg ———————— Ala Thr ——— Ser ——— Asx Ser ———————— Lys ——————————— Ser Arg ———— Ser ——— Tyr Ser Leu
Human λ  Bo     ———————— His ———— Arg ——————————— Val ——— Phe Glu Val ——— Gln Arg Pro Ser ———————— Asp ——————————— Ser Lys ——— Asp Asn Thr Ala Ser Leu
Mouse λ  M104E  Val ———— Pro Asp Lys His Leu Phe Thr Gly ——————— Gly Gly Thr Asn Asn Arg Ala Pro ———————— Ala ——————————— Ser Leu Ile ——— Asn Lys Ala Ala Leu

                                                                      To Cys 23
                                         80                           ↑      90                                   100
Human κ  Roy    Thr Ile Ser Ser Leu Gln Pro Glu Asp Ile Ala Thr Tyr Tyr Cys Gln Gln Phe Asp Asn Leu Pro Leu Thr Phe Gly Gly Gly Thr Lys Val Asp Phe Lys Arg
Mouse κ  M-41   ———————————————— Glu Ser ——————— Phe Val Asp ——— X ——— Leu ——— Tyr Ala Ser Ser ——— Trp ————————————————— Leu Glu Ile ————
Human λ  Bo     ——— Val ——— Gly ——— Arg Ala ——————— Glu ——— Asp ———————— Ser Ser Tyr Val Asp Asn Asn Asn  –  ——— Val Phe ——— Gly Gly Thr Lys Leu Thr Val Leu Arg  –
Mouse λ  M104E  ———— Thr Gly Ala ——— Thr ——————— Glu ——— Ile ——— Phe ——— Ala Leu Trp Tyr Ser Asn His Trp Val ————————————————— Leu Thr Val Leu Gly


                                             CONSTANT REGIONS
                                                                                             To Cys 194
                    110                                120                                      130       ↑                                   140
Human κ  Roy    Thr Val  –  Ala Ala Pro Ser Val Phe Ile Phe Pro Pro Ser Asp Glu Gln Leu Lys Ser Gly Thr Ala Ser Val Val Cys Leu Leu Asn Asn Phe Tyr Pro Arg Glu Ala Lys
Mouse κ  M-41   Ala Asx  –  ———————— Thr ——— Ser ———————————————— Ser ———————— Thr Gly ——— Ser ————————————— Phe ———————————————————— Lys Asp Ile Asn
Human λ  Bo     Gln Pro Lys ——— ( ——————————— Thr)(Leu Thr)(Leu ———— Ser Glx Glx ——) (Gln Ala Asn) Lys ——(Thr Leu) ———————— (Ile Ser Asx ——————— Gly) Val/Ala Val Thr
Mouse λ  M104E  Gln Pro Lys Ser Ser ———————— Thr Leu ——————————— Ser ——— Glu ——— Thr Glu Asn Lys ——— Thr Leu ———————— Thr Ile Thr Asp ——————— Gly Val Val Thr

                         150                                       160                                   170                                180
Human κ  Roy    Val Gln Trp Lys Val Asp Asn Ala Leu Gln Ser Gly Asn Ser Gln Glu Ser Val Thr Glu Gln Asp Ser Lys Asp Ser Thr Tyr Ser Leu Ser Ser Thr Leu Thr Leu Ser Lys
Mouse κ  M-41   ——— Lys ———— Ile ——— Gly Ser Glu Arg Gln Asx Gly Val Leu (Asn ——— Trp ——— Asx Glx) ———————————————————————— Met ———————————————— Thr ——
Human λ  Bo     ——— Ala ———— Ala (—— Gly/Ser Ser Pro Val) Lys Ala (Gly Val  –  ——— Thr Thr ——— Pro Ser) Lys Gln Ser Asx Asx Lys/Asn ——(Ala Ala ———— Tyr)(—— Ser ——— Thr Pro
Mouse λ  M104E  ——— Asp ———————————— Gly Thr Pro Val Thr Gln Gly Met  –  ——— Thr Thr Glu Pro Ser Lys Gln Ser Asn Asn Lys ——— Met Ala ———— Tyr ———————— Thr Arg

                                                     To Cys 134                                                          To H Chain
                                   190               ↑                   200                                    210      ↑
Human κ  Roy    Ala Asp Tyr Glu Lys  –  His Lys Leu/Val Tyr Ala Cys Glu Val Thr His Gln Gly Leu Ser Ser Pro Val Thr Lys Ser Phe Asn Arg Gly Glu Cys
Mouse κ  M-41   Asx Glx ——— Glx Arg  –  ——(Asx Ser) ——— Thr ——— Glx (Ala ———— ) Lys Thr (Ser Thr ———— Ile Val) ——————————— Asn ————
Human λ  Bo     Glx Glx Trp  –  ——— Ser ——— Lys/Arg Ser (—— Ser) ——— Gln (——————— Glx ——— Ser Thr  –   –  ——— Glx) ——— Thr (Val Ala Pro Thr ———— Ser)
Mouse λ  M104E  Ala  –  Trp ——— Arg Ser ——— Ser Tyr Ser Ser ——— Gln ———— (—— Glx ——— His Thr)  –   –  ——— Gln ———— Leu Ser ——— Ala Asp ——— Ser
```

Fig. 4.1

Studies of Bence Jones proteins of type λ have established that these polypeptide chains are structured on the same principle as κ chains; the N-terminal half of the chain (106–108 residues) is variable whereas the remainder is essentially invariant (16–19). The human λ chain also has two intrachain loops, corresponding closely in location to those in κ chains, and another half-cystine residue linking the λ chain to an H chain in the intact molecule. In the λ chain, however, this half-cystine residue is the penultimate rather than the C-terminal amino acid.

Figure 4.1 compares the sequences of a typical human κ chain, a human λ, a mouse κ and a mouse λ chain. Striking features of the sequences are the presence of half-cystine residues, forming intrachain loops at homologous positions in each polypeptide chain, and the presence of identical residues at many positions. The C-terminal half-cystine in κ chains and penultimate half-cystine in λ chains are characteristic of the mouse as well as the human proteins. The degree of sequence homology for the various pairs of L chains is summarized in Table 4.1 and will be discussed later.

Polymorphism with respect to sequence has been demonstrated in the constant region of human λ, as well as κ chains. As indicated in Fig. 4.1, two different residues may appear at positions 143 (Val, Ala), 152 (Ser, Gly), 172 (Lys, Asn), and 190 (Arg, Lys) of λ chains. The different forms of λ chain do not appear to be allelic; the variants at positions 152 and 190 have been found in all individuals studied (20–21a). About one-half of the λ chains in a normal human serum have arginine at position 190; the remainder have a lysine residue. These findings indicate that several nonallelic genes control human C_λ regions.

Proteins with lysine at position 190 are designated Oz(+); those with arginine are Oz(−). This substitution can be detected with an antiserum which gives a positive reaction only with Oz(+) Bence Jones proteins (and with normal sera) (20). A rabbit antiserum which recognizes the presence of glycine at position 152 has also been developed; reactive proteins, designated "Kern(+)," comprised 8 of 38 monoclonal λ chains studied (21a).

Fig. 4.1. Complete amino acid sequences of human and mouse κ and λ chains. For simplicity the Roy ($V_{\kappa I}$) numbering system is used. The gaps, i.e. at position 27, are required to accomodate the λ sequences. References used are: human κ, Roy (4); human λ, Bo (151); mouse κ, M41 (152); and mouse λ, 104E (55). See footnote 1 for description of the conventions used. Allotypic substitutions are shown at position 191 of the human κ chain, and isotypic substitutions at positions 143, 152, 172, and 190 of the human λ chain. In Fig. 4.3, which considers only λ chains, the numbering system of human λ protein "New" is employed. This changes the position numbers of the isotypic substitutions at positions 143 and 152 to 144 and 153, respectively.

TABLE 4.1

AMINO ACID SEQUENCE HOMOLOGIES AMONG IMMUNOGLOBULINS[a]

Comparison made	Percentage homology in sequence	Comparison made	Percentage homology in sequence
		V-Kappa (mouse and human)	
Intrasubgroup (human)			
$V_{\kappa I}$(Roy) vs $V_{\kappa I}$(Ag)	87	m41 vs m70	57
$V_{\kappa I}$(Ag) vs $V_{\kappa I}$(Eu)	74	m41 vs h$V_{\kappa I}$(Ag)	64
$V_{\kappa II}$(Mil) vs $V_{\kappa II}$(Cum)	82	m41 vs h$V_{\kappa II}$(Cum)	49
$V_{\lambda I}$(New) vs $V_{\lambda I}$(Ha)	75	m70 vs h$V_{\kappa I}$(Ag)	60
$V_{\lambda III}$(Kern) vs $V_{\lambda III}$(X)	73	m70 vs $V_{\kappa II}$(Cum)	59
Intersubgroup (human)		Constant regions	
$V_{\kappa I}$(Roy) vs $V_{\kappa II}$(Ti)	61	hC_γ vs hC_κ	30
$V_{\kappa I}$(Eu) vs $V_{\kappa III}$(Ti)	68	h$C_{\gamma I}$ vs hC_λ	25
$V_{\kappa I}$(Roy) vs $V_{\kappa II}$(Cum)	51	h$C_{\gamma I}$ vs hC_μ	33
$V_{\lambda I}$(Ha) vs $V_{\lambda III}$(Kern)	55	hC_κ vs hC_λ	39
$V_{\lambda IV}$(Bo) vs $V_{\lambda V}$(Sh)	60	mC_κ vs mC_λ	35
		h$C_{\gamma I}$ vs rC_γ	67
V-Kappa and V-Lambda (human)		hC_κ vs mC_κ	60
		hC_κ vs mC_λ	23
		hC_λ vs mC_λ	70
$V_{\lambda I}$(Ha) vs $V_{\kappa I}$(Ag)	47	hC_λ vs mC_κ	44
$V_{\lambda I}$(Ha) vs $V_{\kappa II}$(Cum)	50	C_H regions of the four human IgG subgroups	>90
$V_{\lambda III}$(Kern) vs $V_{\kappa III}$(Ti)	43		
$V_{\lambda III}$(Kern) vs $V_{\kappa II}$(Cum)	45		
		Variable and constant regions	
		hC_λ vs h$V_{\lambda I}$(Ha)	12
		hC_λ vs h$V_{\kappa I}$(Ag)	15
		hC_κ vs h$V_{\kappa III}$(Cum)	18

[a] Many of the values presented are from Hood and Talmage (28). Other references are 22, 55, 60, 67, and 90. The letters h, m, and r refer to human, mouse, and rabbit, respectively. Homologies among different domains of the C_H region of IgG1 are presented in reference 2 and in Fig. 1.4. For homologies among C_γ, C_μ, and C_ϵ, see Section VII,B,5; for homologies with rabbit C_κ, see Section VI.

It is of interest that Bence Jones proteins often occur as disulfide bonded L chain dimers; such dimers are linked through the same half-cystine groups which would normally be disulfide bonded to the H chains in an antibody molecule; this reflects a strong tendency of the free —SH groups to form S–S bonds. Moreover, in those Bence Jones proteins which comprise a monomeric L chain, the terminal cysteine is ordinarily joined to another, free cysteine group thus satisfying the tendency of the sulfhydryl to form a disulfide bond (15).

As already noted, a striking feature of the primary structure of all immunoglobulin polypeptide chains is the periodicity of half-cystine residues. In a human κ or λ chain there is one intrachain disulfide bond in the variable and one in the constant region, symmetrically placed within the two regions. Approximately 55–70 amino acid residues are enclosed within each disulfide loop. Such periodic disulfide loops of about the same size are also observed in H chains. This property, and certain sequence homologies between H and L chains, led Hill and collaborators (22) and Singer and Doolittle (23) to propose that a primordial gene encoded an amino acid sequence of about 110 to 115 residues, and that duplication gave rise to a gene controlling the biosynthesis of a complete L chain. Further replications resulted in the larger cistron which controls the biosynthesis of the H chain. The replicated genes then evolved independently. These concepts are discussed at length in Chapter 12. It is now widely believed, however, that separate cistrons control the biosynthesis of the V and C regions. This would imply that the genes controlling the two segments have evolved independently (from a common precursor) and not as a single *V-C* gene.

Edelman *et al.* (2) have proposed the useful term, "domain," to characterize the segments comprising 110 to 120 residues and including a single disulfide loop. (An alternative designation, "homology unit," is also in use.) Edelman *et al.* suggest that each domain in an H or L chain has a unique biological function. The function of the V region is obvious; namely, to provide antibody specificity. Aside from its role in joining the L chain to the H chain through noncovalent and covalent (disulfide) bonds, the biological function of the C region of an L chain is not understood. Possible functions of H chain domains are considered in Chapter 3.

The symmetrical spacing of disulfide bonds suggested that the various domains might have very similar tertiary structures. This view was also supported by homologies in amino acid sequence among domains in the constant region of an H chain, and has been borne out by X-ray crystallographic studies (Chapter 5). The region enclosed within a disulfide loop is a compact, tightly knit structure. Thus, intrachain disulfide bonds are not readily reduced in neutral buffer; the presence of a denaturing agent such as urea, guanidine, or detergent is required. Also, proteolytic enzymes in neutral buffer generally do not attack peptide bonds within a loop. However, L chains can be cleaved between V and C domains, giving rise to large segments corresponding closely to the V_L

and C_L segments (Chapter 9, Section IX). This suggested that the section of the chain joining two segments may be rather loosely folded and therefore subject to enzymatic attack; again, confirmation has come from X-ray crystallographic analysis. Cleavage of H chains between V and C domains has also been accomplished but with greater difficulty.

B. The Nature of the Variability in V Regions of L Chains

1. HUMAN κ CHAINS

Although complete sequences of only a limited number of human κ chains are known, partial sequences, especially in the N-terminal region, of a substantial number of chains have been determined. Most of this work has been done with homogeneous L chains; i.e., Bence Jones proteins or L chains of myeloma proteins; however, data of interest have also been derived from studies of heterogeneous, normal L chains. Two methods of approach are utilized extensively in obtaining partial sequences. One, exploited by Milstein and his collaborators, is to determine sequences in the vicinity of half-cystine residues. Peptides containing cystine are readily identified and separated by the "diagonal electrophoresis" method of Brown and Hartley (24).[3] A second major approach is based on sequential analysis starting from the N-terminus. By successive Edman degradations, using an automatic sequencer, as many as 50 N-terminal residues have been identified, although 20–35 is more typical.

With heterogeneous proteins, the Edman procedure can often permit the identification of multiple residues at a given position in the sequence. For example, at position 3 in a heterogeneous normal human L chain population containing predominantly κ chains, the amino acids identified are glutamine and valine. Most individual Bence Jones proteins of the κ type have one of these two residues at position 3. Besides substantiating the usefulness of the approach, such findings provide strong support for the concept that Bence Jones proteins are normal representatives of the L chain population.

---

[3] If a mixture of peptides is electrophoresed on paper successively in two perpendicular directions under the same conditions, the peptides will necessarily fall in a straight line at 45° to the two directions. If, however, after electrophoresis in one dimension, the peptides are treated with performic acid, cystine groups are converted to the negatively charged cysteic acid. During electrophoresis in the second dimension such peptides will migrate more rapidly toward the anode, to a position above the 45° diagonal line, where they can readily be identified and isolated.

2. VARIABLE REGION SUBGROUPS OF HUMAN κ CHAINS

The variable regions of both κ and λ chains can be divided into subgroups, according to homologies in amino acid sequence. These subdivisions are based on sequences of L chains of myeloma proteins and of Bence Jones proteins. Kappa chains fall naturally into three major subgroups on the basis of the length of the variable region and the presence of certain amino acids at particular positions in the sequence.[4]

Figure 4.2 summarizes partial or complete amino acid sequences of a number of human V_κ regions and shows the division into subgroups. A large proportion of the available data pertains to the N-terminal region of the chain, which is subject to direct analysis in the automatic sequencer when the amino-terminal group is unblocked. Those amino acids which are characteristic of the $V_{\kappa I}$ subgroup are marked with an asterisk in the prototype sequence (the first sequence listed in the subgroup).[5] Many of the subgroup-specific residues identified are among the first 20 in the chain, because of the availability of a large amount of data for this region. It is noteworthy that such characteristic amino acid residues are not restricted to one segment of the chain but appear at various positions along its length. This fact is widely interpreted as indicating that there is at least one germ line gene for each subgroup. It also tends to argue against genetic crossover mechanisms as the basis for the diversity of V region sequences, or at least to limit such crossovers, if they occur, to genes controlling polypeptides within a subgroup. Although subgroup-specific substitutions occur along the length of the chain, the N-terminal sequence of 20 amino acids is generally sufficient to identify the subgroup.

Besides possessing characteristic amino acid residues at various positions, certain insertions and deletions occur with high frequency only in particular subgroups. For example, $V_{\kappa II}$ proteins have six additional amino acid residues between positions 31 and 32 (Roy numbering system);[6] most $V_{\lambda I}$ and $V_{\lambda II}$ proteins require a 3-residue insertion between positions 27 and 28; $V_{\lambda II}$ requires a deletion at position 96 to permit alignment with the $V_{\lambda I}$ subgroup (26,27).

All subgroups of κ chains share the same C_κ regions (including the allotypic variants of C_κ) and, similarly, the various V_λ subgroups share the same C_λ regions, including the Oz and Kern isotypes (21a,28). The

---

[4] A further subdivision of κ_I, into κ_{Ia} and κ_{Ib}, was subsequently suggested (25) and is shown in Fig. 4.2.

[5] It is important to note that even those residues which are characteristic of a subgroup may not occur in every protein belonging to that subgroup.

[6] The extra residues are designated 31a, b, c, d, e, and f.

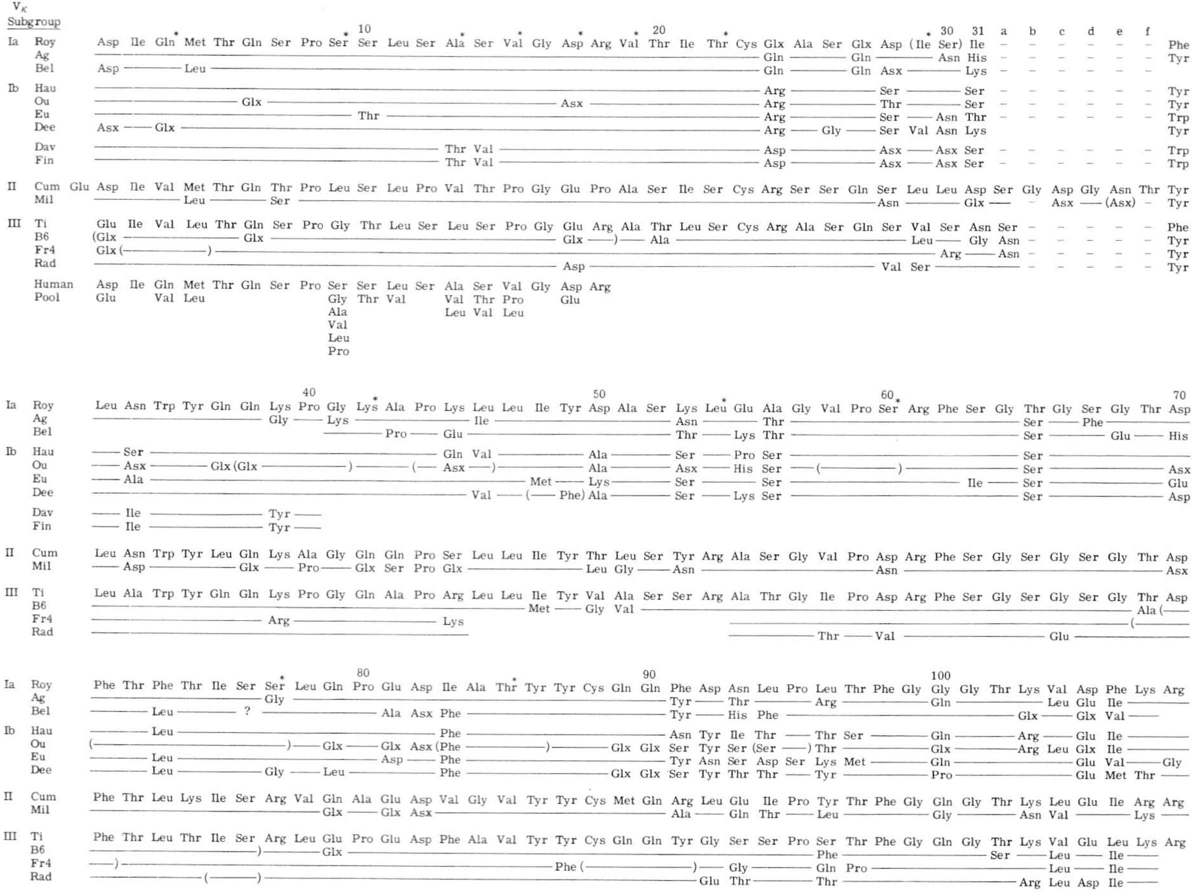
VK Subgroup
Roy Asp Ile Gln Met Thr Gln Ser Pro Ser Ser Leu Ser Ala Ser Val Gly Asp Arg Val Thr Ile Thr Cys Glx Ala Ser Glx Asp (Ile Ser) Ile Phe
Ag — Gln — Gln — Asn His Tyr
Bel Asp — Leu — Gln — Gln Asx — Lys
Hau — Arg — Ser — Ser Tyr
Ou — Glx — Asx — Arg — Thr — Ser Tyr
Eu — Thr — Arg — Ser — Asn Thr Trp
Dee Asx — Glx — Arg — Gly — Ser Val Asn Lys Tyr
Dav — Thr Val — Asp — Asx — Asx Ser Trp
Fin — Thr Val — Asp — Asx — Asx Ser Trp
Cum Glu Asp Ile Val Met Thr Gln Thr Pro Leu Ser Leu Pro Val Thr Pro Gly Glu Pro Ala Ser Ile Ser Cys Arg Ser Ser Gln Ser Leu Leu Asp Ser Gly Asp Gly Asn Thr Tyr
Mil — Leu — Ser — Asn — Glx — Asx — (Asx) Tyr
Ti Glu Ile Val Leu Thr Gln Ser Pro Gly Thr Leu Ser Leu Ser Pro Gly Glu Arg Ala Thr Leu Ser Cys Arg Ala Ser Gln Ser Val Ser Asn Ser Phe
B6 (Glx — Glx — Glx —)— Ala — Leu — Gly Asn Tyr
Fr4 Glx (—) — Arg — Asn Tyr
Rad — Asp — Val Ser — Tyr
Human Pool Asp Ile Gln Met Thr Gln Ser Pro Ser Ser Leu Ser Ala Ser Val Gly Asp Arg
Glu Val Leu Gly Thr Val Val Thr Pro Glu
Ala Leu Val Leu
Val
Leu
Pro
Roy Leu Asn Trp Tyr Gln Gln Lys Pro Gly Lys Ala Pro Lys Leu Leu Ile Tyr Asp Ala Ser Lys Leu Glu Ala Gly Val Pro Ser Arg Phe Ser Gly Thr Gly Ser Gly Thr Asp
Ag — Gly — Lys — Ile — Asn — Thr — Ser — Phe —
Bel — Pro — Glu — Thr — Lys Thr — Ser — Glu — His
Hau — Ser — Gln Val — Ala — Ser — Pro Ser — Ser —
Ou — Asx — Glx (Glx —) — (— Asx —) — Ala — Asx — His Ser — (—) — Ser — Asx
Eu — Ala — Met — Lys — Ser — Ser — Ile — Ser — Glu
Dee — Val — (— Phe) Ala — Ser — Lys Ser — Ser — Asp
Dav — Ile — Tyr —
Fin — Ile — Tyr —
Cum Leu Asn Trp Tyr Leu Gln Lys Ala Gly Gln Gln Pro Ser Leu Leu Ile Tyr Thr Leu Ser Tyr Arg Ala Ser Gly Val Pro Asp Arg Phe Ser Gly Ser Gly Ser Gly Thr Asp
Mil — Asp — Glx — Pro — Glx Ser Pro Glx — Leu Gly — Asn — Asn — Asx
Ti Leu Ala Trp Tyr Gln Gln Lys Pro Gly Gln Ala Pro Arg Leu Leu Ile Tyr Val Ala Ser Ser Arg Ala Thr Gly Ile Pro Asp Arg Phe Ser Gly Ser Gly Ser Gly Thr Asp
B6 — Met — Gly Val — Ala (—
Fr4 — Arg — Lys — (—
Rad — Thr — Val — Glu —
Roy Phe Thr Phe Thr Ile Ser Ser Leu Gln Pro Glu Asp Ile Ala Thr Tyr Tyr Cys Gln Gln Phe Asp Asn Leu Pro Leu Thr Phe Gly Gly Gly Thr Lys Val Asp Phe Lys Arg
Ag — Gly — Tyr — Thr — Arg — Gln — Leu Glu Ile —
Bel — Leu — ? — Ala Asx Phe — Tyr — His Phe — Glx — Glx Val —
Hau — Leu — Phe — Asn Tyr Ile Thr — Thr Ser — Gln — Arg — Glu Ile —
Ou (—)— Glx — Glx Asx (Phe —)— Glx Glx Ser Tyr Ser (Ser —) Thr — Glx — Arg Leu Glx Ile —
Eu — Leu — Asp — Phe — Tyr Asn Ser Asp Ser Lys Met — Gln — Glu Val — Gly
Dee — Leu — Gly — Leu — Phe — Glx Glx Ser Tyr Thr Thr — Tyr — Pro — Glu Met Thr —
Cum Phe Thr Leu Lys Ile Ser Arg Val Gln Ala Glu Asp Val Gly Val Tyr Tyr Cys Met Gln Arg Leu Glu Ile Pro Tyr Thr Phe Gly Gln Gly Thr Lys Leu Glu Ile Arg Arg
Mil — Glx — Glx Asx — Ala — Gln Thr — Leu — Gly — Asn Val — Lys —
Ti Phe Thr Leu Thr Ile Ser Arg Leu Glu Pro Glu Asp Phe Ala Val Tyr Tyr Cys Gln Gln Tyr Gly Ser Ser Pro Ser Thr Phe Gly Gln Gly Thr Lys Val Glu Leu Lys Arg
B6 —)— Glx — Phe — Ser — Leu — Ile —
Fr4 —) — Phe (—)— Gly — Gln Pro — Leu — Ile —
Rad — (—) — Glu Thr — Thr — Arg Leu Asp Ile —

Fig. 4.2

three V_κ subgroups are not allelic; each has been identified in all normal sera examined, when sufficiently sensitive methods were used (29–31).

Antisera have been prepared which can distinguish the three major V_κ subgroups as well as antigenically distinct subdivisions within each subgroup (32,33). This development should facilitate studies of the genetic control of L chain biosynthesis.

Salient features of the variations in V region sequences of L chains have been reviewed and analyzed by a number of authors (e.g., 28,34–39). Figure 4.2 includes the complete sequences of the V regions of seven $V_{\kappa I}$ L chains which serve to illustrate, in part, the nature of the variations. If any two of the six sequences within the $V_{\kappa I}$ subgroup are compared the degree of homology exceeds 70%. This value is typical for sequences within a κ (or λ) subgroup. If two κ chains (or two λ chains) belonging to different subgroups are compared the degree of homology is generally of the order of 50 to 60%. A V_κ sequence exhibits about 40 to 50% homology with a V_λ sequence chosen at random. (See Table 4.1.)

In the seven complete $V_{\kappa I}$ sequences in Fig. 4.2, 58 positions are invariant. The actual number of apparently invariant positions will tend to decrease as more proteins are studied, and it is difficult to estimate the true number. In 22 $V_{\kappa I}$ sequences tabulated up to residues 17–20 by Hood and Talmage (28), 10 of the 20 residues are invariant. However, even these are suspect; for example, 21 of the 22 proteins have isoleucine at position 2, but one protein has valine at this location. Obviously, position 2 would have appeared invariant in a more limited sample. By the same token, additional variants may appear in the future, although some positions are undoubtedly constant.

Four amino acids (glycine, tryptophan, proline, and, particularly, half-cystine) tend to be conserved. The half-cystine residues constituting the intrachain disulfide loops occur at corresponding locations in all human V_κ and V_λ sequences and are used as a basis for alignment. There are 7 glycine residues, at positions 16, 41, 57, 64, 68, 99, and 101 which are present in nearly all κ and λ chains (34).

Fig. 4.2. Amino acid sequences in the variable regions of human κ chains. κ_1 is divided into subgroups, I_a and I_b, according to Milstein and Deverson (25). Amino acids which are characteristic of the $V_{\kappa I}$ subgroup (not necessarily present in all members of the subgroup) are indicated by an asterisk in the prototype sequence. The format used is described in footnote 1. Note that six insertions are needed to provide homology between residues 31 and 32 in $V_{\kappa II}$. References: protein Roy (4); Ag (153); Bel (154); Hau (155); Ou (156); Eu (2); Dee (25); Dav and Fin (42); Cum (157); Mil (158); Ti (159); B6, Fr4, and Rad (160); human pool (29). The subgrouping $V_{\kappa II}$ and $V_{\kappa III}$ is that used by Hilschmann, Capra, and Milstein and Pink; it is reversed in some of the earlier literature. Additional sequences are listed in references 35, 59, and 160a. A solid line represents identity of sequence with the prototype for that subgroup (proteins Roy, Cum, or Ti).

It is easy to understand, from the functional standpoint, the conservation of cystine residues; the disulfide loops are of primary importance in maintaining the appropriate tertiary structure. The relative invariance of certain glycine residues was attributed by Wu and Kabat to the fact that this amino acid, because of the lack of a side chain, lends flexibility to the antibody molecule. Such flexibility might have two important advantages. It could permit a wider variety of amino acid substitutions without disruption of the secondary or tertiary structure, and it could enhance the flexibility of the combining site. This would be important if, by analogy with certain enzymes, interaction with antigen involves an induced fit of amino acids in the active site. There is, however, no clear evidence for flexibility of the combining site.

By X-ray crystallographic analysis Epp *et al.* (39b) and Poljak *et al.* (39a) found that most of the hairpin bends, characteristic of immunoglobulin polypeptide chains, contain an invariant glycine residue, usually as part of a Pro-Gly or Ser(Thr)-Gly sequence. In the λ chain, at positions 99–102, there is a constant Phe-Gly-Gly-Gly sequence which is not part of a bend (39a); the invariance is explained by Poljak *et al.* on the basis that space is so limited around the glycine residues that side chains cannot be accommodated.

Another interesting feature is the conservation of nonpolar residues at specific positions in the amino acid sequence. By contrast, no characteristic conservation of polar sites is apparent. Welscher (40) compared the complete V regions of 15 κ and λ chains, including two mouse κ chains, and found, with appropriate alignment, 63 positions that are consistently occupied by nonpolar amino acids (glycine, alanine, half-cystine, methionine, valine, leucine, proline, phenylalanine, isoleucine, tryptophan, or tyrosine). By analogy with globin chains of different species, Welscher attributed the conservation of nonpolar residues to the fact that in aqueous solution they can form strong hydrophobic bonds which play a major role in the folding of the polypeptide chain; substitution of a polar side chain in certain positions would disrupt the folding pattern, since energy is required to transfer a polar group from an aqueous to a nonaqueous (internal) environment. This conclusion has been confirmed by X-ray analysis (Chapter 5); nonpolar bonds stabilize the internal structure of each domain and are also of primary importance in the interaction of contiguous regions of L and H chains.

Within a subgroup of κ or λ chains about 90% of the observed interchanges (not including the hypervariable regions) can be accounted for by a single base change in the codon; i.e., a single point mutation could account for the substitution. Since most amino acids have multiple codons, relationships in amino acid sequence are arbitrarily analyzed by determining the minimum number of base changes that could account for the observed interchanges. Substitutions in hypervariable regions will be discussed later.

Hood and Talmage (28) have carefully considered the nature of interchanges in the V regions of human κ and λ chains. Most of their discussion is confined to variations within subgroups. Data for the first 20 N-terminal residues were available for 64 L chains, giving a total of about 1300 amino acid residues. Based on the prototype sequences for three κ and five λ subgroups, the total number of intrasubgroup interchanges of amino acids was 63 or about 5%. (Positions 1–20 do not include a hypervariable region.) Of the 63 substitutions, 60 could be attributed to a single base change in a codon. There was a 2:1 ratio of transversions (e.g., purine to pyrimidine) to transitions (e.g., purine to purine). A striking preponderance of substitutions, presumably mutations, involving guanine was noted; this property has also been observed in comparing the cytochromes c of different species. The very large proportion of single base changes noted within a subgroup does not apply when comparisons are made between nonidentical amino acids occupying the same position in two different subgroups. A substantial percentage of such substitutions requires more than one base change in DNA.

The basis for a further subdivision of κ_I into κ_{Ia} and κ_{Ib} (25) is shown by the seven $V_{\kappa I}$ sequences at the top of Fig. 4.2. The positions at which the characteristic differences occur, quite uniformly, are 24, 50, 56, 73, 83, 92, and 100. It is of particular interest that the characteristic differences appear along almost the entire length of the chain. Milstein and Deverson (25) and many other investigators believe that each subgroup must reflect the existence of at least one separate germ line gene (Chapter 12).

3. Amino Acid Sequences in Human λ Chains

The basic pattern of variation observed in κ chains is also seen in λ chains, which have been studied and discussed extensively by Hilschmann, Putnam, Milstein, and their collaborators. References to their work, which includes discussions of the significance of the data, are cited in the legend of Fig. 4.3, which presents a number of amino acid sequences of V regions of λ chains. The sequence data suggest the existence of five subgroups. The basis for the subdivision is not as clear-cut as it is for human κ chains, due in part to the relative paucity of data. It also seems likely that additional subgroups may become evident when more sequence data are reported. Subgroups I and II are characterized

λ

Positions 1–35

Subgroup	1 → 35
I New	Glp Ser Val Leu Thr Gln Pro Pro Ser Val Ser Ala Ala Pro Gly Gln Lys Val Thr Ile Ser Cys Ser Gly Ser Gly Ser Thr[27] Asn[a] Ile[b] Gly[c] — Gly Asn Asn[30] Tyr Val Ser Trp Trp[34] His[35]
Ha	— Ala — — — — — — — — Ala — — — — — — — Arg Gly — — — — — Ser — — — — — Thr — — — — — — Tyr
HBJ7	
HS92	
HBJ11	
II Nei	Glp Ser Ala Leu Thr Gln Pro Ala Ser Val Ser Gly Ser Pro Gly Gln Ser Ile Thr Ile Ser Cys Thr Gly Thr Ser Ser Asp Val Gly — Gly Tyr Asn Tyr Val Ser Trp Tyr
Vil	His — — — — — — — — — — — — — — — — — Leu — — — — — — — — — — — — — — — — — Tyr Phe
HS68	— — — Ser
HS77	
HS70	
III Ker	— Tyr Ala Leu Thr Gln Pro Pro Ser Val Ser Val Ser Pro Gly Gln Thr Ala Arg Ile Thr Cys Ser Gly Asp Ala Leu — — — Glu Lys Phe Thr Val Ser Trp Tyr Cys
X	— Asp — — — — — — — Leu — — — — — — — — — — — — — — — Lys — — — Gly Asp Lys Tyr — — — Cys
Bau	— Gly — Lys — — — Glu Glu Gln Tyr — — — Cys
IV Bo	Glp Ala Leu Thr Gln Pro Pro Ser Val Ser Ala Ala Pro Gly Gln Ser Val Thr Ile Ser Cys Thr Gly Thr Ser Ser Asp Val Gly Val Gly Asp Tyr Val Ser Trp Tyr
V Sh	— Ser Glu Leu Thr Gln Asp Pro Ala Val Ser Val Ala Leu Gly Gln Thr Val Arg Ile Thr Cys Gln Gly Asp Ser Leu — Arg Gly Tyr Asp Ala Ala Trp Tyr

Positions 40–70

Subgroup	40 → 70
I New	Gln His Leu Pro Gly Thr Ala Pro Lys Leu Leu Ile Tyr Glu[50] Asp Asn Lys Arg Pro Ser Gly Ile Pro Asp Arg[60] Phe Ser Gly Ser Lys Ser Gly Thr Ser Ala[70] Thr Leu Gly
Ha	— Gln — — — — — — — — — — — Arg Asp — — — — — — Val — — — — — — — — — — — — — Ser
II Nei	Gln Gln Ala Pro Gly Lys Ala Pro Lys Leu Met Ile Tyr Glu[50] Val Ser Lys Arg Pro Ser Gly Val Ser Asn Arg[60] Phe Ser Gly Ser Lys Ser Gly Asn Thr Ala[70] Ser Leu Thr
Vil	— His — — — — — — — — — — — Ser — — Asn — — — — — — — — — — — — — — — — — — — Asn — —
III Ker	Gln Gln Arg Pro Gly Gln Ser Pro Val Leu Val Ile Tyr His[50] Ser Thr Glu Arg Pro Glu Ile Pro Glu Arg Pro[60] Ser Gly Ser Ser Gly Asn Thr Ala Thr Leu[70] Thr Leu Thr
X	— — Lys — — — — — — — — — Val Asp — — — — — — — — — — — — — — — — Asn — — — — —
Bau	— Lys — — — — — — — — — — His Asp — Gln Ser Lys — — — — Gly Gly — — — — — — — — — — — — —
IV Bo	Gln Gln His Pro Gly Lys Ala Pro Lys Leu Ile Ile Tyr Asp[50] Val Ser Lys Arg Pro Ser Gly Val Ser Asn Arg[60] Phe Ser Gly Ser Lys Ser Gly Asn Thr Ala[70] Ser Leu Thr
V Sh	Gln Gln Lys Pro Gly Gln Ala Pro Val Leu Val Ile Tyr Ser[50] Asn Asp Arg Pro Ser Gly Ile Pro Glu Arg Phe[60] Ser Gly Ser Ser Ser Gly His Thr Ala Ser[70] Leu Thr Thr

Positions 80–109

Subgroup	80 → 109
I New	Ile Thr Gly Leu Arg Thr Gly Asp Glu Ala Asp Tyr Tyr Cys Ala Thr Trp Asp[90] Ser Ser Leu Ser Ala Ala Ala Val Phe[100] Gly Gly Gly Thr Lys Val Thr Val Leu Gly[109] Gln
Ha	— Ser — — Ser Glu His — — — — — His — — — Tyr — Ala — — — — — — — — — — — — — — — — — Gln Leu
II Nei	Ile Ser Gly Leu Gln Val Glu Asp Glu Ala Asp Tyr Tyr Cys Ser Ser Tyr Thr[90] Ser Ser Ser Thr — — — Val Val[100] Phe Gly Gly Gly Thr Lys Leu Thr Val Leu Ser[109] Arg
Vil	— Ala — — — — — — — — — — — — Gly Asn Ser Thr — — — — — — — — — Leu — — — — — — — — — Lys Gly
III Ker	Ile Ser Gly Val Ala Ala Glu Asp Glu Ala Asp Tyr Tyr Cys Gln Ser Tyr Asp[90] Ser Ser Asn His Val Val[100] Phe Gly Gly Gly Thr Lys Leu Thr Val Leu Gly[109] Gln
X	— — — — — — — — — — — — — — — Met Ser Ser Ala Tyr — — — — — — — — — — — — — — — — Gly
Bau	— — — — — — — — — — — — — — — Tyr Ser Tyr Ala Ala — — — — — — — — — — — — — — — — —
IV Bo	Ile Ser Gly Leu Gln Ala Glu Asp Glu Ala Asp Tyr Tyr Cys Ser Ser Tyr Val[90] Ser Ser Ser Thr Arg Val[100] Phe Gly Gly Gly Thr Lys Leu Thr Val Leu Gly[109] Gln
V Sh	Ile Thr Gly Ala Gln Ala Glu Asp Glu Ala Asp Tyr Tyr Cys His Ser Tyr Asp[90] Ser Ser Asn Ser His Val[100] Phe Gly Gly Gly Thr Lys Leu Thr Val Leu Gly[109] Gln

Positions 144, 153, 172, 190

Subgroup	144	153	172	190
I New	Ala	Ser	Lys	Arg
II Nei	Ala	Ser	Lys	Arg
Vil		Gly		Arg
III Ker	Ala	Gly	Lys	Arg
X	Ala	Gly / Ser	Lys	Arg
Bau	Val		Asn	
IV Bo	Ala	Ser	Lys	Arg
V Sh	Ala	Ser	Lys	Arg

Fig. 4.3

by the presence of a blocked N-terminal group (pyrollidonecarboxylic acid) in most proteins. The proteins in subgroup III and the single representative of subgroup V have unblocked N-termini, and a gap must be allowed at the N-terminus to align these sequences with those of the other three subgroups. Intrachain disulfide loops are present in their usual locations and the half-cystine which is disulfide bonded to the H chain is the penultimate residue.

Isotypic amino acid substitutions in C_λ regions, which are apparently present in all individuals, and which have already been mentioned, are shown as an addendum to the figure.

4. HYPERVARIABLE REGIONS IN HUMAN L CHAINS

As we have indicated, certain positions in the amino acid sequence are exceptionally variable. Wu and Kabat (34) defined variability in quantitative terms by means of the following expression: Variability is equal to the number of different amino acids observed at a given position divided by the frequency of occurrence of the most common amino acid which appears at that position.

They then plotted variability in human and mouse κ and λ chains (as a group) as a function of position in the amino acid sequence. A similar plot based only on the nine human $V_{\kappa I}$ sequences (seven complete, two partial) in Fig. 4.2, is presented in Fig. 4.4. It is evident that the regions of major variability are near positions 30, 50, 95, and 106. A similar plot based on a sample which includes two additional κ chains, but not Dav or Fin, was presented by Braun *et al.* (35). Figure 4.4 resembles quite closely the plot of Wu and Kabat, who included both kappa and lambda chains, and the mouse and human species, in their sample.

As mentioned earlier, the generalization that amino acid substitutions within a subgroup can usually be related to a single base change in the nucleotide triplet does not apply to substitutions in hypervariable

---

Fig. 4.3. Variable region sequences of human λ chains. The numbering system of protein New is used. Note the insertions between residues 27 and 28 and the deletions at positions 95 and 96, required to permit maximal alignment of the subgroups. The alternative amino acids found in each protein at positions of isotypic variation in the constant sequence (positions 144, 153, 172, and 190) are shown at the end of the table. In Fig. 4.1, showing comparisons with κ chains, positions 144 and 153 were designated as 143 and 152, respectively. References for individual proteins are: New (5); Ha, Bo, Sh (19,151); Nei (26); Vil (161); Ker (162); X (163); Bau (164); HS68, HS77, HS70 (165); HBJ7, HBJ11 (166). The isotypic variations shown at the end of the table (at positions 144, etc.) are not necessarily restricted to the subgroups shown. There is considerable variation in the literature with respect to subgrouping of these proteins (26,59,160a). Clarification will require additional sequence analyses.

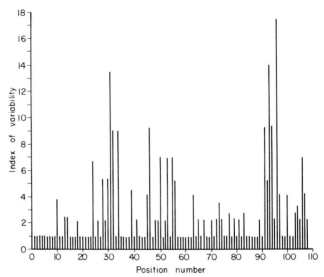

Fig. 4.4. Plot of variability, according to the method of Wu and Kabat (34), for the human $V_{\kappa I}$ sequences shown in Fig. 4.2. The index of variability is defined in the text.

regions. Also, one does not find subgroup-specific amino acid residues in hypervariable regions. On the other hand, deletions and insertions characteristic of a subgroup are often located in or near hypervariable segments of the chain. Note, for example, the insertion of six amino acids next to position 31 in $V_{\kappa II}$ or the deletions in $V_{\lambda III}$ at positions 95 and 96.

An interesting feature is the frequent occurrence of essentially invariant residues on either side of hypervariable regions. In κ chains these include the two half-cystines of the intrachain loop in the V region, glycine residues 99 and 101, and tryptophan at position 35. In λ chains such residues include the corresponding half-cystines, tryptophan 34 and the -Phe-Gly-Gly-Gly-Thr-sequence at positions 99–103.

It has frequently been suggested, for obvious reasons, that hypervariable regions might be directly involved in the formation of the antibody combining site. This conjecture was strongly supported by the results of affinity labeling experiments (Chapter 6), in which the labeling reagent is almost invariably bound to an amino acid in or close to a hypervariable region, and has been proved by X-ray crystallography (Chapter 5).

5. Amino Acid Sequences in Pooled Normal Human κ Chains

Figure 4.2 includes data on normal human L chains (human pool), obtained by Niall and Edman (29). Actually these sequences apply to κ

chains since the pool was partially depleted of λ chains and because most λ chains have a blocked N-terminal group and would not be subject to the Edman degradation. Multiple residues are seen at many positions in the normal sequence, reflecting the heterogeneity of the normal pool. However, most residues have their counterpart among individual monoclonal κ chains. Also, positions which appear invariant in the normal pool are in general also invariant, or nearly so, among the monoclonal chains. This is further evidence that monoclonal proteins are normal, but homogeneous representatives of the L chain population.

C. Human κ Chains with Similar or Identical Amino Acid Sequences

Structural analyses of a large number of human Bence Jones proteins and myeloma light chains failed, initially, to reveal identity of the V regions of any two proteins. For example, Quattrocchi *et al.* (41) examined 102 different monoclonal light chains (κ or λ) and found that each had a distinctive peptide map.

Capra and Kunkel (42) compared L chains of IgG from two individuals with a benign disorder, hypergammaglobulinemic purpura. Such patients have high serum concentrations of antibodies of the IgG class which are generally antiglobulins with specificity for the Fc portion of human IgG. In some instances these anti-antibodies appear homogeneous. They can be purified specifically by exploiting their reactivity with IgG. The L chains of four such proteins from unrelated patients were investigated; two were identical by the criteria of peptide maps and the N-terminal sequence of 40 amino acid residues (proteins Dav and Fin, Fig. 4.2). This of course includes the first hypervariable region. The two identical L chains fit best into the $V_{\kappa I}$ subgroup, but have six amino acids, of the 40 analyzed, that appear unique among known κ_I proteins; only two of the six residues are in a hypervariable region. It is uncertain whether these L chains really constitute a new subgroup or are examples of extreme variability within a subgroup.

Closely related amino acid sequences have also been observed among the L or H chains of homogeneous IgM antiglobulins and among the L chains of certain cold agglutinins. These proteins are discussed in detail in Section II,B of Chapter 11.

These important results suggest that similarities or identities among monoclonal proteins may be found more frequently if they are selected for comparison on the basis of shared antigen-binding specificity. This possibility is supported by studies with mouse myeloma proteins, reviewed later in this chapter.

D. Common Evolutionary Origin of Human κ and λ Chains

A casual inspection of the amino acid sequences of human κ and λ chains (Figs. 4.1–4.3) immediately suggests a common ancestral gene. The chains are of approximately the same length and each has two disulfide loops closely corresponding in size and location. The κ chain has a C-terminal half-cystine which forms an interchain disulfide bond to an H chain, whereas the λ chain has a half-cystine, which serves the same function, as its penultimate residue.

If the amino acid sequences are appropriately aligned, allowing a small number of deletions, the degree of homology, between the C_κ and C_λ sequences is 39% (Table 4.1). The degree of homology between V_κ and V_λ regions will of course vary with the particular pair of Bence Jones proteins chosen for comparison; an average value is about 45 to 50%.

Superficially, the V and C regions of a κ (or λ) chain also bear a striking resemblance in length and in the position of the disulfide loop. However, the degree of sequence homology is actually quite small (about 15%). This suggests that the gene(s) coding V and C regions may have arisen by duplication from a common evolutionary ancestor (22,23) but that this divergence occurred much earlier than that which gave rise to κ and λ chains. The possibility of independent (convergent) evolution of V and C genes cannot, however, be ruled out.

IV. AMINO ACID SEQUENCES IN L CHAINS OF THE MOUSE

Because of the ready availability of myeloma and Bence Jones proteins, a large amount of amino acid sequence data has been accumulated with mouse as well as human immunoglobulins. Comparisons of data on L chains of the two species have improved our understanding of the evolution of immunoglobulins and the nature of the variability in V regions.

The immunoglobulins of normal mouse serum, in contrast to those of the human, contain L chains which are almost exclusively of the κ type; the concentration of λ chains is about 3 to 5% of the total (43,44). This is reflected by the relative infrequency of occurrence of myeloma proteins of type λ (45).

The capacity to maintain a tumor line by continuous passage in mice and the identical structure of the myeloma protein produced by successive implants of the same tumor provide substantial quantities of homogeneous immunoglobulin (46). However, the induction of tumors in mice by intraperitoneal injection of mineral oil or plastics results in a high proportion of IgA myeloma proteins, possibly because of a predominance of IgA-producing cells in the mesentery.

A. Mouse κ Chains

Figure 4.1 shows an essentially complete amino acid sequence of a mouse κ chain and, for comparison, of a human κ chain. The mouse κ chain is similar to that of the human in having a C-terminal invariant segment and an N-terminal variable region which are about equal in length. Other general features of similarity with human κ chains are the length of the polypeptide chain, the location of disulfide loops in the V and C regions, and the presence of a C-terminal half-cystine which is linked to an H chain in a complete immunoglobulin molecule. So far no allotypic differences in mouse L chains have been discerned by immunological methods or by amino acid sequence analysis, although Edelman and Gottlieb have demonstrated polymorphism in the V region by peptide mapping of the L chains of different strains (47).

With proper alignment, the degree of homology between the C regions of mouse and human κ chains is 60% (Table 4.1).

B. V Region Sequences in Mouse L Chains

The fact that mouse κ chains have an unblocked terminal amino group has permitted acquisition, with the automatic sequencer, of a substantial amount of data on N-terminal sequences. Nearly all the results pertain to the proteins of BALB/c mice.

The N-terminal 19 to 23 residues of 44 BALB/c κ chains have been tabulated by Hood *et al.* (48,49). In striking contrast to human κ chains, these do not fall readily into a small number of subgroups. Hood and collaborators believe that, of the 44 sequences, 25 can be considered as belonging to separate subgroups. Some of their data are presented in Fig. 4.5. The first six sequences represent the largest number which can be categorized as belonging to one subgroup. The next three sequences represent another subgroup. The last seven sequences selected are sufficiently unique so that each would represent a separate subgroup.

A comparison of the degree of sequence homology between two members of different subgroups, among the 44 sequences, indicates, on the average, a minimum of nine nucleotide differences in the DNA code (49). If the same frequency of amino acid substitution (40%) were maintained throughout the V region there would be an average difference of about 45 residues between members of different subgroups. This is com-

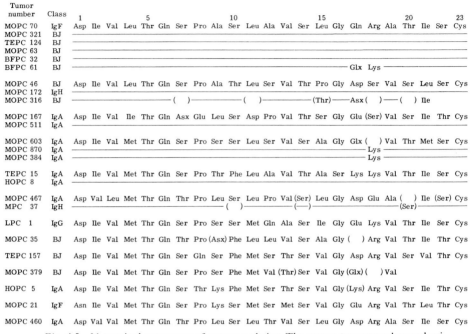

Fig. 4.5. N-terminal sequences of mouse κ chains. The mouse tumor number and origin of the light chain [Bence Jones (BJ) or class of myeloma protein] are given. IgF, IgG, and IgH are subclasses of mouse IgG. Parentheses indicate that a residue is present at that position but has not yet been identified or is uncertain. Sequences are from among 44 compiled by Hood *et al.* (48,49).

parable to the average difference in sequence between two L chains of different human V_κ subgroups. From the data available one cannot estimate an upper limit for the number of mouse V_κ subgroups. When the first 22 sequences were analyzed they comprised nine separate subgroups. The next 22 sequences studied revealed an additional 16 subgroups. So far, then, we are not approaching a plateau.

Hood believes that each subgroup must represent a minimum of one germ line gene, and other investigators, including those who favor the somatic mutation theory, are in agreement with this concept. If this is correct there must be a substantial number of germ line genes encoding V_κ regions of mouse immunoglobulins. The possibility of somatic mutation superimposed on this large array of germ line genes is, of course, not excluded.

There is no obvious explanation for the exceptionally large number of mouse V_κ subgroups. Among possibilities considered by Hood *et al.* are the artificial method of induction of mouse myelomas and their peritoneal origin. Alternatively, there may simply be a greater diversity of κ chains in mouse than in man.

It is instructive to compare the N-terminal sequences of mouse and human κ chains. Figure 4.6, compiled by Hood *et al.* (49), lists the amino acids which appear at each position in the sequence. The similarities are striking. Two of the 23 N-terminal positions are completely invariant with respect both to mouse and human κ chains; these are positions 6 (glutamine) and 23 (half-cystine). Other positions (threonine 5 and glycine 16) are nearly invariant in both species. In addition, the same amino acid predominates in both species at many other positions. At certain positions one can find particular amino acids in one species but rarely in the other. For example, some mouse κ chains, but no human κ chains, have methionine as residue 11. Glycine is present at position 9 in some human κ chains but not in mouse κ chains. Such species-associated residues are enclosed in boxes in Fig. 4.6. On the basis of the theory of multiple germ line genes, one would postulate that the species-specific residues evolved after divergence of the mouse and human evolutionary lines.

When N-terminal sequences are compared, the degree of homology between two mouse κ chains from different subgroups is, on the average,

Position	1	2	3	4	5	6	7	8	9	10	11	12	13	14	15	16	17	18	19	20	21	22	23
Species	1	2	3	4	5	6	7	8	9	10	11	12	13	14	15	16	17	18	19	20	21	22	23
Human	D34	I43	Q27	M31	T45	Q45	S44	P45	S26	S28	L45	S38	A23	S36	V26	G44	D30	R38	V26	T34	I33	T24	C45
	E10	M1	V18	L14			T1		G8	T16		P7	L10	T7	P18	R1	E15	P7	A18	S8	L12	S18	
	K1	V1							L7	P1			V9	V2	L1				I1	A1		A2	
									A4				T2									Z1	
													M1										
BALB/c	D34	I32	V31	M26	T42	Q44	S34	P39	A20	S27	L31	S24	V26	S33	L16	G42	E18	R17	V32	T26	T29	S21	C38
Mouse	E8	V8	Q9	L14	I2		T8	T2	S10	F6	M9	A11	A12	T9	V10	S2	D8	K8	A12	S14	L5	T15	
	N2	T2	T2	I2			B2	E2	L8	T5	D2	P4	M3	A2	I6		Z6	S4			M5		
		N2	L2	V2			Q1	T2	I4	T2	F1	T3	A6		Q5	T2			V1				
								K2	L1		L1		P3		K3	E2							
								B2	Y1		T1		S2		L1	P2							
											V1		T1		B1	Z2							
											Q1					L1							
																B1							

Fig. 4.6. A profile of sequence diversity for the myeloma κ chains of mouse and man. Forty-five human κ chains with known amino-terminal sequences for 22 or more residues were compared against 44 mouse κ chains. The residue alternatives at each position are listed along with their relative frequencies. Major residues (eight or more proteins) present in just one of these species are boxed. Amide or acid assignments were made by homology where possible. The one letter amino acid code is used: A, Ala; B, Asx; C, Cys; D, Asp; E, Glu; F, Phe; G, Gly; I, Ile; K, Lys; L, Leu; M, Met; N, Asn; P, Pro; Q, Gln; R, Arg; S, Ser; T, Thr; V, Val; Y, Tyr; and Z, Glx. Reprinted by permission from Hood *et al.* (49).

comparable to that observed between a mouse κ chain and a randomly selected human κ chain ($\sim$ 50–60%). This seems to reflect a strong evolutionary pressure tending to maintain V region sequences (cf. N-terminal sequences of fish and mammals, Tables 7.2 and 7.3).

Four of the κ chain sequences in Fig. 4.5 (proteins 70, 321, 124, and 63) have identical N-terminal sequences up to position 23. When the complete V region sequences were determined differences were observed (49a). Proteins 321 and 124 differ by three residues, all in hypervariable regions; protein 63 differs from 321 and 124 by eight residues and protein 70 differs from the others in 20–21 positions. Nevertheless, there are striking resemblances, including a 4-residue insertion near position 27. In the same paper, McKean *et al.* tabulate six complete mouse V_κ sequences (49a).

C. Mouse κ Chains with Identical Amino Acid Sequences

As we have seen, in two mouse myeloma proteins selected at random a substantial degree of variation in the L chain sequence is generally observed. When, however, the myeloma proteins are selected on the basis of their capacity to combine with the same antigen, striking resemblances are occasionally seen. The easiest way to predict such similarity is through sharing of unique (idiotypic) antigenic determinants, which sometimes occurs in mouse myeloma proteins which combine with the same antigen. Identity can be established conclusively only through sequence analysis. Potter and Lieberman (50) studied five IgA myeloma proteins with identical idiotypic specificity; each of the proteins reacted with phosphorylcholine or with pneumococcal C carbohydrate, which has phosphorylcholine as a haptenic determinant. Chemical studies (48,49) indicated that two of these proteins, TEPC 15 and HOPC 8, have κ chains with identical peptide maps as well as an identical sequence of 23 amino acids at the N-terminus (Fig. 4.5). Two other myeloma proteins, MOPC 870 and 384, both of which have anti-*Salmonella* activity (51), possess L chains with identical N-terminal sequences (Fig. 4.5), but their peptide maps, although similar, are not identical (48).

Not all BALB/c myeloma proteins with antiphosphorylcholine activity are similar. Some (MOPC 167, MOPC 603) do not share idiotype with other proteins having the same antibody activity and have L chains belonging to unrelated V_κ subgroups. The same principle applies to a myeloma protein with anti-*Salmonella* activity, MOPC 467, whose L chains differ from those of proteins 870 and 384.

Progress toward clarifying these relationships was made by Barstad *et al.* (51a), who determined N-terminal sequences of the L and H chains of five BALB/c myeloma proteins that bind phosphorylcholine (extending the studies mentioned above). Three of the proteins, HOPC 8, TEPC 15, and S107 (Group A), share idiotypic specificity; the other two, MOPC 603 and MOPC 167, differ in idiotype from one another and from the first group. All the proteins have κ chains. The κ chain sequences of the proteins in Group A were identical through position 36, which includes the first hypervariable region. By contrast, the L chain of MOPC 603 differs from this group in 44% of these positions, including several positions in the hypervariable region. The L chain of MOPC 167, which was sequenced to residue 23, differs from the first group in 14 positions (61%). The authors suggest that the V_L region of the three proteins in Group A is encoded by a germ line gene, on the basis that it is unlikely that a random somatic process would generate multiple identical chains in different individuals.

Equally striking are the N-terminal sequences of the H chains of the five proteins. All are identical through position 34 (which includes a hypervariable region) except for a single substitution (valine for leucine) at position 4 of the MOPC 167 H chain. It was concluded that the H chain may play a dominant role in providing specificity against phosphorylcholine. The H chain sequence of the five proteins was not seen in 23 other BALB/c proteins that lacked specificity for phosphorylcholine. It is noteworthy that antiphosphorylcholine antibodies carrying the idiotypic specificity of the Group A proteins are present in normal BALB/c serum (51b).

The frequent appearance of mouse myeloma proteins with anti-phosphorylcholine or anti-*Salmonella* activity may possibly be ascribed to antigenic stimulation, resulting in the presence of substantial numbers of cells making antibody with these specificities and subject to malignant transformation. This implies that the transformation can occur subsequent to magnification of the clone after exposure to antigen.

D. Amino Acid Sequences in Mouse λ Chains

A large preponderance of L chains in normal mouse serum is of the κ type; λ chains represent about 3 to 5% of the total and are very difficult to isolate for chemical studies. Occasionally, however, myeloma or Bence Jones proteins, experimentally produced in BALB/c mice, prove to be λ (52) and can be isolated in good yield.

A significant observation was reported by Appella and Perham who studied the type λ Bence Jones produced independently in two mice (53). Remarkably, these proteins were indistinguishable in their tryptic peptide maps, N-terminal sequences of 10 amino acids, and C-terminal nonapeptides (54). More recently, the complete sequence of one of these proteins was determined (55). In addition, each of the tryptic peptides of the other λ chain was isolated, and compositions and partial sequences of the peptides were analyzed. The tryptic peptides of both proteins were ordered by digestion with another enzyme, thermolysin. By all these criteria the two λ chains were identical (55). The complete sequence is shown in Fig. 4.1.

This work was extended by the important investigations of Weigert *et al.* (56,57) who investigated the amino acid sequences of the variable portions of twelve different λ chains. All the tryptic peptides were aligned and their amino acid compositions determined. A comparison with the sequence reported by Appella permitted the ordering of amino acids. The polypeptide chains sequenced included λ chains isolated from IgA myeloma proteins, as well as urinary Bence Jones proteins from mice with serum myeloma proteins of the IgA, IgM, and IgG2a classes. Two of the proteins were obtained from the transplantable tumors that were used by Appella and Perham.

The V regions of eight of the twelve λ chains appear to have identical amino acid sequences; two differ by one residue from these eight, one protein differs by two residues, and the other by three. Of the variations observed in the four proteins, all occurred at or near positions 25, 52, or 97, which are in or near hypervariable regions of human or mouse κ, and of human λ chains, and which are known to be associated with the antibody combining site.

These results contrast markedly with sequence data obtained with monoclonal human or mouse κ chains, or with human λ chains, where the sequence differences observed between a randomly chosen pair of chains of the same type or subtype are much greater and also involve portions of the V region other than hypervariable segments.

To account for their results, Weigert *et al.* propose that a very small number of germ line genes encode mouse λ chains. The variations are attributed to somatic mutation (occurring during the lifetime of the mouse). The fact that human κ chains of a given subgroup show greater variation in sequence was attributed to the greater life-span of the human which, they believe, would permit a larger number of mutations to occur. A corollary of this hypothesis is that each subgroup of human V_κ regions is encoded by a single, or a very small number of germ line genes.

Several, but not all BALB/c myeloma proteins with identical λ chains also had specific antibody activity directed to $\alpha(1 \to 3)$dextran. It is significant that one of these proteins (J558) is of the IgA class whereas another (MOPC 104E) is IgM; thus the proteins of two different classes can share identical L chains. The idiotypes of J558 and MOPC 104E are similar but not identical (57,58); this suggests the possibility that sequences in the hypervariable regions of the H chains of the two proteins may exhibit homology although they are probably not identical.

It is noteworthy that antibodies produced by normal BALB/c mice in response to immunization with $\alpha(1 \to 3)$dextran are almost exclusively λ and, in addition, share idiotype with protein J558. This supports the possibility that a malignant clone arises through transformation of a cell that has already undergone stimulation by antigen.

V. COMMON EVOLUTIONARY ORIGIN OF κ AND λ CHAINS OF HUMAN AND MOUSE ORIGIN

Table 4.1 includes a summary of the sequence homologies between mouse and human light chains of the κ and λ types. The data suggest a common evolutionary origin of mouse and human C_κ, C_λ, V_κ, and V_λ regions.[7] This is also supported by their general structural similarity; i.e., in length, location of disulfide loops, C-terminal or penultimate half-cystine linked to the H chain. The degree of relatedness between a randomly selected mouse and human V_κ sequence is approximately the same as that existing between two human V_κ sequences of different subgroups (e.g., $V_{\kappa I}$ and $V_{\kappa III}$), although not as great as the degree of similarity of two human V_κ sequences of the same subgroup. Also evident from Table 4.1 is that there is greater similarity between mouse and human C_λ sequences than between human C_λ and human C_κ; this again indicates a separate line of evolution of genes encoding κ and λ chains.

VI. AMINO ACID SEQUENCES IN RABBIT κ CHAINS[8]

We will discuss only briefly the rapidly increasing literature on this subject. Progress in the delineation of sequences of rabbit immunoglobulins has accelerated owing to the availability of homogeneous

---

[7] As indicated earlier, the degree of homology between V and C regions is insufficient to rule out completely the possibility of convergent evolution from different genes.

[8] Allotype-related sequences in rabbit immunoglobulins are discussed in Chapter 9.

```
                    1                                         10                                          20
Rabbit κ_B     Val Glu Val Leu Thr Gln Thr Pro Ser Pro Val Ser Ala Ala Val Gly Gly Thr Val Thr Ile Ser Cys Gln Ser Thr Lys Ser Ile

                   30                                         40                                          50
Rabbit κ_B     Tyr Asx Tyr Leu Ala Trp Tyr Gln Glx Lys Pro Gly Gln Pro Pro Lys Ala Leu Ile Tyr Thr Ala Ser Ser Leu Ala Ser Gly Val

                   60                                         70                                          80
Rabbit κ_B     Pro Ser Arg Phe Thr Gly Ser Gly Ser Gly Thr Glx Phe Thr Leu Thr Leu Ser Asp Val Glx Cys Asp Asp Ala Ala Thr Tyr Tyr

                   90                                        100                                         110
Rabbit κ_B     Cys Gly Gly Ala Asp Tyr Thr Gly Tyr Ser Phe Gly Gly Gly Thr Glu Val Val Val Lys Gly Asx Pro Val Ala Pro Thr Val Leu
Human  C_κ                                                                                            Thr Val Ala ——— Ser ——— Phe
Mouse  C_κ                                                                                            Ala Asx Ala ——— Thr ——— Ser

                  120                                        130                                         140
Rabbit κ_B     Ile Phe Pro Pro Ala Ala Asn Gln Val Ala Thr Gly Thr Val Ile Val Cys Val Ala Asx Lys Tyr Phe Pro Asp Val Thr Val
Human  C_κ         —— Ser Asp Glu ——— Leu Lys Ser ——— Ala Ser Val ——— Leu Leu Asn Asn Phe Tyr ——— Arg Glu Ala Lys
Mouse  C_κ         —— Ser Ser Glu ——— Leu Thr Gly ——— Ser Ala Ser Val ——— Phe Leu Asn Asn Phe Tyr ——— Lys Asp Ile Asn

                  150                                        160                                         170
Rabbit κ_B     Thr Ser Glx Val Gly Thr Trp Val Ser Glx (Asp Gly Thr Thr) Ile Glx Ser Lys Ile Ser Glx Asp Ser Asp Asp Cys Thr Tyr
Human  C_κ     Val Gln Trp Lys Val Asp Asn Ala Leu Gln Ser Gly Asn Ser    Gln Glu Ser Val Thr Glu Gln Asp Ser Lys ——— Ser Thr Tyr Ser
Mouse  C_κ     Val Lys Trp Lys Ile Asp Gly Ser Glu Arg Gln Asx ———  Val Leu (Asn Ser Trp Thr Asx Glx) Asp Ser Lys ——— Ser Thr Tyr Ser

                  180                                        190                       200
Rabbit κ_B     Leu Ser Ser Thr Leu Thr Leu Thr Ser Thr Glx Tyr Asp Ser His Lys Glx Tyr Thr Cys Lys Gly Thr Val Lys Glx (Ser Thr Gly
Human  C_κ                         Ser Lys Ala Asp ——— Glu Lys ———           Leu/Val  Ala ——— Glu Val ——— His Gln Gly Leu Ser Ser
Mouse  C_κ     Met ———             Lys Asx Glx ——— Glx Arg ——— (Asx Ser)               ——— Glx (Ala ——— His) ——— Thr (——— Ser

                  210                214
Rabbit κ_B     Thr Val Val Glx Ser Phe Asn Arg Gly Asx Cys
Human  C_κ     Pro ——— Thr Lys ——— Glu ———
Mouse  C_κ     Pro Ile ——— Lys ——— Asn Glu
```

Fig. 4.7. Amino acid sequence of the L chain derived from rabbit anti-*p*-azobenzoate antibody of restricted heterogeneity [from Appella *et al.* (58a)]. The constant region sequences of human and mouse κ chains are included for comparison.

	1				5					10					15					20					25	
Rabbit V$_{κI}$	Ala	Asp	Ile	Val	Met	Thr	Gln	Thr	Pro	Ala	Ser	Val	Glu	Ala	Ala	Val	Gly	Gly	Thr	Val	Thr	Ile	Lys	Cys	Arg	Ala
V$_{κII}$	Ala	–	Leu	Val	Met	Thr	Glu	Thr	Pro	Ala	Ser	Val	Ser	Ala	Ala	Val	Gly	Gly	Thr	Val	Thr	Ile	Asx	Cys	Glx	Ala
V$_{κIII}$	Ala	–	Val	Glu	Leu	Thr	Gln	Thr	Pro	Ala	Ser	Val	Glx	Ala	Ala	Val	Gly	Gly	Thr	Val	Thr	Ile	Lys	Cys	Glx	Ala
V$_{κIV}$	–	Asp	Val	Val	Met	Thr	Gln	Thr	Pro	Ala	Ser	Val	Ser	Glu	Pro	Val	Gly	Gly	Thr	Val	Thr	Ile	Lys	Cys	Gln	Ala
V$_{κV}$	–	Val	Glu	Val	Leu	Thr	Gln	Leu	Thr	Pro	Ser	Val	Ser	Ala	Ala	Val	Gly	Gly	Thr	Val	Thr	Ile	Ser	Cys	Gln	
V$_{κVI}$	–	Ile	Val	Met	Thr	Gln	Thr	Pro	Ser	Ser	Lys	Ser	Val	Pro	Val	Gly	Asx	Thr	Val	Thr	Ile	Asx	Cys	( )	Ala	
Man V$_{κI}$	–	Asp	Ile	Gln	Met	Thr	Gln	Ser	Pro	Ser	Ser	Leu	Ser	Ala	Ser	Val	Gly	Asp	Arg	Val	Thr	Ile	Thr	Cys	Gln	Ala
V$_{κII}$	–	Glu	Ile	Val	Leu	Thr	Gln	Ser	Pro	Gly	Thr	Leu	Ser	Leu	Ser	Pro	Gly	Glu	Arg	Ala	Thr	Leu	Ser	Cys	Arg	Ala
V$_{κIII}$	Glu	Asp	Ile	Val	Met	Thr	Gln	Ser	Pro	Leu	Ser	Leu	Pro	Val	Thr	Pro	Gly	Glu	Pro	Ala	Ser	Ile	Ser	Cys	Arg	Ser

Fig. 4.8. Prototype N-terminal sequences of six V$_κ$ subgroups of rabbit L chains compared with prototypes for three human V$_κ$ subgroups. Compiled by Braun and Jaton (58c). Light chains in groups V$_{κI}$, V$_{κII}$, V$_{κIII}$, V$_{κIV}$, and V$_{κVI}$ are those of antibodies to bacterial cell wall carbohydrates. The sole representative of V$_{κV}$ is from an anti-*p*-azobenzoate antibody. A total of 24 proteins were included in the compilation. There is considerable uncertainty in the subgrouping of the rabbit L chains, owing to the relatively small number of proteins sequenced and the fact that only partial sequences are available in most instances.

antibodies to streptococcal and pneumococcal carbohydrates and, to a lesser extent, to haptens (Chapter 10).

Figure 4.7 shows the complete amino acid sequence of a rabbit κ chain, reported by Appella *et al.* (58a). The κ chain (allotype b4) was isolated from a homogeneous preparation of rabbit anti-*p*-azobenzoate antibody from an individual rabbit. The constant regions of a human κ chain and a mouse κ chain are included for comparison. Of interest is the fact that no gaps need to be inserted to maximize homology. The degree of sequence homology in the C_κ region is: rabbit versus human, 32%; rabbit versus mouse, 34%; mouse versus human, 59%. A comparison of the rabbit C_κ sequence in Fig. 4.7 with that of normal rabbit L chains of the same allotype (b4) or with b4 L chains from a homogeneous antipneumococcal antibody preparation (58b), showed identity between positions 108 and 164. Differences were noted, however, at positions 165, 166, 169, and 176, suggesting the existence either of isotypes or of subclasses of allotype b4. Twenty-three of thirty residues that appear invariant in human κ chains are present in the V region of the rabbit κ chain. In comparing the rabbit V_κ region with human V_κ subgroups the largest degree of homology (46%) is observed with human $V_{\kappa II}$.

Figure 4.8 shows prototype N-terminal sequences, compiled by Braun and Jaton (58c), for six V_κ subgroups of rabbit L chains from homogeneous antibodies. The prototypes are based on a total of 24 published N-terminal sequences, mainly of antistreptococcal and antipneumococcal antibodies; each subgroup had 1–5 representatives. It seems probable that more subgroups exist. A feature of four of the subgroups is the presence of an additional, N-terminal alanine group, which is also nonhomologous with human or mouse κ chains. Another unique feature of rabbit κ chains (κ_B subtype) is the presence of a third intrachain disulfide bond in the V_κ region (58d) connecting half-cystine residues 80 and 171 in the V and C regions, respectively (58e). Light chains of subtype κ_A have two intrachain disulfide bonds (58d).

VII. AMINO ACID SEQUENCES IN HUMAN AND RABBIT H CHAINS

The technical problems in determining amino acid sequences in H chains are quite different from those encountered with L chains. Because of the large size of an H chain, complete sequence analysis is a formidable problem. Also, the N-terminus in many H chains is blocked; as a result the number of known N-terminal sequences of H chains is relatively small by comparison with L chains. An exception is the V_{HIII}

subgroup of H chains, which is almost always unblocked; a substantial number of N-terminal sequences has been determined. So far the complete sequences of two monoclonal human γ chains and two μ chains have been reported (2,3,59,59a,60), and the sequence of almost the entire C region (about 330 residues) of the rabbit γ-chain has been worked out (61–63). Partial sequences of a number of C_H regions have also been reported, and several human V_{HIII} regions have been completely sequenced (discussed below).

Sequence data on the C region of the H chain can be obtained with the normal immunoglobulin of certain species. This is of particular importance when the species is not susceptible to multiple myeloma. Normal rabbit γ-chains can, for example, be cleaved in the hinge region by various enzymes. The resulting crystallizable Fc fragment is sufficiently homogeneous for sequence studies, which are complicated only by minor allotypic variations. On the other hand, when normal human IgG is cleaved with papain, the resulting Fc fragments are heterogeneous since they are derived from each of the four subgroups; for this reason, it is necessary to work with human myeloma proteins.

A technique that has proved useful as the initial step in determining the sequence of an H chain is cleavage with cyanogen bromide (e.g., 64,65). This reagent selectively attacks peptide bonds adjacent to methionine residues. The methionine is converted to homoserine which then constitutes the C-terminal residue of a fragment. Because of the low methionine content of H chains only a few polypeptides result from the cleavage; these are frequently small enough, however, to permit further sequence analysis by conventional methods, including further degradation with proteolytic enzymes.

In this chapter we will discuss sequences of human H chains, with some reference to H chains of the rabbit.

A. General Structural Features of Human H Chains

Table 3.1 lists the approximate molecular weight and carbohydrate content of H chains of the major human immunoglobulin classes. Exclusive of carbohydrate content the molecular weights of the γ and α chains are approximately equal; the μ, δ, and ϵ chains are somewhat larger. The H and L chain that constitute the basic subunit of each class are linked by an interchain disulfide bond and by noncovalent interactions. [In the $A_2m(1)$ genetic variant of human IgA2, the L chains are bound to H chains only through noncovalent interactions.] The general locations of interchain disulfide bonds in the various classes are indicated by the sketches in Table 3.1. Each H chain is joined to an L chain through a

single disulfide bond, but there is wide variation in the number of interheavy chain disulfide bonds; the largest number, ~15, is found in the
IgG3 molecule (Chapter 3). In each IgG subclass the interheavy chain
disulfide bonds are clustered in the hinge region, near the center of the
chain. In IgM, one of the intrasubunit interheavy chain bonds is located
in the hinge region, the other next to the C-terminus. The half-cystine
which contributes to the disulfide bond joining the H and L chains originates in the hinge region of IgG1 (at position 220) but near position 130[9]
in the other three subclasses of IgG, in the μ-chain, in the rabbit γ-chain
(2,60,66–70), and in a variety of other immunoglobulins. (X-Ray crystallography indicates that residues 130 and 220 are in close proximity.)
Each domain contains an intrachain disulfide loop encompassing about
55 to 70 amino acid residues. There are four domains in the human γ
chain of each subclass, four in the rabbit γ chain, five in human μ and ϵ,
and, probably, five in the human δ chain.

B. Sequences in the Constant Regions of Human and Rabbit H Chains

1. GENERAL CONSIDERATIONS

As in the L chain, the V region of a human H chain occupies a
linear, N-terminal sequence. It comprises approximately 118–124 residues, which makes the segment slightly larger than a V_L domain. The C
region of a human γ chain is about three times as large as a C_L segment.
Different classes of immunoglobulin appear to share the same V_H
regions, reflecting the probable biosynthesis of the complete chain under
the control of two separate genes. Sequences in V_H regions will therefore be discussed independently of the classes of immunoglobulin from
which they were derived.

The various classes and subclasses of human immunoglobulins,
which were initially defined by their antigenic structures, are characterized by distinctive sequences in the C regions of H chains. So far no
definitive evidence has been obtained to indicate that carbohydrate side
chains contribute significantly to the formation of antigenic determinants
which characterize the individual classes. Genetic polymorphism in the
C region, within a class or subclass, is associated with only minor variations in amino acid sequence. In contrast, the number and variability of
V region sequences is very large.

Figure 4.9 tabulates known amino acid sequences in the C regions

---

[9] Numbering system of the γ_1 chain of protein Eu (2).

of human γ chains of the four subclasses, and of the C region of the rabbit γ chain. The amino acid sequence of a μ chain is shown in Fig. 4.10, where it is compared with the C_γ sequence of IgG1, and a partial sequence of the ϵ chain is presented in Fig. 4.13. All the sequences shown, with the exception of that of the rabbit protein, are of myeloma proteins or of a Waldenström macroglobulin. The numbering system used for γ chains is that of Edelman *et al.* (2), who first reported a complete H chain sequence (of protein Eu). The sequences are discussed at some length in the following sections. An obvious and striking feature of the data is the homology of sequence that exists between the C_H regions of all the chains tabulated. The degree of homology between various pairs of chains is listed in Table 4.1.

2. INTERNAL STRUCTURAL HOMOLOGY OF C REGION DOMAINS

The intrachain disulfide loops in each of the H chains are similar in their linear disposition to those in L chains. The presence of one disulfide loop for each 110 to 120 amino acid residues provided the first clue suggesting that there are internal homologies of sequence in the polypeptide chain (22). This was further demonstrated by a comparison of partial sequences in the two halves of the Fc fragment of rabbit IgG (61,71); the Fc fragment comprises two domains (C_H2 and C_H3). The degree of sequence homology between these domains is approximately 30%. In addition, there are many positions in which side chains with similar chemical properties (e.g., isoleucine and valine) are present in the two segments.

A comparison of the three C_H segments of a human IgG1 heavy chain indicates that in a sequence of 100 residues any pair of C_H segments is identical with respect to 29 to 34 residues (70) (Fig. 1.4). Statistical analysis showed that this degree of homology is highly significant. By contrast, a comparison of V_L with C_L, or V_H with a C_H domain, indicated an average degree of homology of about 15%. This, together with the similarity in length, amino acid composition, and disulfide bonded structure suggests a common evolutionary origin, but very early divergence of genes controlling V and C regions.

3. LENGTHS OF AMINO ACID SEQUENCES IN INTRACHAIN DISULFIDE LOOPS; THE HINGE REGION OF IgG

When amino acid sequences of different proteins, or of different domains of a given polypeptide chain, are compared, the half-cystine residues are normally placed in exact alignment. One evidence of the degree of homology, therefore, is the size of the disulfide loop, which de-

Positions 115–150

Protein	115					120					125					130					135					140					145					150
Human γ₁	Val	Ser	Ser	Ala	Ser	Thr	Lys	Gly	Pro	Ser	Val	Phe	Pro	Leu	Ala	Pro	Ser	Ser	Lys	Ser	Thr	Ser	Gly	Gly	Thr	Ala	Ala	Leu	Gly	Cys	Leu	Val	Lys	Asp	Tyr	Phe

To L chain (below position 130)

- γ₂: —— Cys —— Arg —— (—— Glu Ser ——
- γ₃: —L— Cys —L— Arg —— Glu Ser ——
- γ₄: —L— Cys —L— Arg —— Glu Ser ——
- Rabbit γ: Ser Glx Pro Ser Gly —— Ala —— Cys Cys Gly Asp —— Pro Ser Ser —— Val Thr —— Gly —— Leu

Positions 155–180

Protein	155					160					165					170					175					180
Human γ₁	Pro	Glu	Pro	Val	Thr	Val	Ser	Trp	Asn	Ser	Gly	Ala	Leu	Thr	Ser	Gly	Val	His	Thr	Phe	Pro	Ala	Val	Leu	Gln	Ser	Ser	Gly	Leu	Tyr	Ser	Leu	Ser	Ser
Rabbit γ	—— Thr ——							—— Thr ——					—— Asp ——					—— Arg ——					—— Ser ——		—— Arg ——	—— Val Pro ——

Positions 185–215

Protein	185					190					195					200					205					210					215
Human γ₁	Val	Val	Thr	Val	Pro	Ser	Ser	Ser	Leu	Gly	Thr	Gln	Thr	Tyr	Ile	Cys	Asn	Val	Asn	His	Lys	Pro	Ser	Asn	Thr	Lys	Val	Asp	Lys	Arg	Val Glu Pro
γ₂													—— Thr ——					—— Asp ——									H —— Thr ——				Lys Arg
γ₃											(—— Tyr ——					—— Asx ——										H —— Lys)(Cys Thr Pro His) Arg Cys Pro ——						Ser
γ₄											—— Thr ——					—— Asp ——														Arg
Rabbit γ	—— Thr ——	—— Ser ——						—								— Ser Glx Pro (Pro Ser) Thr ——					—— Ala — Thr Asx ——								—— Thr ——		Ala

Positions 220–250

Protein	220					225					230					235					240					245					250
Human γ	Lys	Ser	Cys L	Asp	Lys	Thr	His	Thr	Cys H	Pro	Pro H	Cys H	Pro	Ala	Pro	Glu	Leu	Leu	Gly	Gly	Pro	Ser	Val	Phe	Pne	Pro	Pro	Lys	Pro	Lys	Asp Thr Leu Met Ile
γ₂	—— Cys ——					— — Val Glu ——					H					—— Pro Val Ala														——
γ₃						—— Thr Pro Pro Pro ——					H —— Arg ——																			
γ₄						—— Tyr Gly — — Pro Pro ——					H					—— Ser —— Phe ——													
Rabbit γ	Ser —— Thr —— Ser ——						Thr Met				— — —					—										—— Ile ——				(——)

Positions 255–285

Protein	255					260					265					270					275					280					285
Human γ₁	Ser	Arg	Thr	Pro	Glu	Val	Thr	Cys	Val	Val	Val	Asp	Val	Ser	His	Glu	Asp	Pro	Gln	Val	Lys	Phe	Asn	Trp	Tyr	Val	Asp	Gly	Val	Gln	Val	His	Asn	Ala	Lys	Thr
γ₂																—— Glx Asx ——					—— Glx ——					—— Asx ——					—— Glx ——					Asx
γ₃																—— (——) ——					—— Glx ——															
γ₄																—— Gln —— (——)					—— Glx ——										—— Glu ——					
Rabbit γ																—— (Glu Asp) ——					—— (Glx) ——			Thr		—— Ile ——					—— Asp Glu ——			Arg Thr —— Arg Pro

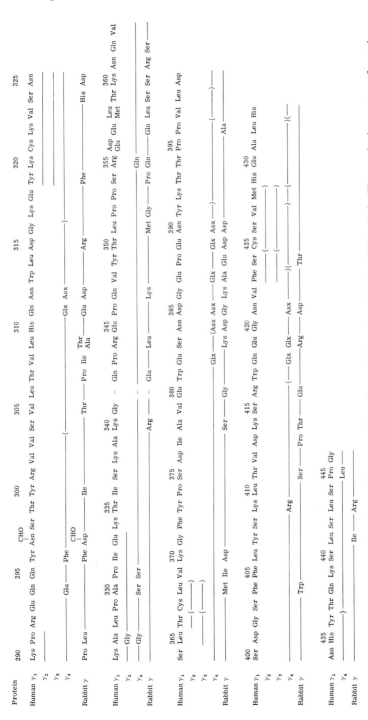

Fig. 4.9. Sequences in the C_H regions of human γ chains (four subclasses) and of the rabbit γ chain. The numbering system of protein Eu (IgG1) is used (2). References for human IgG1 ($γ_1$) are 2, 59, 78, and 92; for IgG2 ($γ_2$): 79, 89, 90, and 168; IgG3 ($γ_3$): 80, 167, and 168; IgG4 ($γ_4$): 88 and 167; rabbit IgG: 71, 61–63, 169. The symbols L or H adjacent to a Cys group indicate a disulfide bond linking that Cys to an L or H chain, respectively. Other Cys residues are involved in intrachain disulfide loops. The symbol, CHO, represents carbohydrate. Allotype-related substitutions, shown in the table, are discussed in Chapter 9.

This page presents a protein sequence alignment (immunoglobulin μ and γ1 heavy chains).

```
    1
μ   Glp Val Thr Leu Thr Glu Ser Gly Pro Ala Leu Val Lys Pro Lys Gln Pro Leu Thr Leu Thr Cys Thr Phe Ser ⌐S
    26                                                                                                     |
    Gly Phe Ser Leu Ser Thr Ser Arg Met Arg Val Ser Trp Ile Arg Gln Pro Pro Gly Lys Ala Leu Glu Trp Leu  ⌐S
    51                                                                                                     |
    Ala Arg Ile Asx Asx Asp Lys Phe Tyr Ser Thr Ser Leu Arg Thr Arg Leu Ser Ile Ser Lys Asn Asp
    76
    Ser Lys Asn Gln Val Val Leu Ile Met Ile Asn Val Asn Pro Val Asp Thr Ala Thr Tyr Tyr Cys Ala Arg Val
```

Variable ⟷ | Constant

```
     101
μ    Val Asn Ser Val Met Ala Gly Tyr Tyr Tyr Tyr Tyr Met Asp Val Trp Gly Lys Gly Thr Thr Val Thr Val Ser
γ1                                                                                                        ──S──      → Light chain

     126
μ    Ser Gly Ser Ala Ser Ala Pro Thr Leu Phe Pro Leu Val Ser Cys Glu Asn Ser (Asx Pro Ser) Ser (Thr) Val Ala
γ1   Ala ──Thr Lys Gly── Ser Val── Ala Pro Ser Ser Lys── Thr Ser Gly Gly── Ala──

     151                            ┌──S──S──┐          To Cys 212
μ    Val Gly Cys Leu Ala Glx Asp Phe Leu Pro Asp Ser Ile Thr Phe Ser Trp Lys Tyr (Asn Asx Ser Asx Lys)
γ1   Leu── Val Lys── Tyr Phe── Glu Pro Val── Val── — — Ser Gly Ala Leu
                                                    (CHO)

     175
μ    Ile Ser Ser Thr Arg Gly Phe Pro Ser Val Leu Arg — Gly Gly Lys Tyr Ala Ala Thr (Ser Glx) Val Leu Leu
γ1   Thr── Gly Val His Thr── Ala── Gln Ser Ser── Leu── Ser Leu Ser── Val── Thr Val

     199                                            Fd'↓
μ    Pro Ser Lys — Asp Val Met Gln Gly Thr Asp Glu His Val Cys Lys Trp Val Gln His Pro Asn Gly Asx Lys
γ1   Ser Ser Leu Gly Thr── Thr Tyr Ile — — Asn — Asn── Lys Pro Ser Asn Thr

     223
μ    Gln Lys Asx Val Pro Leu Pro Val Ile Ala Glu Leu Pro Pro Lys Val Ser Val Phe Val Pro Pro Arg Asx Gly
γ1   — — Asp Lys Arg── Glu Pro Lys Ser Cys

     248                                                                                                ⌐S
μ    Phe Phe Gly Asx Pro Arg Lys Ser Lys Leu Ile Cys Gln Ala Thr Gly Phe Ser Pro Arg Gln Val Trp Ser Leu|
     273                                                                                                ⌐S
     Arg Glu Gly Lys Gln Val Gly Ser Gly Val Thr Thr Asx Glx Val Glx Ala Glx Ala Lys Glx Ser Gly Pro Thr|
     298
     Thr Tyr Lys Val Thr Ser Thr Leu Thr Ile Lys Glx Ser Asp Trp Leu Gly Glu Ser Met Phe Thr Cys Arg Val
```

172

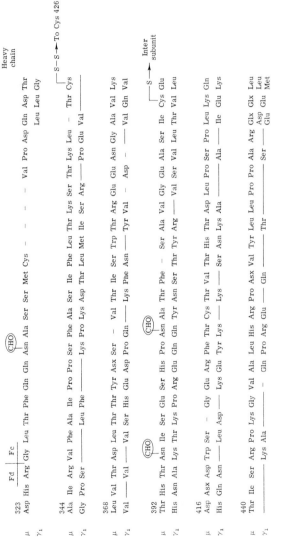

Heavy chain

Fig. 4.10. The complete amino acid sequence of a human μ chain, published by Putnam *et al.* (60). The sequence of the Cμ region resembles closely that of the μ chain of another Waldenström macroglobulin, reported by Watanabe *et al.* (59a). Locations of interchain and intrachain disulfide bonds and of the five carbohydrate groups are shown. The sequence of the C_H region of a γ₁ protein (Eu; reference 2) is included for comparison.

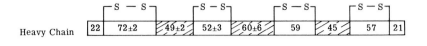

Heavy Chain

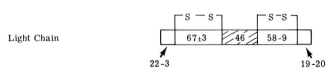

Light Chain

Fig. 4.11. Size variation in the pseudosubunit structures (domains or homology regions) of the H and L chains of human IgG. Lengths of sequence within the disulfide loops and outside disulfide loops are given. The limits of variation shown represent the range of lengths among the IgG subclasses. Reproduced, with permission, from Milstein and Svasti (72).

termines the number of gaps or insertions that are necessary to permit the alignment of cystine residues. Lengths of stretches of amino acids within such loops and between successive loops are shown in Fig. 4.11 (72). It is evident that there is a greater length of sequence between the second (C_H1) and third (C_H2) disulfide loops than between any other successive pair. The number of amino acid residues between the C_H1 and C_H2 disulfide loops is 10–15 residues greater than the number between the C_H2 and C_H3 loops. The extra stretch of sequence is in the hinge region; in IgG1 it comprises residues 221 to 233. This region shows considerable diversity of sequence when two H chains of different classes or subclasses are compared. It is the region in which most interheavy chain disulfide bonds originate and which, in IgG1, contains the half-cystine which is joined to an L chain. The flexibility of this region is believed to be responsible for the mobility of the Fab segment. It is also the site of preferential proteolytic attack by various enzymes. The sequence in the hinge region appears to have evolved independently since it does not have its counterpart elsewhere in the polypeptide chain. Amino acid sequences in the hinge regions of rabbit IgG and the four human IgG subclasses are shown in Fig. 4.12.

In addition to half-cystine, proline is found in unusually high frequency in the hinge regions of rabbit and human γ chains. For example, the γ_1 chain has five prolines between residues 211 and 234. Welscher (73) proposes that the prolines lend rigidity to one segment of the otherwise flexible hinge region and prevent adjacent sequences from folding in such a manner as to make contact with the hinge; the latter is therefore exposed and susceptible to proteolysis.

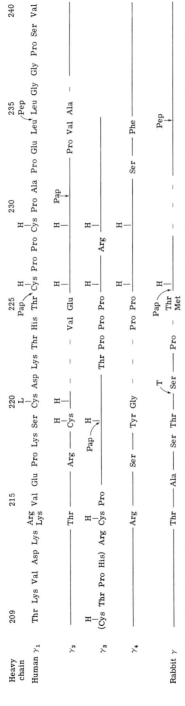

Fig. 4.12. Amino acid sequences and sites of enzymatic cleavage in the hinge regions of human and rabbit γ chains. The symbol H represents the site of an interheavy chain disulfide bond and the symbol L designates the site of a heavy-light chain disulfide bond. The half-cystine at position 220 of the rabbit γ-chain forms an intrachain disulfide loop with Cys 131 or 132. The Eu numbering system is used (2). Pap, Pep, and T refer to cleavage sites for papain, pepsin, and trypsin, respectively. The site of cleavage of the rabbit H chain by papain is that for molecules of allotype d11. Hydrolysis by papain of molecules of allotype d12 is described in the text. Cleavage of the rabbit H chain by trypsin at position 220 occurs only after reduction and aminoethylation (by ethyleneimine) of Cys-220. The symbol CHO represents carbohydrate. References are given in the legend of Fig. 4.9.

4. POSSIBLE HINGE REGION OF IgM

It is difficult to localize a hinge region in the human μ chain, although electron microscopy indicates that the molecule is flexible. One major site of cleavage by trypsin at 65° is at position 325 (μ chain numbering system), which is fairly close to the site of attachment of a carbohydrate group (Fig. 4.10). Paul *et al.* postulate that the hydrophilic carbohydrate tends to be exposed to the aqueous medium, causing this segment of the chain to remain unfolded; this could permit freedom of rotation in this region and account for its susceptibility to enzymatic cleavage (74,74a). [In most rabbit γ chains of allotype d12, a small unbranched oligosaccharide is covalently linked to threonine in the hinge region at position 226; molecules of allotype d11 have methionine, but no carbohydrate, at this position (75–77).] Sequences of the four C_H domains of the μ chain can be aligned without allowing for a hinge region.

5. HINGE REGION OF IgA1 AND IgA2

Frangione and Wolfenstein-Todel isolated and sequenced the hinge regions of IgA1 and IgA2 myeloma proteins (77a). Both contain three half-cystine residues and are rich in proline. Of considerable interest was the finding of a duplication of a small segment of the hinge region in IgA1 but not IgA2; the sequence of the duplicated segment is -Pro-Ser-Thr-Pro-Pro-Thr-Pro-. Carbohydrate is attached to a serine in the hinge region of IgA1 but not IgA2. The authors suggest that the duplication occurred either as a result of tandem duplication or gene insertion, followed by unequal crossing-over. They discuss the possibility of separate genetic control of the hinge region; this will be considered later, after describing deletions observed in proteins associated with "Heavy Chain" disease (this Chapter, Section VII,D).

6. SEQUENCE OF THE HUMAN μ CHAIN

During 1973, the complete sequences of two human μ chains (Gal and Ou) were reported, from the laboratories of N. Hilschmann and F.W. Putnam (59a,60). The C_H region sequences of the two proteins exhibit only minor differences, which may reflect experimental error. (The existence of subclasses of human IgM has not been established.) The complete sequence of protein Ou, as reported by Putnam *et al.* (60), is shown in Fig. 4.10. The protein comprises five domains: one V_H and four C_H; as indicated above, it is difficult to localize a hinge region comparable to that present in IgG. In fact, Watanabe *et al.* (59a) align the sequences of the four C_μ domains with one another, without any major insertions that could represent the hinge region. There is, however, an additional "tail" of 19 amino acids, at the C-terminus of the molecule, which does not have its counterpart in C_H1, C_H2, or C_H3. A homologous C-terminal segment is also seen in IgA (Table 7.5), but not in IgG nor IgE. When the four C_H domains of protein Gal are optimally aligned (allowing gaps where necessary, and not including the 19-residue "tail") the degree of homology is: C_H1 versus C_H2, 18%; C_H1 versus C_H3, 24%; C_H1 versus C_H4, 19%; C_H2 versus C_H3, 24%; C_H2 versus C_H4, 28%; C_H3 versus C_H4, 30%. This, again, can be explained by duplication of a primordial gene encoding one domain. Watanabe *et al.* compared sequences in the γ_1 chain (protein Eu) with those in the μ chain of protein Gal, by aligning $C_\gamma1$ with $C_\mu1$, $C_\gamma2$ with $C_\mu3$, and $C_\gamma3$ with $C_\mu4$. The hinge region of γ_1 (residues 221–223) was omitted. The overall degree of homology found was 33%.

7. PARTIAL AMINO ACID SEQUENCE OF THE ϵ CHAIN

The sequence of the C-terminal domain (118 residues) of the H chain of an IgE myeloma protein, reported by Bennich *et al.* (77b), is shown in Fig. 4.13. The C-terminal sequences of the γ_1 chain and of a portion of the C_H4 domain of the μ chain are included for comparison. (The segment of the μ chain shown represents all but the C-terminal 18 residues, which are not homologous with sequences in γ or ϵ chains.) The 18-residue "tail" is found, however, in the α as well as the μ chain (Table 7.5). A number of gaps are inserted for optimal alignment. The percentage homology, expressed in terms of number of identical amino acids in the sequence, is 27% for ϵ and μ, 37% for ϵ and γ, and 41% for γ and μ. (Gln and Glx are considered identical.) The authors concluded that the ϵ and μ chains diverged prior to the divergence of γ and μ. This is somewhat conjectural since the overall homology between C_γ and C_μ is only 33%.

8. CLEAVAGE OF H CHAINS IN THE HINGE REGION

The types and properties of fragments produced upon enzymatic cleavage of the H chain were described in general terms in Chapter 3. We will concentrate here on specific sites of cleavage with reference to amino acid sequence. In each case discussed, cleavage occurs in or near the hinge region of the H chain.

Figure 4.12 indicates sites of preferential, limited cleavage of H chains by papain, pepsin, or trypsin. Limited cleavage by enzymes occurs only under mild conditions; after reduction of intrachain disulfide bonds, or various other forms of denaturation, extensive enzymatic degradation takes place.

Sequence

438
ε   Met Arg Ser Thr Thr Lys Thr Ser Gly – Pro Arg Ala Ala – Pro Glu Val Tyr Ala Glu Ala Thr Pro Glu Trp
γ₁ Glu Lys Thr Ile Ser Lys Ala Lys Gly Gln – Pro Gln Val Tyr Thr Leu Pro Pro Ser Arg/Gln Glu/Arg
μ   Lys Gln Thr Ile Ser Arg Pro Lys Gly Val Ala Leu His Arg Pro Asx Val Tyr Leu Leu Pro Pro Ala Arg Glx

463
ε   Pro – Gly Ser Arg Asp Lys Arg Thr Leu Ala Cys Leu Ile Gln Asn Phe Met Pro Glu Asp Ile Ser Val Gln
γ₁ Glu – Met Thr Lys Asn Gln Val Ser Leu Thr Cys Leu Val Lys Gly Phe Tyr Pro Ser Asp Ile Ala Val Glu
μ   Glx Leu Asn Leu Arg Glu Ser Ala Thr Ile Thr Cys Leu Val Thr Gly Phe Ser Pro Ala Asp Val Phe Val Glx

488
ε   Trp Leu His Asn Glu Val Gln – Leu Pro Asp Ala Arg His Ser Thr Thr Gln Pro – Arg Lys Thr Lys –
γ₁ Trp Glu Ser Asn Asp Gly Glu Pro – – Glu Asn Tyr Lys Thr Thr Pro Pro Val Leu Asp Ser – Asp –
μ   Trp – Met Gln Arg Gly Glu Pro Leu Ser Pro Gln Lys Tyr Val Thr Ser Ala Pro Met Pro Glu Pro Gln Ala Pro

513
ε   Gly Ser Gly Phe Phe Val Phe Ser Arg Leu Glu Val Thr Arg Ala Glu Trp Gln Glu Lys Asp Glu Phe Ile Cys
γ₁ Gly Ser – Phe Phe Leu Tyr Ser Lys/Arg Leu Thr Val Asp Lys Ser Arg Trp Gln Gln Gly Asn Val Phe Ser Cys
μ   Gly Arg – Tyr Phe Ala His Ser Ile/Leu Leu Thr Val Ser Glu Glu Trp Asn Thr Gly Gln Thr Tyr Thr Cys

537   558
ε   Arg Ala Val His Glu Ala Ala Ser Pro Ser Gln Thr Val Gln Arg Ala Val Ser Val Asn Pro Gly Lys COOH
γ₁ Ser Val Met His Glu Ala Leu His Asn His Tyr Thr Gln – Gln Lys Ser Leu Ser Leu Ser Pro Gly Leu COOH
μ   Val Val Ala His Glu Ala Leu His Asn Arg Tyr Thr Gln Lys Ser Leu Ser Leu Ser Pro Gly Lys

Fig. 4.13. Sequence of the C-terminal region (C_H4 domain) of the human ε chain. From Bennich *et al.* (77b). The C-terminal sequence of the γ1 chain (2) and all but the last 19 residues of the μ chain [which are nonhomologous with ε or γ (59a,60)] are included for comparison. The numbering system is that of the μ chain of protein Ou (60). The μ chain has an additional C-terminal sequence of 19 residues.

a. Papain. In human IgG1, papain selectively hydrolyzes the peptide bond N-terminal to half-cystine 226 or that between His 224 and Thr 225 (Cys 226 participates in an interheavy chain disulfide bond) (78). IgG2 is cleaved first between residues 230 and 231 (Pro-Ala) and later at an indeterminate position in the hinge region on the N-terminal side of the two interheavy chain disulfide bonds (79). After the initial cleavage of IgG2 the Fab fragments are still linked by S–S bonds; i.e., the molecule is bivalent. The subsequent cleavage yields monomeric Fab. In IgG3, proteolysis occurs just N-terminal to a half-cystine (Cys 219) which forms an interheavy chain disulfide bond (80). The H–H disulfide bond at Cys 214 is presumably cleaved by the reducing agent present, resulting in the release of Fab fragments.

Papain initially cleaves the H chain of rabbit IgG of allotype d11, which has methionine as residue 225, between that amino acid and the adjacent half-cystine 226, yielding univalent fragments (76). Additional cleavage toward the N-terminus may occur upon prolonged digestion. When threonine, instead of methionine, is present at position 225 (allotype d12), some proteolysis may still occur between the threonine and cystine, but most molecules are cleaved between residues 220 and 221 (Cys-Ser) or 221 and 222 (Ser-Lys) (76); again univalent fragments are liberated. The relative resistance to papain of the Thr-Cys bond may be caused by steric interference of the carbohydrate which is usually attached to the threonine group (76). (See also, references 81 and 82.)

b. Pepsin. Pepsin, at pH 4, selectively cleaves human IgG1 and rabbit IgG at homologous positions, between the two leucine residues at positions 234 and 235 (78,81). The exact site of cleavage in the other subclasses of human IgG is uncertain, although $F(ab')_2$ fragments are produced. Pepsin degrades the C_H2 domain of each subclass but leaves essentially intact a noncovalently bonded dimer of C_H3, designated pFc'. A similar but slightly smaller fragment is also produced, together with Fc, by proteolysis with papain. These cleavages are discussed in some detail in Chapter 3. Pepsin does not liberate large fragments in good yield from IgM. Paul *et al.* suggest that this may be attributable to the absence in IgM of a Leu-Leu bond corresponding to that in IgG1 (74).

c. Trypsin. The enzyme of choice (83,84) for producing Fab fragments from human IgM is trypsin, which hydrolyzes peptide bonds C-terminal to a lysine or arginine residue. The bond hydrolyzed at 65°C (84) may be exposed through a conformational change at the higher temperature. Digestion at 65°C for a few minutes produces ten Fab fragments and an interesting polymer comprising five Fc fragments, held together by the intersubunit disulfide bonds. Because of its high molecular weight, this pentameric unit is easily separated by gel filtration. It then crystallizes spontaneously (84).

During proteolysis by trypsin at 37°C the peptide bond cleaved is apparently that between Arg 346 and Val 347 (84a). At 60°–65°C the bond cleaved is at Arg 325 (59a,84a) (Fig. 4.10).

Human IgG1 is hydrolyzed by trypsin next to lysine 222 in the hinge region, releasing monovalent, Fab_t fragments (85) (t for trypsin). Rabbit IgG is resistant to trypsin under nondenaturing conditions; lysine 222 in the rabbit protein is followed by proline, which reduces the susceptibility to that enzyme. Fab fragments can be produced, however, from rabbit IgG by tryptic digestion if the half-cystine at position 220 is first reduced and treated with ethyleneimine; these reactions convert cystine to aminoethylcysteine, which is positively charged and provides a site of attack for trypsin. Cleavage then occurs between residues 220 and 221 (81).

d. Cyanogen Bromide. In the presence of 70% formic acid, cyanogen bromide will cleave essentially all polypeptide bonds on the C-terminal side of methionine residues in the denatured protein; methionine is converted to homoserine in the process. This is a very useful reaction in sequence analysis because the methionine content of most proteins is low and only a small number of peptides is produced. Under less drastic conditions, in dilute HCl, methionine residues near the hinge region may be preferentially attacked. Rabbit IgG is cleaved between methionine 252 and isoleucine 253 in the γ chain to produce a bivalent fragment, designated $F(ab'')_2$, which is somewhat larger than $F(ab')_2$ formed by peptic digestion. Subsequent reduction of the single interheavy chain disulfide bond yields monovalent Fab'' fragments (86,81). Sites of cleavage of human IgG1 by cyanogen bromide are discussed in references 86a and 87.

9. COMPARISON OF AMINO ACID SEQUENCES IN THE CONSTANT REGIONS OF RABBIT AND HUMAN H CHAINS

An examination of the sequences in Figs. 4.9 and 4.10 indicates that extensive homology exists among the amino acid sequences of C_H regions of the four subclasses of human IgG, of human IgM, and rabbit IgG. Pink *et al.* (88) compared nearly complete sequences of human IgG1, human IgG4, and rabbit IgG from the hinge region to the C-terminus and found that, with appropriate deletions, the degree of homology between rabbit IgG and human IgG4 is 68% (130 of 190 residues compared are the same). Between rabbit IgG and human IgG1 there is 69% homology (87). Between human IgG1 and IgG4 there are only 14 differences out of 220 known residues (94% homology); subclasses IgG2 and IgG3 show comparable homology to each other and to IgG1 and IgG4 (67,89,90).

These very close similarities among the human IgG subclasses do not apply to their hinge regions (Fig. 4.12). The degree of homology between any two subclasses from residues 208 to 237 is about 60 to 70%, as compared to values greater than 90% in the remainder of the Fc segment of the H chain. Because of this, it has been suggested that successful mutations may have occurred at a more rapid rate in the hinge region than in the remainder of the C_H segment (79). Mutations in the hinge region might be tolerated if this region does not have a biological effector function (such as complement fixation), since it probably does not interact with other segments of the same chain; such interactions, where they occur, may require evolutionary conservatism. The suggestion also occurs repeatedly in the literature that the hinge region may be encoded by a separate gene which is somehow joined or inserted between other genes encoding the H chain.

The close relationship among sequences of the H chains of the four IgG subclasses suggests that their evolutionary divergence is a relatively recent event, as compared to the divergence of IgM and IgG. (The degree of homology between C_γ and C_μ is about 33%.) The fact that rabbit IgG is more closely related than human IgM to human IgG (Table 4.1) indicates that the divergence of IgM from IgG was a relatively early event; it may have occurred at about the time of emergence of the lungfish (Chapter 7).

The sequence of the α chain is currently being studied in two or three laboratories and will undoubtedly be worked out in the near future. The C-terminal sequence of 40 residues, published by Chuang *et al.* (60a) is shown in Table 7.5. (The hinge region was already discussed.) That IgA more closely resembles IgM than IgG is shown by the presence of an additional, homologous 19 residues in the α and μ chains following the termination of γ chains, and by the somewhat greater degree of homology of α and μ, as compared to γ and μ, in the regions where such comparisons can be made. Implications with respect to the evolution of immunoglobulins and the subject of the divergence of IgG subclasses are considered in Chapter 7.

C. Sequences in the Variable Regions of Human H Chains

In contrast to the C region of human H chains, sequences in the V regions are not class-specific. This is illustrated in Fig. 4.14, which shows the complete amino acid sequences of the V_H regions of a number

	1	10	20	30	40	50	60
V_H I							
Eu (γ1)	Z V Q L V E S G A E V K K P G S S V K V S C K A S G G T F S R S A I I - - W V R Q A P G Q G L E W M G G I V P M F G P P
V_H II							
Daw (γ1)	Z V T L R E S G P A L V R P T Q T L T L T C T F S G F S L S G E T M C V A W I R Q P P G E A L E W L A W D I L - N D D K
Ou (μ)	Z — — — T — — — — — — K — P — — — — — — — — — — — — — — — T S R — S — — — — — — — — — — — — — — — R — — K — — — — — — — — — —
He (γ1)	Z — — K — N — — — T — — K — — — — — — — L — — — — — L — — T T D G V A — G — — — — — — — — — — — — — — — G — R — — — — L L Y W
Cor (γ1)	Z — — K — — — — — — — — — K — — — — — — — — — — — — — — — — S T G — — — — G — — — — — — — — — — — — — — — K G — — — — R — D W D
V_H III							
Tei (γ1)	E V Q L V E S G G G L V Q P G G S L R L S C A A S G F T F S T S A V Y - - W V R Q A P G K G L E W V G W R Y E G S S L T
Was (γ1)	— — — — — — — — — — L — — — — — — — — — — — — — — — — S — — — D — M - - — — — — — — — — — — — — — — — A — K — Q E A — N S
Jon (γ3)	D — — — — — — — — — — — — — — — K — — — — — — — — — — — A W M K - - — — — — — — — — — — — — — — — V — V — Q V V E K
Zap (α1)	— — — — — — — — — — — — — — K — — — — — — — — — — — — T S R F - - — — — — — — — — — — — — — — — E F — V Q — A I S
Tur (α1)	— — L — — — — — — — — A — — — — — — — — — — — — — — — R Y L S S - - — — — — — — — — — — — — — — — S G — L N A — N L
Nie (γ1)	Z — Q — — — — — — — — — V — — R — — — — — — — — — — — R Y T I H - - — — — — — — — — — — — — — — — A V M S Y B G B B K
Gal (μ)	— — — — — — — — — — — D — — R — — — — — — — — — — — (B V L B B F) M T - - — — — — — — — — — — — — — — — A N I K Z B G — Z Z
Til (γ2)	— — L — Y V M
Til (μ)	— — L — Y V M

	70	80	90	100	110	120
V_H I						
Eu (γ1)	N Y A Q K F Q G R V T I T A D E S T N T A Y M E L S S L R S E D T A F Y F C A G G Y G I - - - - Y S P E E Y N G G L V
V_H II						
Daw (γ1)	Y - G A S L E T R L A V S K D T S K N Q V V L I M I N V N P V D T A T Y Y C A R V V N S V M A G Y Y M D V W G K G T T V
Ou (μ)	— W S T — R — — — S I — — N D — — — — — — — — — T — T — M D — — — — — — — — — V H R H P R T L — — A F — — — — — — — Q — — K
He (γ1)	R F S P — K S — — T — T R — — — — — — — — — T — — — D — — — — — — — — — I T V I P A P A G — — R — — P —
Cor (γ1)	— Y B T — — — — — T I — — R — — — — — S — N T — G — G — — — — — — — — — S C G — — G — — — — — I L
V_H III						
Tei (γ1)	H Y A V S V Q G R F T I S R N D S K N T L Y L Q M L S L E P Z B T A V V Y Y C A R V T P A A A S L T F S A V W G Q G T L V
Was (γ1)	— F — D T — N — — — — — — — — — — — — — — — — — N R — A — — — — — — — — F R Q P F V Q — — F D — F
Jon (γ3)	A F — N — N — — — — — — — — — — — — — — I — V T — — — — — — — — — V V S T — — — — — F D — — — — — — P
Zap (α1)	— D — A — — — — — — — — — — — — — — — — N T G — A — — — — — — — — T R — G G Y — — — S M D — —
Tur (α1)	— F — A — — — — — — — — — — — — — — — — — — Q A — — — L — — — — — — — L S V T — V — — — A F D —
Nie (γ1)	— D — N — — — — — — — — — — — — — — — — — N — N — — — R — — — — — — — I R D T — M — — — — K
Gal (μ)	B — V D — K — — — D N A — — S — — — — — — — N — R V — — — L — — — — — G W G — — — — G G D Y
Til (γ2)	— N — R A E D — — — — G W G — — — — K G K V S — Y Y F B Y
Til (μ)	— N — R A E D — — — — — — — K G K V S — Y Y F B Y

Fig. 4.14

of proteins, compiled by Capra and Kehoe (90a), in addition to partial sequences of the V_H regions of IgM (Til) and IgG2 (Til), reported by Wang *et al.* (90). The hyphens represent gaps, introduced to maximize homology. It is evident, for example, that the IgM sequence (protein Ou) resembles that of protein Daw more closely than proteins Daw and Eu resemble one another, despite the fact that Daw and Eu are both IgG1. On this basis it was proposed that there are subgroups of V_H regions which are shared by different classes of immunoglobulin (91,92). The existence of V_H subgroups has also been inferred from the observation that the V_H sequences of two IgG1 proteins (Daw and He) closely resemble one another but not the V_H sequence of a third IgG1 protein (Eu) (93). Three subgroups of V regions V_{HI}, V_{HII}, and V_{HIII}, can be recognized (94–98a). The V_H regions vary in length from about 118 to 124 residues. At the amino terminus most V_{HIII} proteins have an unblocked glutamic acid residue which greatly facilitates sequence analysis of the terminal region with an automatic sequencer; this accounts for the relatively large amount of data available for that subgroup. Within the V_{HII} and V_{HIII} subgroups the degree of homology, outside of hypervariable regions, between any protein and the prototype for that sequence is 80–95%; the values are highest for the V_{HIII} proteins. The corresponding result obtained by comparing proteins Daw (V_{HIII}) and Tel (V_{HIII}) is 60%; for proteins Daw (V_{HIII}) and Eu (V_{HI}) the value is 41% (nonhypervariable regions).

Figure 4.14 indicates that the same V_H region sequences can be shared by the various classes of immunoglobulins, which are of course identified by C_H sequences. A plausible and widely discussed explanation of this finding involves translocation of the V_H or C_H gene (99,100). It is assumed that separate genes specify the V_H and C_H regions and, by an unknown mechanism, are brought into juxtaposition. The finding of identical V_H regions in IgG and IgM monoclonal proteins of the same patient, designated Til (Chapter 11), provided strong support for a translocation or "switching" mechanism, and perhaps the best evidence for the two gene-one polypeptide hypothesis. As shown in Fig. 4.14, the V_H regions of Til IgG and IgM are identical with respect to sequences

---

Fig. 4.14. Complete V_H sequences of twelve human myeloma proteins. From Capra and Kehoe (90a). Also included are partial V_H sequences of the H chains of the IgG2 and IgM myeloma proteins of patient Til (90). For the single letter code see the legend of Fig. 4.6. The symbol, Z, at the beginning of a sequence represents pyrollidonecarboxylic acid. The numbering system used by Capra and Kehoe is not that of any single protein since gaps are included in all of the sequences to maximize homology; a minimum number (three gaps) is required for protein He.

so far determined by Wang and Fudenberg. These include segments in three hypervariable regions.

Evidence for translocation in L chains is based in part on the sharing of the various human V_κ subgroups by C regions of different allotype (Inv specificity). A distinction must be made, however, between L and H chains. C_κ regions are always found in combination with V_κ and C_λ regions with V_λ. This difference between H and L chains may be attributable to the fact that the various cistrons controlling C_H regions (of IgG, IgM, etc.) are closely linked while genes controlling C_κ and C_λ, by analogy with the rabbit, may not be linked. Close linkage of C region cistrons may be required to permit the sharing of genes controlling V regions. In the rabbit and mouse it has been shown, in addition, that V_H and C_H genes are closely linked; similar linkage in the human may be inferred.

A question that arose is whether the subgroups of H chains, which are defined by sequences of myeloma proteins, might actually be allelic gene products. This possibility was essentially disproved by the finding that sera from each of 15 normal individuals tested possessed substantial amounts of H chains (15 to 25%) having the V_{HIII} sequence (98). (It is possible to identify sequences of V_{HIII} proteins in the presence of other H chains because of the unique unblocked terminal amino group associated with nearly all V_{HIII} proteins.) The same sera were shown also to possess sequences characteristic of V_{HI} and V_{HII}. We have already discussed data indicating that the V region subgroups of human κ and λ chains are not allelic.

The concentration of V_{HIII} H chains in normal immunoglobulin (15–25% of all H chains) corresponds roughly with the frequency of occurrence of V_{HIII} myeloma proteins (101). This suggests that the conversion of a cell to malignancy is a random event not influenced by the class of immunoglobulin produced by the cell. A roughly similar frequency relationship applies to human κ and λ proteins and to the various human IgG subclasses. [There is, however, a very high frequency (about 75%) of IgA proteins in the V_{HIII} subgroup and a large proportion of IgD myeloma proteins are λ (Chapter 3).]

In the 12 complete sequences shown in Fig. 4.14, 25 positions are invariant. Many of these residues are also correspondingly located and invariant in the V_H regions of mouse, rabbit, and guinea pig immunoglobulins. In the human proteins these include the 2 half-cystines, Trp 38 and 49, 5 of 7 amino acids in positions 92–98, and positions 120, 122, and 123, which are at the junction of the V and C regions. (IgM becomes clearly distinguishable from IgG at position 124 and thereafter.) This relatively invariant sequence at the V/C junction is also conserved in other mammals (90a). Thus, 20% of the positions in the V_H regions are so far invariant, 45% show occasional substitutions, and 35% are in hypervariable regions. Considering only the V_{HIII} subgroup, 23% of the positions are hypervariable.

HYPERVARIABLE REGIONS IN V_H Sequences[10]

From the V_{HII} and V_{HIII} sequences shown in Fig. 4.14, it is evident that there are four hypervariable regions in either subgroup; these comprise residues 31–37, 51–68, 84–91, and 101–110. Within the subgroups the hypervariable regions are similarly, but not identically, located. Outside these regions the pattern of variability resembles that seen within a V region subgroup of κ or λ chains; substitutions are infrequent and one observes examples of identical substitutions in different proteins within a subgroup (for example, leucine for valine at position 5 in V_{HIII}). Within hypervariable regions it is difficult to designate subgroup-specific amino acids; also, in contrast to nonhypervariable regions, multiple base changes in DNA are required to account for many of the amino acid substitutions. This has suggested the possibility that a unique mechanism of mutation may apply to the hypervariable regions. An alternative view is that point mutations accumulate in hypervariable regions. After one mutation, the affected cell is subject to stimulation by a different antigen. When this occurs the population of the clone is increased to such

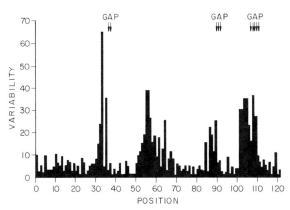

Fig. 4.15. Plot of variability, according to Wu and Kabat (34) of V_H sequences, including those in Fig. 4.14 and other published data. Reprinted by permission from Capra and Kehoe (90a).

[10] N-Terminal V_{HIII} sequences of a number of mammalian H chains have been determined; these and possible relationships to sequences of nonmammalian immunoglobulins are discussed in Chapter 7.

an extent that another point mutation in that gene has a greater probability of taking place. The possibility has also been suggested that DNA segments resembling episomes, which encode hypervariable segments, are inserted in some manner into the immunoglobulin gene.

A plot of variability, according to Wu and Kabat (34), was prepared by Capra and Kehoe (90a) and is reproduced in Fig. 4.15. It is based on the sequences in Fig. 4.15 and a number of additional published sequences. The location of the hypervariable regions are clearly evident. It is of interest that the gaps needed for alignment of amino acid sequences occur exclusively in or very close to hypervariable regions.

D. Sequences of Proteins Associated with "Heavy Chain Disease"

Interesting and informative deletions in human H chain sequences are found in proteins elaborated by patients with a rare lymphoproliferative disorder known as heavy chain disease, which was first described by Franklin *et al.* (102). Monoclonal proteins with antigenic determinants characteristic of the Fc fragment of the H chain of IgG are found, generally in high concentration, in the serum and urine of these individuals. More recently, patients have been described who were producing fragments of the H chain of IgA or IgM, rather than IgG (e.g., 103–106). Depending on the protein synthesized, the terms γ chain, α chain, or μ chain disease are in general usage. In general, the protein comprises a dimer of an incomplete H chain.

These anomalous proteins are not found in association with L chains, and investigations at the cellular level indicate that the lymphoid cells responsible for their biosynthesis do not produce significant quantities of L chains (107–109). The urinary or serum proteins comprise only a segment of the H chain and, when obtained from different patients, usually differ in molecular weight. Radiolabeling experiments have indicated that, at least in some instances, the polypeptides do not result from degradation of complete H chains but are the products of direct biosynthesis (109a).

Partial amino acid sequence analyses have been carried out on several such proteins of the IgG class; schematic diagrams are shown in Fig. 4.16 (110). In three proteins the N- and C-terminal segments of the H chain are present, but there is a large deletion in the N-terminal region. In a fourth protein, designated Mcg, the deletion comprises a major portion of the hinge region of the molecule (residues 216–232) (111,112). In protein Zuc (IgG3), the first 18 N-terminal residues correspond to a normal V_{HI} sequence, but a deletion follows which includes residues 19–215; the sequence then appears to be intact from residues

216 to the C-terminus. In protein Cra (IgG1; V_{HIII}) the deletion comprises residues 12–215. Protein Gif (IgG2) has a deletion starting near residue 100 and, again, extending through residue 215 (113).

Deletions of quite another type were found in two proteins of heavy chain disease investigated by Terry and Ein (114). Each appeared to lack completely the Fd segment; the amino acid sequences were initiated at positions 221 and 225. The authors suggested the possibility that these proteins are products of enzymatic digestion, rather than of *de novo* synthesis. They also point out that protein Cra (Fig. 4.16) is somewhat heterogeneous at the N-terminus and could likewise have been subject to postsynthetic degradation. Certain other proteins of heavy chain disease, such as Zuc, appear homogeneous with respect to amino acid sequence.

The repeated occurrence of a deletion ending at position 216 led Franklin and Frangione (115) to suggest that separate genes may control the Fc region and the constant segment of the Fd region (C_H1), so that

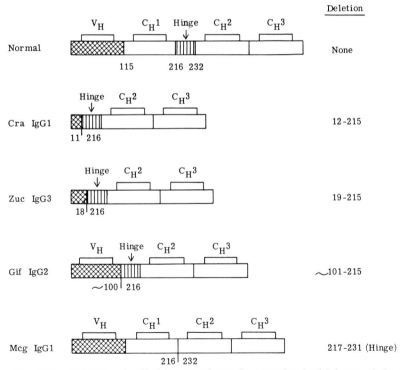

Fig. 4.16. Deletions identified in several proteins associated with heavy chain disease. From Frangione and Franklin (110). The original references are 112 (Mcg), 113 (Gif), 115 (Cra), and 168 (Zuc). The recently determined structure of another such protein (Hal), with a deletion ending at position 252, is discussed in the text.

the deletion only involves the $C_H 1$ gene and part of the V_H gene. The fact that different allotypic markers are localized in the $C_H 1$ and Fc regions of IgG1 proteins lends some support to this notion. If more than one gene does control the C_H region the genes must be very closely linked since genes controlling allotypic markers in the two segments do not segregate independently. If this hypothesis is correct, the H chain would be under the control of at least three genes, with the third encoding the V_H segment. Alternative possibilities involve the deletion of a section of the gene as a result of mispairing the DNA strands during cell division (110) or breakage of DNA strand at a hypothetical branch point and at some place distal to it, with subsequent rejoining back to the branch point (116).

The deletion of the hinge region in protein Mcg, which begins at residue 216, might be interpreted, according to the hypothesis of Frangione and Franklin, as occurring at the end of a separate gene encoding only the $C_H 1$ region. It should be recalled that the hinge region does not show homology with any other segment of the polypeptide chain and differs considerably among human IgG subclasses. It has been suggested that it might be controlled by still another gene (112,115).

Another protein (IgG4; designation Hal) has a deletion starting at position 10 and extending through the Fd segment and the hinge region as well; the IgG4 sequence resumes at methionine 252 and appears to continue normally to the C-terminus. The protein comprises a pair of such chains joined only by noncovalent bonds (116a). The authors make the interesting observation that in prokaryotes, and possibly in eukaryotes, the codon AUG is normally an initiation signal, but codes for methionine when present internally within a cistron. The implication is that in protein Hal the AUG codon was used as a site for reinitiation of the chain and that in the normal individual a separate cistron begins at position 252 (near the beginning of the $C_H 2$ domain). Thus, while highly speculative, the idea is being entertained that two or more C_H domains and the hinge region are encoded by separate genes, which are brought together to form a single functional unit. It is generally accepted that the V_H region is under separate genetic control.

VIII. AMINO ACID SEQUENCE OF β_2-MICROGLOBULIN

In Chapter 3 we discussed properties of β_2-microglobulin, a protein found in low concentration in normal human serum, urine, and cerebrospinal fluids and in higher amounts in patients with certain defects in

```
1                                    10
Ile  Gln  Arg  Thr  Pro  Lys  Ile  Gln  Val  Tyr  Ser  Arg  His  Pro  Ala  Glx  Asx  Gly  Lys  Ser−

21                                   30
Asx  Phe  Leu  Asn  Cys  Tyr  Val  Ser  Gly  Phe  His  Pro  Ser  Asp  Ile  Glu  Val  Asp  Leu  Leu−

41                                   50
Lys  Asp  Gly  Glu  Arg  Ile  Glx  Lys  Val (Asx, His, Ser, Glx)  Leu  Ser  Phe  Ser  Lys  Asn  Ser−

61                                   70
Trp  Phe  Tyr  Leu (Leu, Tyr, Ser)  Tyr  Thr  Glu  Phe  Thr  Pro  Thr  Glu  Lys  Asp  Glu  Tyr  Ala−

81                                   90                                  100
Cys  Arg  Val  Asx  His  Val  Thr  Leu  Ser  Glx  Pro  Lys  Ile  Val  Lys  Trp  Asp  Arg  Asp  Met
```

Fig. 4.17. Amino acid sequence of human β_2-microglobulin. From Smithies and Poulik (116e) and Peterson *et al.* (116f).

kidney secretion. Although its function is unknown it has attracted considerable interest because of an obvious relationship to the immunoglobulins. It is manufactured by a variety of mesenchymal and epithelial human cell lines and is present on the membranes of human lymphocytes. Of considerable interest was the recent observation that each of several HL-A antigens, isolated from human spleen cells by digestion with papain, comprises two subunits, one of which was shown to be β_2-microglobulin (116b,116c,116d). The two subunits are separable by electrophoresis in polyacrylamide gel containing the dissociating agent, sodium dodecyl sulfate. So far the biological significance of this finding has not been ascertained.

β_2-microglobulin has a molecular weight of approximately 11,000 and comprises 100 amino acid residues. The sequence is shown in Fig. 4.17 (116e,116f). Of great interest is the presence of a disulfide loop spanning 57 residues, between positions 25 and 81; the resemblance to a domain of an L or H chain is obvious. Furthermore, the length of the protein is similar to that of an individual homology unit or domain. A comparison of amino acid sequences, after the usual alignment, showed 25–30% identity with human C_κ and C_λ, or with the C_H1, C_H2, or C_H3 homology regions of IgG1. Smithies and Poulik, and Peterson *et al.* stress the relationship to the C_H3 region and discuss various genetic models to account for the evolution of the protein.

IX. AMYLOIDOSIS

Amyloidosis is a general clinical term which refers to extravascular deposition of a homogeneous eosinophilic protein material, which may appear in various organs of the body (117,118). Whether amyloid deposits can occur intracellularly in lymphoid cells is controversial (118a). The amyloid tissue deposits characteristically exhibit birefringence to polarized light, stain with Congo red, and have a fibrillar appearance under the electron microscope. In primary amyloidosis the amyloid deposition is apparently unassociated with another illness. Secondary amyloidosis refers to a condition in which the amyloid deposition is associated with a variety of chronic inflammatory diseases such as rheumatoid arthritis, regional enteritis, leprosy, and many other chronic illnesses, including malignancy. A third clinical form of amyloidosis occurs in association with plasma cell dyscrasias, primarily multiple myeloma. In a fourth type, the amyloid forms small tumors in one of several organs; as in type 1, there is no apparent associated disease state. Isope and Osserman reported the presence of associated amyloidosis in 70 out of a total of 806 cases of plasma cell dyscrasia (119).

The nature of the protein, or more precisely, proteins associated with amyloidosis has been the subject of many investigations and considerable controversy. A number of factors are responsible for the difficulties encountered. One is the insolubility of amyloid in neutral salt solution; the protein can ordinarily be solubilized only by methods which lead to at least partial denaturation. Another problem is contamination of the fibrillar amyloid deposits in extracellular compartments by various substances, including serum proteins. Attempts to identify amyloid by immunofluorescent methods have therefore yielded contradictory results. Serum immunoglobulin, complement, etc., have been associated with amyloid by various investigators.

Major progress in elucidating the structure of amyloid was made by Glenner and his associates when they showed that some amyloid proteins are structurally related to the immunoglobulins. In addition, a number of investigators have now demonstrated that other amyloid proteins are unrelated to immunoglobulins. Glenner's procedure for the solubilization of amyloid consisted of repeated homogenization, extraction with 0.1 N NaOH and reduction of disulfide bonds in 5 M guanidine hydrochloride, followed by gel filtration in 5 M guanidine hydrochloride containing 1 M acetic acid (120). A technique developed by Franklin and Pras involves extraction with dilute HCl for 1 hour at 60°C (121). Principal methods used for characterizing amyloid proteins are antigenic analysis and determination of amino acid sequences.

A. Amyloid Related to Immunoglobulin

In their initial sequence analyses, Glenner *et al.* found that the N-terminal amino acid sequences of two amyloid proteins are related to

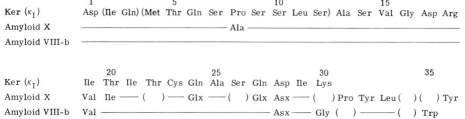

	1			5					10					15			
Ker (κ_I)	Asp	(Ile	Gln)	(Met	Thr	Gln	Ser	Pro	Ser	Ser	Leu	Ser)	Ala	Ser	Val	Gly	Asp Arg
Amyloid X	——————————————— Ala ———————————————
Amyloid VIII-b	———————————————————————————————————

	20				25					30				35
Ker (κ_I)	Ile	Thr	Ile	Thr	Cys	Gln	Ala	Ser	Gln	Asp	Ile	Lys		
Amyloid X	Val	Ile —— ( ) —— Glx ——( ) Glx Asx —— ( ) Pro Tyr Leu ( ) ( ) Tyr
Amyloid VIII-b	Val ——————————————— Asx —— Gly ( ) ——————— ( ) Trp

Fig. 4.18. N-terminal amino acid sequences of two amyloid proteins; that of a human κ chain is included for comparison. From Glenner *et al.* (122). The sequence of protein Ker is from reference 162. Empty parentheses indicate the presence of an unidentified amino acid.

those of human κ chains (122). Their data are shown in Fig. 4.18. In the first 30 positions of the two proteins studied, only two or three residues definitely differed from those of Bence Jones protein "Ker" of the $V_{\kappa I}$ subtype. From these results and the low molecular weight of the amyloid proteins (7,500 and 18,300), the authors concluded that each comprises the N-terminal portion of a κ chain. Following these initial studies, many other amyloid proteins have been shown to be related to κ or λ chains, with the λ type occurring in greater frequency (123,124). Glenner *et al.* have also reported the occurrence in amyloid fibrils of complete L chains, or of a mixture of complete chains and N-terminal fragments (125). The molecular weight of an amyloid protein is generally in the range 5000–30,000 daltons.

Amyloid proteins related to immunoglobulin possess individually specific (idiotypic) antigenic determinants; i.e., such amyloid proteins from different individuals possess unique primary structures. Idiotypic determinants characteristic of a given amyloid protein can sometimes be detected in the serum of the same individual. In addition, however, amyloid proteins of a given type (κ or λ) frequently have shared antigenic determinants (120,124,126). Antiserum directed to an amyloid protein will, in general, cross-react weakly with normal L chains of the same type. It seems likely that these cross-reactions are attributable, in the case of the smaller amyloid proteins, to shared V region sequences.

That amyloid fibrils can be formed from V_L peptides was demonstrated by Glenner *et al.* (127) and by Linke *et al.* (128). Glenner *et al.* treated Bence Jones proteins of types κ and λ with pepsin in such a manner as to cleave the chains into V and C segments (129). During the incubation, precipitates formed in many of the solutions. Under the microscope some of these precipitates (nearly all from λ chains) were seen to consist of fibrils resembling those of amyloid deposits. Furthermore, the X-ray diffraction pattern had a gross appearance characteristic of many amyloid proteins. The artificially produced fibrils were stained by Congo red and exhibited birefringence under polarized light; both properties are characteristic of amyloid deposits. N-terminal sequence analysis and peptide mapping indicated that the fibrillar material consisted of part of the V_λ region of the Bence Jones protein. The molecular weight of the protein in one of the precipitates was 4600 (127), indicating that the peptic digestion had proceeded beyond simple cleavage into V and C regions. In addition, an N-terminal tripeptide had been removed from one of the proteins. Linke *et al.* (128) found that eight of nine λ chains that produced fibrils belonged to the $V_{\lambda I}$ subgroup.

This array of evidence demonstrates convincingly that some amyloid proteins are related to immunoglobulin, and indicates that they generally represent incomplete L chains.

B. Amyloid Unrelated to Immunoglobulin

It now appears that the amyloid deposits occurring in secondary amyloidosis consist largely of a substance unrelated to immunoglobulin (130–134). Husby *et al.* use the convenient designation, AS (amyloid subunit) for this protein. They suggest that protein AS is a fragment of an unknown larger protein. In contrast to the amyloid of immunoglobulin origin, it appears to be very similar or identical in different patients. The protein, which can be solubilized with dilute HCl, has a molecular weight of 8500 (130), and its complete amino acid sequence has been reported (134). The molecule consists of 76 amino acids and lacks cysteine. The sequence (Fig. 4.19) bears no obvious relationship to that of immunoglobulins. Levin *et al.* (134) compared the sequence with partial sequences of the corresponding protein from six other patients,

```
1                5                    10                   15                   20
Arg Ser Phe Phe Ser Phe Leu Gly Glu Ala Phe Asp Gly Ala Arg Asp Met Trp Arg Ala -

                 25                   30                   35                   40
Tyr Ser Asp Met Arg Glu Ala Asn Tyr Ile Gly Ser Asp Lys Tyr Phe His Ala Arg Gly -

                 45                   50                   55                   60
Asn Tyr Asp Ala Ala Lys Arg Gly Pro Gly Gly Ala Trp Ala Ala Glu Val Ile Ser Asn-

                 65                   70                   75
Ala Arg Glu Asn Ile Gln Arg Leu Thr Gly Arg Gly Ala Glu Asp Ser
```

Fig. 4.19. The complete amino acid sequence of an amyloid protein extracted from tissues of a patient with secondary amyloidosis associated with familial Mediterranean fever. The sequence is not related to that of an immunoglobulin. There is some uncertainty at position 53, which may be Arg. From Levin *et al.* (134).

having tuberculosis, rheumatoid arthritis, Hodgkin's disease, bronchiectasis, or familial Mediterranean fever. Only one amino acid substitution (valine for alanine at position 52) was seen.

Levin *et al.* were unable to find any amyloid of nonimmunoglobulin nature in the deposits of three patients with multiple myeloma or macroglobulinemia. However, the converse was not true, since some material related to L chain was found in patients with secondary amyloidosis, whose deposits were mainly nonimmunoglobulin in nature. This immunoglobulin-like material appeared heterogeneous, in contrast to that seen in myeloma patients. Relatively few individuals with secondary amyloidosis have been examined at this writing for the presence of amyloid related to immunoglobulin.

Subsequently, Husby *et al.* detected protein AS in the amyloid deposits of two patients with Waldenström's macroglobulinemia (134a). (Whether amyloid of immunoglobulin origin coexisted was not reported.) In addition, they succeeded in preparing an antiserum which detected protein AS in the sera of nearly all patients with secondary amyloidosis. Of seven patients with amyloidosis associated with lymphoproliferative disease (four with multiple myeloma and three with Waldenström's disease), six possessed a serum component that cross-reacted with protein AS. In addition, a large percentage of patients with multiple myeloma, Waldenström's macroglobulinemia, and with various diseases often associated with secondary amyloidosis had detectable protein AS in their sera, despite the absence of known amyloidosis. It would appear that protein AS is a unique substance (possibly a breakdown product) common to various types of amyloidosis. Antisera to protein AS may prove to be of great importance in the diagnosis and prediction of amyloidosis, particularly since tests can be carried out with the patient's serum.

X. CARBOHYDRATE IN IMMUNOGLOBULINS

A. General Considerations

Virtually all immunoglobulins, including those of primitive vertebrate species, contain significant amounts of carbohydrate; there is, however, considerable qualitative and quantitative variation, even among molecules from the same species and of the same class. Furthermore, an individual myeloma protein may exhibit microheterogeneity with respect to its carbohydrate content. The biological role of the

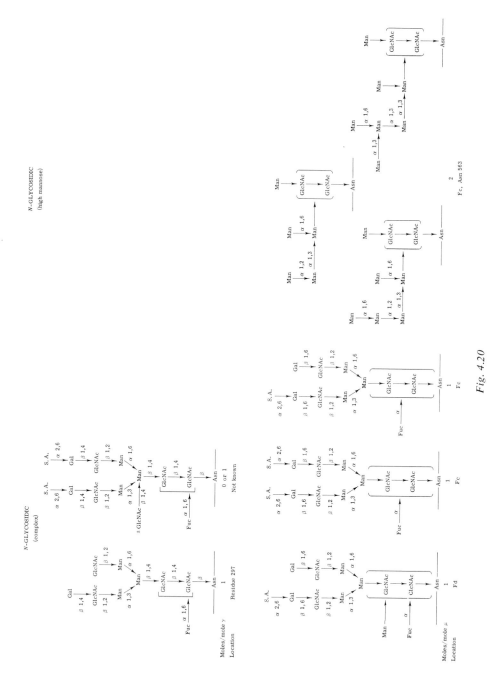

Fig. 4.20

carbohydrate remains to be elucidated. However, there is evidence relating the attachment of carbohydrate to the migration of IgG within the plasma cell and to its secretion. Information is available as to the gross content and composition of the carbohydrate in the immunoglobulins of many species (Chapter 7). We will focus our attention in this section on human immunoglobulins and on those of certain other species for which the data are instructive or of particular interest.

We have listed in Table 3.1 the carbohydrate content of various classes of human immunoglobulin. In discussing composition, the word "average" should be stressed because of variability among molecules of a given class; and there is even microheterogeneity with respect to carbohydrate composition in an individual myeloma protein. Although some L chains and Fd segments contain carbohydrate, the bulk is usually localized in the Fc portion of the H chain. The carbohydrate is covalently attached to asparagine or, occasionally, a threonine or serine side chain. The receptor site for the enzyme, *N*-acetylglucosamine-asparagine transglycosylase, consists of a unique amino acid triplet in which asparagine is the first amino acid and serine or threonine is the third. The second amino acid is quite variable. This pattern is seen in a variety of glycoproteins, in addition to the immunoglobulins (134b,135,136). The enzyme catalyzes the formation of a glycosylamine bond linking the amide group of asparagine to the C-1 carbon of an amino sugar; in immunoglobulins this is usually *N*-acetylglucosamine. Although the Asn, ___, Ser/Thr[11] sequence is required for the reaction, its presence does not make the attachment of carbohydrate mandatory; the sequence has been found in V_L segments without attached carbohydrate (135). A probable explanation is that the sequence of amino acids may occasionally be buried in the interior of the protein molecule, where it is inaccessible to the enzyme. It is, however, noteworthy that the appropriate triplet, when it occurs in the *constant* region of a polypeptide chain, has invariably been associated with carbohydrate.

The larger oligosaccharides are present as a branched chain. Carbohydrate attached to threonine or serine generally occurs as a short oligosaccharide. Carbohydrate structures present in human IgG or IgM, worked out by Dr. Stuart Kornfeld and his associates, are shown in Fig.

[11] The dash represents the second, variable amino acid. The triplet reported sometimes contains aspartic acid rather than asparagine; the possibility of an error in some reports cannot be entirely excluded.

Fig. 4 20. Carbohydrate structures found in monoclonal human IgG and IgM proteins. Both branched and mannose-rich structures are found in IgE, but only the branched type has been identified in IgA. From Baenziger and Kornfeld (139a).

4.20. One recurring structural feature is the successive attachment of two residues of *N*-acetylglucosamine to an asparagine side chain; these residues are followed by a mannose group to which two branches of the chain are attached. Sialic acid, when present, is at the end of a chain. A second major type of carbohydrate chain, found in IgM but not IgG, is rich in mannose (Fig. 4.20). So far only the first of the two types of chain structure has been identified in IgA; both are present in IgE (137,138). An unusual carbohydrate structure, present in the hinge region of IgA, is discussed below in Section X,E.

B. Carbohydrate in the Constant Region of Human γ Chains

The C_H regions of each human IgG subclass contain covalently bound carbohydrate. In IgG1 the appropriate triplet of amino acids comprises residues 297–299 and the carbohydrate is attached to asparagine 297 in each of the two H chains (2). Since this triplet does not appear elsewhere in the C_H region of IgG1, and as the Fc segment of each of a large number of IgG1 myeloma proteins examined contains carbohydrate, it seems likely that an oligosaccharide is consistently attached to asparagine 297. (IgG4 also has the appropriate triplet at positions 297–299, and the carbohydrate is probably attached there.) In rabbit, IgG residue 297 (Eu numbering system) is reported as aspartic acid rather than asparagine; the major carbohydrate chain of the molecule is linked to that position. There is individual variability among IgG1 myeloma proteins in the nature of the carbohydrate attached at position 297; for example, in a large sample of such proteins, the number of hexose groups per mole of fragment Fc varied from 9 to 13 (137,138a).

IgG myeloma proteins of each subclass have been found to contain mannose, galactose, fucose, *N*-acetylglucosamine, and sialic acid (138a). The type of variability found among myeloma proteins is assumed also to be present in the normal immunoglobulin population. Kornfeld *et al.* showed that, with respect to composition, the normal IgG pool falls within the range observed among individual myeloma proteins (137).

In the Fc fragments of each human IgG subclass the same sugars are found, and in roughly the same ratios. There is thus far no evidence for subclass-specific carbohydrate; i.e., one cannot identify the subclass of a human IgG molecule from its carbohydrate content. Of 76 myeloma proteins, comprising representatives of each IgG subclass, examined by Abel *et al.* (138a), 22 contained substantially higher amounts of carbohydrate than the others. The proteins with low carbohydrate content had 9–13 moles of hexose per mole of protein; the others contained 19–37 moles. The excess carbohydrate in the latter group was always localized in the Fab fragment. Examples of proteins with high and low carbohydrate content were found in each IgG subclass and comprised both the κ and λ types; also, there was no evident correlation with allotype. Several myeloma proteins with high carbohydrate content were digested with papain and their Fab fragments isolated and analyzed for sugar content. A typical result, expressed as moles of monosaccharide per mole of Fab fragment is: hexose, 6.9; fucose, 1.0; sialic acid, 1.3; and glucosamine, 5.9. When carbohydrate is present in fragment Fab, the sialic acid content in the two Fab fragments is generally higher than that present in fragment Fc. Glucosamine is almost entirely present as the N-acetyl derivative.

The carbohydrate in the Fab fragment of individual myeloma proteins was found on the L chain, on the Fd fragment, or both. In the latter instance, the total carbohydrate content was correspondingly high. Abel *et al.* did not localize the carbohydrate in the Fab fragment with respect to its position in the amino acid sequence. Since three of the proteins which had carbohydrate in the Fd segment were of the IgG1 subclass, it seems unlikely that carbohydrate was present in the constant segment of Fd, which lacks an appropriate amino acid triplet. This would suggest again that excess carbohydrate is in the V_H region. One can use a similar argument with respect to the L chain and predict that carbohydrate would be found exclusively in the V_L segment; in several instances in which carbohydrate has actually been localized with respect to sequence, this has been found to be the case (92,135,139).

In view of their polar nature, it is probable that all carbohydrate groups are located on the exterior of the molecule.

C. Structure of the Carbohydrate in Human γ Chains

Using enzymes which sequentially degrade oligosaccharides, Kornfeld *et al.* investigated the structure of the carbohydrate attached to H chains of several human IgG myeloma proteins and of IgG from a normal donor (137,139a) (see Fig. 4.20). In each protein the carbohydrate was linked to asparagine; and in one instance where the sequence adjacent to the asparagine was determined, an appropriate triplet, -Asn-Ser-Thr-, was found. The subclass of IgG was not indicated (137) but one would predict that the carbohydrate in each case is linked to an asparagine homologous to residue 297 in IgG1. Although substantial similarities were observed among the myeloma proteins, two types of heterogeneity were noted. First, there were differences among myeloma proteins; second, the myeloma protein from an individual evidenced microheterogeneity in its structure. Microheterogeneity was indicated by the presence of fractional molar concentrations of sialic acid, fucose, or galactose. For example, in one myeloma protein, 9% of the molecules had two sialic acid residues, 31% had one, and 60% of the molecules had none. (For analysis, the corresponding glycopeptides were isolated by high-voltage electrophoresis.) Similarly, the fucose content of the various carbohydrate units varied from 0.6 to 1.0 residue per molecule and the galactose from 0.3 to 2.0. It is noteworthy that microheterogeneity within the molecules of an individual myeloma protein is largely confined to the outer branches of the chain. It is uncertain whether this heterogeneity arises through enzymatic degradation or reflects biosynthetic differences, although the latter seems more likely. Differences among the myeloma proteins could reflect genetic variation in the complement of synthetic enzymes (transferases) controlling the biosynthesis of oligosaccharides. The functional significance, if any, of these variations is unknown.

D. Carbohydrate in Human μ Chains

Davie and Osterland reported that monoclonal IgM proteins from patients with Waldenström's macroglobulinemia can be divided into two classes, which have a carbohydrate content of approximately 11% (Group 1) or 7% (Group 2) (140). About three-fifths of the proteins studied were in Group 1. Proteins of each group contain mannose, galactose, and N-acetylglucosamine, with smaller amounts of fucose and sialic acid. The overall composition of the carbohydrate does not differ greatly except for the presence of a considerably larger amount of sialic acid in Group 1.

Localization with respect to sequence of the carbohydrate in the μ chain and the nature of several of the carbohydrate groups are indicated in Figs. 4.10 and 4.20 (60,136,139a,140a).

E. Carbohydrate in Human α Chains

Most of our information concerning carbohydrate in IgA derives from studies of myeloma proteins. Because of the lack of complete amino acid sequence data, our knowledge of the distribution of carbohydrate along the chain is limited.

An extensive investigation of the carbohydrate composition of IgA myeloma proteins was carried out by Wang and Fudenberg (141). They observed marked differences among IgA proteins; the hexose content varied from 2.5 to 17%. In an individual patient, the IgA monomer and polymer had the same content of carbohydrate.

Dawson and Clamp (141a) demonstrated the presence of three types of carbohydrate groupings, present in a total of six locations in an IgA myeloma protein. One contained galactose and N-acetylgalactosamine (three residues of each) joined to a serine side chain. This oligosaccharide is attached to the hinge region and is present only in IgA1 (142); sugars containing galactosamine are ordinarily not found in IgA2, IgG, or IgM. The absence of this carbohydrate group in IgA2 is attributable to a deletion, as compared to IgA1, of 12 to 13 amino acids in the hinge region (77a). The second type of oligosaccharide identified by Dawson and Clamp contained three mannose, two galactose, and three N-acetylglucosamine residues and was joined to aspartic acid (possibly asparagine). The third type contained mannose and N-acetylglucosamine but lacked galactose; again attachment was through aspartic acid. The three types of oligosaccharide were heterogeneous with respect to their content of fucose and sialic acid. The sequences of these oligosaccharides in IgA are similar to those shown for IgG and IgM in Fig. 4.20 (not including the "mannose-rich" type). Some information on the amino acid sequences immediately surrounding carbohydrate groups was provided by Moore and Putnam (142a).

F. Carbohydrate in V_H Regions of Human Immunoglobulins

Since all immunoglobulin classes appear to share the same V_H subgroups, the carbohydrate content of the V_H region can be considered without reference to class. The available data are limited and are based almost entirely on myeloma proteins. The V_H regions of most H chains lack carbohydrate; when present, however, the carbohydrate is generally attached to asparagine in the usual triplet of amino acids. It has been suggested that, in the V gene, the nucleotide sequence coding for such triplets arises through whatever mechanism of mutation accounts for the general variability and that the attachment of carbohydrate is, therefore, fortuitous and probably without biological significance.

Although carbohydrate has been identified in the V_H regions of a number of myeloma proteins, it has been localized precisely in only a few. In three proteins investigated, two by Spiegelberg *et al.* (139), and one by Press and Hogg (92), the carbohydrate is attached at residues 30, 32, and 62. It is of interest that approximately the same positions in the sequence provide points of attachment in those L chains which have carbohydrate in the V_L segment.

G. Carbohydrate in Human L Chains

As already indicated, most of the carbohydrate of human immunoglobulins is present in H chains. The C regions of κ and λ chains
lack the triplet of amino acids associated with carbohydrate which, as a
consequence, is associated with the V region when it is present. Sox and
Hood (135) carried out carbohydrate analyses on 89 human L chains (71
Bence Jones proteins and 18 L chains from myeloma proteins) and
found carbohydrate in 5. In a similar study, Spiegelberg *et al.* (139) observed a somewhat higher incidence, about 15%. In three instances, the
latter group investigated both the carbohydrate-containing Bence Jones
protein and the corresponding L chain, isolated from the myeloma protein of the same patient. By several criteria the two kinds of L chain
from an individual appeared very similar, as is generally observed. However, in each patient the Bence Jones protein contained considerably
more sialic acid than the L chain from the myeloma protein. As a
consequence, the Bence Jones protein also had a greater anodal electrophoretic mobility. The Bence Jones proteins exhibited heterogeneity
with respect to mobility, which the authors attributed to microheterogeneity in sialic acid content. This was established through removal
of sialic acid by treatment with neuraminidase; the multiple electrophoretic bands of the Bence Jones protein were replaced by a single
band.

As in the case of H chains, differences in composition are seen in
the carbohydrate attached to human L chains from different sources. In
several Bence Jones proteins or L chains from myeloma proteins, studied by Sox and Hood (135), the range of composition was approximately
as follows (values are expressed as moles per mole of L chain); *N*-ace-
tylglucosamine, 2.3–3.4; *N*-acetylgalactosamine, 0.3–1.8; neutral sugar,
6.5–10; sialic acid, 1.3–1.5 (only two proteins tested). Fractional values
are indicative of microheterogeneity within a single L chain population.
Those L chains which do have carbohydrate contain a rather high percentage (about 10% by weight). Peptide mapping indicated that glycopeptides are confined to the V region.

Sox and Hood also localized the carbohydrate within the amino acid
sequence of three mouse L chains. The asparagine to which carbohydrate is attached was found at positions 26 and 28 in two proteins and
was either at position 65 or 70 (possibly both) in the third. The same two
regions of the sequence were found to contain carbohydrate in the case
of two human λ and two human κ chains investigated by Spiegelberg
et al.; a fifth L chain had carbohydrate attached at position 91. The regions of sequence around positions 27 and 70 have also been found to

be associated with carbohydrate in the case of the V regions of human H chains, discussed below. Since only a minority of L chains, as well as V_H regions, contains carbohydrate, it seems unlikely that it has a significant biological function when present in those regions.

H. Carbohydrate in the Rabbit γ Chain

Since the rabbit is not susceptible to multiple myeloma, data on carbohydrate content are obtained with normal immunoglobulins. If, as would be anticipated, there is microheterogeneity with respect to carbohydrate, the results we will discuss must represent average values. In overall composition the carbohydrate is similar to that found in human IgG. The major oligosaccharide, present in all or nearly all molecules or rabbit IgG, is linked to an asparagine in the Fc region at position 297 (143) (numbering system of human IgG1 myeloma protein Eu); this is also the position of attachment of carbohydrate in human IgG1. The oligosaccharide comprises five glucosamine (probably acetylated), two galactose, five mannose, and approximately one fucose and one sialic acid residue. A second carbohydrate group, present in about 40% of rabbit γ chains, is joined covalently to a threonine in the hinge region at position 225 (77).

$$-Pro-Thr-Cys-Pro-Pro-Pro-Glu-$$
$$\uparrow$$
$$CHO$$

This threonine is associated with allotype d12; in molecules of allotype d11 it is replaced by methionine (Chapter 9). The carbohydrate group is small, consisting of one galactosamine (probably the *N*-acetyl derivative), which is attached to the threonine, a galactose, and two sialic acid residues. Fanger and Smyth made the interesting observation that an individual IgG molecule appears to be asymmetrical with respect to this carbohydrate, which is joined to only one H chain (77). A possible explanation is that the first carbohydrate group attached interferes sterically with the transferase enzyme. The negative charge conferred by sialic acid permits physical separation, by electrophoresis, of those IgG molecules possessing the carbohydrate group.

About 15% of the H chains of normal rabbit IgG possess a third carbohydrate group, which is small and contains glucosamine. Its location is uncertain, but its presence on a small fraction of the molecules would suggest that it is the V_H segment (144).

Melchers has shown that a major carbohydrate unit is attached to asparagine or aspartic acid in the Fc segment of each H chain of a mouse IgG1 myeloma protein (144a).

I. Assembly of the Carbohydrate on Immunoglobulin Molecules

The available evidence indicates that immunoglobulin biosynthesis takes place largely on polyribosomes bound to membrane surfaces in the rough endoplasmic reticulum of lymphoid cells (145–147); the polyribosomes are present in the microsomal fraction isolated from a cell homogenate. The possibility that some biosynthesis may occur on free polyribosomes has not been rigorously excluded. After release from the polyribosome an immunoglobulin molecule traverses the membrane into the cisternal compartment where it travels to the smooth endoplasmic reticulum (devoid of polyribosomes) and to the Golgi vesicles, prior to its release from the cell.

Pulse-labeling experiments (147a,148–150), using radioactive sugars, indicate that the attachment of the first carbohydrate groups, N-acetylglucosamine and mannose, is initiated in the rough endoplasmic reticulum, soon after separation of the molecule from the polyribosome. The attachment of galactose, fucose and sialic acid, present on the branches (Fig. 4.20), occurs mainly in the smooth endoplasmic reticulum and Golgi complex. Some incorporation of N-acetylglucosamine also takes place in the smooth endoplasmic reticulum; it is uncertain whether this includes the N-acetylglucosamine attached to the asparagine of the polypeptide, or only that present on the branches. The attachment of fucose occurs shortly before secretion of the molecule from the cell.

The role of carbohydrate in the transport of the immunoglobulin molecule within the cell and with respect to its secretion is not clearly understood. The secretion of light chains lacking carbohydrate, frequently observed in multiple myeloma, argues against an essential role, but does not disprove the necessity for carbohydrate in the transport of complete Ig molecules. The fact that a full complement of carbohydrate residues is not essential for secretion was shown by Melchers, who used 2-deoxy-D-glucose to inhibit the growth of the carbohydrate chain of an IgG1 mouse myeloma protein (150a). Molecules lacking fucose or sialic acid, normally present on the branches of the chain, were secreted from the plasma cell in the usual manner. 2-Deoxy-D-glucose did, however, inhibit migration of completed chains within the cell; this was attributed either to the lack of carbohydrate on the IgG or, alternatively, to an induced defect in some other glycoprotein, which is required for intracellular transport.

REFERENCES

1. Potter, M. (1972). *Physiol. Rev.* **52**, 631.
2. Edelman, G.M., Cunningham, B.A., Gall, W.E., Gottlieb, P.D., Rutishauser, U., and Waxdal, M.J. (1969). *Proc. Nat. Acad. Sci. U.S.* **63**, 78.
3. Cunningham, B.A., Gottlieb, P.D., Pflumm, M.N., and Edelman, G.M. (1971). *In* "Progress in Immunology" (Bernard Amos, ed.), p. 3. Academic Press, New York.
4. Hilschmann, N. (1967). *Hoppe-Seyler's Z. Physiol. Chem.* **348**, 1077.
5. Langer, B., Steinmetz-Kayne, M., and Hilschmann, N. (1968). *Hoppe-Seyler's Z. Physiol. Chem.* **349**, 945.
6. Edelman, G.M. and Gally, J.A. (1962). *J. Exp. Med.* **116**, 207.
7. Putnam, F.W. (1962). *Biochim. Biophys. Acta* **63**, 539.
8. Hilschmann, N. and Craig, L.C. (1965). *Proc. Nat. Acad. Sci. U.S.* **53**, 1403.
9. Putnam, F.W. and Easley, C.W. (1965). *J. Biol. Chem.* **240**, 1626.
10. Milstein, C. (1966). *Nature (London)* **209**, 370.
11. Baglioni, C., Alescio-Zonta, L., Cioli, D., and Carbonara, A. (1966). *Science* **152**, 1517.
12. Milstein, C. (1966). *Biochem. J.* **101**, 338.
13. Putnam, F.W., Titani, K., and Whitley, E., Jr. (1966). *Proc. Roy. Soc. Ser. B* **166**, 124.
14. Putnam, F.W., Titani, K., Wikler, M., and Shinoda, T. (1967). *Cold Spring Harbor Symp. Quant. Biol.* **32**, 9.
15. Milstein, C. (1964). *J. Mol. Biol.* **9**, 836.
16. Milstein, C., Clegg, J.B., and Jarvis, J.M. (1967). *Nature (London)* **214**, 270.
17. Wikler, M., Titani, K., Shinoda, T., and Putnam, F.W. (1967). *J. Biol. Chem.* **242**, 1668.
18. Ponstingl, H., Hess, M., Langer, B., Steinmetz-Kayne, M., and Hilschmann, N. (1967). *Hoppe-Seyler's Z. Physiol. Chem.* **348**, 1213.
19. Putnam, F.W., Shinoda, T., Titani, K., and Wikler, M. (1967). *Science* **157**, 1050.
20. Appella, E. and Ein, D. (1967). *Proc. Nat. Acad. Sci. U.S.* **57**, 1449.
21. Gibson, D., Levanon, M., and Smithies, O. (1971). *Biochemistry* **10**, 3114.
21a. Hess, M., Hilschmann, N., Rivat, L., Rivat, C., and Ropartz, C. (1971). *Nature New Biol.* **234**, 58.
22. Hill, R.L., Delaney, R., Fellows, R.E., Jr., and Lebovitz, H.E. (1966). *Proc. Nat. Acad. Sci. U.S.* **56**, 1762.
23. Singer, S.J. and Doolittle, R.F. (1966). *Science* **153**, 13.
24. Brown, J.R. and Hartley, B.S. (1963). *Biochem. J.* **89**, 59p.
25. Milstein, C.P. and Deverson, E.V. (1971). *Biochem. J.* **123**, 945.
26. Garver, F.A. and Hilschmann, N. (1971). *FEBS Lett.* **16**, 128.
27. Garver, F.A. and Hilschmann, N. (1972). *Eur. J. Biochem.* **26**, 10.
28. Hood, L. and Talmage, D.W. (1970). *Science* **168**, 325.
29. Niall, H.D. and Edman, P. (1967). *Nature (London)* **216**, 262.
30. Milstein, C. (1967). *Nature (London)* **216**, 330.
31. Grant, J.A. and Hood, L. (1971). *Immunochemistry* **8**, 63.
32. Solomon, A. and McLaughlin, C.L. (1969). *J. Exp. Med.* **130**, 1295.
33. Solomon, A. and McLaughlin, C.L. (1971). *J. Immunol.* **106**, 120.
34. Wu, T.T. and Kabat, E. (1970). *J. Exp. Med.* **132**, 211.
35. Braun, M., Leibold, W., Barnikol, H-U., and Hilschmann, N. (1972). *Hoppe-Seyler's Z. Physiol. Chem.* **353**, 1284.

36. Lennox, E.S. and Cohn, M. (1967). *Annu. Rev. Biochem.* **36**, 365.
37. Milstein, C. and Munro, A.J. (1970). *Annu. Rev. Microbiol.* **24**, 335.
38. Edelman, G.M. and Gall, W.E. (1969). *Annu. Rev. Biochem.* **38**, 415.
39. Putnam, F.W. (1969). *Science* **163**, 633.
39a. Poljak, R.J., Amzel, L.M., Chen, B.L., Phizackerley, R.P., and Saul, F. (1974). *Proc. Nat. Acad. Sci. U.S.* **71**, 3440.
39b. Epp, D., Colman, P., Fehlhammer, H., Bode, W., Schiffer, M., and Huber, R. (1974). *Eur. J. Biochem.* **45**, 513.
40. Welscher, H.D. (1969). *Int. J. Protein Res.* **1**, 267.
41. Quattrocchi, R.D., Cioli, D., and Baglioni, C. (1969). *J. Exp. Med.* **130**, 401.
42. Capra, J.D. and Kunkel, H.G. (1970). *Proc. Nat. Acad. Sci. U.S.* **67**, 87.
43. McIntire, K.R. and Potter, M. (1964). *J. Nat. Cancer Inst.* **33**, 631.
44. McIntire, K.R. and Rouse, A.M. (1970). *Fed. Proc. Fed. Amer. Soc. Exp. Biol.* **29**, 704.
45. Potter, M., Dreyer, W.J., Kuff, E.L., and McIntire, K.R. (1964). *J. Mol. Biol.* **8**, 814.
46. Potter, M. and Lieberman, R. (1967). *Advan. Immunol.* **7**, 91.
47. Edelman, G.M. and Gottlieb, P.D. (1970). *Proc. Nat. Acad. Sci. U.S.* **67**, 1192.
48. Hood, L.E., Potter, M., and McKean, D.J. (1970). *Science* **170**, 1207.
49. Hood, L., McKean, D., Farnsworth, V., and Potter, M. (1973). *Biochemistry* **12**, 741.
49a. McKean, D., Potter, M., and Hood, L.E. (1973). *Biochemistry* **12**, 760.
50. Potter, M. and Lieberman, R. (1970). *J. Exp. Med.* **132**, 737.
51. Potter, M. (1970). *Fed. Proc. Fed. Amer. Soc. Exp. Biol.* **29**, 85.
51a. Barstad, P., Rudikoff, S., Potter, M., Cohn, M., Konigsberg, W., and Hood, L. (1974). *Science* **183**, 962.
51b. Lieberman, R., Potter, M., Mushinski, E.B., Humphrey, W. Jr., and Rudikoff, S. (1974). *J. Exp. Med.* **139**, 983.
52. McIntire, K.R., Asofsky, R.M., Potter, M., and Kuff, E.L. (1965). *Science* **150**, 361.
53. Appella, E. and Perham, R.N. (1967). *Cold Spring Harbor Symp. Quant. Biol.* **32**, 37.
54. Appella, E. and Perham, R.N. (1968). *J. Mol. Biol.* **33**, 963.
55. Appella, E. (1971). *Proc. Nat. Acad. Sci. U.S.* **68**, 590.
56. Weigert, M.G., Cesari, I.M., Yonkovich, S.J., and Cohn, M. (1970). *Nature (London)* **228**, 1045.
57. Cesari, I.M. and Weigert, M.G. (1973). *Proc. Nat. Acad. Sci. U.S.* **70**, 2112.
58. Blomberg, B., Geckeler, W.R., and Weigert, M. (1972). *Science* **177**, 178.
58a. Appella, E., Roholt, O.A., Chersi, A., Radzimski, G., and Pressman, D. (1973). *Biochem Biophys. Res Commun.* **53**, (1122).
58b. Strosberg, A.D., Fraser, K.J., Margolies, M.N., and Haber, E. (1972). *Biochemistry* **11**, 4978.
58c. Braun, D.G. and Jaton, J.C. (1973). *Immunochemistry* **10**, 387.
58d. Rejnek, J., Appella, E., Mage, R.G., and Reisfeld, R.A. (1969). *Biochemistry* **8**, 2712.
58e. Strosberg, A.D., Margolies, M.N., and Haber, E. (1974). *Fed. Proc. Fed. Amer. Soc. Exp. Biol.* **33**, 726.
59. Gally, J.A. and Edelman, G.M. (1972). *Annu. Rev. Genet.* **6**, 1.
59a. Watanabe, S., Barnikol, H.U., Horn, J., Bertram, J., and Hilschmann, N. (1973). *Hoppe-Seyler's Z. Physiol. Chem.* **354**, 1505.
60. Putnam, F.W., Florent, G., Paul, C., Shinoda, T., and Shimizu, A. (1973). *Science* **182**, 287.

60a. Chuang, C-Y., Capra, J.D., and Kehoe, J.M. (1973). *Nature (London)* **244**, 158.
61. Lebovitz, H.E., Delaney, R., Fellows, R.E., Jr., and Hill, R.L. (1968). *J. Biol. Chem.* **243**, 4197.
62. Fruchter, R.G., Jackson, S.A., Mole, L.E., and Porter, R.R. (1970). *Biochem. J.* **116**, 249.
63. Appella, E., Chersi, A., Mage, R.G., and Dubiski, S. (1971). *Proc. Nat. Acad. Sci. U.S.* **68**, 1341.
64. Givol, D. and Porter, R.R. (1965). *Biochem. J.* **97**, 32c.
65. Hill, R.L., Delaney, R., Lebovitz, H.E., and Fellows, R.E. (1966). *Proc. Roy. Soc. B* **166**, 159.
66. Frangione, B. and Milstein, C. (1968). *J. Mol. Biol.* **33**, 893.
67. Frangione, B. and Milstein, C. (1969). *Nature (London)* **221**, 145.
68. Frangione, B. and Milstein, C. (1967). *Nature (London)* **216**, 939.
69. O'Donnell, I.J., Frangione, B., and Porter, R.R. (1970). *Biochem. J.* **116**, 261.
70. Edelman, G.M. (1970). *Biochemistry* **9**, 3197.
71. Hill, R.L., Lebovitz, H.E., Fellows, R.E., Jr., and Delaney, R. (1967). *3rd Nobel Symp.*, p. 109. Wiley (Interscience), New York.
72. Milstein, C. and Svasti, J. (1971). *In* "Progress in Immunology" (Bernard Amos, ed.), Vol. I, p. 35. Academic Press, New York.
73. Welscher, H.D. (1970). *Nature (London)* **228**, 1236.
74. Paul, C., Shimizu, A., Köhler, H., and Putnam, F.W. (1971). *Science* **172**, 69.
74a. Putnam, F.W., Shimizu, A., Paul, C., and Shinoda, T. (1972). *Fed. Proc. Fed. Amer. Soc. Exp. Biol.* **31**, 193.
75. Prahl, J.W., Mandy, W.J., and Todd, C.W. (1969). *Biochemistry* **8**, 4935.
76. Smyth, D.S. and Utsumi, S. (1967). *Nature (London)* **216**, 332.
77. Fanger, M.W. and Smyth, D.G. (1972). *Biochem. J.* **127**, 767.
77a. Frangione, B. and Wolfenstein-Todel, C. (1972). *Proc. Nat. Acad. Sci. U.S.* **69**, 3673.
77b. Bennich, H., Milstein, C., and Secher, D.S. (1973). *FEBS Lett.* **33**, 49.
78. Steiner, L.A. and Porter, R.R. (1967). *Biochemistry* **6**, 3957.
79. Wang, A.C. and Fudenberg, H.H. (1972). *Nature New Biol.* **240**, 24.
80. Milstein, C. and Pink, J.R.L. (1970). *Progr. Biophys. Mol. Biol.* **21**, 209.
81. Givol, D. and DeLorenzo, F. (1968). *J. Biol. Chem.* **243**, 1886.
82. Prahl, J.W. and Porter, R.R. (1968). *Biochem. J.* **107**, 753.
83. Miller, F. and Metzger, H. (1965). *J. Biol. Chem.* **240**, 3325.
84. Plaut, A.G. and Tomasi, T.B., Jr., (1970). *Proc. Nat. Acad. Sci. U.S.* **65**, 318.
84a. Shimizu, A., Paul, C., Köhler, H., Shinoda, T., and Putnam, F.W. (1971). *Science* **173**, 629.
85. Gall, W.E., Cunningham, B.A., Waxdal, M.J., Konigsberg, W.H., and Edelman, G.M. (1968). *Biochemistry* **7**, 1973.
86. Cahnmann, H.H., Arnon, R., and Sela, M. (1966). *J. Biol. Chem.* **241**, 3247.
86a. Waxdal, M.J., Konigsberg, W.H., Henley, W.L., and Edelman, G.M. (1968). *Biochemistry* **7**, 1959.
87. Rutishauser, U., Cunningham, B.A., Bennett, C., Konigsberg, W.H., and Edelman, G.M. (1970). *Biochemistry* **9**, 3171.
88. Pink, J.R., Buttery, S.H., De Vries, G.M., and Milstein, C. (1970). *Biochem. J.* **117**, 33.
89. Milstein, C. and Frangione, B. (1971). *Biochem. J.* **121**, 217.
90. Wang, A.C., Gergely, J., and Fudenberg, H.H. (1973). *Biochemistry* **12**, 528.
90a. Capra, J.D. and Kehoe, J.M. (1975). *Advan. Immunol.*, in press.

91. Wikler, M., Köhler, H., Shinoda, T., and Putnam, F.W. (1969). *Science* **163**, 75.
92. Press, E.M. and Hogg, N.M. (1970). *Biochem. J.* **117**, 641.
93. Gottlieb, P.D., Cunningham, B.A., Waxal, E.A., Konigsberg, W.H., and Edelman, G.M. (1968). *Proc. Nat. Acad. Sci. U.S.* **61**, 168.
94. Köhler, H., Shimizu, A., Paul, C., Moore, V., and Putnam, F.W. (1970). *Nature (London)* **227**, 1318.
95. Kaplan, A.P., Hood, L.E., Terry, W.D., and Metzger, H. (1971). *Immunochemistry* **8**, 801.
96. Capra, J.D. (1971). *Nature New Biol.* **230**, 62.
97. Kehoe, J.M. and Capra, J.D. (1971). *Proc. Nat. Acad. Sci. U.S.* **68**, 2019.
98. Wang, A.C., Fudenberg, H.H., and Pink, J.R.L. (1971). *Proc. Nat. Acad. Sci. U.S.* **68**, 1143.
98a. Capra, J.D., Wasserman, R.L., and Kehoe, J.M. (1973). *J. Exp. Med.* **138**, 410.
99. Nisonoff, A., Wilson, S.K., Wang, A.C., Fudenberg, H.H., and Hopper, J.E. (1971). *In* "Progress in Immunology" (B. Amos, ed.), Vol. 1, p. 61. Academic Press, New York.
100. Symposium, "2 genes, 1 polypeptide chain" (1972). *Fed. Proc. Fed. Amer. Soc. Exp. Biol.* **31**, 206.
101. Pink, J.R.L., McNally, M.P., Wang, A.C., and Fudenberg, H.H. (1972). *Immunochemistry* **9**, 84.
102. Franklin, E.C., Lowenstein, J., Bigelow, B., and Meltzer, M. (1964). *Amer. J. Med.* **37**, 332.
103. Seligmann, M., Danon, F., Hurez, D., Milhaesco, E., and Preud'homme, J.L. (1968). *Science* **162**, 1396.
104. Forte, F.A., Prelli, F., Yount, W.J., and Franklin, E.C. (1970). *Blood* **36**, 137.
105. Seligmann, M., Milhaesco, E., Hurez, D., Milhaesco, C., Preud'homme, J.L., and Rambaud, J.C. (1969). *J. Clin. Invest.* **48**, 2374.
106. Lee, S.L., Rosner, F., Ruberman, W., and Glasberg, S. (1971). *Ann. Intern. Med.* **75**, 407.
107. Ein, D., Buell, D.N., and Fahey, J.L. (1967). *J. Clin. Invest* **48**, 785.
108. Buxbaum, J., Franklin, E.C., and Scharff, M.D. (1970). *Science* **169**, 770.
109. Ellman, L.L. and Bloch, K.J. (1968). *New Engl. J. Med.* **278**, 1195.
109a. Buxbaum, J.M. and Preud'homme, J.L. (1972). *J. Immunol.* **109**, 1131.
110. Frangione, B. and Franklin, E.C. (1973). *Sem. Hematol.* **10**, 53.
111. Deutsch, H.F. and Suzuki, T. (1971). *Ann. N.Y. Acad. Sci.* **190**, 472.
112. Fett, J.W., Deutsch, H.F., and Smithies, O. (1973). *Immunochemistry* **10**, 115.
113. Cooper, S.M., Franklin, E.C., and Frangione, B. (1972). *Science* **176**, 187.
114. Terry, W.D. and Ein, D. (1971). *Ann. N.Y. Acad. Sci.* **190**, 467.
115. Franklin, E.C. and Frangione, B. (1971). *Proc. Nat. Acad. Sci. U.S.* **68**, 187.
116. Smithies, O., Gibson, D.A., Fanning, E.M., Perry, M.E., Parr, D.M., and Connell, G.E. (1971). *Science* **172**, 574.
116a. Frangione, B., Lee, L., Haber, E., and Bloch, K.J. (1973). *Proc. Nat. Acad. Sci. U.S.* **70**, 1073.
116b. Nakamura, N., Tanagaki, N., and Pressman, D. (1973). *Proc. Nat. Acad. Sci. U.S.* **70**, 2863.
116c. Poulik, M.D., Bernocco, M., Bernocco, D., and Ceppellini, R. (1973). *Science* **183**, 1352.
116d. Peterson, P.A., Rask, L., and Lindblom, J.B. (1974). *Proc. Nat. Acad. Sci. U.S.* **71**, 35.
116e. Smithies, O. and Poulik, M.D. (1972). *Science* **175**, 189.

116f. Peterson, P.A., Cunningham, B.A., Berggard, I., and Edelman, G.M. (1972). *Proc. Nat. Acad. Sci. U.S.* **69**, 1697.

117. Magnus-Levy, A. (1931). *Z. Klin. Med.* **116**, 510.

118. Osserman, E.F., Takatsuki, K., and Talal, N. (1964). *Sem. Hematol.* **1**, 3.

118a. Franklin, E.C. and Zucker-Franklin, D. (1972). *Advan. Immunol.* **15**, 249.

119. Isope, T. and Osserman, E.F. (1971). *Ann. N.Y. Acad. Sci.* **190**, 507.

120. Glenner, G., Harada, M., Isersky, C., Cuatrecasas, P., Page, D., and Keiser, H. (1970). *Biochem. Biophys. Res. Commun.* **41**, 1013.

121. Franklin, E.C. and Pras, M. (1969). *J. Exp. Med.* **130**, 797.

122. Glenner, G.G., Terry, W., Harada, M., Isersky, C., and Page, D.L. (1971). *Science* **172**, 1150.

123. Kimura, S., Guyer, R., Terry, W.D., and Glenner, G.G. (1972). *J. Immunol.* **109**, 891.

124. Isersky, C., Ein, D., Page, D.L., Harada, M., and Glenner, G.G. (1972). *J. Immunol.* **108**, 486.

125. Glenner, G.G., Terry, W.D., and Isersky, C. (1973). *Sem. Hematol.* **10**, 65.

126. Husby, G. and Natvig, J.B. (1972). *Clin. Exp. Immunol.* **10**, 635.

127. Glenner, G.G., Ein, D., Eanes, E.D., Bladen, H.A., Terry, W.D., and Page, D.L. (1971). *Science* **174**, 713.

128. Linke, R.P., Tischendorf, E.W., Zucker-Franklin, D., and Franklin, E.C. (1973). *J. Immunol.* **111**, 24.

129. Solomon, A. and McLaughlin, C.L. (1969). *J. Biol. Chem.* **244**, 3993.

130. Benditt, E.P., Eriksen, N., Hermodson, M.A., and Ericsson, L.H. (1971). *FEBS Lett.* **19**, 169.

131. Franklin, E.C., Pras, M., Levin, M., and Frangione, B. (1972). *FEBS Lett.* **22**, 121.

132. Ein, D., Kimura, S., and Glenner, G.G. (1972). *Biochem. Biophys. Res. Commun.* **46**, 498.

133. Husby, G., Sletten, K., Michaelson, T.E., and Natvig, J.B. (1972). *Nature New Biol.* **238**, 187.

134. Levin, M., Franklin, E.C., Frangione, B., and Pras, M. (1972). *J. Clin. Invest.* **51**, 2773.

134a. Husby, G., Natvig, J.B., Michaelson, T.E., Sletten, K., and Host, H. (1973). *Nature (London)* **244**, 362.

134b. Eylar, E.H. (1965). *J. Theoret. Biol.* **10**, 89.

135. Sox, H.C., Jr., and Hood, L. (1970). *Proc. Nat. Acad. Sci. U.S.* **66**, 975.

136. Shimizu, A., Putnam, F.W., and Paul, C. (1971). *Nature New Biol.* **231**, 73.

137. Kornfeld, R., Keller, J., Baenziger, J., and Kornfeld, S. (1971). *J. Biol. Chem.* **246**, 3259.

138. Baenziger, J., Kornfeld, S., and Kochwa, S. (1974). *J. Biol. Chem.* **249**, 1889.

138a. Abel, C.A., Spiegelberg, H.L., and Grey, H.M. (1968). *Biochemistry* **7**, 1271.

139. Spiegelberg, H.L., Abel, C.A., Fishkin, B.G., and Grey, H.M. (1970). *Biochemistry* **9**, 4217.

139a. Baenziger, T. and Kornfeld, S. (1974). *J. Biol. Chem.* **249**, 7270.

140. Davie, J.M. and Osterland, C.K. (1968). *J. Exp. Med.* **128**, 699.

140a. Hurst, M.M., Niedermeyer, W., Zikan, J., and Bennett, J.C. (1973). *J. Immunol.* **110**, 840.

141. Wang, A.C. and Fudenberg, H.H. (1970). *J. Immunol.* **105**, 1286.

141a. Dawson, G. and Clamp, J.R. (1968). *Biochem. J.* **107**, 341.

142. Grey, H.M., Abel, C.A., and Zimmerman, B. (1971). *Ann. N.Y. Acad. Sci.* **190**, 37.

142a. Moore, V. and Putnam, F.W. (1973). *Biochemistry* **12**, 2361.

143. Fanger, M.W. and Smyth, D.G. (1972). *Biochem. J.* **127**, 757.
144. Hinrichs, W.A. and Smyth, D.G. (1970). *Immunology* **18**, 759.
144a. Melchers, F. (1971). *Biochemistry* **10**, 653.
145. Scharff, M. and Uhr, J.W. (1965). *Science* **148**, 646.
146. Askonas, B.A. and Williamson, A.R. (1966). *Proc. Roy. Soc.* **B166**, 232.
147. Norton, W.L., Lewis, D., and Ziff, M. (1965). *Proc. Nat. Acad. Sci. U.S.* **53**, 851.
147a. Melchers, F. (1970). *Biochem. J.* **119**, 765.
148. Uhr, J.W. and Schenkein, I. (1970). *Proc. Nat. Acad. Sci. U.S.* **66**, 952.
149. Sutherland, E.W., Zimmerman, D.H., and Kern, M. (1972). *Proc. Nat. Acad. Sci. U.S.* **69**, 167.
150. Choi, Y.S., Knopf, P.M., and Lennox, E.S. (1971). *Biochemistry* **10**, 668.
150a. Melchers, F. (1973). *Biochemistry* **12**, 1471.
151. Wikler, M. and Putnam, F.W. (1970). *J. Biol. Chem.* **245**, 4488.
152. Gray, W.R., Dreyer, W.J., and Hood, L. (1967). *Science* **155**, 465.
153. Titani, K., Shinoda, T., and Putnam, F.W. (1969). *J. Biol. Chem.* **244**, 3550.
154. Milstein, C.P. (1969). *In* "Proceedings of the Fifth FEBS Symposium" (F. Franek and D. Shugar, eds.), Vol. 15, p. 43. Academic Press, New York.
155. Watanabe, S. and Hilschmann, N. (1970). *Hoppe-Seyler's Z. Physiol. Chem.* **351**, 1291.
156. Köhler, H., Shimizu, A., Paul, C., and Putnam, F.W. (1970). *Science* **169**, 56.
157. Hilschmann, N. (1967). *Hoppe-Seyler's Z. Physiol. Chem.* **348**, 1718.
158. Dreyer, W.J., Gray, W.R., and Hood, L. (1967). *Cold Spring Harbor Symp. Quant. Biol.* **32**, 353.
159. Suter, L., Barnikol, H.U., Watanabe, S., and Hilschmann, N. (1972). *Hoppe-Seyler's Z. Physiol. Chem.* **353**, 189.
160. Milstein, C.P. (1969). *FEBS Lett.* **2**, 301.
160a. Smith, G.P., Hood, L., and Fitch, W.M. (1971). *Annu. Rev. Biochem.* **40**, 969.
160b. Dayhoff, M.O. (1972). "Atlas of Protein Structure," Vol. 5. The National Biomedical Research Foundation, Silver Spring, Maryland.
161. Ponstingl, H. and Hilschmann, N. (1969). *Hoppe-Seyler's Z. Physiol. Chem.* **350**, 1148.
162. Ponstingl, H., Hess, M., and Hilschmann, N. (1968). *Hoppe-Seyler's Z. Physiol. Chem.* **349**, 867.
163. Milstein, C., Clegg, J.B., and Jarvis, J.M. (1968). *Biochem. J.* **110**, 631.
164. Baczko, K., Braun, D.G., Hess, M., and Hilschmann, N. (1970). *Hoppe-Seyler's Z. Physiol. Chem.* **351**, 763.
165. Hood, L. and Ein, D. (1968). *Nature (London)* **220**, 764.
166. Hood, L., Grey, W.R., Sanders, B.G., and Dreyer, W.J. (1968). *Cold Spring Harbor Symp. Quant. Biol.* **32**, 133.
167. de Preval, C., Pink, J.R.L., and Milstein, C. (1970). *Nature (London)* **228**, 930.
168. Frangione, B. and Milstein, C. (1969). *Nature (London)* **224**, 597.
169. Fleischman, J.B. (1973). *Immunochemistry* **10**, 401.

5

The Three-Dimensional Structure of Immunoglobulins

I. X-RAY CRYSTALLOGRAPHY

In 1942, Northrop succeeded in crystallizing a preparation of trypsin-treated horse diphtheria antitoxin (1). The crystals were grown from a solution containing protein having a molecular weight of 90,500 and antibody activity. It seems likely that the preparation consisted of F(ab')$_2$ fragments. Crystallization of human macroglobulins (IgM) was first reported by Kratochvil and Deutsch (2) and by Caputo and Appella (3). Crystals possessing antibody activity were prepared from a specifically purified preparation of anti-p-azobenzoate antibody (IgG) obtained from a rabbit producing it in very high concentrations (4). Initially, crystallization took place from neutral buffer at a protein concentration of 60 mg/ml, but recrystallization could be carried out at concentrations as low as 5 mg/ml. The purified protein behaved as a cryoglobulin; i.e., it was much less soluble at 0° than at room temperature. Evidence for homogeneity included the shape of the hapten-binding curve and the fact that the antibody possessed only one allotypic marker at a locus for which the rabbit was heterozygous. The crystals did not give an X-ray diffraction pattern suitable for detailed analysis.

A. X-Ray Crystallography of Intact Immunoglobulins

Only a few intact immunoglobulins have been subjected to extensive X-ray crystallographic analysis, and these studies have not yet attained high resolution. Terry *et al.* (5) crystallized a human myeloma protein, designated "Dob" [IgG1 (κ)], which was analyzed by Sarma *et al.* (6); protein "Dob" is a cryoglobulin. At the highest resolution obtainable, 6 Å, the overall shape of the molecule could be estimated; studies at higher resolution have been precluded so far by the sensitivity of the crystals to irradiation. Of possible models that fit the data the authors favored a T-shaped configuration with the two Fab fragments comprising the arms of the T   The horizontal length of the T is 142 Å and the verticle dimension is 85 Å. The distance of 142 Å between the ends of the

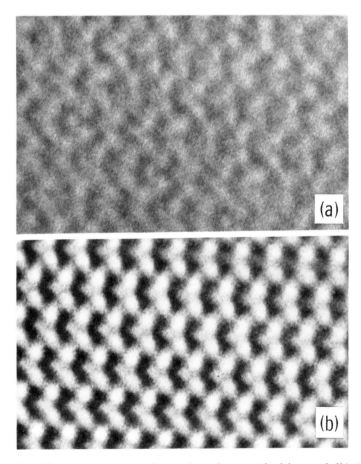

Fig. 5.1. Electron micrograph of a section of a crystal of human IgG1 (protein "Dob"), 400–900 Å in thickness. The thin section was stained by immersion first in saturated aqueous uranyl acetate, followed by lead citrate solution. Photograph (a) was obtained by a technique of "optical averaging," applied to the original photograph, (b) was obtained by optical averaging of (a). The IgG molecule is seen to be composed of three segments (see text). Reprinted from Labaw and Davies (8).

Fab fragments is somewhat greater than that obtained by electron microscopy ($\sim$ 120 Å) (7,8). The molecule was found to possess a twofold axis of symmetry, corresponding to the vertical axis of the T, which passes through the middle of the Fc fragment and defines two half-molecules.

A T-like configuration can be clearly seen in the electron micrographs of Labaw and Davies (8) (Fig. 5.1); the arms of the T make a slight angle so that the shape is actually intermediate between that of a T and a Y. The average dimensions of each arm (Fab fragment) in the photograph are 60 × 30 Å.

Preliminary X-ray crystallographic analyses have been carried out on another human myeloma protein [protein "Mcg," IgG1(λ)] by Edmundson *et al.* (9). This protein has the interesting characteristic that a portion of each H chain is deleted; the deletion comprises 15 residues in the hinge region. The protein was shown to possess a twofold axis of symmetry, with the asymmetric unit consisting of one L and one H chain. The Bence Jones protein (λ chain dimer) of this patient was also crystallized and subjected to X-ray analysis (Section I,E).

B. X-Ray Crystallography of Fc Fragments

Following the discovery by Porter (10) that fragment Fc crystallizes from a papain digest of rabbit IgG, the corresponding fragment was crystallized from the IgG of a number of species (e.g., 11,12). Goldstein *et al.* examined crystals of the Fc fragment of a human IgG1 myeloma protein (13). A twofold axis of symmetry was detected, which is consistent with the presence of two H chain segments. The fragment can be enclosed in a parallelepiped of dimensions 50 × 40 × 70 Å.

Preliminary studies have indicated the feasibility of carrying out X-ray analysis on the Fc fragment of normal rabbit IgG (14). In an initial investigation, no differences in intensities of the diffraction patterns or in cell dimensions were noted between Fc fragments of IgG preparations differing in allotype at the *a* and *b* loci, which control V_H regions and L chains, respectively. This is not surprising since the corresponding sets of markers are located in the Fab fragments.

C. Crystallization of Fab and Fab′ Fragments

The number of proteins that yield crystals, and the stability of the crystals, appear to be considerably greater when Fab or Fab′ fragments of human IgG myeloma proteins, rather than the intact proteins, are used (15,16). Also, the smaller molecular size of either fragment facilitates detailed analysis by X-ray crystallography. Myeloma proteins used for the preparation of fragments are first fractionated by ion-exchange chromatography to remove most of the nonspecific IgG present. After digestion with papain, or by pepsin followed by reduction, the Fab or Fab' fragments are isolated by ion-exchange chromatography and gel filtration, and are crystallized in the presence of ammonium sulfate; the optimal pH varies for individual proteins. About one-half of the myeloma proteins investigated have yielded crystals of Fab or Fab'. One preparation [from protein New, IgG1(λ)] has been studied extensively by X-ray analysis in the laboratory of R.J. Poljak. This work and that of D.R. Davies and his collaborators with the Fab' fragment of a mouse myeloma protein will be described next. In both studies the investigators succeeded in localizing the site of binding of a ligand of low molecular weight.

D. X-Ray Crystallographic Analysis of an Fab' Fragment of Human IgG

A detailed investigation of the Fab' fragment[1] of protein New was undertaken in 1969 by R.J. Poljak and his associates. This work resulted, first, in a model at 6 Å resolution (17) and, more recently, at 2.8 Å (18).

Poljak et al., have also worked out the complete amino acid sequence of the V_λ segment of the protein (Fig. 5.2). From the electron density map, the known sequences of the λ chain and the C_H1 region of IgG1, and published V_H sequences, they were able to trace both the L chain and the Fd' segment of the H chain throughout their lengths. All residues in the L chain and many in the Fd region, particularly those with bulky side chains, were identified.

A photograph of their 2.8 Å model is shown in Fig. 5.3. The two domains of both the L chain (in green) and the H chain (in red) are readily distinguishable; the V domains are to the left of the figure. The long yellow rods are approximate twofold axes of symmetry; i.e., there is a very close structural resemblance between the C_L and C_H1 domains and, to a somewhat lesser degree, between the V_L and V_H domains. The two

---

[1] The Fab and Fab' fragments give indistinguishable diffraction patterns and have therefore been used interchangeably, despite the extra stretch of 10 amino acids at the C-terminal end of the Fd' fragment in Fab'. This suggests that the extra length of polypeptide is flexible and varies in its conformation within the crystal; this possibility would be consistent with the fact that this segment is in the hinge region, which is believed to be a loosely folded portion of the chain.

```
 1                        10                      20                27  27a
(Glp, Ser, Val) Leu Thr Gln Pro Pro Ser Val Ser Gly Ala Pro Gly Gln Arg Val Thr Ile Ser Cys Thr Gly Ser Ser Ser Asn

27b 27c
Ile Gly Ala Gly Asn His Val Lys Trp Tyr Gln Gln Leu Pro Gly Thr Ala Pro Lys Leu Leu Ile Phe His Asn Asn Ala Arg

54
 –   –   –   –   –  Phe Ser Val Ser Lys Ser Gly Ser Ser Ala Thr Leu Ala Ile Thr Gly Leu Gln Ala Glu Asp

82
Glu Ala Asp Tyr Tyr Cys Gln Ser Tyr Asp Arg Ser Leu Arg  –   –  Val Phe Gly Gly Gly Thr Lys Leu Thr Val Leu Arg
```

Fig. 5.2. Sequence of the V_1 region of λ chain New. The numbers, 27a, b, and c and gaps in positions 54–60 and 96–97 are introduced to maximize homology with other human λ chains. Glp, pyrollidonecarboxylic acid. [From Poljak *et al.* (18).]

V domains also resemble the C domains, but the former have an additional loop of polypeptide chain (see Fig. 5.4). The middle of each chain, where the C region begins (switch region), is marked by a tag (one tag is in the upper right corner). A large cleft is apparent in the center of the molecule. The approximate dimensions of the molecule are $80 \times 50 \times 40$ Å; the maximum dimension of each domain is approximately 40 Å. Each domain has a compact globular structure which is quite independent of the other domain. Major structural features also include a hydrophobic core and the presence of a substantial amount of the antiparallel β-pleated sheet conformation. In agreement with physicochemical measurements, little α-helix can be discerned. The switch region is loosely folded and accessible as compared to the compact internal structure of the molecule.

The four intrachain disulfide bonds, symmetrically disposed in the four domains, are indicated by pairs of white spheres in Fig. 5.3. These are buried in the hydrophobic core, which accounts for their resistance to reducing agents in the undenatured molecule. The spheres at the extreme right mark the interchain (H–L) disulfide bond. Very close to each of the disulfide bonds is a tryptophan residue, shown in blue. These tryptophan residues are a common, almost invariant feature of immunoglobulins.

A representation of the folding of the polypeptide chains within a domain is shown in Fig. 5.4. The folding patterns of the four individual domains are very similar, except for the presence of an extra segment in each V domain. In the C_L domain, four antiparallel chains form a β pleated sheet, while three other antiparallel chain segments form another β-pleated sheet. The two sheets are held together by a strongly hydrophobic region. Each of the four domains in the Fab fragment is built on a similar pattern (18a). The β-pleated sheet conformation is inferred from the spacings between chain segments and orientation of carbonyl and amino groups, which are appropriate to permit formation of

---

Fig. 5.3. View of the 2.8 Å resolution model of Fab' New. The backbones of the L and Fd' (H) polypeptide chains are shown in green and red, respectively. The V (left) and C (right) domains are separated by a central cleft. Labels show the "switch regions" at the junction of V and C domains, near the midpoints of both chains. The approximate local twofold axes of symmetry are indicated by two yellow rods. The four intrachain disulfide bonds and the interchain disulfide bond (extreme right) are marked by white spheres. Yellow tapes connect the α-carbon positions of residues that form disulfide bonds in other immunoglobulin molecules. The numbered labels at the left end of the model indicate the hypervariable positions; circular tags are on L chains, rectangular tags on H chains. Blue tags mark the homologous tryptophan residues near the intrachain disulfide bonds in each of the four subunits. Arrows at the right end of the model point to Ser 154 and Lys 191, Kern(−) and Oz(+) serological markers, respectively. From Poljak *et al.* (18).

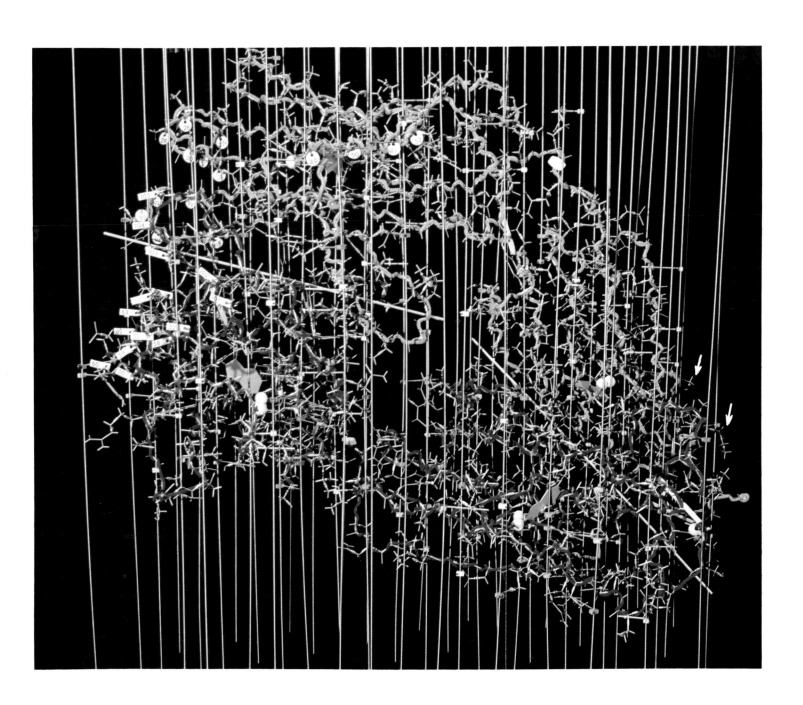

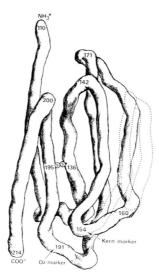

Fig. 5.4. Diagram showing the folding of the constant region of the λ chain of protein New. Position 110 is the N-terminal amino acid of the C region. The C_H1 domain, which interacts with C_L to form the C module of the Fab fragment, has virtually the same three-dimensional structure. The dotted line indicates the additional loop of polypeptide chain present in the V_L and V_H domains. From Poljak *et al.* (18).

multiple hydrogen bonds between adjacent chain segments. The authors point out that homology of amino acid sequence should be reflected in homology of three-dimensional structure, and that is the case with respect to the four domains. They predict, on this basis, a similar three-dimensional structure for β_2-microglobulin. Note that positions 154 and 191, which determine the Kern and Oz allotypic markers, are localized on the exterior of the molecule where they are accessible to an antibody.

Nearly all the sharp bends in the polypeptide chains include glycine residues, which are essentially invariant. A proline, serine, or threonine residue generally occupies the position on the N-terminal side of the glycine. Glycine residues 100–102 are believed to be invariant because amino acids with large side chains would interfere sterically with the close packing in that region. The invariance of a number of hydrophobic residues is explained by their presence in the hydrophobic core, responsible for holding together two β-pleated sheets.

1. COMPARISON OF PATTERNS OF DISULFIDE BONDS IN PROTEIN NEW AND OTHER IMMUNOGLOBULINS

From data on amino acid sequences the arrangement of disulfide bonds in different immunoglobulins might appear to be quite distinct. As one example, the L–H disulfide bond in human IgG1 involves half-cystine 220 in the hinge region of the γ_1 chain, whereas in the other subclasses of human IgG, in human IgM, rabbit IgG, mouse IgG2a and IgG2b, and in guinea pig IgG2a, the L chain is disulfide bonded to a half-cystine in the H chain at a position homologous to position 131 of the human γ_1 chain.[2] The crystallographic model of protein New shows, however, that positions 131 and 220 in the γ_1 chain are in very close proximity, so that the alternative disulfide bonds could be formed without disrupting the three-dimensional structure. An extra intrachain disulfide bond in rabbit κ_B chains, linking residue 80 in the V_L domain to residue 171 in the C_L domain (19,19a) is similarly consistent with the structure of protein New; i.e., the two positions are in close proximity even though protein New does not possess these half-cystines. The same principle applies to an "extra" intrachain disulfide bond in the rabbit γ chain, joining positions 130 or 132 and 221 (human γ_1 numbering system) (20). Poljak et al. conclude that the three-dimensional structures of κ chains, λ chains, and the V_H and C_H domains of a variety of immunoglobulins are all very similar. This is consistent with the hypothesis that a primordial gene encoded a polypeptide the size of one domain (Chapter 12).

2. Region of the Combining Site

A striking feature of the structural model is the clustering of amino acids present in hypervariable regions of both the H and L chains into one portion of the three-dimensional structure, which is almost entirely exposed to the solvent. These residues are tagged in Fig. 5.3. An exception is the stretch of amino acids, 49–52, which extends to the right of the cluster in the figure. However, even these amino acids would be within that region if it were not for the deletion of residues 55–61 in the λ chain of protein New (Fig. 5.2). Also, the third hypervariable region of the H chain (identified so far in V_{HIII} proteins, at positions 85–90), does not fall within the same region of the molecule. The size of the cluster of hypervariable residues is quite substantial; the maximum distance separating two such residues is about 25 Å. Among these amino acids are several tyrosine groups. That this part of the molecule is indeed responsible for antigen binding is shown by the interaction of protein New with ligands (to be discussed later). The model confirms the conclusion, reached earlier from studies of affinity labeling and the requirement of both chains for full antibody activity, that the combining site comprises

---

[2] Numbering system of protein Eu (IgG1).

amino acids from both the L and the H chain. The "contact area" in the H chain appears larger than that in the L chain.

No deep cavity can be observed in the combining region. It does, however, contain a shallow groove, $15 \times 6 \times 6$ Å, which can accommodate a hapten of moderate size; both chains contribute to the formation of the groove. It would appear that if protein New were, for example, an antiprotein antibody, it might combine with the antigen by face-to-face contact rather than by a lock-and-key type of fit.

The large number of amino acids in the combining region, and their hypervariability, could apparently yield an almost infinite variety of combining sites. This would account, also, for the uniqueness of idiotypic determinants and the fact that the region of the combining site is generally one of the most important idiotypic determinants of the molecule (21–24). The interference of a specific hapten with binding by antiidiotypic antibody, when the ligand is an antihapten antibody, might well be accounted for simply by steric blocking of the region of the active site; there appears to be no need to postulate that the idiotypic determinant is distal from the combining site and is altered by an allosteric type of transition when hapten enters the site. (This does not imply that no conformational change occurs when hapten is bound, but only that the region of the active site itself is an idiotypic determinant; the observation that most hypervariable residues are exposed to the solvent further supports this hypothesis, since such residues could interact with an antibody.)

The fact that many of the residues in hypervariable regions are on the surface of the molecule is in accord with the great variability of sequence in these regions; restrictions are not imposed by the necessity for appropriate interaction with other segments of the molecule. In contrast, many of the hydrophobic residues buried in the interior of the molecule are either invariant or are replaced in known sequences by other hydrophobic amino acids. Residues on the surface of the molecule, but outside the hypervariable regions, include amino acids with both hydrophobic and polar side chains.

Since affinity labeling generally takes place in hypervariable regions (Chapter 2), the labels would be present in the combining region indicated by the crystallographic model. Exceptions are tyrosine 85 in the L chain (Fig. 5.2) and tyrosine 94 in the H chain; these residues are in the core of the molecule and not readily accessible from the hypervariable region. Yet the corresponding tyrosine groups, in mouse or rabbit anti-2,4-dinitrophenyl antibodies, appear to be affinity labeled by the reagent, [^{3}H]m-nitrobenzenediazonium fluoroborate (25,26).

3. BINDING OF A HYDROXYL DERIVATIVE OF VITAMIN K_1 BY
   THE Fab' FRAGMENT OF PROTEIN NEW

It is possible to prepare difference Fourier maps, with and without ligand in the active site of a crystallized protein, and determine the precise location of the ligand with respect to the amino acids that make up the site. This is perhaps the strongest and most direct experimental approach to the determination of the structural basis of specificity, the size of the contact area, and the nature of the forces operating to bind a ligand to the protein molecule. It can also provide information as to the occurrence of a conformational change as a consequence of the interaction. The possibility that a conformational change is responsible for complement fixation, or for triggering the differentiation of a B lymphocyte upon interaction of surface receptors with antigen, has often been considered but not proved.

A large number of small molecules were tested for their capacity to interact with the Fab' fragment of protein New (27). The strongest binding ($K_0 = 2 \times 10^5$ M^{-1}) was observed with a γ-hydroxyl derivative of vitamin K_1 (vitamin K_1OH):

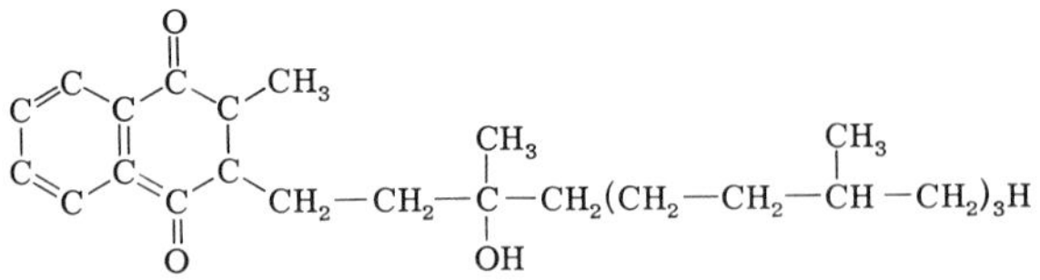

It was possible to introduce vitamin K_1OH by allowing it to diffuse into the Fab' crystal structure. A difference Fourier map, calculated at a resolution of 3.5 Å, showed that vitamin K_1OH occupies a position in the hypervariable region. A photograph indicating the nature of the fit is shown in Fig. 5.5. The quinone portion of the molecule occupies the shallow groove, mentioned earlier, which is bounded by amino acids from both the H and L chains, is 6 Å deep, and 15 × 6 Å in length and width. The hydrocarbon "tail" of vitamin K_1OH extends downward about 10 Å, terminating near residue 57 of the H chain. That this portion of vitamin K_1OH contributes to the energy of interaction is shown by the lower binding affinity ($K_0 = 1 \times 10^3$ M^{-1}) of 2-methyl-1,4-naphthoquinone, which resembles vitamin K_1OH but lacks the hydrocarbon chain. From the difference in K values the tail would appear to contribute 3 kcal/mole to the standard free energy of interaction of vitamin K_1OH (~7.2 kcal/mole) with Fab' New. The smaller compound was found to bind to the same position of the Fab' molecule as the quinone portion of vitamin K_1OH; it makes contact with the aromatic

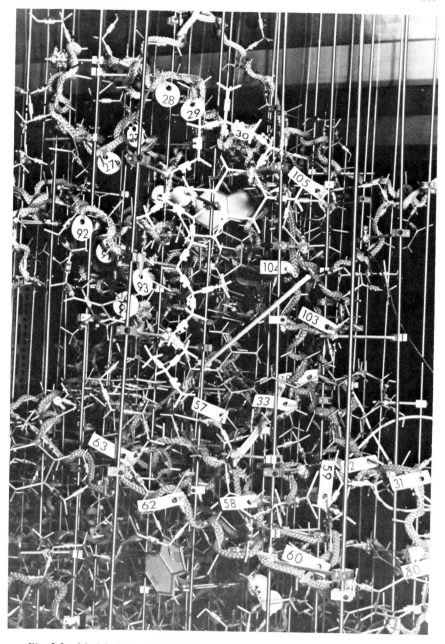

Fig. 5.5. Model of vitamin K₁OH (in white) bound to Fab' of protein New. Hyper-variable positions in L and H chains are designated by round and rectangular tags, respectively. From Amzel *et al.* (27).

side chain of tyrosine 90 at the bottom of the shallow groove, and with two or three other amino acids as well. The hydrocarbon tail makes very close contact with several amino acids in both the L and H chain; at least ten amino acids of the protein are direct contact residues. A complete description of the fit will be possible when the H chain sequence is worked out.

4. ABSENCE OF A DETECTABLE CONFORMATIONAL CHANGE ASSOCIATED WITH BINDING OF VITAMIN K_1OH

The difference Fourier map failed to reveal any structural alterations in the Fab' molecule as a consequence of binding vitamin K_1OH. This finding would not rule out minor alterations in the positions of side chains, or the possibility that binding in solution, as opposed to the crystalline state, might be associated with a conformational change. It does suggest, however, that a major conformational change is not a prerequisite for binding at the active site. A similar finding was made by other investigators in their studies of crystallized Fab' fragment of a mouse myeloma protein with antihapten activity (Section I,F).

Poljak (18a) does not rule out the possibility of a conformational change upon interaction with a ligand that makes contact with a larger segment of the hypervariable region (e.g., a protein antigen rather than a hapten). He notes that the flexibility in the switch region of the Fd segment could permit some extension of the molecule, exposing more of the side chains in the H chain to the solvent and resulting in a slight elongation of the Fab' fragment. He tends to exclude such movement in the L chain because the V_L domain is disulfide bonded to C_L in rabbit κ_B chains; this would prevent any appreciable movement of the domains relative to one another.

E. Structure of a Bence Jones Protein (Human λ Chain Dimer) at 3.5 Å Resolution

The structure of a λ chain dimer has been solved at high resolution in the laboratory of A.B. Edmundson (28,29). Results of this study were published at about the same time as the 2.8 Å model of the Fab' fragment of protein New. Many of the conclusions concerning immunoglobulin structure drawn from the two investigations are identical although each molecule has certain distinctive features. The myeloma protein from the patient ("Mcg"), who provided the Bence Jones protein, has a deletion of 15 residues in the hinge region of each H chain

(30). Results of preliminary X-ray analysis of the intact myeloma protein were mentioned earlier.

In addition to the customary isomorphous heavy metal derivatives, a mercury atom was inserted between the half-cystine groups which form the interchain disulfide bond (31) in the Bence Jones protein (λ-S-Hg-S-λ) by a method devised by Steiner and Blumberg (32): the disulfide bond is reduced with mercaptoethanol, excess reducing agent is removed by gel filtration, and mercuric acetate is then added. The disulfide bond which is reduced originates at the half-cystine adjacent to the C-terminal residue of each λ chain in the dimer.

Although the amino acid sequence of this protein has not yet been reported, the sequence of the C_L region is known from the literature, as are the locations of a number of relatively invariant residues in the V_L region. Furthermore, some bulky amino acid side chains could be identified from the electron density maps. From these data the authors were able to trace the course of both polypeptide chains in the dimer and to identify nearly all of the amino acids in the C region and many in the V region, including the half-cystine residues. Sketches of their crystallographic model are reproduced in Figs. 5.6 to 5.11. The numbering system they used is that of λ chain "Bo" of Wikler and Putnam (33).

The disulfide bonds of the molecule are clearly defined, as is the "switch" position in each of the polypeptide chains (position 111, Figure

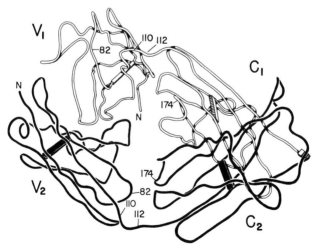

Fig. 5.6. Model of the Bence Jones dimer from patient Mcg. The photograph was taken facing the C_λ domain of monomer 2. The cleft lined by amino acids in hypervariable regions is in the upper left corner. From Schiffer *et al.* (29).

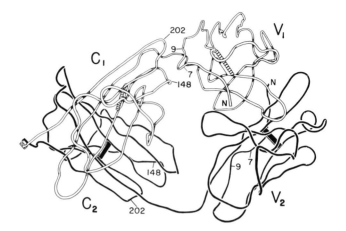

Fig. 5.7. Photograph of the model of the Bence Jones dimer from patient Mcg. The photograph was taken facing the C_λ domain of monomer 1. The cleft lined by amino acids in hypervariable regions is in the upper right corner. Note that residues 9 and 202, and 7 and 148, interact in monomer 1 but are widely separated in monomer 2. From Schiffer *et al.* (29).

5.6). This amino acid is part of an extended length of polypeptide chain connecting the two globular domains of each polypeptide chain. The cleft, or hollow region in the center of the molecule closely resembles that in Fab fragment of protein New. Since the two λ chains do not have the same spatial configuration in the dimer one is designated monomer 1 and, the other, monomer 2 (Fig. 5.6 to 5.8).[3]

If one considers the four domains as separate entities, V_1 and V_2 are found to be virtually identical in size and conformation, as are C_1 and C_2, but the conformations of the V and C domains differ somewhat; for example, the stretch comprising residues 48–60 in the V domain has several bends (Fig. 5.8); it does not have its counterpart in the C domain. The loop adjacent to residue 26 is also unique to the V domain. Both of these sequences are in hypervariable regions.

The arrangement in space of the V and C domains, relative to one another, differs markedly in the two polypeptide chains; i.e., despite the fact that the two monomeric λ chains are identical in sequence they adopt different spatial configurations. To illustrate this point, the distance between the intrachain disulfide bonds in the V and C domains in monomer 1 (Figs. 5.6 and 5.7) is 25 Å; the corresponding distance in monomer 2 is 43 Å. Schiffer *et al.*, deduce that monomer 2 corresponds

---

[3] The corresponding domains in monomer 1 and monomer 2 have the same three-dimensional structure. The domains are, however, arranged differently in space in the two monomers.

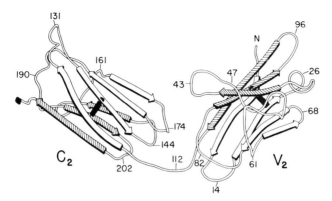

Fig. 5.8. Schematic drawing of monomer 2 (see Fig. 5.6). The arrows point in the C-terminal direction of the polypeptide chain. The white arrows are in the "4-chain layers" (see text) and the shaded arrows are in the "3-chain layers." The solid bars represent the intrachain disulfide bonds. From Schiffer *et al.* (29).

in its configuration to the L chain in an Fab fragment and monomer 1 to the Fd segment of the H chain. This conclusion is based first on the fact that position 147 in the C region lies so close to the V region in monomer 1 (Fig. 5.7) that it could not readily accommodate the valine side chain which has occasionally been found there in λ chains (in place of the usual alanine); in monomer 2 position 147 is on the surface and presents no difficulties. Second, residues corresponding to numbers 82 and 174 in the Mcg λ chain form an intrachain disulfide bond in rabbit κ_B chains (Chapter 8). These residues are in very close proximity in monomer 2 but not in monomer 1 (Fig. 5.6), again suggesting that monomer 2 plays the role of the L chain in the dimer, whereas monomer 1 has the conformation normally assumed by the H chain. The conclusion that monomer 1 has adopted the structural role of the H chain is supported by the model of the Fab' fragment (Fig. 5.3). (Note, for example, the greater distance separating the two intrachain disulfide bonds in the L chain as compared to the H chain.) It is of interest that the two L chains in the IgG molecule (protein Mcg) appear to be identical in structure. The adoption of two different configurations is therefore unique to the L chain dimers.

Perhaps the most remarkable feature of the λ chain dimer is that the hypervariable regions of the two L chains come together at one corner of the molecule and produce a cavity which might well act as a combining site for an appropriate ligand. This can be seen in the upper left corner of Fig. 5.6 and, in more detail, in Fig. 5.9. The cavity is cone-shaped with a diameter of 15 Å at the mouth and a depth of 10 Å. It is

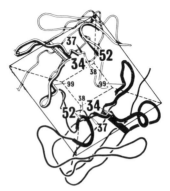

Fig. 5.9. View into the cavity between the V_λ domains of the Bence Jones dimer (patient Mcg). The hypervariable regions (residues 23–36, 51–55, and 91–100) are indicated by thickened chains. The side chains of residues 34 and 52, in positions homologous to those which are affinity labeled in murine anti-DNP antibodies, are represented by large numbers protruding into the cavity. The floor of the cavity is shown as a square array of four residues, two (residues 38 and 99) from each monomer. The invariant tryptophan residue at position 37 is also indicated. From Schiffer *et al.* (29).

bounded by residues in the three hypervariable segments of both chains. The floor of the cavity consists of four aromatic side chains, tyrosine 38 and phenylalanine 99 from each monomer. These are variable, but not hypervariable positions. There appear to be ten aromatic side chains in the cavity or its immediate vicinity. The size of the cavity formed by the L chain dimer is much greater than that in the Fab' fragment of protein New.

This significant finding indicated that an L chain dimer might act as an effective antibody in the absence of an H chain, and that an ancestral immunoglobulin might have consisted only of L chains. However, in forming a dimer an L chain would be restricted to one specificity whereas one L chain can presumably generate antibodies of different specificities by combining with a variety of H chains. Thus, 100 H and L chains can conceivably generate 10^4 specificities by forming H–L pairs, but 200 L chains can form only 200 homologous dimers. (So far there is no evidence that nonhomologous L chain dimers can form an active site.) Positions 34 and 52 around the cavity correspond to residues which have been affinity labeled in mouse immunoglobulins. Schiffer *et al.* agree with Poljak *et al.* that a tyrosine residue which has been affinity labeled in mouse immunoglobulins (corresponding to position 88 in the Mcg λ chain) is not readily accessible from the active site.

Schiffer *et al.* note that each domain comprises a layer of antiparallel segments containing four chain-segments and another layer

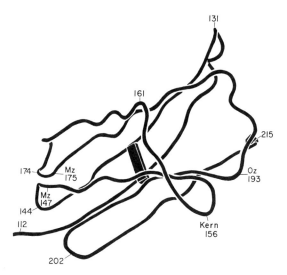

Fig. 5.10. Outline of the polypeptide chain in the C domain of monomer 2 (Fig. 5.8). Note the interior location of the intrachain disulfide bond (solid bar) and the exposed locations of the Kern and Oz antigenic markers (Chapter 4). The Mz substitutions are valine for alanine 147 and asparagine for lysine 175 (32). From Schiffer *et al.* (29).

containing three segments (Fig. 5.8). Each intrachain disulfide bond connects the middle section in the three-chain layer to a parallel segment in the four-chain layer. In the two C domains of the dimer the three-chain layers provide the outside surfaces of the molecule. In the V domains these two layers face one another and form the cavity which resembles the combining site of an antibody. Other aspects of the structure of the dimer are shown in Figs. 5.10 and 5.11. The three-dimensional structures of the individual domains are very similar to those determined by Poljak *et al.* (18) for a human Fab′ fragment.

F. X-Ray Crystallography of Fab′ Fragment of a Mouse Myeloma Protein

Rudikoff *et al.* (34,35) are applying X-ray crystallography to Fab′ fragments of a mouse myeloma protein (McPC 603), which specifically binds phosphorylcholine, and have determined its structure to a resolution of 4.5 Å.

The overall dimensions of the fragments are approximately $40 \times 50 \times 80$ Å, which are precisely the same as those reported for the Fab or Fab′ fragments of human protein New. In other important structural features as well, the mouse protein closely resembles that of the human. The V and C regions are compact and distinct globular units

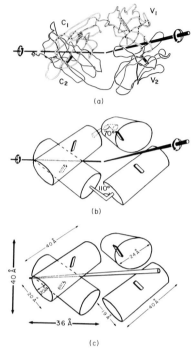

Fig. 5.11. (a) Local pseudo-twofold axes of rotation in the Bence Jones dimer. The axis on the right runs through the center of the cavity between the V domains (lined by hypervariable residues) and intersects the twofold axis between the C domains at an angle of about 120°. (b) Schematic representation of the dimer. The long axes through the cylinders representing the V_1 and C_1 domains make an angle of about 70°; the corresponding angle in monomer 2 is ~110°; thus monomer 2 has a more extended configuration. (c) Dimensions of the Bence Jones dimer and its constituent domains. A "particle axis," defined as a line through the centers of the two modules, is included in the drawing. The length of the dimer, measured along this axis, is 77 Å, a value very close to that of the Fab fragment of protein New. The thicker arrows indicate dimensions of the small module (on the left), as distinguished from individual domains. The third dimension of the small module (41 Å) is normal to the page. From Schiffer *et al.* (29).

with a region of low electron density separating them. Although the course of the polypeptide chains was not completely traced at 4.5 Å resolution, the electron density map is entirely in accord with the expectation that one globular unit comprises the V_L and V_H domains and the other the C_L and C_H1 domains.

The hapten-binding site was localized by using the phosphorylcholine derivative, 2-(5'-acetoxymercury-2'-thienyl)-ethyl phosphorylcholine. When soaked in a solution of this hapten the crystallized protein binds two molecules per Fab' fragment, but only one molecule is displaced by *p*-nitrophenyl phosphorylcholine; the latter is assumed to occupy the active site since the crystals bind only one mole of phosphorylcholine per mole of Fab'. From the difference in electron density patterns in the presence and absence of the mercury derivative of phosphorylcholine, and with the knowledge as to which part of the difference is due to binding in the active site, the site was localized to one end of the molecule, at a position corresponding to that of the active site in protein New. (This experiment also served to identify the V region.) The hapten was present in a cleft between the two regions of high electron density which evidently correspond to the V_L and V_H domains. The cleft appears to be deeper than that in protein New and would apparently accommodate molecules much larger than the hapten used in the study.

Another finding of interest was the absence of detectable electron density changes when hapten was added. This argues, again, against any substantial conformational change (at least in the crystal) associated with binding of the hapten. The authors suggest the possibility that the protein crystallizes in a conformation characteristic of the presence of bound hapten, owing to the presence of sulfate ion in the active site; in other words, that the conformational change had already occurred when the protein was crystallized. The simpler interpretation is that there is little conformational change upon interaction with hapten. The structure of the Fab' fragment has now been determined in great detail and will be described in forthcoming publications.

G. Structure of a Human V_κ Dimer

Epp *et al.* (35a) have worked out the crystal structure of a Bence Jones protein (Rei) which proved to be a symmetrical dimer of a $V_{\kappa I}$ domain, lacking a C_L region; the molecular weight of the protein is 25,000. The C-terminal residue is arginine 108 and the electron density map, at 2.8 Å resolution, could be followed through isoleucine 106. The approximate dimensions of the dimer are $40 \times 25 \times 28$ Å. The authors had available the complete amino acid sequence to aid in their structural analysis. The general folding pattern of the V_κ domain closely resembles that of the V_λ domain in proteins New or Mcg. The only major difference is in the first hypervariable region where the λ chains have an additional, small helical segment which accommodates three "extra" residues. Thus, virtually the same structural pattern appears in the V and C regions of mouse κ, and human λ and γ chains. The results of Epp *et al.* indicate that the V domain acquires the same conformation, whether or not a C domain is present. As in Fab' of protein New there is a great deal of β-pleated sheet structure, involving about 50% of the amino acid residues, with many hydrophobic residues buried in the core. A detailed map of the hydrogen bonding pattern within the pleated sheets is given in reference 35a.

One portion of the V_κ dimer resembles the combining region of the Fab' fragment. It consists of a cavity surrounding the axis of twofold symmetry at one end of the molecule which is lined by amino acids from all three hypervariable regions of both chains. As in protein New and the Mcg λ chain dimer this region is rich in tyrosine residues. The cavity could accommodate a hapten molecule containing an aromatic ring with polar substituents. Thus, a V_κ dimer, as well as a λ chain dimer, might have served as a primitive antibody molecule.

II. PHYSICOCHEMICAL INVESTIGATIONS RELATING TO THREE-DIMENSIONAL STRUCTURE

We will describe briefly some of the general conclusions concerning three-dimensional structure that have been derived from measurements other than X-ray crystallography. (The topological arrangement of poly-peptide chains in various classes of human immunoglobulins is discussed in Chapter 3.) Among reviews of this topic are those by Dorrington and Tanford (36), Metzger (37), and Haber and Cathou (38).

Studies of optical rotatory dispersion (ORD) have consistently failed to detect appreciable amounts of α-helix in immunoglobulins (39–42). This is in accord with the X-ray crystallographic models of the proteins studied so far. The ORD spectra of IgM and IgA are quite similar to that of IgG in their general properties (43,44) although distinctive features are also present in each class. It should be noted that spectra are not readily interpretable in terms of detailed molecular structure. Steiner and Lowey (42) found that the ORD spectrum of a papain digest of rabbit IgG was identical to that of the intact protein; this suggests that the cleavage does not significantly alter the internal conformation of the Fab or Fc fragments. Similarly, Dorrington and Tanford (44) noted that reduction of IgM to produce the IgMs (four-chain) subunit does not change the ORD spectrum.

Steiner and Lowey (42) did observe small differences, localized in the Fab fragment, between the ORD spectra of specifically purified rabbit antidinitrophenyl antibodies and nonspecific rabbit IgG. The authors speculated that a specific antibody may have a unique conformation in at least one portion of the Fab fragment, whereas the remainder of the molecule is invariant; this would be in accord with the limited data available from crystallographic studies, which are indicative of some variability in conformation in the region of the active site.

Measurements of circular dichroism, as well as ORD, are consistent with the presence of little α-helix (45–47). Cathou *et al.* interpreted a negative band at 217 nm in the circular dichroic spectrum of the Fab fragment of nonspecific rabbit IgG or of rabbit antidinitrophenyl antibody as indicative of the presence of a substantial amount of β structure; the band was more pronounced in the Fab fragment of the antibody than in the Fab fragment of IgG. An alternative possibility, that the band is due to aromatic structures, was considered less probable. As indicated above, there is a very substantial amount of β-pleated sheet structure in each of the four domains of an Fab' fragment or in the two domains of a V_κ dimer. This confirms the interpretation of data on circular dichroism favored by Cathou and co-workers.

The X-ray crystallographic model of an Fab fragment (Fig. 5.3) shows the individual V and C domains of both the L chain and the Fd fragment of the H chain as compact globular structures, with the V and C segments of each chain linked by an exposed stretch of polypeptide chain. A number of earlier findings had predicted such a structure in general terms. For example, Givol and co-workers prepared an "Fv" fragment, consisting only of the variable segments of the H and L chain by proteolysis of mouse IgA; the fragment was found to retain its ability to react with ligand and also its idiotypic specificity (48,49). It is possible to cleave L chains preferentially in the "switch region" with proteolytic enzymes (50,51) or by mild acid hydrolysis (52). The resulting V_L and C_L fragments retain their compact globular structures (53,54) and the circular dichroic spectrum of a mixture of the fragments is similar to that of the intact L chain (55). In the Fc region, rabbit (56,57) and human (58–62) IgG can be cleaved by proteolytic enzymes, under appropriate conditions, between the C_H2 and C_H3 domains (as well as in the hinge region) without disrupting the globular structure of the C_H3 domain. Finally, either the isolated V_L or C_L segment of an L chain has been shown to combine *in vitro* with an intact H chain; this would suggest that each segment retains much or all of its globular structure (63).

Flexibility of the Immunoglobulin Molecule

1. ELECTRON MICROSCOPY

Evidence that immunoglobulins are flexible comes from electron microscopy and, to a lesser degree, from physicochemical studies. The

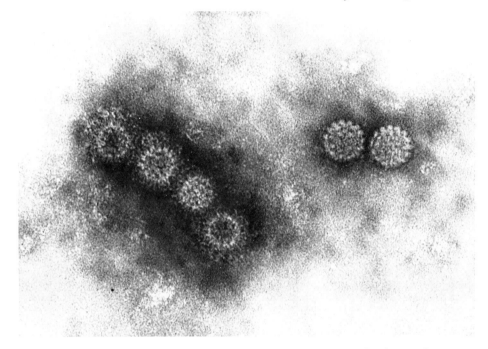

Fig. 5.12. Electron micrograph showing a mixture of wart and polyoma virus to which antipolyoma virus antiserum had been added. The polyoma virus (at the left) is coated with antibody molecules which cross-link the particles, while the wart virus is free of antibody. The diameters of the polyoma and wart viruses are approximately 450 and 550 Å, respectively. A suspension of virus containing 1.5% phosphotungstic acid was dehydrated on a carbon-Formvar coated grid in the electron microscope. Reprinted by permission of Dr. B. Cinader from reference 65.

technique of negative staining has proven to be the most effective for electron microscopy; shadow-casting after spraying a solution onto freshly cleaved mica has also been used (64). Almeida *et al.* (65) and Lafferty and Oertilis (66) were the first to demonstrate that antibody molecules can be visualized by the negative staining technique when present on the surface of a virus particle. Some of their micrographs are shown in Figs. 5.12–5.16. Individual antibody molecules (IgG) are seen to occur both in an extended form, joining two virus particles, or as "horseshoes," with both combining sites attached to the same particle; the latter is favored by addition of antibody to the virus in small increments (66). Bivalent attachment to a single particle, such as a bacterium or virus, is of biological significance since it results in a greatly increased strength of binding, or avidity.

   The width of the molecule appears to be about 35 Å, a value in

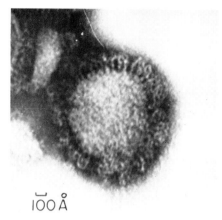

Fig. 5.13. Influenza A virus particle coated with rabbit antibody molecules, many of which are in the "horseshoe" configuration characteristic of bivalent attachment to a single virus. The number of such molecules was maximized by adding the antibody in small increments; addition of excess antibody all at once favors monovalent binding. Reprinted by permission, from reference 66.

good agreement with that obtained earlier by spraying a suspension of antibodies onto mica, then shadowing with heavy metal (64). It is difficult to estimate the length from the appearance of an individual molecule selected at random since it is generally not fully extended. The maximum length noted by Almeida *et al.* (65) was somewhat greater than the currently accepted value of 140 to 150 Å.

Valentine and Green examined purified rabbit anti-2,4-dinitrophenyl (anti-DNP) antibodies of the IgG class, complexed with univalent hapten, by electron microscopy and could see only small globular

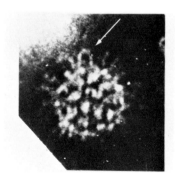

Fig. 5.14. Electron micrograph showing an antibody molecule joined to a single particle of wart virus through both of its combining sites. The virus has a diameter of approximately 550 Å. Reprinted by permission, from reference 65.

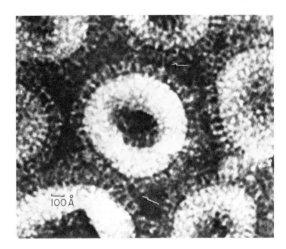

Fig. 5.15. Aggregate of influenza B virus with rabbit antibody. One can see antibody molecules which appear to be in an extended conformation and to link two virus
particles. Reprinted by permission of Dr. K.J. Lafferty, from reference 66.

masses of irregular shape (7). However, when the antibody was first
mixed with bivalent hapten [DNP—NH—$(CH_2)_n$—NH—DNP, with
$n \geqslant 8$], well-defined structures were observed. Prior to electron microscopy the mixture of antibody and hapten was centrifuged and gel fil-
tered, and the soluble protein in the void volume was studied. Electron
micrographs (Fig. 5.17) show the formation of closed structures, com-

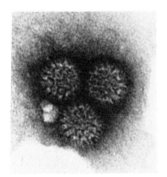 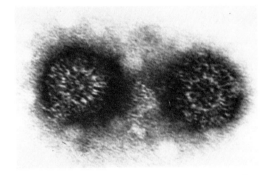

Fig. 5.16. The three particles at the left are polyoma virus coated with univalent,
Fab fragments of rabbit antibody. Numerous V's can be seen, suggesting attachment of
two Fab fragments to individual capsomeres on the virus. At the right are two particles of
polyoma virus treated first with univalent rabbit antibody, then with bivalent goat antibodies directed to the rabbit antibody. The width of the combined antibody layer is about
300 Å. Reprinted by permission, from reference 67.

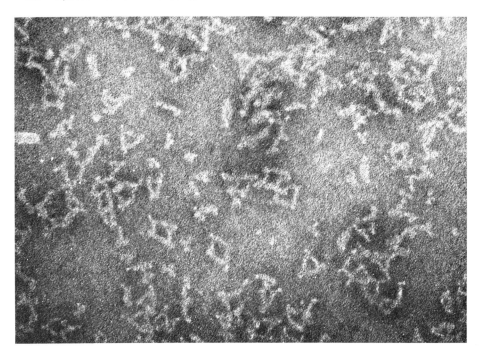

Fig. 5.17. Electron micrograph, prepared by the negative staining technique, of a mixture of specifically purified rabbit anti-2,4-dinitrophenyl (anti-DNP) antibody and a bivalent hapten (see text). The length of a typical linear segment in one of the many closed structures is about 120 Å. From Valentine and Green (7).

prising cyclic dimers, trimers, tetramers, and pentamers; the hapten is, of course, too small to be seen. The author's interpretation of these structures is shown by the representation of a trimer in Fig. 5.18. The fact that the segments appear in the micrograph as almost straight lines, without distortion, suggested that the combining sites are at the ends of the Fab fragments; if they were, for example, near the center the apparent width would be increased where the sites on two different molecules came together. A striking feature is the wide variation with respect to the angle that Fab fragments make with one another, depending on the number of units in a polymer. This confirmed an earlier suggestion of Feinstein and Rowe as to the flexibility of the molecule, which was based on electron microscopy of ferritin–anti-ferritin complexes (68). The sum of the lengths of two Fab fragments, 120 Å, agrees fairly well with, but is somewhat less than, that deduced from X-ray crystallography (140–150 Å). The cross section of 35 Å is in good agreement with other data.

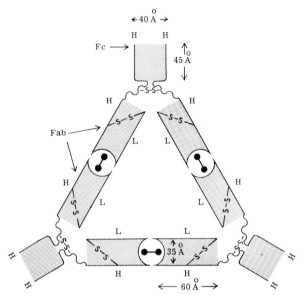

Fig. 5.18. Schematic diagram of a trimer of anti-DNP antibody and bivalent hapten (●—●), based on the electron micrograph in Fig. 5.17. The sum of the lengths of two Fab fragments, linked by hapten, varies from 117 to 123 Å. The widths of the Fab and Fc fragments varied over a maximum of ± 10 Å from the mean values of 35 and 40 Å, respectively. From Valentine and Green (7).

Protuberances can be seen at the corners of the structures in Fig. 5.17. According to the authors' interpretation these represent fragment Fc. Evidence that this is indeed the case was obtained by digesting the complexes with pepsin, which removes and degrades fragment Fc, prior to electron microscopy. This resulted in removal of the protuberances, as predicted from the model, but did not otherwise disturb the regular structures.

The swiveling points for the rotation of Fab fragments are believed to be in the hinge regions of the two H chains. This would be consistent with the electron micrographs, which indicate that rotation occurs at or near the junction of the Fab and Fc fragments. The hypothesis that the hinge region serves this function is supported by evidence indicating that it is a loosely folded segment of the chain (41). The region is, for example, the site of preferential cleavage by various proteolytic enzymes or by cyanogen bromide. Also, the single interheavy chain disulfide bond, which is located in the hinge region of rabbit IgG, is the most labile disulfide bond in the molecule (69).

In testing the series of bivalent haptens described above, the shortest chain that permitted bridging of two antibody molecules had eight

—CH$_2$— groups. This would be consistent with the notion that the antibody combining site is a crevice whose depth is half the length of the bivalent hapten containing eight —CH$_2$— groups (half of 25 Å); then, steric interference would prevent cross-linking by a shorter hapten. (See also, Chapter 2, Section VI,D.) It would be hazardous to generalize as to the size of such crevices, since different molecules studied by X-ray crystallography appear to vary with respect to the depth of invagination at the active site.

2. OTHER EVIDENCE RELATING TO FLEXIBILITY OF IMMUNOGLOBULINS

Data relating to flexibility which are derived from measurements other than electron microscopy appear somewhat inconclusive. Measurements of X-ray scattering have suggested that the IgG molecule in solution is an extended molecule (70) and may have a greater maximum length (200 Å) in solution than in the crystal state or the dried form used for electron microscopy; this would be suggestive of flexibility. Measurements of the intrinsic viscosity of IgG and its Fab and Fc fragments (36,71) are consistent with models in which the IgG molecule is rigid but more elongated than its component fragments or, alternatively, in which the compact fragments are joined by a flexible segment of polypeptide chain. Data on relaxation times of IgG or its Fab fragments have been interpreted as being consistent with the presence of rigid fragments joined by flexible segments (72). The interpretation of such data is rather complex and other laboratories had arrived at a different conclusion (reviewed in references 36 and 73).

Recent studies of resonance energy transfer between the two combining sites of rabbit IgG indicate that the molecule in solution prefers an extended form (74); this does not preclude the possibility that the sites can come closer together upon interaction with an appropriate antigen. Thus, much but not all of the data obtained by physicochemical measurements are consistent with flexibility. In any event the evidence for flexibility of an antibody molecule, based on electron microscopy, seems highly convincing. Whether structural changes occur *within* a domain upon interaction with antigen or hapten is an unsettled question.

REFERENCES

1. Northrop, J.A. (1942). *J. Gen. Physiol.* **25**, 465.
2. Kratochvil, C.H. and Deutsch, H.F. (1956). *J. Biol. Chem.* **222**, 31.
3. Caputo, A. and Appella, E. (1960). *Arch. Biochem. Biophys.* **91**, 201.

4. Nisonoff, A., Zappacosta, S., and Jureziz, R. (1967). *Cold Spring Harbor Symp. Quant. Biol.* **32,** 89.
5. Terry, W.D., Matthew, B.W., and Davies, D.R. (1968). *Nature (London)* **220,** 239.
6. Sarma, V.R., Silverton, E.W., Davies, D.R., and Terry, W.D. (1971). *J. Biol. Chem.* **246,** 3753.
7. Valentine, R.C. and Green, N.M. (1967). *J. Mol. Biol.* **27,** 615.
8. Labaw, L.W. and Davies, D.R. (1971). *J. Biol. Chem.* **246,** 3760.
9. Edmundson, A.B., Wood, M.K., Schiffer, M., Hardman, K.D., Ainsworth, C.F., and Ely, K.R. (1970). *J. Biol. Chem.* **245,** 2763.
10. Porter, R.R. (1959). *Biochem. J.* **73,** 119.
11. Kern, M., Helmreich, E., and Eisen, H.N. (1961). *Proc. Nat. Acad. Sci. U.S.* **47,** 767.
12. Hershgold, E.J., Cordoba, F., Charache, P., and Gillin, D. (1963). *Nature (London)* **199,** 284.
13. Goldstein, D.J., Humphrey, R.L., and Poljak, R.J. (1968). *J. Mol. Biol.* **35,** 247.
14. Poljak, R.J., Dintzis, H.M., and Goldstein, D.J. (1967). *J. Mol. Biol.* **24,** 351.
15. Rossi, G. and Nisonoff, A. (1968). *Biochem. Biophys. Res. Commun.* **31,** 914.
16. Rossi, G., Choi, T. K., and Nisonoff, A. (1969). *Nature (London)* **223,** 837.
17. Poljak, R.J., Amzel, L.M., Avey, H.P., Becka, L.N., and Nisonoff, A. (1972). *Nature New Biol.* **235,** 137.
18. Poljak, R.J., Amzel, L.M., Avey, H.P., Chen, B.L., Phizackerley, R.P., and Saul, F. (1973). *Proc. Nat. Acad. Sci. U.S.* **70,** 3305.
18a. Poljak, R.J. (1974). Personal communication.
19. Strosberg, A.D., Fraser, K.J., Margolies, M.N., and Haber, E. (1972). *Biochemistry* **11,** 4978.
19a. Strosberg, A.D., Margolies, M.N., and Haber, E. (1974). *Fed. Amer. Soc. Exp. Biol.* **33,** 726.
20. O'Donnell, I.J., Frangione, B., and Porter, R.R. (1970). *Biochem. J.* **116,** 261.
21. Brient, B.W. and Nisonoff, A. (1970). *J. Exp. Med.* **132,** 951.
22. Brient, B.W., Haimovich, J., and Nisonoff, A. (1971). *Proc. Nat. Acad. Sci. U.S.* **68,** 3136.
23. Sirisinha, S. and Eisen, H.N. (1971). *Proc. Nat. Acad. Sci. U.S.* **69,** 3130.
24. Sher, A. and Cohn, M. (1972). *J. Immunol.* **108,** 176.
25. Thorpe, N.O. and Singer, S.J. (1969). *Biochemistry* **11,** 4253.
26. Singer, S.J., Martin, N., and Thorpe, N.O. (1971). *Ann. N. Y. Acad. Sci.* **190,** 342.
27. Amzel, L.M., Poljak, R.J., Saul, F., Varga, J.M., and Richards, F.F. (1974). *Proc. Nat. Acad. Sci. U.S.* **71,** 1427.
28. Ely, K.R., Girling, R.L., Schiffer, M., Cunningham, D.E., and Edmundson, A.B. (1973). *Biochemistry* **12,** 4233.
29. Schiffer, M., Girling, R.L., Ely, K.R., and Edmundson, A.B. (1973). *Biochemistry* **12,** 4620.
30. Fett, J.W., Deutsch, H.F., and Smithes, O. (1973). *Immunochemistry* **10,** 115.
31. Milstein, C., Frangione, B., and Pink, J.R.L. (1967). *Cold Spring Harbor Symp. Quant. Biol.* **32,** 31.
32. Steiner, L.A. and Blumberg, P.M. (1971). *Biochemistry* **10,** 4725.
33. Wikler, M. and Putnam, F.W. (1970). *J. Biol. Chem.* **245,** 4488.
34. Rudikoff, S., Potter, M., Segal, D.M., Padlan, E.A., and Davies, D.R. (1972). *Proc. Nat. Acad. Sci. U.S.* **69,** 3689.
35. Padlan, E.A., Segal, D.M., Spande, T.F., Davies, D.R., Rudikoff, S., and Potter, M. (1973). *Nature New Biol.* **245,** 165.
35a. Epp, O., Colman, P., Fehlhammer, H., Bode, W., Schiffer, M., and Huber, R. (1974). *Eur. J. Biochem.* **45,** 513.

36. Dorrington, K.J. and Tanford, C. (1970). *Advan. Immunol.* **12**, 333.
37. Metzger, H. (1970). *Annu. Rev. Biochem.* **39**, 889.
38. Haber, E. and Cathou, R. (1972). *Proc. 8th Meeting Fed. Eur. Biochem. Soc. Amsterdam*, p. 61. North-Holland, Amsterdam.
39. Jirgensons, B. (1961). *Arch. Biochem. Biophys.* **94**, 59.
40. Winkler, M. and Doty, P. (1961). *Biochim. Biophys. Acta* **54**, 448.
41. Noelken, M.E., Nelson, C.A., Buckley, C.E., and Tanford, C. (1965). *J. Biol. Chem.* **240**, 218.
42. Steiner, L.A. and Lowey, S. (1966). *J. Biol. Chem.* **241**, 231.
43. Dorrington, K.J. and Rockey, J.H. (1968). *J. Biol. Chem.* **243**, 6511.
44. Dorrington, K.J. and Tanford, C. (1968). *J. Biol. Chem.* **243**, 4745.
45. Cathou, R.E., Kulczicki, A., Jr., and Haber, E. (1968). *Biochemistry* **7**, 3958.
46. Ross, D.L. and Jirgensons, B. (1968). *J. Biol. Chem.* **243**, 2829.
47. Ikeda, K., Hamaguchi, K., and Migita, S. (1968). *J. Biochem. (Tokyo)* **63**, 654.
48. Inbar, D., Hochman, J., and Givol, D. (1972). *Proc. Nat. Acad. Sci. U.S.* **69**, 2659.
49. Wells, J.V., Fudenberg, H.H., and Givol, D. (1973). *Proc. Nat. Acad. Sci. U.S.* **70**, 1585.
50. Solomon, A. and McLaughlin, C.L. (1969). *J. Biol. Chem.* **244**, 3393.
51. Karlsson, F.A., Peterson, P.A., and Berggard, I. (1969). *Proc. Nat. Acad. Sci. U.S.* **64**, 1257.
52. Poulsen, K., Fraser, K.J., and Haber, E. (1972). *Proc. Nat. Acad. Sci. U.S.* **69**, 2495.
53. Karlsson, F.A., Peterson, P.A., and Berggard, I. (1972). *J. Biol. Chem.* **247**, 1065.
54. Bjork, I., Karlsson, F.A., and Berggard, I. (1971). *Proc. Nat. Acad. Sci. U.S.* **68**, 1707.
55. Ghose, A.C. and Jirgensons, B. (1971). *Biochim. Biophys. Acta* **251**, 14.
56. Utsumi, S. and Karush, F. (1965). *Biochemistry* **4**, 1766.
57. Utsumi, S. (1969). *Biochem. J.* **112**, 343.
58. Heimer, R., Schnoll, S.S., and Primack, A. (1967). *Biochemistry* **6**, 127.
59. Turner, M.W. and Bennich, H. (1968). *Biochem. J.* **107**, 171.
60. Turner, M.W., Bennich, H., and Natvig, J.B. (1970). *Clin. Exp. Immunol.* **7**, 603.
61. Turner, M.W., Bennich, H., and Natvig, J.B. (1970). *Clin. Exp. Immunol.* **7**, 627.
62. Natvig, J.B. and Turner, M.W. (1971). *Clin. Exp. Immunol.* **8**, 685.
63. Smith, B.R. and Dorrington, K.J. (1972). *Biochem. Biophys. Res. Commun.* **46**, 1601.
64. Hall, C.E., Nisonoff, A., and Slayter, H.S. (1959). *J. Biophys. Biochem. Cytol.* **6**, 407.
65. Almeida, J., Cinader, B., and Howatson, A. (1963). *J. Exp. Med.* **118**, 327.
66. Lafferty, K.J. and Oertilis, S. (1963). *Virology* **21**, 91.
67. Almeida, J.D., Cinader, B., and Naylor, D. (1965). *Immunochemistry* **2**, 169.
68. Feinstein, A. and Rowe, A.J. (1965). *Nature (London)* **205**, 147.
69. Hong, R. and Nisonoff, A. (1965). *J. Biol. Chem.* **240**, 3883.
70. Pilz, I., Puchwein, G., Kratky, O., Herbst, M., Haager, O., Gall, W.E., and Edelman, G. (1970). *Biochemistry* **9**, 21.
71. Nisonoff, A., Wissler, F.C., and Woernley, D.L. (1960). *Arch. Biochem. Biophys.* **88**, 241.
72. Yguerabide, J., Epstein, H.F., and Stryer, L. (1970). *J. Mol. Biol.* **51**, 573.
73. Gally, J.A. (1973). *In* "The Antigens" (M. Sela. ed.), Vol. 1, p. 161. Academic Press, New York.
74. Werner, Y.C., Bunting, J.R., and Cathou, R.E. (1972). *Proc. Nat. Acad. Sci. U.S.* **69**, 705.

6

Properties and Interactions of the Light and Heavy Chains of Immunoglobulins

I. INTRODUCTION

This chapter describes methods of separating and recombining H and L chains and considers some of the physical and biochemical properties of the individual chains. The contribution of each chain to the antigen-binding capacity and to the formation of an active site will be discussed. Other topics included are the preferential recombination of H and L chains derived from the same molecule, such as a myeloma protein or antibody from an individual animal, the separation and recombination of univalent half-molecules, each comprising a complete L and H chain, and the formation of hybrid antibody molecules through recombination of half-molecules of different specificity. Interactions of chain segments, produced by proteolysis, are also considered.

Because of interspecies variation it is difficult to make generalizations that may not prove to have exceptions. A large part of our discussion will refer specifically to rabbit and human immunoglobulins, which have been studied extensively, but will be applicable to the immunoglobulins of many other species as well. Only a fraction of the literature in this area will be covered, but an effort will be made to illustrate the more important principles.

As indicated in Chapter 5, X-ray crystallographic analysis has demonstrated that the hypervariable regions of H and L chains come together at one tip of the Fab fragment to form the antibody combining site. The site includes a cleft or groove in the molecule, which is lined with residues from both L and H chains. Amino acids in hypervariable segments are also present immediately adjacent to the cleft. It seems possible that a fairly large part of this region comprising hypervariable amino acids may contribute to specificity in the case of a macromolecular antigen but that the cleft itself may be the most significant site with respect to interactions with small haptens. This is, however, conjectural.

II. SEPARATION OF LIGHT AND HEAVY CHAINS

The polypeptide chains of immunoglobulin molecules are held together by noncovalent interactions and by interchain disulfide bonds (1–3). Cleavage of interchain disulfide bonds, which can ordinarily be accomplished under nondenaturing conditions, generally does not result in a decrease in molecular weight, or in destruction of antibody combining sites (3). However, the chains can then be separated by treatment with reagents such as detergents, concentrated urea, or guanidine that disrupt noncovalent interactions in proteins (2–7). The mildest reagents adequate for the separation of H and L chains of the immunoglobulins of many species are 0.5–1 M acetic or propionic acids (3).[1] The fact that hydrochloric acid at the same pH ($\sim$2.5) is much less effective suggests that the slight detergent action of the hydrocarbon portion of the fatty acid is significant. This, in turn, would imply the participation of hydrophobic bonds in the noncovalent interaction of H and L chains; it does not, however, exclude an additional role for other types of noncovalent forces, such as electrostatic or hydrogen bonds. X-Ray crystallographic analysis suggests that both types of interaction participate in holding the H and L chains together in the Fab fragment (Chapter 5).[2]

A number of reagents have been used for selective cleavage of interchain disulfide bonds. Those most commonly employed are reducing agents, such as 2-mercaptoethanol, 2-mercaptoethylamine, dithiothreitol, or sulfite. Sulfite is generally used together with an oxidizing agent; this converts each sulfur atom to $-S-SO_3^-$. Interchain bonds can be reduced in neutral buffer solution with a moderate concentration of reducing agent, e.g., 0.2 M 2-mercaptoethanol or 0.01 M dithiothreitol. Under these conditions most (not necessarily all) intrachain disulfide bonds remain intact, and the polypeptide chains do not undergo extensive conformational changes. Reduction of most or all intrachain bonds,

[1] The additional presence of 4.5 M urea is required for mouse IgA or IgG (3a).

[2] In the IgA of BALB/c mice and in human IgA2 of allotype $A_2m(1)$ L chains are not disulfide bonded to the H chains. These exceptions are discussed in Chapters 8 and 3, respectively.

which is accompanied by extensive denaturation, requires the presence of a reagent, such as detergent, concentrated urea, or guanidine, which causes unfolding of the protein structure. To prevent reoxidation during subsequent handling, the sulfhydryl groups liberated during reduction are usually alkylated with iodoacetic acid or iodoacetamide (Fig. 6.1). For details of these procedures the reader may consult references 2–4, 6, and 7.

On an analytical scale, one can separate the L and H chains, after cleavage of interchain disulfide bonds, by zone electrophoresis in the presence of a dissociating agent, e.g., concentrated urea or detergent (2,8). (For example, in urea-starch gel at low pH, L chains move more rapidly than H chains toward the cathode.) Conventional or disc electrophoresis in polyacrylamide gel has also been used frequently for analytical purposes (9,10).

Separation of L and H chains on a preparative scale is best accomplished by gel filtration, often on Sephadex G-100 with 1 M propionic acid as solvent. A typical pattern of elution from Sephadex is shown in Fig. 6.2. The double peak in the H chain region is attributed to the presence of a small amount of undissociated IgG or H chain aggregates (frequently both) in the leading peak.

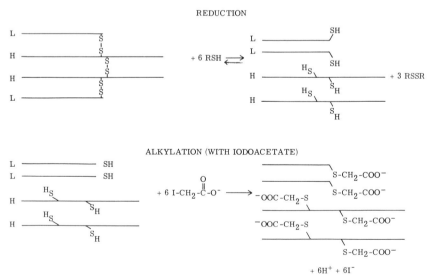

Fig. 6.1. Reduction and alkylation of interchain disulfide bonds in immunoglobulins. In the absence of dissociating agents (urea, guanidine, etc.) most intrachain bonds remain intact. The reduction with mercaptan is reversible and a large excess of the reagent is therefore employed. The alkylation is essentially irreversible.

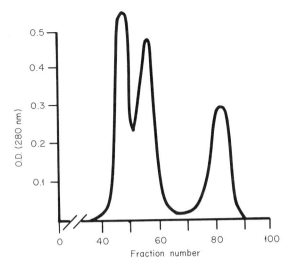

Fig. 6.2 Separation of H and L chains of reduced, alkylated rabbit IgG on Sephadex G-100. The eluent is 1 *M* propionic acid. The leading portion of the double H chain peak is attributable to the tendency of H chains to aggregate and, possibly, to the presence of undissociated H–L pairs. A human IgG fraction will ordinarily give a similar pattern. O.D., optical density.

III. SOLUBILITY AND CONFORMATIONAL PROPERTIES OF THE ISOLATED CHAINS

Both H and L chains are, of course, soluble in the reagents (1 *M* propionic acid, 8 *M* urea, etc.) used to separate them. Upon dialysis against neutral buffer, L chains remain in solution but H chains of many immunoglobulins form a precipitate which can be redissolved in the dissociating solvent.[3] In such solvents the polypeptide chains undergo significant conformational changes.

Many investigations of the physical and biological properties of isolated chains have been reported. For such studies, H chains may be solubilized by working at pH 5.5 or below (11,12) or by the attachment of polyalanyl side chains (13,14). At pH 5.5, rabbit or human H chains exist as a dimer of approximate molecular weight 100,000; monomers are separated in the presence of 6 *M* guanidine hydrochloride (15). Light chains at neutral pH generally comprise a mixture of monomers and dimers; the latter are readily dissociated by exposure to low pH or to denaturing reagents. Measurements of optical rotatory dispersion in-

[3] We should emphasize that these generalizations apply to human and rabbit immunoglobulins and that interspecies variability exists; for example, mouse kappa chains isolated from IgG may be only sparingly soluble in neutral buffer.

dicate that isolated H and L chains retain ordered structures which, however, differ markedly from those in the native protein (15,16).

When the IgG molecule or its Fab fragment is exposed to a reducing agent in the presence of 6 *M* guanidine hydrochloride, all disulfide bonds are reduced, native conformation is lost, and the separated chains acquire the configuration of a random coil (17). Despite this complete loss of ordered structure a substantial amount of antibody activity can be recovered if the H and L chains are allowed to renature and recombine under appropriate conditions (17,17a). Since this occurs in the absence of antigen, these important experiments provided the first conclusive evidence that antibody specificity is determined by primary amino acid sequences, which, in turn, specify the final tertiary structure of the folded molecule.

IV. ANTIBODY ACTIVITY IN ISOLATED CHAINS AND IN RECOMBINANTS OF HEAVY AND LIGHT CHAINS

Most investigations of this type utilize polypeptide chains which are separated under minimal denaturing conditions. In general, interchain disulfide bonds are reduced in neutral buffer, in the absence of dissociating agents (3). (The relatively great lability of interchain disulfide bonds makes this procedure feasible.) The polypeptide chains can then be separated by gel filtration, as described above. When recombinants are prepared the H and L chains are ordinarily mixed while still in the organic acid solution and the mixture is dialyzed against water or very dilute acid prior to final dialysis against neutral buffer. These procedures are reviewed by Porter and Weir (18). On occasion the chains have been allowed to renature at pH 5.5 prior to neutralization (11,12). Recombination occurs through noncovalent interactions, since the sulfhydryl groups released from interchain bonds on reduction are inactivated by alkylation. However, recombination is feasible even if the H chains are first dimerized through disulfide bonding (omitting alkylation). In contrast, L chain dimers will generally not combine with H chains (11).

From studies of this type one can obtain answers to questions such as the following:

1. Will a given H chain combine with its autologous L chain, with L chain from antibody of a different specificity, or with an L chain of nonspecific IgG?

2. Can activity be restored by recombining the H and L chains of an antibody?

3. Do recombinants in which the H and L chains are derived from two different antibodies, or from an antibody and nonspecific IgG, have antibody activity?

4. If the H and L chains are isolated from antibody of the same specificity, but from different animals of the same species will they recombine to form molecules with antibody activity?

5. Will an H chain, presented with a mixture of its autologous L chains and L chains from a different molecule, preferentially recombine with the autologous chain?

6. Do isolated (unrecombined) polypeptide chains have appreciable antibody activity or specificity?

A. Capacity of H and L Chains to Recombine through Noncovalent Interaction

The physical recombination of H and L chains has been demonstrated by a number of different techniques. Evidence indicative of recombination was obtained by Fleischman *et al.* (19), who showed that the presence of L chains greatly increases the solubility of H chains at neutral pH. Olins and Edelman (20) separated H and L chains of nonspecific human IgG, labeled one chain with ^{131}I and the other with ^{125}I, and then prepared recombinants. Reassociation of the chains was demonstrated by density gradient centrifugation and gel filtration. An example of their experimental data is shown in Fig. 6.3. The exact coincidence of the H and L chain peaks, sedimenting with a velocity of approximately 7 S, indicates reformation of four-chain molecules. It was also found that interchain disulfide bonds, joining the H chains to one another and to L chains, could be reformed by reoxidation after the noncovalent association of polypeptide chains into 7 S molecules. The correct juxtaposition of sulfhydryl groups in recombinant molecules provided striking evidence that the native conformation had been largely restored. The 7 S reconstituted molecules showed antigenic identity with native IgG, as indicated by Ouchterlony analysis with anti-IgG. Similar experiments demonstrating a close structural similarity of recombinants and native molecules, were carried out by recombining and then reoxidizing half-molecules, each comprising an L and an H chain (21) (Section VIII). Physicochemical studies indicating close similarity in conformation of native and reconstituted molecules were reported by Björk and Tanford (12).

Many other investigators have demonstrated the recombination of L and H chains. In general, the major product, when IgG is the starting

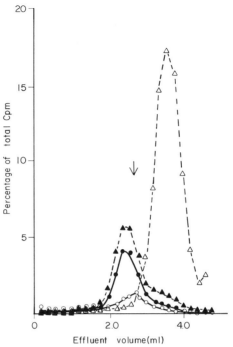

Fig. 6.3. Sucrose density gradient centrifugation of L chains and H chains of human IgG or of a mixture of the two chains. Mass ratio of recombinants: H/L = 6.1. △---△, Labeled L chains centrifuged alone; ○—○, labeled H chains centrifuged alone; ▲---▲, reconstructed mixture of labeled L chains and unlabeled H chains; ●—●, reconstituted mixture of labeled H chains and unlabeled L chains; ↓, position of alkaline phosphatase marker (~ 6 S). Reprinted by permission from Olins and Edelman (20).

material, is a 7 S molecule; almost invariably, however, smaller and larger components are observed, reflecting incomplete recombination and a certain amount of aggregation. The 7 S component can be isolated from the mixture by gel filtration. Frequently, a molar excess of L chains is used in recombination experiments to ensure complete reassociation of the H chains. The absence of insoluble material, after neutralization, provides some assurance that this has been accomplished; more direct proof is available when the H chains carry a radioactive label which can be followed during subsequent gel filtration or sedimentation velocity measurements.

RECOMBINATION OF H CHAINS OF DIFFERENT CLASSES

There appears to be a strong tendency of H chains of the same class to recombine preferentially. Zimmerman and Grey observed virtually no formation of hybrid molecules containing one α chain and one γ chain when IgA and IgG were dissociated into H and L chains, mixed, and allowed to recombine (21a). Similarly, they were unable to produce mixed molecules containing one γ and one μ chain. There was, however, substantial hybridization with respect to H chains when a similar experiment was carried out using an IgGl and an IgG4 myeloma protein. Eden *et al.* observed preferential autologous recombination of H chains from guinea pig IgGl and IgG2 although some hybrid molecules were found. L chains combined randomly with the γ_1 and γ_2 chains (22).

These findings may have biological implications. If a cell at some stage produces molecules of two classes simultaneously (Chapter 11), the physicochemical properties of the Ig molecules may prevent the formation of mixed molecules.

B. Restoration of Antibody Activity by Recombination of H and L Chains

Before discussing the antibody activity of recombinants, we shall briefly mention activity in the individual, separated chains, a topic to be reviewed in more detail later. Isolated L chains generally have no activity detectable by conventional means but in a few instances have been shown by sensitive methods to combine with antigen, although with low affinity. The activity of H chains is somewhat difficult to study owing to their insolubility at neutral pH and also because of possible contamination with L chains. Various devices, including solubilization by recombination with nonspecific L chains or by attachment of polyalanyl side chains, have been employed to circumvent the problem of insolubility. The antibody activity of solubilized H chains, while often quite significant, is usually diminished in comparison to that of the intact molecule, as evidenced by a decrease in affinity for the antigen (see below).

A substantial proportion of the initial antigen-binding capacity can be restored if H and L chains from a given antibody population are allowed to recombine. Experiments of this type were first reported by Edelman *et al.* (23) and have since been carried out in many laboratories. An excellent representative is shown in Table 6.1 which presents data obtained by Roholt *et al.* (24,25). It is evident that reduction and alkylation of interchain disulfide bonds caused little decrease in antibody activity; thus, noncovalent forces are sufficient to maintain the integrity of the antibody combining site. When the H and L chains were separated by gel filtration in 1 M propionic acid, then recombined and gradually brought to neutrality, more than one-half of the hapten-binding capacity was restored. In contrast, recombinants of H chains of the antibody with nonspecific L chains, or antibody L chains with nonspecific H chains, exhibited very little activity (discussed below).

TABLE 6.1

RECOVERY OF ANTIGEN-BINDING ACTIVITY OF SPECIFICALLY PURIFIED RABBIT
ANTI-*p*-AZOBENZOATE IgG ANTIBODY AFTER RECOMBINATION OF H AND L
CHAINS ISOLATED FROM THE ANTIBODY OF AN INDIVIDUAL RABBIT[a]

Antibody preparation	Treatment	Relative hapten-binding capacity[b]
Rabbit A	Untreated	100
	Reduced and alkylated	93
	Reduced and alkylated; chains separated, then recombined[c]	51
Rabbit B	Untreated	100
	Reduced and alkylated; chains separated, then recombined[c]	59

[a] Data taken from Roholt *et al.* (24,25).
[b] Measured by equilibrium dialysis. Refers to concentration of hapten bound with a fixed free hapten concentration.
[c] Chains separated on Sephadex G-100 equilibrated with 1 *M* propionic acid.

In view of the heterogeneity of ordinary rabbit antihapten antibodies, it seems quite remarkable that as much as half of the activity was restored; one might expect that random recombination of H and L chains, from molecules with different structure but having the same specificity, might yield inactive recombinants. The answer is that recombination does not occur at random; there is preferential pairing of autologous chains (see below).

From these results, the question arises as to the amount of activity that would be recovered in a recombinant of H and L chains prepared from a structurally homogeneous population of antibody molecules. The discovery of myeloma proteins with antihapten activity provided an avenue of approach to this question. Bridges and Little (3a), working with a mouse myeloma protein with specificity for the 2,4-dinitrophenyl (Dnp) group, found that virtually 100% of the original hapten-binding activity was restored in a recombinant of H and L chains. Activity was described in terms of both the number of hapten-binding sites recovered and the equilibrium constant for the binding reaction. A large degree of recovery of activity was also reported by Sher *et al.* in similar studies of mouse myeloma proteins with specificity for the phosphorylcholine hapten group (26).

Up to 70–80% restoration of activity in recombinants was obtained by Klinman (27), who utilized homogeneous anti-Dnp antibodies synthesized by splenic foci; the latter were obtained by injection of a small number of cells from one mouse into a recipient irradiated mouse. Each focus is thought to be derived from a single cell; this would explain the production of antibodies of uniform structure.

MacDonald *et al.* (28) found that substantial amounts of activity could be recovered in recombinants prepared from the chains of specifically purified anti-*p*-azobenzoate antibodies isolated from the serum of an individual rabbit at widely spaced intervals of time. Thus the H chain isolated from one bleeding recombined with the L chain isolated from a much later bleeding to yield a product having a substantial amount of antibenzoate activity. This was taken as evidence for the presence of molecules with similar or identical structures over a long period of time in the serum of an individual animal. These results are considered in Chapter 11 together with data on idiotypy which later provided support for the same conclusion.

1. Recombination of H and L Chains from Antibodies of the Same Specificity but from Different Animals

In this section we will describe experiments in which recombinants were prepared from H and L chains derived from antihapten antibody of the same specificity but from different rabbits. Results of two such investigations by Roholt *et al.* (24,29) are summarized in Table 6.2. It is evident that little antibody activity was restored in recombinants in which the H and L chains came from different rabbits, despite the fact that both chains were isolated from specifically purified anti-*p*-azobenzoate antibodies. A large fraction of the initial activity was restored in autologous recombinants. Roholt *et al.* obtained very similar results when Fd fragments were substituted for intact H chains (29).

There is an interesting set of circumstances in which a large amount of activity was restored when the H and L chains came from different animals (26). The investigation utilized myeloma proteins that had arisen in different mice but had specific antibody activity directed to the same hapten (phosphorylcholine) and shared idiotypic specificity. A large amount of hapten-binding activity (comparable to that of an autologous recombinant) was restored when the H chains were derived from one such myeloma protein and the L chains from another. When myeloma proteins had the same antigen-binding specificity but were of different idiotype, little or no antibody activity was recovered in heterologous recombinants. Restoration of activity was also observed with pairs of mouse myeloma proteins having antidextran activity and shared idiotype (30). Evidence based on amino acid sequences for close similarity or identity of mouse myeloma proteins with shared idiotype is discussed in Chapter 11.

TABLE 6.2

RECOVERY OF ANTIGEN-BINDING ACTIVITY OF SPECIFICALLY PURIFIED RABBIT
ANTI-*p*-AZOBENZOATE ANTIBODY AFTER RECOMBINATION OF H AND L CHAINS
ISOLATED FROM THE ANTIBODIES OF DIFFERENT RABBITS[a]

Antibody preparation	Treatment	Relative K value[b]
A[c]	Untreated	100
B[c]	Untreated	100
C[c]	Untreated	100
D[d]	Untreated	100
H(A) + L(A)[e]	Recombined[f]	82
H(B) + L(B)	Recombined	78
H(A) + L(B)	Recombined	9
H(B) + L(A)	Recombined	11
H(C) + L(D)	Recombined	6
H(C) + L(C)	Recombined	59
H(D) + L(C)	Recombined	7

[a] The data are from Roholt *et al.* (24,29).

[b] Measured by equilibrium dialysis.

[c] Individual rabbit.

[d] Antibody from a pool of sera of 24 rabbits.

[e] The letters in parentheses indicate the source of the H or L chains.

[f] Antibody preparations were reduced and alkylated, dialyzed against 1 M propionic acid, and passed through Sephadex G-100 in that solvent to separate H and L chains. Appropriate pairs of chains were mixed at low pH. Recombination occurred when the mixtures were dialyzed against a buffer at neutral pH.

2. PREFERENTIAL RECOMBINATION OF AUTOLOGOUS H AND L CHAINS

We will use the phrase "autologous chains" to denote H and L chains derived from a given population of antibody molecules (not necessarily homogeneous) or from one myeloma protein. The question at issue is whether autologous chains recombine preferentially in a competitive situation in which a polypeptide chain from another antibody or myeloma protein is also present.

One may interpret the degree of preferential recombination as providing an indication of the free energy of interaction between the V regions of the H and L chains. X-Ray crystallographic data (Chapter 5) indicate that in the Fab fragment the V_H and V_L regions are in contact, and that the C_L region is in contact with the C_H1 segment of the H chain. This, in turn, would suggest that there may be approximately the same energy of interaction in the C region for any H chain of a given class and subclass and L chain of a given type. Differences in affinity between pairs of chains would then reflect differences in noncovalent bonding energy in the V regions. The data to be discussed below demonstrate that, in general, autologous chains do indeed recombine preferentially. In a typical competition experiment, 3 to 10 times as much of the autologous L chain, as compared to a competing L chain, will combine with an H chain.

Despite these apparently large differences, the following considerations suggest that the differences in combining energy in the V region between two pairs of chains may be relatively small in relation to the total free energy of interaction of the H and L chain. At neutral pH and with a protein concentration of 10^{-5} M, no spontaneous separation of reduced and alkylated rabbit antibody into separate chains can be detected; a high concentration of dissociating agent such as urea or guanidine is required. If the degree of spontaneous dissociation of H and L chains is less than 1%, the association constant for the reaction $H + L \rightleftharpoons HL$ exceeds 10^9 M^{-1} This would correspond to a free energy release for the reaction of > 12 kcal/mole. Next, suppose that preferential recombination occurs in a ratio of 10 to 1. This would signify a difference between the free energy of binding of an H chain with two different L chains of 1.3 kcal/mole, or less than 15% of the total energy of interaction. Thus, relatively small differences in free energy of interaction can result in a significant degree of preferential recombination. This, in turn, suggests that energies of interaction in V regions may not vary markedly.

Direct competition experiments were carried out by Grey and Mannik (31) with L and H chains from monoclonal proteins. In a typical experiment L chains from two myeloma proteins were labeled with two different isotopes of iodine, ^{125}I and ^{131}I, which can be quantified simultaneously in a mixture because of differences in the energies of their gamma emissions. Unlabeled H chains of a myeloma protein were added to a mixture containing an equimolar quantity of autologous L chains and L chains from another myeloma protein. The total molar concentration of L chains was twice as great as that of the H chains and, therefore, a maximum of only one-half of the L chains could combine with H chains. After recombination, the mixture was subjected to density gradient centrifugation and the positions of the two L chains in the gradient were ascertained by measurements of radioactivity. L chains which had recombined with H chains sedimented with a velocity corresponding to that of IgG (or IgA), whereas free L chains migrated more slowly.

A representative example of their data is shown in Table 6.3, which indicates that there is preferential recombination of autologous chains. In only one instance (L chains from protein Fe) did the heterologous L chain recombine to a greater extent than the autologous L chain. An-

TABLE 6.3

Competitive Recombination of IgG Myeloma Protein H Chains
with Autologous and Heterologous L Chains[a]

Autologous chains (H and L) used for recombination[b]	Competing L chain[c]	Weight ratio of autologous to heterologous L chains in 7 S peak after recombination
Mu IgGl(κ)	Ku IgGl(λ)	10.4
	Ne IgG2(λ)	8.4
	Gr IgG1(κ)	4.3
	Di IgM(λ)	4.3
	Ke IgG1(κ)	3.4
	Ge IgG4(κ)	2.9
	Sz IgG1(λ)	1.8
	Met IgG1(λ)	1.3
Ke IgGl(κ)	Mer IgG1(κ)	6.5
	Di IgM(λ)	6.4
	Ge IgG4(κ)	5.5
	Ne IgG2(λ)	4.5
	Ku IgG1(λ)	4.0
	Sz IgG1(λ)	2.4
	Met IgG1(λ)	2.4
	Gr IgG1(K)	2.1
	Am IgA(λ)	2.1
	Ro IgG4(κ)	2.0
	Fe IgG3(κ)	0.48

[a] The data presented are from Grey and Mannik (31).

[b] Although only the L chains were used as competitors, the subclass of the H chain present in the myeloma protein is also given. The abbreviations (Mu, etc.) represent the name of the patient.

[c] Equal weights of autologous and competing chains were used.

other major conclusion was that the source of the heterologous L chain did not correlate with effectiveness of recombination with a given H chain; i.e., an L chain derived from a myeloma protein whose H chain was of the IgG class did not show any special affinity for other γ chains as compared, say, to α chains. Also, no correlation with IgG subclass was noted.

Another type of experiment illustrating preferential recombination of autologous chains was reported by Roholt *et al.* (32). They took advantage of the fact that H chains of rabbit antibenzoate antibody express very little antibody activity after recombination with nonspecific L chains, or even with L chains of antibenzoate antibody from another

TABLE 6.4

COMPETITION BETWEEN NONSPECIFIC L CHAINS AND AUTOLOGOUS (ANTIBODY)
L CHAINS FOR RECOMBINATION WITH H CHAINS OF SPECIFICALLY PURIFIED
ANTI-*p*-AZOBENZOATE ANTIBODY[a]

Equivalents of each chain[b]			Relative hapten-binding activity[c]
H	L	L(N)	
1	1	0	0.79
1	5	0	0.78
1	1	1	0.63
1	1	2	0.55
1	1	3	0.49
1	1	6	0.38
1	1	9	0.35

[a] Data are from Roholt *et al.* (32).

[b] H and L chains were prepared from specifically purified antibenzoate antibody derived from an individual rabbit; L(N), light chains isolated from normal serum.

[c] Relative to untreated anti-*p*-azobenzoate antibody. Refers to relative concentration of hapten bound with the free hapten concentration held at a constant value.

rabbit. A large fraction of the original hapten-binding activity is, however, recovered upon recombination with autologous antibenzoate L chains. On the basis of this information, they permitted recombination of antibenzoate H chains with autologous L chains to take place in the presence of increasing concentrations of nonspecific L chains; the results are summarized in Table 6.4. In the presence of a ninefold excess of nonspecific L chains the amount of antibody activity recovered was about 45% of that observed in the absence of nonspecific, competing L chains (as compared to the value, 10%, expected if there were no preferential recombination). These results, again, are consistent with a strong preference of H chains for autologous L chains.

V. INTERACTION OF V_L OR C_L SEGMENTS OF LIGHT CHAINS WITH INTACT HEAVY CHAINS

Smith and Dorrington demonstrated that either V_L or C_L segments of human L chains are capable of combining with isolated, monomeric H chains (33). The V_L segment was prepared by enzymatic cleavage of a myeloma κ chain and the C_L segment from a λ chain. Heavy chains were isolated from pooled human IgG and from several myeloma proteins. Using radiolabeled L chain segments it was found that, in the presence of excess H chains, 5–88% of the V_L fragments were bound; surprisingly, there was no preferential recombination with autologous H chains. The recombination of C_L fragments was relatively weak but was considerably enhanced in the presence of V_L fragments. High ionic strength favored each of these interactions. Similar experiments were reported at the same time by Karlsson, who also noted the importance of high ionic strength (33a). Both V_L and C_L segments of human IgG recombined with intact H chains although the interaction was much stronger when an intact L chain was employed. These data suggest that the V_L and C_L segments are independently capable of acquiring conformations similar to those in the intact L chain and reinforce the concept of the relative independence of structure of separate domains. A direct demonstration of the ability of isolated, denatured C_L and V_L segments to refold into their native conformations was reported by Karlsson *et al.*, who measured the optical rotatory dispersion, circular dichroism, fluorescence spectra, and antigenic properties of the refolded segments (33b).

VI. STABILITY OF FRAGMENTS CONSISTING ONLY OF V DOMAINS

That a stable fragment can comprise only V regions is shown by the work of Inbar *et al.*, who prepared such a fragment by digestion of a mouse IgA myeloma protein with pepsin (34). The protein, MOPC 315, has specificity for the ϵ-Dnp-L-lysine hapten group. The fragment, liberated by pepsin and designated Fv, comprises a V_H and a V_L domain. It retains full (univalent) hapten-binding activity and has all the idiotypic determinants of the intact molecule (35). Many immunoglobulins have proven to be resistant to the preparation of Fv fragments, although such a fragment has been prepared from IgM by peptic digestion (36). V_L and C_L domains are much more readily obtained. The preparation of C_H domains by proteolysis is discussed in Chapter 3. A fragment, designated Fb, which consists of the C domains of a human Fab fragment, was prepared by Gall and D'Eustachio (37).

Epp *et al.* (38) have determined the crystal structure of a stable Bence Jones protein, which proved to comprise only a dimer of the V_κ domain, held together by noncovalent interactions. A striking feature of this protein, held in common with a λ-chain dimer whose three-dimensional structure is also known (39), is the clustering of hypervariable residues in the region of the combining site (Chapter 5).

VII. EFFECT OF HAPTEN ON THE STRENGTH OF INTERACTION OF H AND L CHAINS

Several types of experiments have demonstrated that the presence of hapten stabilizes the interaction of H and L chains. Antibodies to the 2,4-dinitrophenyl (Dnp) group have been of particular value because they combine with specific hapten even at the low pH required to separate H and L chains (40).

Metzger and Singer (41) reduced and alkylated specifically purified rabbit anti-Dnp antibodies and subjected them to gel filtration on Sephadex G-75 in 1 M propionic acid solution. A typical elution pattern was obtained; the yields of H and L chains were 75 and 25%, by weight, respectively. If, however, the specific hapten, ϵ-2,4-dinitrophenyl-L-lysine (ϵ-Dnp-L-lysine) was present at a concentration of 6×10^{-6} M during gel filtration, the first peak contained 82–84% of the protein. This indicated that the hapten had reinforced the noncovalent interactions between the H and L chains, rendering them less dissociable in propionic acid solution. From readings of optical density at 360 nm it was evident that the hapten, which absorbs at this wavelength, was present in the first peak (H plus L chains) but not in the second peak (L chains). This observation provided evidence for the absence of specific binding activity, or a very low K value, in L chains of anti-Dnp antibody.

A related experiment was reported by Metzger and Mannik (42), who allowed H chains from rabbit anti-Dnp antibody to combine with a competing mixture of L chains from anti-Dnp antibody and nonspecific rabbit IgG, respectively. The two types of L chain were labeled with different isotopes of iodine to permit their identification. The presence of 2×10^{-5} M hapten, Dnp-6-aminocaproic acid, substantially increased the ratio of specific to nonspecific L chains that recombined with antibody H chains.

A stabilizing effect of hapten on rabbit anti-Dnp antibody has also been demonstrated by determining its effect on changes in optical rotatory dispersion of the antibody in the presence of a strong denaturing agent, 4 M guanidine hydrochloride (43). The increase in levorotation, characteristic of denaturation by guanidine, was much less pronounced in the presence of the specific hapten, ϵ-Dnp-L-lysine. This was particularly true of the Fab fragment, which was almost completely stabilized, according to this criterion, when hapten was present. The authors interpreted this result as indicating that amino acid residues involved in the binding site are widely separated in the amino acid sequence and are brought into close proximity in the folded structure of the molecule; the hapten makes direct contact with these amino acids and helps to stabilize the tertiary structure. This conclusion concerning the folded structure has been confirmed by X-ray crystallography (Chapter 5).

VIII. CONTRIBUTION TO ANTIBODY ACTIVITY OF ISOLATED H AND L CHAINS

A. General Considerations

The antigen-binding capacity of individual polypeptide chains has been studied in many laboratories; only a few of the more illustrative experiments will be described. Whereas L chains from many sources are quite soluble and therefore relatively easy to investigate, H chains generally have a strong tendency to aggregate and form a precipitate. Methods used to circumvent this difficulty include recombination of antibody H chains with nonspecific L chains or solubilization of H chains by attachment of polyalanyl groups of moderate length; such polyalanyl side chains are joined to the ϵ-amino groups of lysine residues. Another problem that arises is the difficulty of obtaining H chains completely free of L chains. Repeated recycling on Sephadex is necessary, and sensitive analytical methods (which have been infrequently employed) are required to prove the absence of L chains from the final preparation. The absence of L chains can be demonstrated by immunological analysis, using sufficiently sensitive techniques, or by quantitative analysis for N-terminal amino acids characteristic of the L chains.

B. Antibody Activity in L Chains

In most investigations, L chains have been found to possess little or no antibody activity (e.g., 4,19,23,24,44). Among the few reports of a substantial degree of antigen-binding activity are those of Raynaud and Mangalo (45,46) who found that about 10% of the L chains from horse diphtheria antitoxin are coprecipitable with antigen and intact antibody; in addition, L chains were reported to have toxin-neutralizing activity. Specific activity in L chains derived from rabbit antiphage antibody was reported by Goodman and Donch (47), who used a very sensitive viral neutralization assay.

The method of fluorescence enhancement was used by Yoo *et al.* (48) to demonstrate binding activity of the L chains of rabbit antibody specific for a fluorescent hapten, 4-azonaphthalene-1-sulfonate. The binding affinity, K_0, was found to be very low (approximately $10^2 \, M^{-1}$); the method does not yield a value for the number of binding sites per L chains. Since the binding by L chains is very weak, the possibility was considered that it could be accounted for by the presence of a small amount of contaminating H chains, interacting with L chains to form half or whole molecules. This was essentially ruled out in subsequent experiments of Nakamure *et al.*, who showed, again by the method of fluorescence enhancement, that L chains are capable of interacting weakly with a hapten, even after immunoabsorption to remove residual H chains (49). The L chains were shown to react specifically with haptens related to the immunogen, but the relative K values for different haptens differed considerably from those of the native molecule. In contrast, isolated H chains, which had a binding affinity about 10% as great as that of the native antibody, appeared to have specificity similar to that of the original antibody molecule.

Binding of ϵ-Dnp-lysine to L chains of specifically purified rabbit anti-Dnp antibody was measured by the method of equilibrium dialysis (50). Because of the very low binding affinity, a high concentration of L chains (36 mg/ml) was employed. The data were corrected for binding by nonspecific L chains. An average equilibrium constant of 2×10^2 to $5 \times 10^2 \, M^{-1}$ was observed and the maximal binding capacity was, roughly, 0.5 mole of hapten per mole of L chain (or 1 mole per mole of L chain dimer). Corrections to the data for binding by nonspecific L chains were large, amounting to 50 to 60% of the total binding at each free hapten concentration. Additional data on nonspecific binding of Dnp derivatives by L chains from other antibodies would be useful to establish specificity.

C. Antibody Activity in H Chains

The first clear demonstration of such activity was reported by Fleischman *et al.* (19). Heavy chains isolated from horse anti-rabbit IgG coprecipitated when mixed with rabbit IgG and the untreated horse antibody. The degree of coprecipitation indicated that a large percentage of the antibody H chains had specific activity. In a second system, specific activity of H chains from horse antidiphtheria toxoid was revealed by their capacity to inhibit specific precipitation of horse antibodies and diphtheria toxoid; i.e., the H chains behaved as if they were univalent. In neither set of experiments did the L chains have demonstrable antibody activity. Another early demonstration of antibody activity in H chains was that of Utsumi and Karush (4), who isolated the polypeptide

chains from specifically purified rabbit antibody directed to the
p-azophenyl-β-lactoside hapten group. Their method consisted in reduction of interchain disulfide bonds, followed by gel filtration on Sephadex G-200 in 0.05 *M* sodium decyl sulfate. The H chains, which
remained soluble after dialysis, bound specific hapten with an affinity
about one-eighth as great as that of untreated antibody; L chains
were inactive. Nearly all H chains appeared to possess an active site.

Porter and Weir (18) quantitatively assessed the antibody activity of
the H and L chains of horse antidiphtheria toxoid by using ^{125}I-labeled
toxoid and a direct assay. H and L chains retained 20 and 5%, respectively, of the binding capacity of the intact molecule; after recombination
of the H chains with nonspecific L chains the value was increased to
40%. The measurements were designed to provide information as to
binding capacity rather than binding affinity. Very similar results, with
respect to activity in isolated chains and in their recombinants, were
obtained by Franek *et al.,* who worked with bovine anti-Dnp antibodies (51).

In certain investigations the binding affinity of H chains has been
found to be much lower, relative to that of intact antibody.For example,
Edelman *et al.* (23) observed very little residual activity in either the H
or L chains of antibodies to bacteriophage f1 or f2, whereas recombination of autologous chains resulted in some restoration of activity. Also,
the work of Roholt and Pressman *et al.* (24,25,29,32,52) showed that
the isolated H chains of rabbit antibenzoate antibody have minimal
hapten-binding activity, and Hong and Nisonoff (44) found only a small
fraction of the original hapten-binding activity in recombinants consisting of the H chains of rabbit anti-Dnp antibody and nonspecific L
chains.

One of the most careful investigations of this question is that by
Haber and Richards (13), who utilized purified rabbit antibodies specific
for the 2,4-dinitrophenyl (Dnp) and 2,4,6-trinitrophenyl (Tnp) groups. In
contrast to many studies of this type, precautions were taken to ensure
that the separated H chains were free of L chains, and analyses for
purity were carried out. The H chains were recycled through Sephadex
G-100 until they were essentially free of L chains by two criteria: failure
to react with antiserum to L chains and the absence of the N-terminal
alanine characteristic of rabbit L chains, as measured by a sensitive
isotope-dilution assay. Light chains of antibody, either alone or combined with nonspecific H chains, possessed no activity detectable by the
method of fluorescence quenching. By contrast, a large percentage of the
H chains, polyalanylated or in combination with nonspecific L chains,
were able to bind hapten specifically, but with reduced affinity. Some of

TABLE 6.5

<small>Hapten-Binding Activity of Derivatives and Recombinants
of Anti-Dnp and Anti-Tnp Antibodies[a]</small>

Derivative[b] or recombinant	Relative number of binding sites remaining intact (%)[c]
Anti-Dnp (untreated)	100
Ala-H(Dnp)	23
Ala-L(Dnp)	0
H(Dnp) + L(Dnp)	49
H(Dnp) + L(NIgG)	58
H(NIgG) + L(Dnp)	0
Anti-Tnp (untreated)	100
H(Tnp) + L(Tnp)	80
H(Tnp) + L(NIgG)	66
H(NIgG) + L(Tnp)	0
NIgG	0
H(NIgG) + L(NIgG)	0

[a] Data are from Haber and Richards (13).

[b] Abbreviations: Ala, polyalanylated; Dnp, 2,4-dinitrophenyl; Tnp, 2,4,6-trinitrophenyl; N, derived from normal serum. Designations in parentheses show the source of H or L chains used in the recombinant molecule.

[c] Measured by fluorescence quenching.

their data are reproduced in Tables 6.5 and 6.6. The hapten-binding affinity of H chains, whether polyalanylated or recombined with nonspecific L chains, is less than 5% as great as that of the intact molecule for one or more haptens, but most of the binding sites are retained. Despite this decreased activity, the average K value for the isolated H chains of anti-Dnp antibody ($\sim 6 \times 10^6$ M^{-1}) was still respectable since the original antibodies were of high affinity. Although binding affinities of H chains were much lower than those of the corresponding antibodies, the energy of binding of hapten by H chain represented a large fraction of the binding energy of the intact molecule, since the free energy of binding is proportional to log K.

Binding affinities of polyalanylated H chains of anti-Dnp antibody were investigated also by Jaton *et al.* (14). In rather close agreement with the findings of Haber and Richards, they observed about a 100-fold decrease in binding affinity of H chains, relative to that of the intact molecule. About one-fourth of the H chains still possessed active hapten-binding sites.

TABLE 6.6

ASSOCIATION CONSTANTS OF ANTIBODIES AND RECOMBINANTS[a] $(M^{-1} \times 10^{-6})$

Hapten	Anti-Dnp[b]	H(Dnp) + L(IgG)	H(Dnp) + L(Dnp)	Ala-H(Dnp)	Anti-Tnp	H(Tnp) + L(NIgG)	H(Tnp) + L(Tnp)
ε-Dnp-lysine	370[c]	15	260	6.2	1.5	0.16	—
Dnp-OH	4.1	0.24	0.48	3.3	0.013	0.01	0.11
Tnp-OH	2.8	0.14	0.2	1.1	18	0.2	0.73
ε-Tnp-lysine	97	0.28	1.1	—	~100	0.74	1.3

[a] Values determined by fluorescence quenching with the exception noted below. Data are from Haber and Richards (13).

[b] Abbreviations are the same as those in Table 6.5. In this table, Dnp-OH and Tnp-OH correspond to 2,4-dinitrophenol and 2,4,6-trinitrophenol, respectively.

[c] Value determined by equilibrium dialysis.

Haber and Richards also noted that the specificity of H chains, in terms of relative degree of reactivity with different Dnp and Tnp derivatives, was qualitatively similar to that of the corresponding intact antibody, although marked quantitative differences were evident (13).

These experiments suggest that the role of L chains in anti-Dnp or anti-Tnp antibodies consists principally in enhancing the binding energy of H chains, without greatly altering their specificity. This has important implications with respect to the number of genes needed to encode all the antibodies present in an animal. If specificity were determined by both the H and L chain, the number of different specificities could approach the product of the number of genes encoding L and H chains. Haber and Richards (13) suggest that this may not be the case for the two antibodies investigated, since H chains alone appeared to determine specificity. In certain other systems, however, isolated H and L chains have been found to possess little antigen-binding activity, suggesting a greater cooperative role for both chains. Since both H and L chains participate in the structuring of the active site it seems to us highly probable that the presence of an appropriate L chain can modify the specificity of the molecule, as well as alter its affinity for particular antigenic determinants.

More recently, Stevenson (52a) confirmed the existence of weak but specific binding activity in H and L chains of rabbit antibody to the Dnp and 4-azobenzene-1-sulfonate hapten groups. For either type of chain the dimeric but not the monomeric form was active. The author postulated that a pair of identical chains can combine in such a manner as to produce a site with hapten-binding activity. (See also Chapter 5.)

D. Affinity Labeling as an Indication of Participation of a Chain in the Combining Site

Convincing evidence indicating that the L chain, as well as the H chain, participates directly in the formation of an active site of an antibody first came from studies of affinity labeling, which showed that the labeling reagent may become covalently attached to amino acid residues in either the H or the L chain. Such investigations are discussed at length in Chapter 2. X-Ray crystallographic analyses are in complete accord with this conclusion.

Careful studies of the amino acid composition of antibodies of different specificities, and of their H and L chains, indicated that differences in composition associated with specificity are localized in both the L and H chains (53). These data were correctly interpreted as indicating the participation of both chains in the active site.

IX. HALF-MOLECULES OF IgG

Half-molecules of rabbit IgG, consisting of one complete H chain and one L chain, can be prepared by selective reduction of the H–H disulfide bond, followed by acidification. Half-molecules recombine spontaneously at neutral pH through strong noncovalent forces acting between the Fc segments of the two H chains; therefore, they remain as half-molecules only under dissociating conditions, such as low pH or the presence of detergent (54,55–57).

Half-molecules are prepared from rabbit IgG by taking advantage of two properties of the molecule. First, the disulfide bond joining the two H chains (H–H bond) is more labile than the H–L bonds and, in fact, is the most labile disulfide bond in the molecule; in the presence of 0.01 M 2-mercaptoethanol nearly all H–H disulfide bonds, but very few H–L bonds, are reduced (56). Second, the noncovalent forces joining the two H chains are weaker than those linking H and L chains. Thus, even if all interchain disulfide bonds are reduced and alkylated, and the molecule is then exposed to HCl solution at pH 2.5, half-molecules, rather than free H and L chains, are liberated because the noncovalent interactions between H and L chains are not disrupted (56). (Separation of H from L chains requires more drastic dissociating conditions.) In practice, then, half-molecules are produced by reduction with 0.01 M to 0.02 M 2-mercaptoethanol, followed by alkylation of sulfhydryl groups and exposure to HCl-NaCl, pH 2.5 (54,55). The separation can be monitored in the ultracentrifuge or by gel filtration. Half-molecules have a molecular weight of 75,000 at pH 2.5 but recombine in good yield (up to 80%) at neutral pH to form 7 S molecules which can be purified by filtration on Sephadex G-200. Methods have not been devised to prevent half-molecules from reassociating at neutral pH. The reassociation of half-molecules necessarily takes place through noncovalent interaction, rather than reformation of disulfide bonds, since sulfhydryl groups are inactivated by alkylation.

Hybridization of Half-Molecules from Different Sources

Evidence that half-molecules are univalent was obtained by an indirect procedure (55,57). When half-molecules of specifically purified rabbit antiovalbumin were allowed to recombine at neutral pH, a large fraction of the original precipitating activity was restored. If, however, the half-molecules of the antibody were mixed at low pH with a large excess of half-molecules of nonspecific IgG and then neutralized, the 7 S product specifically blocked the precipitin reaction of the antigen with untreated antiovalbumin, indicating the presence of univalent, hybrid molecules, each comprising a half-molecule of antibody and a half-molecule of nonspecific IgG.

The recombination of half-molecules of purified antibody with half-molecules of nonspecific IgG was studied quantitatively, using radioactive labels, and was found to be a random process (55). This was not unexpected since half-molecules are linked through noncovalent interactions in the Fc region, whose structure is independent of antibody specificity. The formation and mode of action of hybrid molecules is illustrated in Fig. 6.4. Hybrid molecules produced from Fab' fragments are discussed in Chapter 8.

Univalent, hybrid molecules of antiovalbumin and nonspecific IgG failed to fix guinea pig complement in the presence of ovalbumin, indicating that bivalence is essential (58). Although univalent fragments produced by papain also do not fix complement, this conceivably could be due to the absence of fragment Fc; this alternative explanation would not apply in the case of 7 S univalent molecules.

Bivalent antiovalbumin molecules reconstituted from half-molecules of specifically purified antibody were able to fix guinea pig complement, although the activity was somewhat diminished as compared to that of the untreated antibody (58).

When a mixture of half-molecules of rabbit IgG differing in allotype (at either the *a* or *b* locus) was allowed to reassemble, there was no pref-

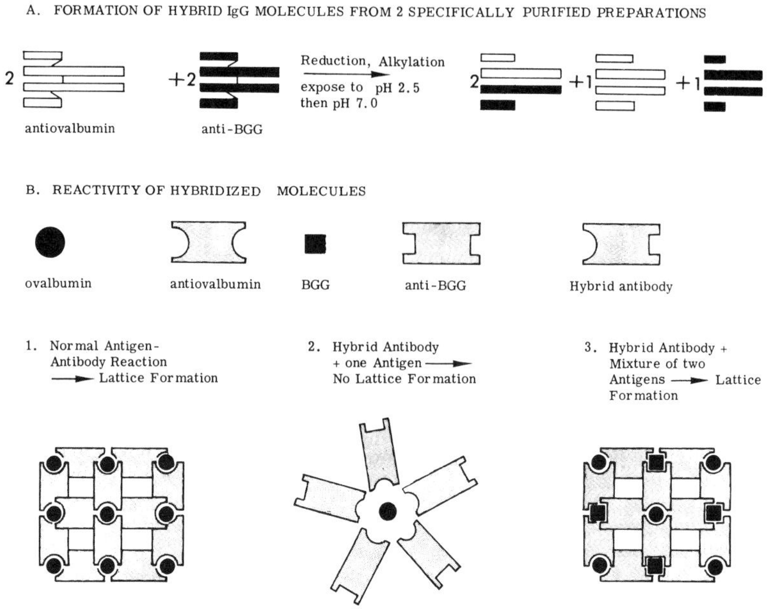

A. FORMATION OF HYBRID IgG MOLECULES FROM 2 SPECIFICALLY PURIFIED PREPARATIONS

B. REACTIVITY OF HYBRIDIZED MOLECULES

Fig. 6.4. Mechanism of formation and mode of action of hybrid antibody molecules produced from half-molecules of rabbit IgG.

erential recombination of half-molecules of the same allotype (59). Hybrid molecules of mixed allotype, produced artificially by this procedure, do not occur naturally, presumably because a given cell synthesizes only one species of L chain and H chain. Actually, one would not anticipate an effect of allotype on the recombination, since rabbit allotypic determinants are localized in the Fab fragment whereas half-molecules are joined through noncovalent interactions in the Fc segment of the H chain (60). Recombination of isolated L and H chains (rather than half-molecules) to form allotypically asymmetrical molecules can also be accomplished *in vitro* (61).

The relative labilities of the H–H and H–L disulfide bonds vary among immunoglobulins. Human IgG4 resembles the rabbit in that H–H bonds are reduced most readily while in the other human IgG subclasses the interchain disulfide bonds are randomly reduced (62).

REFERENCES

1. Edelman, G.M. (1959). *J. Amer. Chem. Soc.* **81**, 3155.
2. Edelman, G.M. and Poulik, M.D. (1961). *J. Exp. Med.* **113**, 861.

3. Fleischman, J.B., Pain, R., and Porter, R.R. (1962). *Arch. Biochem. Biophys. Suppl.* **1**, 174.
3a. Bridges, S.H. and Little, J.R. (1971). *Biochemistry* **10**, 2525.
4. Utsumi, S. and Karush, F. (1964). *Biochemistry* **3**, 1329.
5. Marler, E., Nelson, C.A., and Tanford, C. (1964). *Biochemistry* **3**, 279.
6. Pain, R.H. (1963). *Biochem. J.* **88**, 234.
7. Franek, F. (1961). *Biochem. Biophys. Res. Commun.* **4**, 28.
8. Scharff, M.D. and Uhr, J.W. (1965). *Science* **148**, 646.
9. Cohen, S. and Gordon, S. (1965). *Biochem. J.* **97**, 460.
10. Reisfeld, R.A. and Small, P.A. (1966). *Science* **152**, 1253.
11. Stevenson, G.T. and Dorrington, K.J. (1970). *Biochem. J.* **118**, 703.
12. Björk, I. and Tanford, C. (1970). *Biochemistry* **10**, 1289.
13. Haber, E. and Richards, F.F. (1966). *Proc. Roy. Soc. Ser. B.* **166**, 176.
14. Jaton, J.C., Klinman, N.R., Givol, D., and Sela, M. (1968). *Biochemistry* **7**, 4185.
15. Björk, I. and Tanford, C. (1970). *Biochemistry* **10**, 1271.
16. Björk, I. and Tanford, C. (1970). *Biochemistry* **10**, 1280.
17. Haber, E. (1964). *Proc. Nat. Acad. Sci. U.S.* **52**, 1009.
17a. Whitney, P.L. and Tanford, C. (1965). *Proc. Nat. Acad. Sci. U.S.* **53**, 524.
18. Porter, R.R. and Weir, R.R. (1966). *J. Cell. Physiol. Suppl.* **67** (Part II), 51.
19. Fleischman, J.B., Porter, R.R., and Press, E.M. (1963). *Biochem. J.* **88**, 220.
20. Olins, D.E. and Edelman, G.M. (1964). *J. Exp. Med.* **119**, 789.
21. Stein, S.R., Palmer, J.L., and Nisonoff, A. (1964). *J. Biol. Chem.* **239**, 2872.
21a. Zimmerman, B. and Grey, H.M. (1971). *J. Immunol.* **107**, 1788.
22. Eden, A., Lamm, M.E., and Nussenzweig, V. (1972). *J. Immunol.* **108**, 1605.
23. Edelman, G.M., Olins, D.E., Gally, J.A., and Zinder, N.D. (1963). *Proc. Nat. Acad. Sci. U.S.* **50**, 753.
24. Roholt, O., Radzimski, G., and Pressman, D. (1965). *Science* **147**, 613.
25. Roholt, O., Onoue, K., and Pressman, D. (1964). *Proc. Nat. Acad. Sci. U.S.* **51**, 173.
26. Sher, A., Lord, E., and Cohn, M. (1971). *J. Immunol.* **107**, 1226.
27. Klinman, N.R. (1971). *J. Immunol.* **106**, 1330.
28. MacDonald, A.B., Alescio, L., and Nisonoff, A. (1969). *Biochemistry* **8**, 3109.
29. Roholt, O., Radzimski, G., and Pressman, D. (1966). *J. Exp. Med.* **123**, 921.
30. Carson, D. and Weigert, M. (1973). *Proc. Nat. Acad. Sci. U.S.* **70**, 235.
31. Grey, H.M. and Mannik, M. (1965). *J. Exp. Med.* **122**, 619.
32. Roholt, O.A., Radzimski, G., and Pressman, D. (1965). *J. Exp. Med.* **122**, 785.
33. Smith, B.R. and Dorrington, K.J. (1972). *Biochem. Biophys. Res. Commun.* **46**, 1061.
33a. Karlsson, F.A. (1972). *J. Immunol.* **109**, 110.
33b. Karlsson, F.A., Björk, I., and Berggård, I. (1972). *Immunochemistry* **9**, 1129.
34. Inbar, D., Hochman, J., and Givol, D. (1972). *Proc. Nat. Acad. Sci. U.S.* **69**, 2659.
35. Wells, J.V., Fudenberg, H.H., and Givol, D. (1973). *Proc. Nat. Acad. Sci. U.S.* **70**, 1585.
36. Kakimoto, K. and Onoue, K. (1974). *J. Immunol.* **112**, 1373.
37. Gall, W.E. and D'Eustachio, P. (1972). *Biochemistry* **11**, 4621.
38. Epp, O., Colman, P., Fehlhammer, H., Bode, W., Schiffer, M., and Huber, R. (1974). *Eur. J. Biochem.* **45**, 513.
39. Schiffer, M., Girling, R.L., Ely, K.R., and Edmundson, A.B. (1973). *Biochemistry* **12**, 4620.
40. Velick, S.F., Parker, C.W., and Eisen, H.N. (1960). *Proc. Nat. Acad. Sci. U.S.* **46**, 1470.
41. Metzger, H. and Singer, S.J. (1963). *Science* **142**, 674.

42. Metzger, H. and Mannik, M. (1964). *J. Exp. Med.* **120,** 765.
43. Cathou, R.E. and Haber, E. (1967). *Biochemistry* **6,** 513.
44. Hong, R. and Nisonoff, A. (1966). *J. Immunol.* **96,** 622.
45. Raynaud, M. and Mangalo, R. (1967). *Ann. Inst. Pasteur, Paris* **113,** 549.
46. Raynaud, M. and Mangalo, R. (1968). *Bull. Soc. Chim. Biol.* **50,** 1041.
47. Goodman, J.W. and Donch, J.J. (1965). *Immunochemistry* **2,** 351.
48. Yoo, T.J., Roholt, O.A., and Pressman, D. (1967). *Science* **157,** 707.
49. Nakamura, H., Grossberg, A.L., and Pressman, D. (1973). *Immunochemistry* **10,** 485.
50. Painter, R.G., Sage, H.J., and Tanford, C. (1972). *Biochemistry* **11,** 1327.
51. Franek, F.O., Simek, L., and Zikan, J. (1965). *Proc. Symp. Prague, June, 1964,* p. 128, Publ. House of Czech. Acad. of Sci. Academic Press, New York.
52. Roholt, O., Radzimski, G., and Pressman, D. (1963). *Science* **141,** 726.
52a. Stevenson, G.T. (1973). *Biochem. J.* **133,** 827.
53. Koshland, M.E., Englberger, F.M., and Shapanka, R. (1966). *Biochemistry* **5,** 641.
54. Palmer, J.L., Nisonoff, A., and Van Holde, K.E. (1963). *Proc. Nat. Acad. Sci. U.S.* **50,** 314.
55. Nisonoff, A. and Palmer, J.L. (1964). *Science* **143,** 3605.
56. Hong, R. and Nisonoff, A. (1965). *J. Biol. Chem.* **240,** 3883.
57. Nisonoff, A. and Hong, R. (1964). *Brookhaven Nat. Lab. Symp. No.* **17,** p. 204.
58. Fudenberg, H.H., Hong, R., and Nisonoff, A. (1965). *Science* **148,** 91.
59. Seth, S.K., Nisonoff, A., and Dray, S. (1965). *Immunochemistry* **2,** 39.
60. Inman, F.P. and Nisonoff, A. (1966). *J. Biol. Chem.* **241,** 322.
61. Mannik, M. and Metzger, H. (1965). *Science* **148,** 383.
62. Virella, G. and Parkhouse, R.M.E. (1973). *Immunochemistry* **10,** 213.

7

Evolution of the Immunoglobulins

I. INTRODUCTION

Molecules identifiable as immunoglobulins have been found in all vertebrate species investigated, with the possible exceptions of the hagfish and lamprey. Despite the presence of certain types of adaptive immunity in invertebrates, the existence of molecules related to the immunoglobulins, with respect to specificity or structure, has not been shown. There is a widespread feeling that proteins of a transitional nature may exist in invertebrates, and a number of investigators have, without success, sought to identify such molecules. Although invertebrate immunity appears to be mediated largely by cells, humoral factors of broad specificity have also been identified. Many invertebrates have been found to possess natural agglutinins, active against protozoa, bacteria, and the red blood cells of various invertebrate and vertebrate species (1–5). There is evidence that these agglutinins are capable of acting as opsonins (6–9), but they do not appear to have the narrow specificity characteristic of immunoglobulins; for example, a mussel hemagglutinin was shown to be cross-absorbed by each of a variety of vertebrate red blood cells (10). Many vertebrates, including such a primitive species as the lamprey, also have natural hemagglutinins, but as yet there are no data which establish an evolutionary pattern or which clearly relate the agglutinins of vertebrates and invertebrates structurally. A relationship of invertebrate proteins to the immunoglobulins is, at this stage, conjectural (11,12). Recent studies on invertebrate immunity are summarized in reference 12a. A recent review of the evolution of the immunoglobulins is presented in reference 5.

Figure 7.1 shows an abbreviated phylogenetic tree of the vertebrates, including a few representative species (13). In all vertebrate species studied, with the possible exception of the lamprey and the hagfish, immunoglobulin molecules comprise one or more subunits, each consisting of two H and two L chains. The chains are linked by noncovalent interactions and in most, but not all instances, by interchain disulfide bonds. Assignment of an immunoglobulin to a particular class is made

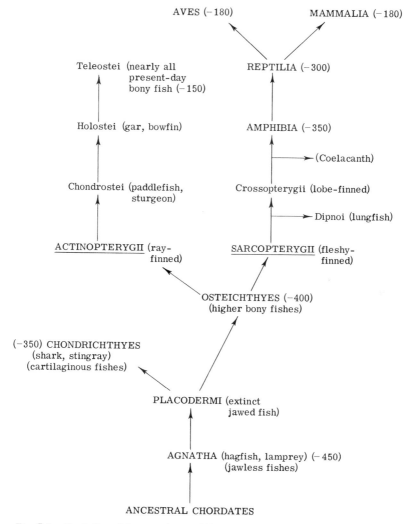

Fig. 7.1. Evolution of the vertebrates. The numbers in parentheses show the approximate time of emergence during evolution (years ×10⁻⁶). Data from Romer (13).

by comparison with mammalian or, more specifically, with human immunoglobulins. Ideally, the assignment should be based on amino acid sequences; however, the relevant data from nonmammalian species are at present quite limited. Also, it is not certain that a knowledge of the amino acid sequence of the C_H region would immediately permit identification of the class to which the immunoglobulin of a primitive species belongs. Even if, for example, the gene controlling the C_μ region of human IgM evolved directly from a corresponding gene in fish, the divergence in sequence may prove to be so great as to make a definite assignment difficult. A clear-cut decision may be possible if sequences are determined for selected species along the evolutionary scale and a pattern emerges.

Other useful criteria include the following: (a) Arrangement of 4-chain disulfide bonded monomers (e.g., the pentameric structure characteristic of IgM), and carbohydrate content; (b) the number of domains in the H chain; (c) the presence of a secretory component (for IgA) or J chain (IgM and polymeric IgA); synthesis by a secretory immune system associated with epithelial tissues (for IgA); (d) heat lability, sensitization of skin with a relativity long latent period, prolonged persistence in skin, and a molecular weight somewhat greater than that of IgG (for IgE); (e) attachment to mast cells and basophilic leukocytes (IgE).

A convincing criterion for classification is immunological cross-reactivity with the corresponding human immunoglobulin class. This has proven very useful for mammals but of limited value for more primitive species, because antigenic cross-reactivity with mammalian immunoglobulins has rarely been observed. An exception is avian IgM (see below). The absence of cross-reactivity, of course, does not disprove evolutionary relatedness. Since, for example, mammals diverged from reptiles about 2×10^8 years ago, it is not surprising that antigenic cross-reactivity among their immunoglobulins has not been reported.

On the basis of the data at hand the following tentative conclusions can be drawn: (a) a homolog of mammalian IgM is probably present in all classes of vertebrates; (b) the presence of IgG in vertebrates other than mammals has not been established, although an immunoglobulin of low molecular weight, differing antigenically from IgM of the corresponding species, and having a lower carbohydrate content, is present in the lungfish, higher amphibia, reptiles, and birds. It is conceivable that the immunoglobulin of low molecular weight arose just once during evolution or, alternatively, that it evolved independently (perhaps from IgM) in two or more classes of vertebrate. Data on amino acid sequences might resolve this question. Since the amount of sequence homology between human γ and μ chains is only 30%, the two structural genes must have diverged very early in evolution; i.e., they probably coexisted in classes lower than mammals. It would not be surprising, then, if the γ gene has been retained in one or more nonmammalian classes. (c) The counterpart of mammalian IgA exists in birds, but its presence has not been demonstrated in other vertebrate classes. (d) A class similar to human IgE has been identified in many mammalian species. A heat-labile molecule with reagenic properties has been demonstrated in birds, but its relationship to human IgE is conjectural. The small degree of homology between the ϵ and μ chain suggests very early divergence. (e) A homolog of human IgD appears, by antigenic analysis, to be present in some mammalian species but has not been identified in lower vertebrates. (f) Subclasses of IgG, found in many mammals, appear from their amino acid sequences and antigenic relatedness to be products of recent evolutionary events; therefore, all could not have evolved directly from lower vertebrates. (g) There appears to be a direct line of evolution of L chains from the most primitive vertebrate species to man. An apparent precursor of human κ chains is present in the nurse shark, and polypeptides resembling human λ chains are found in birds. The degree of homology between human C_κ and C_λ sequences (about 40%) strongly suggests a common precursor. The molecular weight of the L chain ($\sim 23,000$) has remained remarkably constant throughout evolution.

II. UNIVERSALITY OF IgM-LIKE MOLECULES IN VERTEBRATES

Molecules comparable in certain properties to mammalian IgM have been found in all classes of vertebrate. For example, the dogfish shark, a very primitive species, has an immunoglobulin with a sedimentation coefficient of 17 S and high carbohydrate content (14,15). In common with human IgM, the molecule comprises five IgMs subunits which separate upon mild reduction; each contains two H and two L chains with approximate molecular weights of 70,000 and 22,000, respectively. The mobility of the H chain during starch gel electrophoresis is similar to that of human or rabbit μ chain. Circumstantial evidence therefore suggests that the shark immunoglobulin is the counterpart of human IgM. Further evidence for the close similarity of fish and human IgM is the pentameric structure of the 18 S immunoglobulin of the stingray (another elasmobranch), as seen in the electron microscope (16). It would, of course, be useful to show that the C_μ regions of the IgM of fish and human IgM exhibit sequence homology which is

TABLE 7.1

COMPARISON OF AMINO ACID COMPOSITION AMONG IMMUNOGLOBULIN
HEAVY POLYPEPTIDE CHAINS OF VERTEBRATE SPECIES[a]

	Lamprey μ	Catfish μ	Gar μ	Paddlefish μ	Dogfish μ	Stingray μ	Human μ	Human α	Human γ
Lamprey μ	0								
Catfish μ	31	0							
Gar μ	70	26	0						
Paddlefish μ	41	17	21	0					
Dogfish μ	46	12	20	14	0				
Stingray μ	40	17	27	27	13	0			
Human μ	27	14	18	19	15	14	0		
Human α	57	44	37	55	48	45	26	0	
Human γ	64	26	25	36	29	35	21	48	0

[a] The data are values of $S\Delta Q$, defined by the relationship, $S\Delta Q = (X_{ij} - x_{kj})^2$, where i and k designate the two proteins being compared and X_j or x_j are the content (residues per 100) of a given amino acid of type j. Reprinted by permission from Marchalonis (17).

greater than that observed upon comparison of the shark protein with other human H chain classes.

Although less definitive, data on the amino acid composition of H chains indicate that the immunoglobulins of high molecular weight from primitive species are more closely related to mammalian IgM than to mammalian IgG. A summary of data on amino acid compositional differences and a statistical analysis have been presented by Marchalonis (17) (Table 7.1). The data support a closer resemblance of the immunoglobulins of the most primitive vertebrates to human IgM than to human IgG or IgA. Marchalonis notes that the differences in composition among the immunoglobulins of high molecular weight from various species are remarkably small, reflecting evolutionary conservatism in the IgM molecule.

That the 19 S protein of the chicken is indeed homologous to mammalian IgM is shown by the fairly strong immunological cross-reaction observed between the chicken and human proteins; the tests were carried out with antiserum specific for human μ chains (18). No cross-reaction could be detected between human IgG and the chicken immunoglobulin of comparable molecular weight.

Although an IgM-like molecule is present in nearly all vertebrates its structure is somewhat variable. In most species the molecule comprises five subunits, each containing two H and two L chains. (This conclusion is based on electron microscopy and/or molecular weights of the 19 S and 7 S forms.) One important exception is the subclass of bony fishes, the Actinopterygii (Fig. 7.1) which comprise nearly all the present-day bony fishes. In each of several species studied so far (carp, gar, catfish, paddlefish, and goldfish) the IgM appears to exist as a tetramer ($\sim$ 14 S), rather than a pentamer of the basic 4-chain subunit (19–21). In *Xenopus laevis*, the clawed toad, which is a very primitive amphibian, IgM occurs as a hexamer of the basic 4-chain subunit (22). Whether this is true of the IgM of other amphibia is uncertain; molecular weight data on bullfrog IgM and its subunits suggest a pentameric form (23). A small proportion of the molecules of a mouse IgM myeloma protein also appeared, by electron microscopy, to have six discernible subunits, although the majority of the molecules were pentameric (22). It remains to be determined whether this is also true of normal mouse IgM. Electron micrographs of chicken IgM also show the pentameric structure (24). The number of electron microscopic studies carried out so far is quite limited; that the 5-subunit structure prevails in most species is inferred from data on molecular weights of IgM and of the IgMs (7 S), 4-chain subunit. On the basis of the available data marked interspecies variability may be anticipated. In most mammals, however, it seems probable from their molecular weights that IgM molecules will generally prove to be pentameric.

III. IMMUNOGLOBULINS OF FISH

Fish are not only the most primitive vertebrates extant but also the most numerous. The vast majority of present-day fish are teleosts, the highest order of bony fish. Relatively few examples of more primitive bony fishes are still in existence; these include the sturgeon and paddlefish (Chondrostei), the bowfin and gar (Holostei), and the coelacanth (Crossopterygii).

On the line of ascent to mammals is the subclass Sarcopterygii (Fig. 7.1) which includes the lungfish and coelacanth, the latter representing the closest relative to man among existing fish. Lungfish resemble amphibians in many anatomic features, and a resemblance will become evident also with respect to their immunoglobulins, but they are off the direct line of ascent. The coelacanth was thought to be extinct until 1939, when a specimen was captured off the coast of South Africa; since then a number of additional coelacanths have been caught and studied. Their immunoglobulins have not, however, been investigated.

The class Chondrichthyes, or cartilaginous fish, represented by sharks, skates, and rays, diverged from the main line of ascent to man at

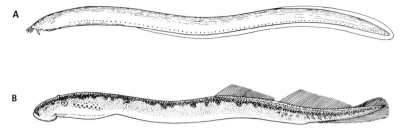

Fig. 7.2.   The hagfish (A) and lamprey (B). From Romer (13).

the latter part of the Devonian period, about 350×10^6 years ago. Present-day genera of sharks whose immunoglobulins have been studied appeared from 30 to 130×10^6 years ago. Immunoglobulins of sharks have been studied rather intensively and provide some of the best evidence for the continuity of evolution of immunoglobulin molecules.

The most primitive fish in existence are the hagfish and lamprey, which are Agnathan (jawless) cyclostomes (Fig. 7.2). Each has a cartilaginous skeleton and a notachord which persists into adulthood, but lacks a stomach. The immunoglobulins of these species have received some attention and will be considered first.

A. Immunoglobulins of the Hagfish

The hagfish, which is the most primitive vertebrate extant, is capable of mounting an immune response. Although earlier studies had suggested that the species does not exhibit cellular or humoral immunity, Hildemann and Thoenes (25) were able to demonstrate that the animal exhibits first- and second-set rejection of skin allografts, with rejection times of 72 and 28 days, respectively. The very slow rejection of the first-set graft could be due to a weak histocompatability barrier or to a poorly developed immune mechanism. The authors favor the former hypothesis on the basis of the hyperacute reaction which is observed if the second graft is applied very soon after rejection of the first.

Humoral antibodies were formed by the hagfish after 2 or 3 months, in response to immunization either with sheep red blood cells or keyhole limpet hemocyanin (25,26). Antibodies to the former antigen were demonstrated by direct hemagglutination and to the latter by passive hemmagglutination or gel diffusion methods. The titer of antibody to sheep red blood cells was comparatively low, reaching a maximum of 128 in some specimens and 1024 in others, as compared to values exceeding 10,000 that are readily obtained in the rabbit. The antibody to sheep red blood cells did not cross-react with burro red blood cells, thus indicating a degree of specificity. The activity was localized to a globulin fraction of high molecular weight, with a sedimentation coefficient of 23 S. Immunization with keyhole limpet hemocyanin, intramuscularly or into the coelomic cavity, resulted after 5 to 10 weeks in passive hemagglutination titers as high as 1024.

Because of the limited amount of physicochemical data available, the identification of hagfish immunoglobulin as IgM is uncertain, although its high molecular weight, chromatographic behavior, and electrophoretic mobility provide suggestive evidence. In contrast to many other fish, the hagfish has not been shown to synthesize an immunoglobulin of low molecular weight. Linthicum and Hildemann note that, by analogy with the shark, such an immunoglobulin might possibly be produced after extensive immunization (27). This has so far not been possible because of the great difficulty of keeping hagfish alive and healthy in captivity; the fish rarely survive for more than 3 months and do not tolerate repetitive bleeding. The difficulty experienced by earlier workers in demonstrating an immune response is attributed by Hildemann to the poor viability of the hagfish.

B. Immunoglobulins of the Lamprey

The lamprey is a somewhat more advanced cyclostome than the hagfish and is the most primitive species known to have thymic and splenic tissue. Cells with the morphology of small lymphocytes are found in all vertebrates, including the hagfish and lamprey; the lamprey, but not the hagfish also has cells similar to medium and large lymphocytes (28). Tissue resembling the thymus was identified in the lamprey, but not in the hagfish (28).

The nature of the immunoglobulins of the lamprey is controversial. Marchalonis and Edelman were able to induce the formation of antibody capable of neutralizing bacteriophage f2 in about three-fifths of the lampreys they immunized, but observed poor responses to sheep red blood cells and none to hemocyanin 1 month after challenge (29). (In view of experiences with other primitive fish, it would appear that a more prolonged immunization schedule might be successful.) The antiphage activity was localized in globulin fractions sedimenting with velocities of 14 S and 6.6 S, with the 6.6 S component predominating. The fractions of high and low molecular weight showed antigenic similarity or identity, suggesting that the 14 S molecule is a polymeric form of the smaller molecule. Upon gel filtration of 6.6 S molecules in 1 M propionic acid, subunits of molecular weight 70,000 and 25,000 were separated in roughly equimolar amounts. There was no requirement for prior reduction, which indicated the absence of interchain disulfide bonds linking H chains to L chains.

Contrasting findings were reported subsequently by Litman et al. (30), who were unable to find typical H and L chains in the lamprey immunoglobulin molecule. They prepared antibody to human red blood cells by prolonged immunization and localized it in a globulin fraction having a molecular weight of 320,000 and a sedimentation coefficient of 9 S, which differs from that of either component isolated by Marchalonis and Edelman. Upon storage, the molecule dissociated into antigenically identical components, with molecular weights of 150,000 and 75,000, which were devoid of hemagglutinating activity. Reduction and alkylation, followed by gel filtration in 1 M propionic acid failed to liberate a subunit resembling L chains, although a smaller, unidentified polypeptide was produced in low yield when the reduction was carried out in 6 M guanidine.

Additional work will be needed to resolve the conflicting findings of the two groups of investigators. It may be relevant that neither laboratory showed that the entire fraction with antibody activity is immunoglobulin. It is conceivable that immunoglobulin is present only in low concentration in the antibody-containing fractions, isolated by gel filtration. Experiments with specifically purified antibody, which could resolve this question, are difficult because of the low titers produced in these primitive species. Marchalonis and Edelman (29) did show that rabbit antibody to a lamprey 6.6 S fraction could neutralize lamprey antibody; but this result could be obtained even if the fraction were a mixture containing immunoglobulin and, principally, nonimmunoglobulin molecules.

C. Immunoglobulins of Sharks

Among the most primitive vertebrates are the various species of sharks, which are members of the elasmobranch subclass of the Chondrichthyes (cartilaginous fishes). Sharks can respond to a broad spectrum of antigens, including proteins, bacteria, viruses, and haptens conjugated to protein. There is no clear-cut evidence that their antibodies are less heterogeneous than those of higher species. There is some controversy as to the number of classes of immunoglobulin that sharks can synthesize. Marchalonis and Edelman (14,15), and Small et al. (31) reported the presence in several species of shark of 7 S and 19 S immunoglobulins, which appear to be antigenically identical and are therefore believed to represent a single class of immunoglobulin. Gitlin *et al.*, on the other hand, observed multiple precipitin bands with antiimmunoglobulin antisera, when tested by immunoelectrophoresis against the sera of several sharks, and concluded that the species they studied (which overlap with those investigated by Edelman and by Clem), possess two to four classes of immunoglobulin (32). Differences in antigenicity were localized to H chains. So far these classes have not been separated or further characterized, and much more work is needed to substantiate the existence of multiple classes and their antigenic relationships.

The initial studies on shark immunoglobulins were carried out by Marchalonis and Edelman, who prepared antibodies to hemocyanin in the smooth dogfish shark (*Mustelus canis*) and also investigated the normal immunoglobulins of the species (14,15). As already indicated they observed only one class of immunoglobulin, which they designated IgM on the basis of its high molecular weight, carbohydrate content, amino acid composition, and electrophoretic mobility. Molecules antigenically identical to the 17–19 S IgM also appeared in a low molecular weight form (7 S). A high carbohydrate content was found in the 7 S as well as the 19 S molecule and, indeed, is characteristic of all immunoglobulins of fish that have been studied. The 7 S and 17–19 S molecules also yield similar peptide maps. The 7 S protein can be produced *in vitro* from the 19 S molecule by reduction under nondenaturing conditions; thus the subunits are linked only by disulfide bonds and not by strong noncovalent forces. There is no evidence that this transformation occurs extracellularly *in vivo* (31); i.e., the 7 S molecule appears to be a product of direct synthesis. The 19 S, but not the 7 S immunoglobulin of the leopard shark contains J chain (Section III,C,2).

For the IgM of the dogfish shark, Marchalonis and Edelman reported molecular weights of 980,000 (19 S) and 198,000 (7 S) (15). After reduction, alkylation, and exposure to 8 *M* urea, H chains (mol. wt. 72,000) and L chains (26,000) were liberated in equimolar amounts. Very similar results were obtained with the immunoglobulin of the leopard shark (33). In addition, it has been shown that the N-terminal sequence of six amino acids is the same for the H chains of the 7 S and 19 S forms (34). The N-terminal residue is glutamic acid, rather than cyclized glutamic acid; this was the first of many demonstrations of an unblocked amino-terminus in an H chain. (It is now known that some of the H chains of the shark have a blocked N-terminal group.)

The existence of a 19 S pentamer and a homologous 7 S, 4-chain monomer has also been demonstrated in nurse, lemon, and horned sharks (31,35,36); molecular weights of the polypeptide chains are in agreement with those of the dogfish shark. Newborn sharks were found to possess only the 19 S form of IgM, but in the mature animal the concentration of 7 S IgM (~ 9 mg/ml) exceeded that of the 19 S protein (~ 6 mg/ml) (31). An appreciable extravascular distribution of 7 S IgM but not of 19 S IgM was noted. This ability to penetrate extravascular spaces suggests a possible biological advantage associated with possession of an immunoglobulin of low molecular weight (such as the IgG of higher species). The half-lives of 7 S and 19 S IgM were about the same in the lemon shark (4–5 days); in the nurse shark the half-life of the 7 S IgM was somewhat greater (12 versus 6 days). The rate of synthesis of immunoglobulin, per unit body weight, was calculated to be higher in the shark (100 to 150 mg/kg/day) than the rate of total immunoglobulin biosynthesis in man (~ 80 mg/kg/day). Thus the apparent deficiency of the shark with respect to the number of classes of immunoglobulin it can synthesize is not reflected by the overall synthetic rate (31).

Shulkin *et al.* (37) prepared antibodies to *Salmonella typhi* in adult nurse sharks. Both 19 S and 7 S antibodies were elicited; the 7 S antibodies did not appear, however, until almost a year after the start of immunization. Investigations with specifically purified antibodies showed that the 19 S form is about 100 times as effective, on a weight basis, as the 7 S form in the agglutination of *Salmonella*. Also, the 19 S antibody, but not the 7 S, was bactericidal in the presence of bovine complement.[1]

Voss *et al.* (42) found no differences between the average binding affinities or the shape of the hapten-binding curves for 7 S and 18 S anti-2,4-dinitrophenyl (anti-Dnp) antibodies isolated from the antiserum of nurse sharks. K_0 values were of the order of 10^5 M^{-1}, a value considerably smaller than that of anti-Dnp antibodies produced by prolonged immunization of mammalian species. From the binding data, valences of 5 and 1, respectively, were calculated for the 18 S and 7 S antibodies. The 18 S antibody was able to agglutinate red cells coated with Dnp groups and to form precipitates with protein-Dnp conjugates; negative results were obtained in both tests with the 7 S antibody, even at concentrations much higher than those at which the 18 S anti-Dnp antibody was active.

These results would suggest that the 7 S antibody of the nurse shark is monovalent. Contrasting results, however, were obtained by Clem *et al.* who also worked with the nurse shark and found that 7 S antibodies

---

[1] A greater agglutinating or hemolytic capacity of 19 S antibody as compared to IgG is also observed in higher species. It is attributable to the greater binding energy associated with multivalent attachment and possibly to a superior capacity of the multivalent 19 S molecule for steric accommodation to the antigenic determinants on the bacterial surface (38–41).

to BSA are capable of specific precipitation with the antigen (43). Precipitating activity was similarly observed in 7 S anti-BSA antibodies of the lemon shark (35). In addition, 7 S antibodies to hemocyanin, prepared in the leopard shark, are capable of forming specific precipitates (33). Each of these three investigations is consistent with bivalence of the 7 S molecule. The hapten-binding study, which suggests a valence of 1 for the 7 S antibody, could be reconciled with data indicating that the antibody can form specific precipitates if some of the 7 S antibody combining sites are of such low affinity ($K < 10^4 M^{-1}$) that they are not readily detected in the binding assay but are capable of participating in the formation of the lattice which constitutes the immune precipitate.

This possibility was supported by an investigation in which nurse sharks were subjected to prolonged immunization with 2,4-dinitrophenyl-hemocyanin and the affinities of the anti-Dnp antibodies produced were measured (44). Both 7 S and 19 S antibodies were elicited, with the latter predominating. At first, both the 7 S and 19 S antibodies had K_0 values of $2 \times 10^5 M^{-1}$, which remained virtually unchanged during 16 months of immunization. The apparent valences of the antibodies were 1 and 5, respectively. By the end of 30 months, however, the K_0 of the 7 S molecule had increased by a factor of 100 to 1000 while that of the 19 S species increased only by a factor of 10. At the same time, valences rose to 2 and 10, respectively, for the smaller and larger molecule. This careful study demonstrates the very slow maturation of the immune response in sharks and suggests that the valence of the immunoglobulin is compatible with the number of H–L pairs, provided the K values of some of the sites are not too low to be measured. The results also reflect the difficulty of demonstrating a secondary response in sharks (43). It seems possible that a similar explanation may apply to reports that 6.4 S anti-Dnp antibodies of the grouper are monovalent (45) and that the 19 S antibodies of the snapper have a valence of 5 (46). (The 16 S anti-Dnp antibody of the grouper was found to have a valence of 8, which is compatible with its tetrameric structure.) It is relevant that early studies failed to reveal the decavalence of rabbit IgM antihapten antibody, owing to the presence of combining sites of low affinity (Chapter 8, Section V,C).

1. LIMITED PROTEOLYSIS OF SHARK IMMUNOGLOBULINS

The 7 S antibodies of the dogfish shark and of the lamprey are almost unaffected by treatment with papain in neutral buffer (29). Klapper *et al.* investigated the effects of papain and trypsin on the 19 S and 7 S immunoglobulins of the lemon shark, and on 7 S molecules obtained by mild reduction of the 19 S protein (47). Upon treatment with papain or trypsin in neutral buffer, the sedimentation coefficient of the naturally occurring 7 S protein (mol. wt. 180,000) was decreased to 6 S (mol. wt. 110,000). After subsequent mild reduction, the sedimentation coefficient and molecular weight were lowered to 4.5 S and 60,000, respectively. The 6 S molecule, if derived from anti-*Salmonella* antibody, completely retained the capacity to agglutinate the bacteria, but this activity was lost upon mild reduction, yielding the 4.5 S form. The antibody-combining sites appeared to be intact in the 4.5 S fragments, as shown by their capacity to bind to *Salmonella*. Treatment of the naturally occurring 7 S immunoglobulin of the lemon shark with trypsin results in the same series of events; i.e., production of a bivalent 6 S molecule which is cleaved by mild reduction into univalent 4.5 S fragments (47). This behavior is very reminiscent of that observed upon peptic digestion, followed by mild reduction, of the IgG of many mammalian species. After treatment with pepsin, the IgG is reduced in size [to F(ab')₂ fragments] but remains bivalent; it is then separated into monovalent Fab' fragments by reduction of interchain disulfide bonds.

Upon prolonged digestion with trypsin, the 4.5 S shark molecule is further degraded to 3.5 S fragments, which are stable to further digestion and still retain univalent antibody activity (47). The 3.5 S univalent fragments seem to correspond to the Fab (or Fab') fragments that have been thoroughly characterized in higher species. Besides being functionally univalent they contain L chains, as shown by antigenic analysis. Furthermore, as in higher species, the 3.5 S fragments possess only a small fraction (20%) of the carbohydrate present in the native molecule. The bulk of the carbohydrate appears to be attached in the region between the points of early and late cleavage by trypsin.

2. J Chain in Shark Immunoglobulins

An investigation by Klaus *et al.* indicated the presence of J chain in the 19 S immunoglobulin of the leopard shark (48). It was not found in the naturally occurring 7 S immunoglobulin, which shows antigenic identity with the 19 S protein. Evidence for the presence of J chain was the release, after complete reduction and alkylation, of an electrophoretically homogeneous peptide of low molecular weight, having high anodal mobility. The molecular weight was estimated by gel filtration to be about the same as that of an L chain. That the chain is found only in 19 S, but not in the 7 S immunoglobulin, is another indication of homology with mammalian J chain. Although these properties are characteristic of the J chain of higher species, data on amino acid sequences should be very informative.

Weinheimer *et al.* (49) failed to detect J chain in the 19 S IgM of the paddlefish, gar or nurse shark, but a protein component of low molecular weight (12,000), which may be J chain, was noted by Klapper and Clem upon gel filtration in guanidine solution of the IgM of the nurse shark (50). J chain is present in the IgM of the pheasant, marine toad, catfish, chicken, and each of a large variety of mammals (49,51). It is also present in the polymeric IgA of the chicken and of various mammals (51). J chain is thus found throughout the phylogenetic scale. It remains to be determined whether it was not detected in the IgM of certain primitive species because the properties of the J chain vary, or simply because it is absent.

3. Amino Acid Sequences in Shark Immunoglobulins

The common origin of the immunoglobulins of all vertebrates is most convincingly illustrated by a comparison of amino acid sequences of mammalian immunoglobulins with those of the shark. A sequence of six residues at the N-terminus of the unblocked H chains of leopard shark immunoglobulin was determined by Suran and Papermaster (34). The 7 and 19 S forms were found to have the same principal sequence: Glu-Ile-Val-Leu-Thr-Gln-. This identity was taken as further evidence that the 19 and 7 S molecules in the shark are of the same class; but this probably would no longer be accepted as relevant, since the various H chain classes in higher species share the same V_H genes.

Suran and Papermaster made the remarkable observation that in five of these positions the amino acids present are also commonly found in human κ chains. These studies were extended by Klaus *et al.* (52) who showed, first, that there are some blocked (by pyrrolidonecarboxylic acid) as well as unblocked H and L chains in leopard shark immunoglobulins. Most of their sequence data were, however, obtained with unblocked H chains or L chains. Sequences up to position 10 showed homology of shark L chains with human κ and λ chains and impressive homology of shark and human H chains. Of the first 10 positions, eight residues present in the highest proportion in shark H chains are also found at the same position in some human H chains.

Subsequently, Sledge *et al.* (53) determined the sequence of 28 N-terminal residues of the L and H chains, isolated from antibodies of restricted heterogeneity from individual nurse sharks. The antibody was specific for the carbohydrate of Group A-variant streptococci. The N-terminal sequence of the L chains from a normal serum pool was also reported. L chain sequences from the antibodies of two sharks were virtually identical up to position 28 and were greatly restricted in their heterogeneity. The sequences are shown in Table 7.2 together with that of

TABLE 7.2

Comparison of the Unblocked N-Terminal Amino Acid Sequences of L Chains[a]

Sequences	1	10	20	28	No. of identities with shark 225 L[c]
Shark L (antibody 225)[a,b]	Asp Ile Thr Met Thr Glu Ser Pro Pro Val Leu Ser Val Gly Leu Gly Gln Thr Ala Thr Ile Thr Cys Thr Ala Ser – Ser				
	Val Lys				
Shark L (antibody Francis)[a,b]	Asp Ile Thr Met Thr Glu Ser Pro Pro Val Leu Ser Val Gly Leu Gly Gln Thr Ala Ser Ile Thr Cys Thr Ala Ser Glx Ser				26
	Val Lys Leu				
Shark L (normal pool)	Asp Ile Thr Met Thr Glu Ser Pro Pro Val Leu Ser Val Gly Leu Gly Gln Thr Ala Thr Ile Thr Cys Thr Ala Ser Glx Ser				26
	Val Leu				
Human κ_I (protein Ou)	Asp Ile Gln Met Thr Gln Ser Pro Ser Ser Leu Ser Ala Ser Val Gly Asp Arg Val Thr Ile Thr Cys Arg Ala Ser Glx Thr				15
Human λ_{II} (protein Vil)	His Ser Ala Leu Thr Gln – Pro Ala Ser Val Ser Gly Ser Leu Gly Gln Ser Ile Thr Ile Ser Cys Thr Gly Thr Ser Ser				10
African lungfish I	Asp – – Leu Thr Glx Asx Gly Ser Met				3/8
	Ala Leu				
Chicken λ	– – Ala Leu Thr Glx Pro Ala Ala Val				3/8

[a] See references 52 and 53 for sequence data and original sources.
[b] Specifically purified antistreptococcal antibody of the nurse shark.
[c] To position 26 of antibody 225.

L chains from nonspecific IgM prepared from a pool of serum. Aside from the isoleucine-valine interchange at position 2 and the heterogeneity of antibody "Francis" at position 4, both of the antibody L chains appear homogeneous through position 28. Remarkably, this is true also of the nonspecific L chains. Furthermore, the three sequences are nearly identical. A comparison of the sequences with those of human L chains is also shown in Table 7.2. The authors conclude that the shark L chain is somewhat more homologous to mammalian κ than to mammalian λ chains. In comparing the shark sequences with those of human κ_I, κ_{II}, and κ_{III} and with three mouse κ subgroups 9 to 15 differences were noted in the first 28 positions; with respect to four human, one mouse, and one pig λ subgroup the number of differences, 13–19, is somewhat greater. Of perhaps greater significance is the fact that no gaps are necessary in aligning the various κ sequences, whereas one or two gaps had to be permitted in the mammalian λ sequences.

The virtual identity in sequence of the L chains of the specific shark antistreptococcal antibodies and normal L chains is of great interest. It suggests, first, that the L chains of many shark antibodies will prove to have similar sequences for the first 28 residues. [Normal shark L chains are, nevertheless, quite heterogeneous as shown by their electrophoretic patterns (54); this heterogeneity evidently exists mainly beyond position 28.] In fact, the L chains from the normal pool and from antibody Francis both appeared quite heterogeneous from position 29–36, reflecting the onset of the first hypervariable region. It should be of interest to ascertain whether nurse shark L chains from other antibodies have similar sequences in the first 28 positions. [The L chains of the leopard shark appear considerably more heterogeneous in the first 10 positions (52).]

Shark H chains similarly show significant homology with human H chains. A comparison with a human V_{HIII} sequence is shown in Table 7.3. (The H chains of the shark antistreptococcal antibodies are unblocked at the N-terminus.) In comparing the shark H chain sequence with prototypes for human V_{HI}, V_{HII}, and V_{HIII}, the number of differences observed in the first 28 positions are 17, 13, and 14, respectively (53).

Since the shark H chains are more closely related to mammalian H chains than to shark L chains, Sledge *et al.* concluded that the V_L and V_H genes must have been in existence before the divergence of elasmobranchs from the path leading to present-day mammals ($\sim 400 \times 10^6$ years ago). Although the shark H chains are unblocked, they bear no more resemblance to the unblocked human V_{HIII} subgroup than to the other human V_H subgroups. Another point of interest is that shark and human H chains differ about as much as shark and human L chains,

TABLE 7.3

N-Terminal Amino Acid Sequences of H Chains[a]

Sequence	1		10		20			No. of identities with shark 225 H
Shark H (antibody 225)[b]	Glu Val Thr Leu Thr Glx Pro Glx Ala Glx Asp Ser Glx Pro Gly Gly Ala Leu Thr Leu Thr Cys Glx Val – Gly Ser Ser							28
Human V_III (Protein Ou)	Glp Val Thr Leu Thr Glu Ser Gly Pro Ala Leu Val Lys Pro Lys Gln Pro Leu Thr Leu Thr Cys Thr Phe Ser Gly Phe Ser							13
Rabbit H (Aal)	Glp – Ser Val Glu Glu Ser Gly Gly Arg Leu Val Thr Pro Thr Pro Gly Leu Thr Leu Thr Cys Thr Val Ser Gly Phe Ser Ala							10
Paddlefish H	Asp Val Val Leu Thr Val							3/5

[a] See references 52 and 53 for sequence data and original sources.
[b] Specifically purified antistreptococcal antibody of the nurse shark.

suggesting a similar rate of evolution for H and L chains. The data of Sledge *et al.* suggested that most normal shark L and H chains are unblocked at the N-terminus; however, a small proportion of the H chains appear to be blocked (52). Sledge *et al.* note that shark L chains are about as closely related to mammalian L chains as mammalian V_κ subgroups are to one another; thus, the divergence of the V_κ genes into subgroups may have occurred at about the same period as the divergence of elasmobranchs and mammals.

Tables 7.2 and 7.3 also include partial amino acid sequences of immunoglobulins of a few other species; the obvious homologies further illustrate the common evolutionary origin of the immunoglobulins. The similarity in sequence of paddlefish H chains to those of the shark is of interest since the IgM of the paddlefish (its only class of immunoglobulin) is a tetramer, rather than a pentamer, of the 4-chain subunit and because its H chain has an unusually low molecular weight (55).

The common origin of immunoglobulins is strikingly illustrated by a highly conserved amino acid sequence (Arg or Lys-Phe-Ser-Gly-Ser-) which was detected in the V_L regions, at positions 68–72, of a wide range of species; these include the nurse shark, chicken, duck, turkey, and a number of mammals (56). It is also present in mouse and human myeloma proteins; only an occasional substitution is seen. The same sequence is found in κ and λ chains. Its structural role is, as yet, unknown. A homologous but more variable sequence is found in the H chains of several mammals; lower species have not yet been examined.

4. Versatility of the Immune Response of Sharks

So far there appears to be no major restrictions on the capacity of sharks to respond to various antigens, although prolonged immunization is sometimes required and titers are often not high. Antibodies have been produced against bacteria, bacteriophage, protein antigens, and haptens, and typical secondary responses are observed. Upon challenge with a Dnp–protein conjugate, moderate concentrations of anti-Dnp antibody were elicited, which increased to about 0.3 to 0.4 mg/ml after prolonged immunization (57). Comparable concentrations of antibody were developed in the nurse shark in response to *Salmonella typhi* O antigens (37). In the smooth dogfish shark maximum passive hemagglutination titers of about 2000 were obtained after immunization with keyhole limpet hemocyanin (14). This figure is lower by an order of magnitude than titers obtainable in rabbits. As indicated above, antibodies of restricted heterogeneity were produced in nurse sharks by immunization with a vaccine derived from Group A-variant streptococci (54). The antibodies were present in high titer (~ 7 mg/ml) and were exclusively 19 S, even after prolonged immunization.

D. Immunoglobulins of the Stingray

The immunoglobulins of sharks can be compared with those of another group of elasmobranchs, the stingrays. Two species of stingray, *Dasyatis americana* and *Dasyatis centroura*, both possess the 19 S class of immunoglobulin and also have a smaller immunoglobulin, which appears antigenically identical to the molecule of higher molecular weight (16,58); in these respects, stingrays resemble sharks. In *Dasyatis centroura*, however, the smaller molecule has a molecular weight of 360,000 and appears to comprise a dimer of the basic 4-chain structure.

E. Immunoglobulins of the Actinopterygii

Three major orders of this subclass (ray-finned bony fish) are in existence; the Chondrostei (paddlefish, sturgeon); Holostei (gar, bowfin); and the Teleostei, which constitute the most advanced order and comprise the vast majority of present-day fishes; the number of nonteleost species of bony fish is very limited.

All the Actinopterygii studied to date have an IgM-like immunoglobulin of high molecular weight. An antigenically related protein of low molecular weight has been demonstrated in the giant grouper (a teleost) (59) and in the bowfin (60) which is a member of the Holostei, but not in several other bony fishes investigated so far (61). In each species studied (paddlefish, gar, channel catfish, carp, grouper, and goldfish) the IgM appears to exist as a tetramer, rather than a pentamer, of the basic 4-chain subunit. (The six species listed include members of each of the three orders of the Actinopterygii.) A tetrameric structure is indicated by the molecular weight (630,000–700,000) and, more convincingly, by electron microscopy which shows four arms attached to a central region in carp or paddlefish immunoglobulin (19,20,55). (See Fig. 7.3.) The carbohydrate moieties of paddlefish, gar, and catfish IgM are comparable in concentration to that found in human IgM but differ strikingly in composition from the human protein. Whereas in human IgM the molar ratio of mannose to galactose is 3 : 1, there is somewhat more galactose than mannose in the IgM of the three species of fish (20). (See also Section VII.)

There is some uncertainty as to the molecular weight of the H chain

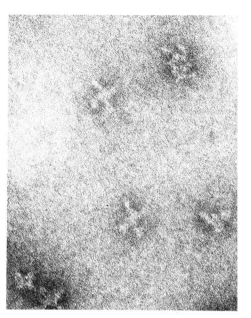
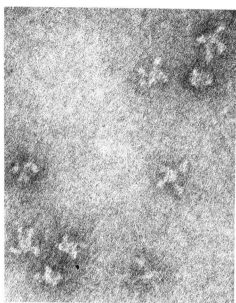

Fig. 7.3. Two electron micrographs of molecules of IgM of the paddlefish (*Polyodon spathula*). The molecules span a total of about 380 to 480 Å. The diameter of the central region is about 100 Å. Reprinted from reference 20 through the courtesy of Dr. Emma Shelton. The IgM of the carp appears virtually identical (19).

of the IgM of the various Actinopterygii. Clem (59) and, initially Acton *et al.* (20) reported the typical molecular weight of 70,000. This was subsequently modified, for the paddlefish, to 58,000 (55). Special properties of a low molecular weight immunoglobulin are described below.

In view of the tetrameric structure, the difference in carbohydrate composition as compared to human IgM, and possible differences in molecular weight of the H chain, one might again raise the question as to the validity of designating the immunoglobulin of the Actinopterygii as IgM. Perhaps the best supporting evidence is based on its polymeric disulfide-linked structure and amino acid composition, which more closely resembles that of the IgM than the IgG of higher species (Table 7.1).

F. IgM of the Giant Grouper

A study of this IgM protein suggests that one cannot generalize concerning the immunoglobulins that may occur in an individual species on the basis of those found in closely related species (59). The normal serum of the grouper, a teleost, has 16 and 6.4 S immunoglobulins, both in substantial concentrations. The L chains of the two proteins show antigenic identity but the H chain of the 16 S protein has all the antigenic determinants of the H chain of the 6.4 S molecule and additional determinants as well. The molecular weight of the H chain of the 6.4 S immunoglobulin was found to be only 40,000 whereas that of the H chain of the 16 S protein is 70,000. In addition the carbohydrate content of the H chain of the 6.4 S molecule is substantially lower. These observations, together with peptide maps, indicate that the smaller H chain is only a segment of the larger chain, and probably comprises only three domains (59). It is uncertain whether the difference in size results during biosynthesis or as a consequence of subsequent enzymatic cleavage. The occurrence of H chains of unusually low molecular weight in the more slowly sedimenting (6 S) immunoglobulin, has also been noted in certain higher species, such as the turtle and duck. In the latter two species, however, these molecules appear to belong to a separate class, which may possibly be related to mammalian IgG.

Thus, the limited data at hand suggest that the H chains of IgM in various species of Actinopterygii have from three to five domains (see Table 7.4).

TABLE 7.4

PROBABLE NUMBER OF DOMAINS OF IMMUNOGLOBULIN
HEAVY CHAINS OF SEVERAL SPECIES[a]

	High mol. wt. IgM	Low mol. wt. IgM	Low mol. wt. non-IgM	References
Paddlefish	4 or 5	—	—	55
Giant grouper	5	3[b]	—	59
Australian lungfish	5	—	3	64, 66
Turtle, duck	5	—	3 and 5[c]	{ For references see Sections V and VI

[a] It is assumed that one V_H domain is always present although there are little direct data bearing on this point for the lower species. Light chains invariably have a molecular weight of about 22,000 to 23,000.

[b] The IgM of low molecular weight in this species is antigenically deficient to that of high molecular weight.

[c] The H chain (non-IgM) of the turtle and duck that is believed to have three domains is antigenically deficient as compared to the H chain with five domains, i.e., it shares some but not all determinants. The non-IgM immunoglobulin of low mol. wt. in the chicken probably has five domains.

G. Immunoglobulins of the Carp, Goldfish, and Gar

As indicated above, each of these teleost fishes possesses a tetrameric, 14 S IgM. There is some question, however, as to whether they can synthesize monomeric (4-chain, 7 S) antibodies. As is true of the grouper, the serum of the carp or goldfish contains antigenically cross-reactive material of low molecular weight. Antibody activity was not found, however, in a low molecular weight fraction upon immunization with protein antigens or, in the case of goldfish, with protein–hapten conjugates, although such activity was readily demonstrated in the fraction of high molecular weight (21,61). The response of the gar to protein antigens, red blood cells, and bacteria consisted exclusively of 14 S IgM (62,63). Differing results were obtained with another teleost, the grouper; anti-Dnp antibodies were readily detected in a 6.4 S fraction by the precipitin reaction (59). One should recall in this context that prolonged immunization of sharks may be required before 7 S antibodies appear; differences among teleosts might be attributable in part to differences in rapidity of response.

H. The Lungfish; Emergence of an Antigenically Distinct Immunoglobulin of Low Molecular Weight

The lungfish is the only surviving member of the Sarcopterygii, which are on the direct line of ascent to mammals; the lungfish itself, however, is not a direct ancestral form. (The coelacanth, which is the only extant species of the order Crossopterygii, is considered to be a direct ancestor of mammals.) Lungfish require air, can survive for months in a nonaqueous environment, and have a number of the physiological characteristics of amphibia.

Because of the rarity of the species, immunoglobulins of coelacanths have not been studied. Investigations have been carried out, however, with African and Australian lungfish. These are the most primitive species that have clearly been shown to possess two antigenically distinct classes of immunoglobulin of different molecular weight; both classes display antibody activity. (All vertebrates investigated that are higher than fish on the evolutionary scale, with the possible exception of the most primitive amphibia, similarly have at least two antigenically distinct immunoglobulin classes, including one of high and one of low molecular weight.)

In both the Australian and African lungfish, the larger molecule has a sedimentation coefficient of about 19 S and is probably a pentamer of a 4-chain subunit, which comprises two H and two L chains (64,66); it

thus has the characteristics of IgM. In contrast to sharks and other primitive fish, the lungfish does not have a readily detectable 7 S immunoglobulin that is antigenically identical to the 19 S molecule. It does,
however, possess a 5.8 S immunoglobulin having unique antigenic determinants and comprising two H and two L chains. In both the Australian
and African lungfish the molecular weight of the H chain of the immunoglobulin of smaller size is only 38,000, which suggests that it may
have only three domains (Table 7.4). The H chain of the 19 S molecule
has a molecular weight of 70,000, a value typical of IgM and consistent
with the presence of five domains. In the African lungfish, the N-terminal residue of the H chain of the 5.8 S molecule is blocked and presumably is pyrrolidonecarboxylic acid. About 70% of the L chains are
similarly blocked. Automatic sequence analysis was carried out on the
unblocked 30% of the L chain population and the first 9 residues were
determined (65; Table 7.2). Obvious homology with L chains of various
species was observed; however, the data do not yet permit the designation of lungfish L chains as κ or λ. In order to demonstrate homologies
with other species it is necessary to assume a deletion of two residues
near the N-terminus of lungfish L chains (Table 7.2). Whether the immunoglobulin of low molecular weight in the lungfish is a predecessor of
mammalian IgG is unknown.

IV. IMMUNOGLOBULINS OF AMPHIBIA

A. Anurans

Two orders of amphibia have been studied: the Anura (frogs, toads)
and Urodela or Caudata (tailed amphibia, including salamanders and
newts). The urodeles are the more primitive of the two orders.

The antibodies of the bullfrog, *Rana catesbiana,* occur as molecules
of high (18 S) and low (7 S) molecular weight, which, as in the lungfish,
represent two separate classes. The larger molecules are readily broken
down into 7 S subunits upon reduction (23,67), but this product is antigenically distinguishable from the induced 7 S antibodies (23,68). Marchalonis and Edelman (23) inoculated bullfrogs once with bacteriophage
f2 and assayed for antibody by phage neutralization. The earliest serum
antibodies (15 days) were found exclusively in an 18 S fraction. After 35
days both 6.7 S and 18 S antibodies were present, and after 58 days the
6.7 S form predominated, although the 18 S antibody concentration had
not diminished. The H chains of the two classes of antibody share some
antigenic specificities but each possesses unique determinants as well

(23,68). Equimolar amounts of H and L chains were isolated from either class of immunoglobulin. The H chains of the 18 S and 6.7 S fractions have molecular weights of 72,000 and 53,000, values corresponding to the presence of five and four domains, respectively. The data on molecular size and antigenic differences suggest but do not prove that the two classes may be homologous to human IgM and IgG. Measurements of carbohydrate content provided some supporting evidence; the concentrations were found to be 10.8 and 2.1% for the 18 S and 6.7 S immunoglobulins, respectively. In addition, the electrophoretic mobilities in starch gel of the H chains of the 18 S and 6.7 S classes correspond fairly well to those of human μ and γ chains, although the H chains of the 6.7 S protein have a somewhat lower mobility toward the anode than human γ chain (23). Data on amino acid composition provide further suggestive evidence for the same homologies but are not in themselves convincing because of the rather small differences between the two classes. It is noteworthy, however, that the overall amino acid compositions of bullfrog and human immunoglobulins are quite similar. On the basis of their data, Marchalonis and Edelman tentatively designated the two classes of bullfrog as IgM and IgG. A knowledge of amino acid sequences in the constant region of the H chain will be necessary to support the validity of this conclusion, particularly with respect to IgG. If the differences in sequence between human and bullfrog H chains prove to be great, a decision may require sequence data on intermediate species as well. Investigations on other anurans have substantiated the generality of the observation that there are two distinct immunoglobulin classes, differing in size (69–71). This applies as well to the clawed toad, a primitive representative of the order.

The intensity of the immune response in amphibia is comparable to that of mammals, and in general greater than that of fish, in terms of rapidity of the response, strength of the secondary response, and the ultimate antibody titer. Most, but not all, antigens give rise to both 7 S and 19 S antibodies (71). Plasma cells synthesizing immunoglobulins in the marine toad (*Bufo marinus*) are morphologically very similar to the plasma cells of higher species, by the criteria of light and electron microscopy (72).

The immune response of the marine toad (*Bufo marinus*) was found to be temperature-dependent (73). Upon challenge with flagellin of *Salmonella adelaide*, antibody-forming cells and humoral antibodies appeared much more promptly at 37° than at 22°C. At the higher temperature, antibody-producing cells first appeared at 3 days, and the number peaked at 7 days; at 22°, the corresponding values were 7 and 14 days, respectively. A similar delay in the appearance of humoral antibodies was seen at the lower temperature. The antibody titers ultimately attained were, however, about the same.

Serum fractions containing either the high or the low molecular weight antibodies of the bullfrog are capable of fixing guinea pig complement in the presence of antigen (74). Interestingly, frog antisera fixed guinea pig complement at least as effectively as they fixed frog complement.

The amphibia are of interest also because their development includes a free-living larval stage, the tadpole. Marchalonis demonstrated the presence in the tadpole of IgM, which appears 18 days after hatching and which is antigenically similar to that of the adult frog, *Rana pipiens* (75). Geczy *et al.* were able to identify, in addition, small amounts of immunoglobulins of low molecular weight that had the antigenic characteristics of the smaller immunoglobulin molecules of the adult frog. Immunoglobulins of low molecular weight were found in three different species of ranid tadpoles and frogs. The corresponding classes of immunoglobulin in the tadpole and frog are evidently identical with respect to antigenic characteristics and subunit structure. The two major immunoglobulin classes thus appear before metamorphosis (68,76).

B. Urodeles

The urodeles, an order of tail-bearing amphibia which includes salamanders and newts, are believed to be more primitive than the anurans (frogs and toads). Marchalonis and Cohen (77) isolated a fraction containing immunoglobulin by zone electrophoresis and gel filtration from the serum of a salamander, *Necturus maculosis*. A molecule with the properties of IgM was identified (mol. wt. 900,000; H and L chains, 70,000 and 22,000, respectively). The protein was related antigenically to IgM of the toad. Of primary interest was the absence of detectable immunoglobulin of low molecular weight. This was in accord with an earlier investigation of the immune response in urodeles (78). By contrast, Ching and Wedgewood (79) reported that *Siredon mexicanum,* a urodele, can synthesize antibodies of low as well as high molecular weight against bacteriophage ϕX174. However, quantitative data were not presented, and antigenic analyses to determine whether different classes exist were not carried out.

Possible interpretations of the existing data are: (a) an immunoglobulin class of low molecular weight arose subsequent to the appearance of the earliest amphibians and is the precursor of the IgG of higher animals; (b) an immunoglobulin of low molecular weight arose independently in different classes of vertebrate. One can only speculate as to why a class of low molecular weight is present in lungfish but (probably) not in urodeles.

V. IMMUNOGLOBULINS OF REPTILES

Turtles possess two antigenically distinguishable immunoglobulin classes (18 and 7.5 S) and a third class (5.7 S) which is antigenically deficient with respect to the 7.5 S class and may lack a portion of the Fc region (80–84) (Table 7.4). The 18 S molecule, which resembles mammalian IgM, has the characteristic pentameric structure, as evidenced by electron microscopy, a molecular weight of about 900,000, and a total carbohydrate content of 5 to 7% (82); the latter value is relatively low for IgM. The mannose : galactose ratio is considerably lower than that in mammalian IgM. The H chain of the 17 S protein has the typical molecular weight of 70,000 (82–84).

The 7.5 S and the antigenically related 5.7 S protein are sometimes referred to as IgG although the relationship to mammalian IgG is inferred and tenuous. The molecular weights of the two classes are 180,000 and 120,000, respectively; this difference is reflected in the molecular weights of their H chains (67,000 and 35,000). The larger H chain has all the antigenic determinants of the smaller, and additional determinants as well (84). It thus appears that the H chain of the 7.5 S molecule may have two domains in addition to those present in the H chain of the 5.7 S protein. The 7.5 S molecule is also richer in carbohydrate. Both the 5.7 S and 7.5 S classes are present in substantial concentration in the serum of the adult turtle (84). It has not been determined whether the smaller protein is a product of enzymatic degradation of the larger; however, in ducks, which have a similar pair of immunoglobulin molecules, this has been shown not to be the case (Section VI,B). In general, during an immune response antibodies of low molecular weight appear later than those of high molecular weight.

In response to the antigen, Dnp-bovine IgG, antihapten antibodies of all three classes appeared in the serum of a turtle 6 weeks after immunization. Only the 5.7 S class was found in an extract of the yolk of turtle eggs, which suggests that this class may have a selective advantage in its ability to pass through certain membranes (84).

Snapping turtles respond to immunization with *Brucella abortus* or human erythrocytes with the production of agglutinating antibodies of high and low molecular weight. Both classes of immunoglobulin are capable of interaction with frog complement (81). In common with many other species, the earliest antibodies produced during immunization of turtles appear to be of the 19 S form; antibodies of lower molecular weight frequently appear later (80).

The presence of yet another class of turtle immunoglobulin, intermediate in size between 7 S and 19 S, is suggested by the investigation of Coe, who employed density gradient centrifugation for separating immunoglobulins of different sizes (85).

Alligators and tuataras, which are primitive reptiles, possess antigenically distinct immunoglobulin classes of high and low molecular weight (18 S and 7 S) (86,87). The 5.8 S class has not been identified.

VI. IMMUNOGLOBULINS OF BIRDS; APPEARANCE OF IgA

In common with the lungfish, certain amphibia, and all higher classes, avian species possess a class of immunoglobulin with the properties of IgM, plus an antigenically distinct class of smaller size.[2] Two varieties of immunoglobulin of low molecular weight are present in ducks. In addition, birds synthesize an immunoglobulin that appears homologous to mammalian IgA.

The most extensive studies on avian immunoglobulins have been carried out with the domestic chicken. Physicochemical investigations have been hampered by the tendency of both the high and low molecular weight forms of chicken immunoglobulins to aggregate in neutral buffers. In dissociating solvents, the sedimentation coefficients of the serum immunoglobulins are 7 S and 17 S and the molecular weights of their H chains are 67,000 and 71,000, respectively (88). As shown by antigenic analysis, the 7 S and 17 S forms represent distinct classes, having unique antigenic determinants on their H chains. Both classes possess equimolar amounts of L and H chains (88). The 17 S molecule has a hexose content of approximately 3%, a value considerably smaller than that of mammalian IgM. The hexose content of the 7 S molecule is 2.2%, which is comparable to that of mammalian IgG. The molecular weight of the 17 S protein is 890,000 (88); that of the 7 S molecule has been variously reported as 165,000–206,000, with most values (for chicken, quail, and pheasant) in the vicinity of 170,000 (reviewed in reference 89). This would be consistent with a molecular weight for the H chain of about

[2] We should reiterate that the term "antigenically distinct" does not imply that no antigenic determinants are shared. Within a species the various classes of immunoglobulin share determinants present in L chains, and cross-reactivity attributable to shared V_H regions has been observed.

62,000, as compared to the experimental value of 67,000 mentioned above.

The molecular weight of the H chain of the avian 7 S immunoglobulin is thus higher than that of mammalian IgG and is consistent with the possible presence of a fifth domain. (As already indicated, the 7 S protein is not a simple monomer of IgM.) Because of these considerations, Leslie and Clem are reluctant to use the term IgG to refer to the 7 S class and prefer to designate it as IgY. Other investigators have, however, called the 7 S molecule IgG and we will use this designation for convenience. As noted earlier, Mehta *et al.* failed to observe immunological cross-reactions between the Fc segments of human IgG and the chicken 7 S protein (18); this, of course, does not prove that the two proteins are not homologous. Chicken IgM, on the other hand, does share antigenic determinants with human IgM (18).

The rate of biosynthesis of immunoglobulins in chickens, per unit body weight, is comparable to that observed in man. The half-lives of chicken IgM and IgG are 1.7 and 4.1 days, respectively, values one-third and one-fifth of those of the corresponding human proteins (90,91).

It has long been known that chicken antibodies to many antigens require a high salt concentration in order to form specific precipitates. A physicochemical basis for this property is suggested by the finding that chicken IgG, but not rabbit IgG, aggregates in the presence of 1.5 M NaCl and sediments with a velocity of 14 S, as compared to 7 S in 0.15 M NaCl (92). There are at least two mechanisms whereby aggregation might enhance the precipitability of the antibody molecule. The aggregation of IgG caused by the higher salt concentration suggests that there may be electrostatic repulsion among the immunoglobulin molecules, which is overcome by high salt concentration; the same factor may operate in the case of soluble antigen–antibody complexes, enhancing their growth to a size sufficient for precipitation. Second, aggregated antibody is effectively multivalent; attachment to a single antigen through more than one combining site corresponds to a higher effective energy of interaction even though, as shown by Voss and Eisen, the energy of interaction of a single site with hapten is not affected by increased salt concentration (93). The aggregation of chicken IgG at high salt concentration involves interactions in the Fc portion of the molecule (94).

A. Avian IgA

Evidence for the presence of an avian immunoglobulin corresponding to mammalian IgA was first reported by Lebacq-Verheyden *et al.* (95), and by Orlans and Rose (96). In one investigation (95) rabbit antibodies were prepared against intestinal secretions of the chicken and against purified serum IgM and IgG (95). After absorbing the antiserum to intestinal secretions with IgM and IgG, a precipitating antibody remained which reacted with a component of the secretions that migrates in the gamma region. The reactive antigen, which also possessed antigenic determinants of L chains, was found in serum, but at a far lower concentration. The observations that the component is antigenically distinct from IgM and IgG and is present in much higher concentration in secretions than in serum, suggest its correspondence with mammalian IgA (95,96). Further evidence that this chicken protein indeed corresponds to mammalian IgA was obtained by Bienenstock et al., who showed that the putative serum IgA is capable of combining with human secretory component (97). Chicken IgG was incapable of binding the component and only a very weak interaction was observed with chicken IgM. The evidence is thus convincing that a class corresponding to mammalian IgA is present in chickens.

The sedimentation coefficient of different preparations of chicken sIgA, isolated from secretions, varied from 11 S to 16 S (98). IgA has also been identified by Leslie and Martin (99) in chicken serum, where it is present at low concentration. The serum protein, which reacts with antiserum to chicken sIgA, exists mainly in a polymeric form but is transformed into the "monomer" (mol. wt. 175,000) upon mild reduction. The molecular weight of the chicken α chain is about 70,000. IgA from chicken bile contains an additional antigenic determinant, as compared to serum IgA, which might be present on secretory component or J chain (99).

B. Duck Immunoglobulins

The duck differs from the chicken in possessing two major serum immunoglobulins of low molecular weight, in addition to an antigenically distinct, typical IgM (100) (Table 7.4). The smaller molecules have sedimentation coefficients of 5.7 S and 7.8 S; the former is antigenically deficient with respect to the latter. Because the 5.7 S molecule does not possess unique determinants, its assignment as a separate class is questionable. However, experiments in which radiolabeled 7.8 S protein was injected into ducks failed to reveal breakdown in vivo to the 5.7 S form (101), suggesting that the smaller molecule is not simply derived from the larger by enzymatic fragmentation. When the 5.7 S molecule is reduced at neutral pH it dissociates into half-molecules (3.5 S). Thus the half-molecules appear to be linked only by one or more disulfide bonds and not by noncovalent interactions. In this respect they closely resemble the 5 S fragments derived from rabbit or human IgG by peptic digestion; pepsin removes the Fc fragment, in which the H chains are joined through noncovalent interactions, and thus permits dissociation after reduction of interheavy chain disulfide bonds.

This and other observations indicate that the 5.7 S protein lacks a large portion of the Fc region of the 7.8 S molecule. It has a very low carbohydrate content (0.6%) as compared to 5.0% for the 7.8 S molecule. The molecular weights of the H chains of the 5.7 S and 7.8 S proteins are 35,000 and 62,000, respectively (102). Antibody specific for the H chain of chicken IgG cross-reacts strongly with duck 7.8 S immunoglobulin but hardly at all with duck 5.7 S protein; this is consistent with the possibility that the cross-reactions involve Fc determinants. Finally, the 7.8 S, but not the 5.7 S molecule, is able to fix duck complement (100,101).

On the basis of their molecular weights it was postulated that the H chain of the 7.8 S molecule comprises five domains (1 V_H + 4 C_H), whereas the H chain of the 5.7 S molecule consists of only three domains (102).

Grey observed that each of three varieties of duck possesses a low molecular weight immunoglobulin in addition to IgM. After prolonged immunization a large proportion of the low molecular weight antibody, in two of the three varieties, was of the 5.7 S form (100).

VII. CARBOHYDRATE CONTENT OF IMMUNOGLOBULINS FROM VARIOUS SPECIES ON THE PHYLOGENETIC SCALE

Acton *et al.* carried out extensive studies of carbohydrate (CHO) content and composition in the H and L chains of immunoglobulins from a variety of species. These ranged from the shark to the human and included representatives of each of the five major classes of vertebrate (103). Immunoglobulins of both high and low molecular weight were investigated.

Mannose, galactose, glucosamine, and sialic acid were found in the immunoglobulins of all species studied. At least small amounts of fucose were present in each of the immunoglobulins, except for duck IgM and the catfish immunoglobulin of low molecular weight. In all species the bulk of the CHO was present in the H chains, with L chains in many species containing only fractional amounts (expressed as mole per mole of L chain) of each type of carbohydrate residue. The authors point out that some of the carbohydrate present in L chains isolated from immunoglobulin of high molecular weight might have been due to contamination by J chains, which are relatively rich in carbohydrate (7–8%).

In the H chains of many species, fucose and sialic acid were found in amounts less than one residue per molecule, but the sum of the two approached unity; the authors suggested that fucose and sialic acid may substitute for one another in the synthesis of the CHO; an alternative explanation would simply invoke microheterogeneity.

A striking feature of the data is that the mannose to galactose ratio was greater than one (~ 3–5) in mammals and birds but is about one or less in lower species, thus indicating an evolutionary trend with respect to CHO composition. The CHO contents of the immunoglobulins of high and low molecular weight were similar in fish and also in birds; as indicated elsewhere, mammalian and amphibian IgM has a higher CHO content than does IgG (or the non-IgM of low molecular weight in amphibia).

VIII. PHYLOGENY OF IgA, IgE, IgG SUBCLASSES, LIGHT CHAIN TYPES, AND THE V_{HIII} SUBGROUP

A. Evolution of IgA

Characteristics of an immunoglobulin which contribute toward its designation as IgA are the following (not all criteria need be fulfilled): Immunological cross-reactivity with mammalian human IgA; existence in a polymeric form (4-chain monomers may also be present); a relatively high concentration in secretory fluids as compared to serum;[3] an association with plasma cells in mucosal areas; the presence in the polymeric, but not the monomeric molecule of secretory component and J chains. Data on comparative amino sequences, when they become available, should represent the most definitive criterion for identification of a protein as IgA, particularly if there should prove to be large differences among the C_H regions of IgA and other immunoglobulin classes. (This seems quite possible since there is only about 30% homology between human C_γ and C_μ chains.)

Immunological cross-reactivity with human IgA was demonstrated initially for the serum and secretory immunoglobulins of the dog, cat, horse, cow, sheep, pig, goat, hedgehog, rabbit, and mouse, as well as of primates. The use of chicken rather than mammalian antiserum proved particularly valuable for demonstrating cross-reactions (105). No cross-

---

[3] In many mammalian species, with the man and mouse as notable exceptions, IgA is found almost exclusively in secretory fluids, and at much lower concentration in serum.

reactivity was demonstrated between human IgA and secretory proteins of the hamster or, a nonmammalian species, the chicken (104,105).

A more extensive investigation of immunological cross-reactivity of mammalian IgA's was subsequently reported by Neoh *et al.* (105a), who utilized in their tests sheep, goat, rabbit, and chicken antisera specific for human IgA. A protein cross-reacting with human IgA was identified in the plasma of nearly all of the more than 90 mammalian species tested. The chicken antiserum was especially useful for demonstrating reactivity of nonprimate IgA. Among the relatively few species whose sera failed to react with anti-IgA were several artiodactyls (big horned sheep, antelope, etc.). In view of the diversity of mammalian species in which IgA has been identified it seems reasonable to extrapolate to the conclusion that it may be present in all mammals (104).

We have discussed evidence for the presence of an IgA-like molecule in chickens. In brief, the chicken protein has antigenic determinants not shared by IgG or IgM, is found in relatively high concentration in secretory fluids, and is selectively synthesized by plasma cells in the lamina propria of the gut. In addition, this protein, alone among chicken immunoglobulins, is capable of binding human secretory piece (97).

So far IgA-like proteins have not been reported in species lower than birds, and they could not be detected in mucus secretions of catfish (106) or of plaice (107), another teleost fish. Since IgA is very frequently present in very low concentration in serum, many investigations of lower species have probably not been relevant to its detection, and it would seem premature to rule out its occurrence.

B. Structural Evidence Suggesting that IgA Evolved from IgM Subsequent to the Appearance of IgG

On the basis of limited but informative amino acid sequence analysis, Chuang *et al.* have proposed that IgA is more closely related to IgM than to IgG and have speculated as to the approximate time of its divergence from IgM during evolution (108). They determined the amino acid sequence of the C-terminal 40 residues of a human α chain and compared it with the known C-terminal sequences of human μ and γ_1 chains. Their data are shown in Table 7.5. The most striking observation is the presence of an additional 19 residues in both μ and α chains that extend beyond the C-terminus of the γ_1 chain. The degree of homology between α and μ in the 40-residue sequence is 55% and, of the 18 positions at which α and μ differ, 14 can be explained by a single base change in a codon. In comparison, the overall homology between

TABLE 7.5

Comparison of C-Terminal Amino Acid Sequences of Human Heavy Chains[a]

Sequence	426	430	440	450
IgA1	Met	*Val* Gly *His Glu Ala* Leu *Pro* Leu *Ala* Phe *Thr Gln Lys Thr* Ile *Asp* Arg *Leu Ala Gly Lys Pro Thr* His *Val Asx Val Ser*		
IgM	Val	*Val Val Ala His Glu Ala* Leu *Pro* Asn *Arg* Val *Thr Gln* Arg *Thr* Val *Asp Lys Ser Thr Gly Lys Pro Thr* Leu Tyr *Asx Val Ser*		
IgG1	Ser	*Val* Met *His Glu Ala* Leu *His* Asn *His* Tyr *Thr Gln Lys* Ser *Leu* Ser *Leu Ser* Pro *Gly*		

Sequence	455	460
IgA1	Val Glu *Met* Ala Glu Val Asp *Gly Thr Cys Tyr*	
IgM	Leu Val *Met* Ser Asp Thr Ala *Gly Thr Cys Tyr*	

[a] The data on IgA are from Chuang *et al.* (108). The numbering system is based on that of the H chain of the IgG1 protein Eu (109).

human μ and γ chains is about 32%, although it is somewhat higher near the C-terminus.

Chuang *et al.* propose that the α chain (as well as the γ chain) evolved from the μ chain, but that the α chain arose more recently. On the basis of the approximate rates of evolution of other immunoglobulin polypeptide chains they estimated that the α chain appeared about 200×10^6 years ago. This would be consistent with its presence in birds and animals and its (presumed) absence in reptiles, amphibia, and fish. The interesting question remains as to how both the α and γ chains independently lost one of the four C_H domains present in the human μ chain.

C. Evolution of IgE

The IgE class is generally defined on the basis of the properties of the human protein. (For reviews see references 110, 111, and 111a.) For the purpose of discussing its evolution we will briefly mention some of its principal properties. (See Chapter 3 for a more detailed discussion.) IgE is the primary human homocytotropic antibody, i.e., antibody capable of persisting in human tissue and mediating reactions of immediate hypersensitivity. The cell targets in the human are mast cells and basophilic leukocytes. IgE is able to fix to cutaneous tissue and various membranes and to mediate reactions of immediate hypersensitivity by initiating the release of the humoral factors, histamine, and SRS-A (slow-reacting substance). It has the typical 4-chain structure and is bivalent, but its H chain, with a molecular weight of 75,000 to 80,000, is larger than that of other human immunoglobulins. The reaginic activity of the molecule is labile at 56°C and is sensitive to reducing agents under conditions which cleave interchain disulfide bonds. The migration of IgE during electrophoresis is, on the average, anodal to that of IgG. IgE antibodies can persist for long periods of time after exposure to antigen and are pharmacologically active at minute concentrations. Radiolabeled IgE, injected into skin sites, can still be detected after many weeks. Its adherence to cells is mediated through the Fc fragment, which must be essentially intact. IgE does not fix human complement by the normal pathway, but an aggregated IgE myeloma protein is capable of fixing complement through the alternate pathway which involves an initial interaction with C3 proactivator (112). Antisera to human IgE have been prepared in large quantities by using IgE myeloma proteins as the antigens.

In general, the most convincing criteria for identification of the immunoglobulin of a nonhuman species as IgE are its skin-sensitizing properties, particularly in relation to optimal latent period (2–3 days), duration of sensitization (2–3 weeks), lability at 56°C, and neutralizability by antiserum to L chains but not by antiserum to other known H chain classes of that species (113). Homocytotropic antibodies with the general characteristics of IgE have been found in many mammalian species and may be present in all mammals. Antigenic cross-reactivity with human IgE was reported initially for monkey (114), dog (115), and rat (116) homocytotropic antibodies. An extensive study was subsequently carried out by Neoh *et al.* (105a), who utilized anti-IgE prepared against human myeloma proteins in a sheep and in several chickens. Cross-reacting protein was identified in the sera of nearly all primates but only in a few other mammalian species of the many investigated.

The presence of an evolutionary precursor of IgE has not been demonstrated. Homocytotropic antibodies have, however, been identified in lower species. For example, a pigeon hyperimmune to BSA responded to intracutaneous injection of the antigen with an immediate hypersensitivity reaction characterized by increased capillary permeability to a dye (117). Responsiveness was passively transferred to a nonimmune pigeon, and the responsible serum factor was heat labile. The minimal latent period after passive transfer varied among pigeons from 24 to 72 hours; reactions could be detected as much as 14 days later (117).

On the basis of homocytotropic activity alone, one cannot designate a molecule as IgE, particularly since certain mammalian species produce homocytotropic antibodies of another class as well as IgE. In the guinea pig and mouse, such activity is found in the IgGl subclass and it is a property of IgGa in the rat (113).[4] These homocytotropic antibodies are distinguishable from IgE, which is also present, by the greater resistance of their reaginic activity to heat and to reducing agents, by a shorter latent period required for cellular sensitization (hours instead of days), and by their more rapid disappearance from tissues after sensitization.

With this information in mind we can reconsider the classification of the pigeon immunoglobulin. On the basis of its heat lability, latent period, and persistence it appears to be more closely related to IgE than to the other homocytotropic classes of mammalian immunoglobulin. A definite assignment, however, will probably require structural studies.

Homocytotropic antibodies have also been observed in the duck, where it was found in a 7.8 S fraction (111). There is, at present, insufficient evidence to establish a direct relationship to mammalian IgE.

---

[4] The original sources are cited in reference 113.

D. Evolution of L Chains

It is sometimes suggested that during evolution L chains appeared before H chains, but the evidence for this conjecture is not very strong. It is based to a large extent on the fact that the L chain is smaller than the H chain; since the L chain contains only a single constant region domain, it is conceivable that genes controlling C_H regions arose by duplication and subsequent mutation of a C_L gene. Data on amino acid sequences are in accord with this possibility, since there is considerable structural homology between the C region of an L chain and that of an H chain of the same species. The degree of homology is greater, for example, than the very limited homology that exists between the V and C regions of a typical polypeptide chain (either H or L). This suggests that if all immunoglobulin genes are derived from a common ancestor the divergence of C from V genes occurred prior to the divergence of C_H and C_L genes.

Kappa and Lambda Chains

The extent of sequence homology between human κ and λ chains (about 39%; Chapter 4) is sufficient to suggest strongly a common evolutionary origin. Both types comprise two domains, with correspondingly located disulfide loops. The amount of sequence homology in C regions between human κ and mouse κ chains ($\sim 60\%$) exceeds that which exists between human κ and human λ (39%) or mouse κ and mouse λ chains (35%) (Table 4.1); this indicates that the two types of L chain have evolved independently. Such interspecies resemblances also make it possible to identify the L chains of many species as κ or λ and should eventually yield a precise outline of the evolution of the two types of chain.

A significant point of distinction is that in many mammalian species most λ, but few κ chains, are blocked at the N-terminus, i.e., have a terminal residue of pyrrolidonecarboxylic acid.[5] Also, human and mouse κ chains are distinguishable from λ by the presence of a half-cystine residue at the C-terminal position of κ chains; in λ chains the terminal sequence is -Cys-Ser. In each case, the cysteine residue forms a disulfide bond with the H chain. This feature cannot be generalized to all species since L chains of the chicken, which are of the λ type according to sequence analysis (118), have a terminal half-cystine group (and an unblocked amino terminus) (118,119). Interestingly, the L chains of the

---

[5] About 20% of human λ chains belong to the $V_{\lambda III}$ and $V_{\lambda V}$ subgroups, which have unblocked N-terminal residues (in the few examples that have been characterized).

TABLE 7.6

COMPARISON OF C-TERMINAL AMINO ACID SEQUENCES OF L CHAINS[a]

Species	Kappa type	Lambda type
Human	—Gly Glu Cys	—Thr Glu Cys Ser
Rabbit	—Gly Asp Cys	—Thr Glu Cys Ser
Mouse	—Asn Glu Cys[b]	—Ala Asp Cys Ser[c]
Pig	—Asx Glx Cys Glx Ala	—Ser Glu Cys Ser
Guinea pig	—Ser Glu Cys	—Ser Glu Cys Ser
Rat	—Asn Glu Cys	—
Chicken	—	—Ser Glu Cys[d]
Turkey	—	—Ser Glu Cys Ser[d]
Dog	—	—Ala Glu Cys Ser
Horse	—	—Ser Glu Cys Pro

[a] Except where indicated, data are from Hood *et al.* (120).
[b] Gray *et al.* (121).
[c] Appella (122).
[d] Grant *et al.* (118).

turkey, which are also λ and closely resemble those of the chicken in amino acid sequence, have -Cys-Ser as the terminal peptide. C-terminal sequences of the L chains of several species are shown in Table 7.6.

Lambda chains are also distinguishable by deletions or insertions (as compared with κ chains) occurring at characteristic positions in the amino acid sequence (Chapter 4). These represent a striking structural feature because many of the same deletions and insertions have been seen in all λ chains studied, including those of the chicken as well as several mammalian species (118). Thus, deletions or insertions, once established, may be almost irreversible evolutionary events, probably because they cause important structural alterations. Their presence provides a strong basis for characterizing a polypeptide chain of a species under investigation as κ or λ.

Another highly conserved structural feature of λ chains is the sequence between residues 104–111 (123), which is very similar or identical in various mammalian species and in chickens. Hood refers to this sequence as a "switch peptide" since it occurs at the end of the V_λ region.

The precise point of divergence of κ and λ chains on the evolutionary scale is difficult to pinpoint with the available data. Although sharks appear to have κ chains (See Section III,C,3), it is uncertain whether the blocked L chains which occur in sharks, and other fish as well, might more closely resemble λ chains. In alligators, two antigenically distinct classes of L chain have been demonstrated, but these

TABLE 7.7

DISTRIBUTION OF LIGHT CHAIN TYPES AMONG VARIOUS SPECIES[a]

Order	Common species	Percentage light chain distribution	
		Kappa	Lambda
Lagomorpha	Rabbit	70–90	10–30
Rodentia	Mouse	95	5
	Rat	>95	<5
	Guinea pig	70	30
Primates	Human	70	30
	Rhesus	50	50
	Baboon	50	50
Cetacea	Whale	10	90
Carnivora	Dog	10	90
	Cat	10	90
	Mink	<5	>95
Artiodactyla	Pig	50	50
	Cow	<5	>95
	Goat	<5	>95
	Sheep	<5	>95
Perissodactyla	Horse	<5	>95
	Mule	<5	>95
Avian	Chicken	<5	>95
	Turkey	<5	>95

[a] From Grant *et al.* (118) and Hood *et al.* (123).

have not been identified as κ and λ (86). It is clear, however, that birds possess λ chains; and since κ chains are present in sharks, the divergence of the two types must have occurred at least 250×10^6 years ago (118).

The distribution of κ and λ types among different species is highly variable, with some species having a strong predominance of one type and others a mixture of the two. Table 7.7 presents data, compiled by Hood and co-workers, on κ–λ distribution in a number of species (118,123). It is noteworthy that in most primate species a single type predominates and that closely related species have a similar distribution of κ and λ chains.

E. Evolutionary Relationship of Mammalian IgG and IgM

In making these comparisons, we will confine our discussion to C regions of the polypeptide chains, inasmuch as the different H chain classes appear to share the same repertory of V_H region sequences. (This is a consequence of the contribution of two genes to the biosynthesis of a single polypeptide chain.)

The degree of sequence homology between mammalian IgG and IgM is rather small. With respect to sequences so far determined in human IgG1 and IgM, approximately 32% of the residues are identical when the necessary insertions and deletions are made for the purpose of the comparison (124). In addition to major differences in sequence, the two classes are distinguished by the presence of four, rather than three, C_H domains in human IgM, and by the high carbohydrate content and the presence of J chain in IgM. These important differences reflect the early divergence of IgG from IgM, which may have occurred with or prior to the appearance of the lungfish (Fig. 7.1). Actually, the small degree of homology between human C_μ and C_γ sequences is the strongest current evidence for their early divergence, since the existence of a homolog of mammalian IgG has not been established in a non-mammalian species.

One can contrast the low degree of similarity of the C_H regions of human γ and μ chains with the much greater homology ($\sim 65\%$) that exists between human and rabbit γ chains. This implies a linear and separate evolution of genes controlling the C_H regions of IgG and IgM, at least in mammals.

F. Evolution of Subclasses of Human IgG

The separation of human IgG into subclasses appears to be a relatively recent evolutionary event. Thus, the amino acid sequences of the C_H regions of IgG1 and IgG4 exhibit more than 90% homology (125). More limited sequence data on IgG2 and IgG3 suggest a similar degree of relatedness among all four subclasses (126). On the basis of the number of differences in the Fc sequence between IgG1 and IgG4, Pink et al. estimate that the IgG subclasses began to diverge about 20 to 30×10^6 years ago (125). This interesting calculation is based on the number of differences in sequence among the C regions of mouse, human, and rabbit immunoglobulin polypeptide chains; from these data Pink et al. compute a rate of mutation corresponding to 1 amino acid residue per 100 per 4 to 5×10^6 years (a mutation rate considerably higher than that of cytochrome c or of hemoglobin). This rate and the differences in amino acid sequences among the IgG subclasses were used to estimate the time at which they diverged. If the authors are correct, this did not occur much before the appearance of *Homo sapiens*.

The rough calculation of Pink *et al.* is supported by studies of Gm allotypic markers and subclass-specific antigenic determinants in the immunoglobulins of primates. The specific antigenic determinants of human IgG2 appear to be present in nearly all nonhuman primates (127); however, the determinants specific to human IgG1, IgG3, and IgG4 are found only in Old-World monkeys and apes. (See Fig. 7.4.) It is of considerable interest that H chains of IgG of Old-World monkeys contain a peptide which is intermediate with respect to its amino acid sequence between that of a short peptide sequence characterizing the Gm(a) and the Gm(non-a) determinants in human IgG (128).

Position in human γ_1 chain: 356 357 358 359 360
Gm(a) peptide: Asp Glu Leu Thr Lys
Old-World monkey peptide: <u>Glu</u> Glu Leu Thr Lys
Gm(non-a) peptide: <u>Glu</u> Glu <u>Met</u> Thr Lys

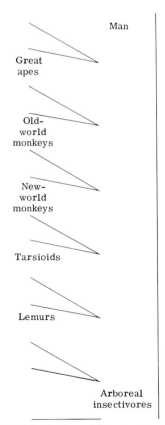

Fig. 7.4. A simplified family tree of the primates. From Romer (13).

Obviously, serological cross-reaction does not provide a positive means of identification; it is conceivable, for example, that an IgG1 counterpart might be present in earlier primates but not be detectable by the antisera employed. If, however, one accepts antigenic analysis at face value, it would indicate that IgG1, IgG3, and IgG4 appeared between the time of divergence of the New-World and the Old-World monkeys, about 10×10^6 years ago.

This conclusion is also consistent with studies of Gm allotypic markers characteristic of human IgG1, which are detectable, among other primates, only in the serum of the great apes (129). In addition, allotypic markers characteristic of human IgG3 are found in the great apes and Old-World monkeys but not in the New-World monkeys (130).

It is noteworthy that IgG2, which according to these antigenic analyses may have evolved before the other subclasses, is also the predominant IgG subclass present on the membranes of circulating human lymphocytes, despite its relatively low concentration in normal serum (131). IgG1 and IgG3 are also represented on cell surfaces but in lower concentrations.

G. Evolution of the V_{HIII} Subgroup

In humans, about 20% of H chains belong to the V_{HIII} subgroup, which is found in many but not all mammalian species. It is readily identified by analysis of an H chain pool in the automatic sequencer since, in general, only V_{HIII} proteins have an unblocked N-terminus (132–134). At this point the data on nonmammalian species are limited, but it appears that sequences homologous to mammalian V_{HIII} are present in avian H chains (101). The chicken has a substantial proportion of unblocked H chains. Of the first 20 residues of an unblocked chicken H chain, 14 were identical to those of a human V_{HIII} protein; this compares with 8, 11, and 10 positions of identity of the unblocked chicken H chain with examples of blocked human V_{HI}, V_{HII}, or V_{HIV} proteins, respectively (135).

Extensive studies of the N-terminal sequences of mammalian V_{HIII} proteins were reported by Capra *et al.* (132). All H chains that were unblocked at the N-terminus proved to be highly homologous to human V_{HIII} in sequence. The percentage of unblocked H chains in a normal pool ranged from zero (pig, cow, sheep, goat, mouse, horse, whale) to > 95% (opossum, dog, mink, cat, sea lion, seal). Other species studied have 19–29% unblocked H chains (man, monkey, rat, mouse, guinea pig). Closely related species generally have similar percentages of unblocked V_{HIII} chains. Except for hypervariable regions the sequence within a species tends to be remarkably homogeneous; at most such positions more than 95% of the V_{HIII} molecules in a normal pool have the same residue; this as well as the unblocked N-terminus greatly facilitates sequence analysis of the N-terminal region. There are also striking similarities among different mammalian species; the average degree of homology, when V_{HIII} is present, appears to exceed 80%, and it is even greater among closely related species. The presence of species-specific or (a term the authors prefer), phylogenetically associated residues, at certain positions is discussed by Capra *et al.* (132) and is of significance in relation to theories of the genetic control of antibody variability (Chapter 12).

A schematic outline of the evolution of various genes controlling immunoglobulins is shown in Fig. 7.5.

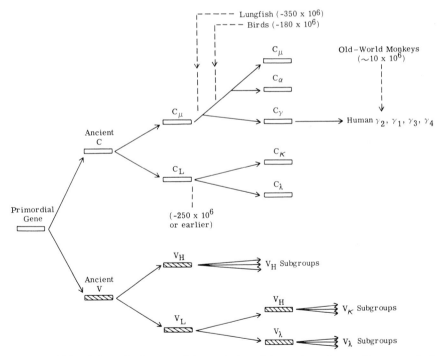

Fig. 7.5. Schematic diagram of the evolution of the various classes of genes controlling the immunoglobulins.

IX. SELECTIVE ADVANTAGES IN THE EVOLUTION OF IMMUNOGLOBULIN CLASSES

This discussion will necessarily be speculative since the primary basis for the evolution of a new class may be related to early environmental conditions that are unknown to us. Nevertheless, there are various teleological factors that can be considered. We will make the assumption that IgM was the primordial immunoglobulin and list selective advantages that appear to be associated with the evolution of other classes.

The question can be considered at two levels, one concerned with the antigen-binding properties of the molecules and the other with biological properties associated with the class-specific regions of the protein (C regions) and with parameters such as size and charge.

Since the various H chain classes share essentially the same V region sequences and the same repertory of L chains, they are not, in general, distinguishable on the basis of the types of antigenic determinants with which they can combine. However, overall size can enter into this question. The large IgM molecule may be capable of interacting with a partially buried antigenic determinant on a particulate surface and cross-linking it to a similar determinant on another particle. Also, a multiplicity of binding sites is associated with greater avidity in the interaction of an immunoglobulin with a multivalent antigen (38,39). Through such mechanisms, molecules of different classes with identical combining sites may have different immunologic potential.

Perhaps a more important basis for differences in biological activity is the amino acid sequence and (possibly) the carbohydrate content of the constant region of the polypeptide chain. These may control such diverse functions as complement fixation, passage through the placenta or yolk sac, opsonization, homocytotropic activity, and attachment to a variety of cellular membranes. For simplicity, we will discuss in this context only the human immunoglobulins.

A. IgG

A number of significant properties that are not common to IgM are associated with this class. Each of the subclasses of IgG can cross the human placenta, and thus afford protection to the fetus and to the newborn child prior to maturation of its own immune system. This property is associated with the Fc, or class-specific region of the molecule and is therefore related to the evolution of a unique amino acid sequence.

In contrast to IgM, IgG is capable of passing into extravascular fluids and secretions. This characteristic may well be a function of the smaller size of the molecule, rather than its chemical structure, since 7 S shark IgM, which is antigenically identical to the 19 S shark protein, is similarly distributed in both compartments, whereas the 19 S molecule is restricted to intravascular spaces. The extravascular presence of immunoglobulins probably represents an important defense mechanism.

Human macrophages possess receptor sites for IgG1 and IgG3, but apparently not for IgM (136). Molecules of these subclasses are therefore superior to IgM as opsonins.

Hyperimmunization of experimental animals is often associated with the appearance of high concentrations of IgG (but not IgM) of high affinity. This could represent a significant biological advantage.

Another important biological property, shared by all subclasses of human IgG and by IgA, but not IgM, is the capacity, in an aggregated form or as an antigen–antibody complex, to cause the degranulation of circulating neutrophils, liberating pharmacologically active amines and lysosomal enzymes which are responsible for the active inflammatory process (137).

B. IgA

The IgA class, which has been identified in birds and mammals, is distinguishable by its relatively high concentration in secretory fluids. It is not yet clear why other classes could not have served a similar function, although one might speculate that the interaction with secretory component confers some unique biological property. This could relate, for example, to the ability of IgA to cross epithelial membranes. The fact that secretory IgA is more resistant than monomeric IgA to proteolytic enzymes may also be of great significance, with respect to conferring stability in the presence of bacterial enzymes. Although IgA apparently can fix complement through the alternate pathway, beginning with C3, it cannot do so by the conventional route. This could be a biological advantage under certain circumstances, for example, in minimizing cytolytic effects on host cells during antigen–antibody reactions on tissue surfaces. The multivalence of IgA in its dimeric form may be biologically significant, since multivalent attachment to a single particulate antigen increases the avidity of an antibody molecule.

We will not attempt to discuss the various types of secretory fluids and the importance of antibodies in these fluids to host defense. The reader is referred to reviews on this subject (104,138–140).

C. IgE

This class, which has so far been shown to be present in mammals and possibly in birds, is associated with reactions of immediate hypersensitivity, which it mediates through its capacity to bind to mast cells and basophilic leukocytes; this response is often detrimental to the host. What biological advantages IgE may confer are somewhat conjectural. It has been suggested that the cytophilic property of IgE provides a mechanism for immobilizing antigens and permitting their phagocytosis. Also, the very rapid release of histamine and SRS-A that occurs when antigen encounters cell-bound IgE antibody on mucosal surfaces may be important in invoking immediate local inflammatory responses, which bring other immunoglobulins as well as cells into the area. IgE may be significant in host defense against parasitic invasion. Such infections are sometimes associated with chronic hyperemia of the bowel wall, which is believed to be caused by histamine and SRS-A; the hyperemia may be important in containing parasitic infections (113).

The fact that IgE is active in minute concentrations may in effect provide prolonged immunological memory to tissue sites; in this context it may also be relevant that the half-life of IgE injected into skin sites is 2–3 weeks, as compared to 2 to 3 days for injected IgG (113). (The half life of IgE in human serum is, however, only 2–3 days.)

REFERENCES

1. Bang, F.B. (1967). *Fed. Proc. Fed. Amer. Soc. Exp. Biol.* **26,** 1680.
2. Johnson, H.M. (1964). *Science* **146,** 548.
3. Tyler, A., and Metz, C.B. (1945). *J. Exp. Zool.* **100,** 387.
4. Pauley, G.B., Granger, G.A., and Krassner, S.M. (1971). *J. Invertebr. Pathol.* **18,** 207.
5. Kubo, R.T., Zimmerman, B., and Grey, H.M. (1973). *In* "The Antigens" (M. Sela ed.), p. 417. Academic Press, New York.
6. Sindermann, C.J. (1970). "Principal Diseases of Marine Fish and Shellfish," p. 369. Academic Press, New York.
7. Pauley, G.G., Krassner, S.M., and Chapman, F.A. (1971). *J. Invertebr. Pathol.* **18,** 227.
8. Prowse, R.H., and Tait, N.N. (1969). *Immunology* **17,** 437.
9. McKay, D., and Jenkin, C.R. (1970). *Aust. J. Exp. Biol. Med. Sci.* **48,** 139.
10. Jenkin, C.R., and Rowley, D. (1970). *Aust. J. Exp. Biol. Med. Sci.* **48,** 129.
11. Marchalonis, J.J., and Edelman, G.M. (1968). *J. Mol. Biol.* **32,** 453.
12. Fernandez-Moran, H., Marchalonis, J.J., and Edelman, G.M. (1968). *J. Mol. Biol.* **32,** 467.
12a. Acton, R.T. (ed.). (1972). "Invertebrate Immune Defense Mechanisms." MSS Information Corp., New York.

13. Romer, A.S. (1970). "The Vertebrate Body," 4th ed. Saunders, Philadelphia, Pennsylvania.
14. Marchalonis, J.J., and Edelman, G.M. (1965). *J. Exp. Med.* **122,** 601.
15. Marchalonis, J.J., and Edelman, G.M. (1966). *Science* **154,** 1567.
16. Johnston, W.H., Jr., Acton, R.T., Weinheimer, P.F., Niedermeir, W., Evans, E.E., Shelton, E., and Bennett, J.C. (1971). *J. Immunol.* **107,** 782.
17. Marchalonis, J.J. (1972). *Nature New Biol.* **236,** 84.
18. Mehta, P.D., Reichlin, M., and Tomasi, T.B., Jr. (1972). *J. Immunol.* **109,** 1272.
19. Shelton, E., and Smith, M. (1970). *J. Mol. Biol.* **54,** 615.
20. Acton, R.T., Weinheimer, P.F., Hall, S.J., Niedermeier, W., Shelton, E., and Bennett, J.C. (1971). *Proc. Nat. Acad. Sci. U.S.* **68,** 107.
21. Everhart, D.L. (1972). *Immunology* **22,** 503.
22. Parkhouse, R.M.E., Askonas, B.A., and Dourmashkin, R.R. (1970). *Immunology* **18,** 575.
23. Marchalonis, J.J., and Edelman, G.M. (1966). *J. Exp. Med.* **124,** 901.
24. Feinstein, A., and Munn, E.A. (1969). *Nature (London)* **224,** 1307.
25. Hildemann, W.H., and Thoenes, G.H. (1969). *Transplantation* **7,** 506.
26. Thoenes, G.H., and Hildemann, W.H. (1970). "Developmental Aspects of Immunoglobulin Synthesis," Vol. II, p. 711. Academic Press, New York.
27. Linthicum, D.S., and Hildemann, W.H. (1970). *J. Immunol.* **105,** 912.
28. Finstad, J., Papermaster, B.W., and Good, R.A. (1964). *Lab. Invest.* **13,** 490.
29. Marchalonis, J.J. and Edelman, G.M. (1968). *J. Exp. Med.* **127,** 891.
30. Litman, G.W., Frommel, D., Finstad, J., Howell, J., Pollara, B.W., and Good, R.A. (1970). *J. Immunol.* **105,** 1278.
31. Small, P.A., Jr., Klapper, D.G., and Clem, L.W. (1970). *J. Immunol.* **105,** 29.
32. Gitlin, D., Perricelli, A., and Gitlin, J.D. (1973). *Comp. Biochem. Physiol.* **44B,** 225.
33. Tarail, M.H., Suran, A.A., and Papermaster, B.W. (1967). *J. Immunol.* **99,** 679.
34. Suran, A.A., and Papermaster, B.W. (1967). *Proc. Nat. Acad. Sci. U.S.* **58,** 1619.
35. Clem, L.W., and Small, P.A., Jr. (1967). *J. Exp. Med.* **125,** 893.
36. Frommel, D., Litman, G.W., Finstad, J., and Good, R.A. (1971). *J. Immunol.* **106,** 1234.
37. Shulkin, M.L., Robbins, J.B., and Clem, L.W. (1972). *Nature New Biol.* **230,** 182.
38. Greenbury, C.L., Moore, D.H., and Nunn, L.A.C. (1965). *Immunology* **8,** 420.
39. Klinman, N.R., Long, C.A., and Karush, F. (1967). *J. Immunol.* **99,** 1128.
40. Robbins, J.B., Kenney, K., and Suter, E. (1965). *J. Exp. Med.* **122,** 385.
41. Talmage, D.W., Freter, G.G., and Taliaferro, W.H. (1956). *J. Infect. Dis.* **98,** 300.
42. Voss, E.W., Jr., Russell, W.J., and Sigel, M.M. (1969). *Biochemistry* **8,** 4866.
43. Clem, L. W., DeBoutand, F., and Sigel, M. M. (1967). *J. Immunol.* **99,** 1226.
44. Sigel, M.M., Voss, E.W., Jr., and Rudikoff, S. (1972). *Comp. Biochem. Physiol,* **42A,** 249.
45. Clem, L.W., and Small, P.A., Jr. (1970). *J. Exp. Med.* **132,** 385.
46. Russell, W.J., Voss, E.W., Jr., and Sigel, M.M. (1970). *J. Immunol.* **105,** 262.
47. Klapper, D.G., Clem, L.W., and Small, P.A., Jr. (1971). *Biochemistry* **10,** 645.
48. Klaus, G.G.B., Halpern, M.S., Koshland, M.E., and Goodman, J.W. (1971). *J. Immunol.* **107,** 1785.
49. Weinheimer, P.F., Mestecky, J., and Acton, R.T. (1971). *J. Immunol.* **107,** 1211.
50. Klapper, D.G., and Clem, L.W. (1972). *Comp. Biochem. Physiol.* **42A,** 241.
51. Kobayashi, K., Vaerman, J-P., Baxim, H., Lebacq-Verheyden, A-M., and Heremans, J.F. (1973). *J. Immunol.* **111,** 1590.
52. Klaus, G.G.B., Nitecki, D.E., and Goodman, J.W. (1971). *J. Immunol.* **107,** 1250.

53. Sledge, C., Clem, L.W., and Hood, L. (1974). *J. Immunol.* **112**, 941.
54. Clem, L.W., and Leslie, G.A. (1971). *Proc. Nat. Acad. Sci. U.S.* **68**, 139.
55. Acton, R.T., Weinheimer, P.F., Dupree, H.K., Russell, T.R., Wolcott, M., Evans, E.E., Schrohenloher, R.E., and Bennett, J.C. (1971). *J. Biol. Chem.* **246**, 6760.
56. Stanton, T., Sledge, C., Capra, J.D., Wood, R., Clem, W., and Hood, L.E. (1974). *J. Immunol.* **112**, 633.
57. Voss, E.W., Jr., and Sigel, M. (1971). *J. Immunol.* **106**, 1323.
58. Marchalonis, J.J., and Schonfeld, S.A. (1970). *Biochim. Biophys. Acta* **221**, 604.
59. Clem, L.W. (1971). *J. Biol. Chem.* **246**, 9.
60. Litman, G.W., Frommel, D., Finstad, J., and Good, R.A. (1971). *J. Immunol.* **106**, 747.
61. Marchalonis, J.J. (1971). *Immunology* **20**, 161.
62. Legler, D.W., Acton, R.T., Weinheimer, P.F., and Dupree, H.K. (1971). *Immunology* **20**, 1009.
63. Bradshaw, C.M., Clem, L.W., and Sigel, M.M. (1969). *J. Immunol.* **103**, 496.
64. Marchalonis, J.J. (1969). *Aust. J. Exp. Biol. Med. Sci.* **47**, 405.
65. Litman, G.W., Wang, A.C., Fudenberg, H.H., and Good, R.A. (1971). *Proc. Nat. Acad. Sci.* **68**, 2321.
66. Litman, G.W., Frommel, D., Chartrand, S.L., Finstad, T., and Good, R.A. (1971). *Immunochemistry* **8**, 345.
67. Uhr, J.W., Finklestein, M.S., and Franklin, E.C. (1962). *Proc. Soc. Exp. Biol. Med.* **111**, 13.
68. Geczy, C.L., Green, P.C., Gaydas, K.C., and Steiner, L.A. (1972). *Fed. Proc. Fed. Amer. Soc. Exp. Biol.* **31**, 750.
69. Hadjii-Azimi, I. (1971). *Immunology* **21**, 463.
70. Acton, R.T., Evans, E.E., Weinheimer, P.F., Niedermeier, W., and Bennett, J.C. (1972). *Biochemistry* **11**, 2751.
71. Marchalonis, J.J., Allen, R.B., and Saarni, E.S. (1970). *Comp. Biochem. Physiol.* **35**, 49.
72. Cowden, R.R., Dyer, R.F., Gebhardt, B.M., and Volpe, E.P. (1968). *J. Immunol.* **100**, 1293.
73. Diener, E., and Marchalonis, J.J. (1970). *Immunology* **18**, 279.
74. Romano, E.L., Geczy, C.L., and Steiner, L.A. (1973). *Immunochemistry* **10**, 655.
75. Marchalonis, J.J. (1971). *Develop. Biol.* **25**, 479.
76. Geczy, C.L., Green, P.C., and Steiner, L.A. (1973). *J. Immunol.* **111**, 1261.
77. Marchalonis, J.J., and Cohen, N. (1973). *Immunology* **24**, 395.
78. Ambrosius, H., Hemmerling, J., Richter, R., and Schimke, R. (1970). *In* "Developmental Aspects of Antibody Formation and Structure" (J. Sterzl and I. Riha, eds.), p. 727. Academic Press, New York.
79. Ching, Y.C., and Wedgewood, R.J. (1967). *J. Immunol.* **99**, 191.
80. Grey, H.M. (1963). *J. Immunol.* **91**, 819.
81. Chartrand, S.L., Litman, G.W., LaPointe, N., Good, R.A., and Frommel, D. (1971). *J. Immunol.* **107**, 1.
82. Acton, R.T., Weinheimer, P.F., Shelton, E., Niedermeier, W., and Bennett, J.C. (1972). *Immunochemistry* **9**, 421.
83. Lykakis, J.J. (1968). *Immunology* **14**, 799.
84. Leslie, G.A., and Clem, L.W. (1972). *J. Immunol.* **108**, 1656.
85. Coe, J.E. (1972). *Immunology* **23**, 45.
86. Saluk, P.H., Krauss, J., and Clem, L.W. (1970). *Proc. Soc. Exp. Biol. Med.* **133**, 365.

87. Marchalonis, J.J., Ealey, E.H., and Diener, E. (1969). *Aust. J. Exp. Biol. Med. Sci.* **47,** 367.
88. Leslie, G.A., and Clem, L.W. (1969). *J. Exp. Med.* **130,** 1337.
89. Leslie, G.A., and Benedict, A.A. (1969). *Immunochemistry* **6,** 762.
90. Leslie, G.A., and Clem, L.W. (1970). *Proc. Soc. Exp. Biol. Med.* **134,** 195.
91. Waldmann, T.A., and Strober, W. (1969). *Progr. Allergy* **13,** 1.
92. Hersh, R.T., and Benedict, A.A. (1966). *Biochim. Biophys. Acta* **115,** 242.
93. Voss, E.W., Jr., and Eisen, H.N. (1972). *J. Immunol.* **109,** 944.
94. Kubo, R.T., and Benedict, A.A. (1969). *J. Immunol.* **102,** 1523.
95. Lebacq-Verheyden, A., Vaerman, J.P., and Heremans, J.F. (1972). *Immunology* **22,** 165.
96. Orlans, E. and Rose, M.E. (1972). *Immunochemistry* **9,** 833.
97. Bienenstock, J., Percy, D.Y.E., Gauldie, J., and Underdown, B.J. (1972). *J. Immunol.* **109,** 403.
98. Bienenstock, J., Perey, D.Y.E., Gauldie, J., and Underdown, B.J. (1973). *J. Immunol.* **110,** 524.
99. Leslie, G.A., and Martin, L.N. (1973). *J. Immunol.* **110,** 1.
100. Grey, H.M. (1967). *J. Immunol.* **98,** 811.
101. Grey, H.M. (1967). *J. Immunol.* **98,** 820.
102. Zimmerman, B., Shalatin, N., and Grey, H.M. (1971). *Biochemistry* **10,** 482.
103. Acton, R.T., Niedermeier, W., Weinheimer, P.F., Clem, L.W., Leslie, G.A., and Bennett, J.C. (1972). *J. Immunol.* **109,** 371.
104. Heremans, J.F., and Vaerman, J.P. (1971). *In* "Progress in Immunology" Vol. I, (B. Amos, ed.), p. 875. Academic Press, New York.
105. Orlans, E., and Feinstein, A. (1971). *Nature (London)* **233,** 45.
105a. Neoh, S.H., Jahoda, D.M., Rowe, D.S., and Voller, A. (1973). *Immunochemistry* **10,** 805.
106. DiConza, J.I., and Halliday, W.J. (1971). *Aust. J. Exp. Biol. Med. Sci.* **49,** 517.
107. Fletcher, T.C., and Grant, P.T. (1969). *Biochem. J.* **115,** 65p.
108. Chuang, C-Y., Capra, J.D., and Kehoe, J.M. (1973). *Nature New Biol.* **244,** 158.
109. Edelman, G.M., Cunningham, B.A., Gall, W.E., Gottlieb, P.D., Rustishauser, U., and Waxdal, M.J. (1969). *Proc. Nat. Acad. Sci. U.S.* **63,** 78.
110. Bennich, H., and Johannson, S.G.O. (1971). *Advan. Immunol.* **13,** 1.
111. Ishizaka, K., and Ishizaka, T. (1971). *Ann. N.Y. Acad. Sci.* **190,** 443.
111a. Ishizaka, K. (1973). *In* "The Antigens" (M. Sela, ed.), Vol. I, p. 479. Academic Press, New York.
112. Ishizaka, T., Sian, C.M., and Ishizaka, K. (1972). *J. Immunol.* **108,** 848.
113. Ishizaka, K., and Ishizaka, T. (1971). *In* "Progress in Immunology" (B. Amos, ed.), Vol. I, p. 859. Academic Press, New York.
114. Ishizaka, K., Ishizaka, T., and Tada, T. (1969). *J. Immunol.* **103,** 445.
115. Halliwall, R.E.W., Schwartzman, R.M., and Rockey, J.H. (1972). *Clin. Exp. Immunol.* **10,** 399.
116. Kanyerezi, B., Jaton, J.C., and Bloch, K.J. (1971). *J. Immunol.* **106,** 1411.
117. Guttman, R.M., Tebo, T., Edwards, J., Barboriak, J.J., and Fink, J.N. (1971). *J. Immunol.* **106,** 392.
118. Grant, J.A., Saunders, B., and Hood, L. (1971). *Biochemistry* **10,** 3123.
119. Kubo, R.T., Rosenblum, I.Y., and Benedict, A.A. (1970). *J. Immunol.* **105,** 534.
120. Hood, L., Gray, W.R., Saunders, B.G., and Dreyer, W.J. (1967). *Cold Spring Harbor Symp. Quant. Biol.* **32,** 133.

121. Gray, W.R., Dreyer, W.J., and Hood, L. (1967). *Science* **155**, 465.
122. Appella, E. (1971). *Proc. Nat. Acad. Sci. U.S.* **68**, 590.
123. Hood, L., Grant, J.A., and Sox, H.C., Jr. (1969). *In* "Developmental Aspects of Antibody Formation and Structure" (J. Sterzl and I. Riha, eds.), Vol. I, p. 283. Academic Press, New York.
124. Putnam, F.W., Florent, G., Shinoda, P.T., and Shimizu, A. (1973). *Science* **182**, 287.
125. Pink, J.R.L., Buttery, S.H., DeVries, G.M., and Milstein, C. (1970). *Biochem. J.* **117**, 33.
126. Frangione, B., Milstein, C., and Pink, J.R.L. (1969). *Nature (London)* **221**, 145.
127. van Loghem, E., and Litwin, S.D. (1972). *Transplantation Proc.* **4**, 129.
128. Wang, A-C., Shuster, J., and Fudenberg, H.H. (1969). *J. Mol. Biol.* **41**, 83.
129. van Loghem, E., Shuster, J., and Fudenberg, H.H. (1968). *Vox Sang.* **14**, 81.
130. Shuster, J., Warner, N.L., and Fudenberg, H.H. (1969). *Ann. N.Y. Acad. Sci.* **162**, 195.
131. Froland, S.S., and Natvig, J.B. (1971). *In* "Progress in Immunology" (B. Amos, ed.), Vol. I, p. 109. Academic Press, New York.
132. Capra, J.D., Wasserman, C.L., and Kehoe, J.M. (1973). *J. Exp. Med.* **138**, 410.
133. Wang, A.-C., Pink, J.R.L., Fudenberg, H.H., and Ohms, J. (1970). *Proc. Nat. Acad. Sci. U.S.* **66**, 657.
134. Wang, A.-C., and Fudenberg, H.H. (1972). *J. Human Evolution* **1**, 617.
135. Kubo, R.T., Rosenblum, I.Y., and Benedict, A.A. (1971). *J. Immunol.* **107**, 1781.
136. Abramson, N., Gelfand, E.W., Jandl, J.H., and Rosen, F.S. (1970). *J. Exp. Med.* **132**, 1207.
137. Henson, P.M. (1971). "Progress in Immunology" (B. Amos, ed.), Vol. I, p. 155. Academic Press, New York.
138. Tomasi, T.B., Jr., and Bienenstock, J. (1968). *Advan. Immunol.* **9**, 2.
139. Vaerman, J.P. (1973). *Res. Immunochem. Immunobiol.* **3**, 91.
140. Tomasi, T.B., and Grey, H.M. (1972). *Prog. Allergy* **16**, 81.

8

Immunoglobulins of the Rabbit, Mouse, Guinea Pig, and Horse

I. INTRODUCTION

In this chapter we shall describe properties of immunoglobulins of four mammalian species that have been studied quite extensively: the rabbit, mouse, guinea pig, and horse. Human immunoglobulins are considered in Chapter 3 and the pattern of evolution of immunoglobulins in vertebrates in Chapter 7. Allotypy of immunoglobulins is reviewed in Chapter 9 and will not be considered here. Because of the extensive body of information available on amino acid sequences and allotypes a more complete understanding of the structure of the immunoglobulins of these species will require reference to Chapters 4 and 9.

II. GENERAL CONSIDERATIONS

Before listing special properties of Ig classes of the individual species we will note some general similarities. Each of the four species to be considered possesses the IgM, IgG, and IgA classes, which are defined by analogy to the corresponding human immunoglobulin classes. IgE has been identified in the rabbit, mouse, and guinea pig. The evidence for homology to human IgE is indirect since the serum concentration of IgE is too low to permit purification; this evidence will be discussed below. A class corresponding to human IgD has been identified in the guinea pig, but not, so far, in the other three species[1]. The classes

[1] A molecule resembling human IgD in some of its properties has recently been identified on the surface of mouse spleen cells (1).

are, as in all species, characterized by their C_H regions, either through antigenic or sequence analysis, and share the same library of V_H regions and L chains; the latter always have a molecular weight of 22,000 to 23,000. Kappa and lambda chains are distributed as follows (1a-8):[2]

	$\kappa(\%)$	$\lambda(\%)$
Rabbit	70–90	10–30
Mouse	95–97	3–5
Guinea pig	70	30
Horse	< 5	> 95

A protein is designated κ or λ on the basis of sequence homology to the corresponding human chain.

The proportions of κ and λ chains may change during immunization. For example, anti-2,4-dinitrophenyl (anti-Dnp) antibodies synthesized by guinea pigs 2 weeks after immunization with a bovine γ-globulin–Dnp conjugate contain over 99% κ chains (9), and several strains of mice produce antibodies to $\alpha(1 \rightarrow 3)$dextran that are almost exclusively λ (10), despite the paucity of λ chains in normal mouse serum.

In each species IgM is characterized by its high carbohydrate content ($\sim 10\%$), pentameric structure comprising ten H and ten L chains, the relatively high molecular weight of its H chain ($\sim 70,000$), its appearance early in ontogeny, and the presence of J chain attached in the Fc_μ region. An electron micrograph of a mouse IgM myeloma protein is shown in Fig. 8.1 (10a). The pentameric structure is clearly visible in many of the molecules; a few appear to be hexamers.

IgA occurs in many secretory fluids as sIgA and, in serum, as the 4-chain "monomer" or polymers thereof. Secretory IgA comprises four H and four L chains, secretory component (SC; mol. wt. 70,000 ± 10,000), and J chain (15,000). The J chains and SC's of various mammalian species are similar in their general properties to the corresponding human protein (Chapter 7). Depending on the species, varying amounts of SC can be released upon exposure to concentrated guanidine hydrochloride without prior reduction. J chain is disulfide bonded to the Fc portion of the molecule. Whether it actually serves to join monomeric units has not as yet been conclusively established. References 11 to 13a are reviews of the properties of IgA from various species.

The nature of the subclasses of IgG is variable among species and

[2] For the κ/λ distribution in other species see Table 7.7.

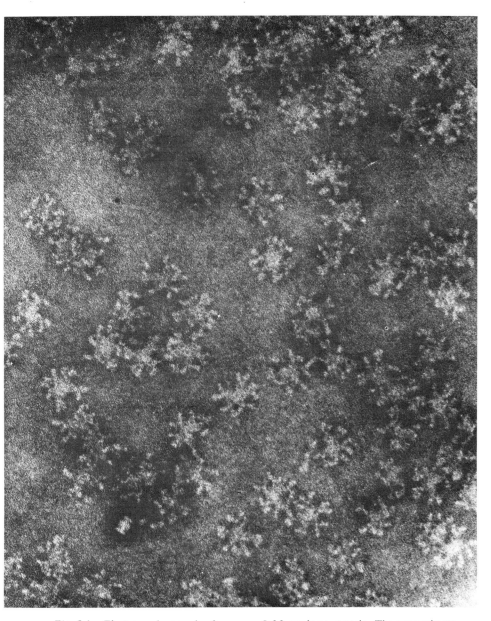

Fig. 8.1. Electron micrograph of a mouse IgM myeloma protein. The approximate magnification in this reproduction is 500,000×. The sample was prepared by a negative staining procedure using phosphotungstate. Molecules consist of a central core to which Y-shaped subunits are attached in a radial arrangement. Each fork of a Y is believed to comprise an Fab segment. The length of a fork is 60–80 Å, and the overall diameter of the molecule is 300–375 Å. Five, or in a few instances, six subunits appear to be present in each molecule. Reprinted, by permission, from Parkhouse *et al.* (10a). (The section shown here overlaps with the authors' Fig. 1.)

TABLE 8.1

SUBCLASSES OF IgG IN FOUR MAMMALIAN SPECIES

Species	IgG subclasses[a]	Disulfide bonded structure	Approximate concentration in normal adult serum[b] (mg/ml)	Half-Life in serum (days)	Complement fixation[c]
Rabbit	IgG		10–15	5.5–8	+
	IgG1 (minor component)				
Guinea pig[d]	IgG1		0.3–1	7	−
	IgG2		5–10	5	+
Mouse	IgG1		0.3–4	2.5	−

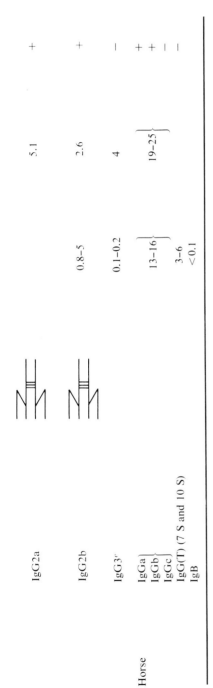

IgG2a		5.1	+
IgG2b	0.8–5	2.6	+
IgG3″	0.1–0.2	4	−
Horse IgGa	13–16 }	19–25 }	+
IgGb			+
IgGc			−
IgG(T) (7 S and 10 S)	3–6		−
IgB	<0.1		

a The carbohydrate content of the various IgG subclasses of each species is relatively low (2–3%) and all possess the typical four-chain structure. Half-lives of immunoglobulins of classes other than IgG may be found in reference 190.

b Relative concentrations of the subclasses may be greatly altered upon immunization.

c Guinea pig complement; conventional pathway.

d A minor IgG subclass with skin sensitizing activity and rapid anodal mobility may also be present (41). Recent data of J. Cebra indicate that IgG1 has one interheavy chain disulfide bond.

e There are probably two interheavy chain disulfide bonds in IgG3 (150). Data in this table are taken in part from the following references: 7, 12, 13, 47, 138, 150, 156, 169, 185, 190–197.

will be taken up in some detail. In most instances the nomenclature of the IgG subclasses reflects average electrophoretic mobility; for example, the average anodal electrophoretic mobility of guinea pig IgG1 is greater than that of IgG2 at slightly alkaline pH. In the normal heterogeneous population there is overlap among the subclasses with respect to mobility. The marked variation among species with respect to the nature of their IgG subclasses reflects recent evolutionary divergence of the subclasses, possibly having occurred within the species itself, or in some relatively recent ancestor. This is suggested also by the high degree of antigenic cross-reactivity among the H chains of different IgG subclasses. (By definition, each subclass also has unique determinants.)

In most, but not all immunoglobulins, one disulfide bond joins an H chain to an L chain. There are marked variations, however, with respect to H–H disulfide bonds. The number of such bonds, where known, is indicated by the diagrams in Table 8.1. An unusual chain structure, analogous to that found in the $A_2m(1)$ allotype of human IgA2 (14,15) is observed in the IgA of BALB/c (16,16a,17) but not NZB mice (18); the L chains are disulfide bonded to one another, as are the H chains, but there are no H–L disulfide bonds. The H and L chains are therefore separable in the presence of a a dissociating agent such as 1 M acetic acid, without prior reduction of disulfide bonds.

The relative serum concentrations of the immunoglobulin classes vary among species. Some of these values are included in Table 8.1. Many of these immunoglobulins have been studied with respect to cleavage by proteolytic enzymes. As in the case of human immunoglobulins, large fragments, some of which have active binding sites, can readily be obtained. The prototype for such investigations, rabbit IgG, will be discussed in some detail and the enzymatic cleavage of a few other immunoglobulins will be described.

III. ANTIGENIC RELATIONSHIPS

One reliable method for identifying a class as homologous to that of a human immunoglobulin is antigenic cross-reactivity. Amino acid sequence homologies, which are more definitive, are also available in some instances.

Mehta *et al.,* using the method of quantitative complement fixation, carried out extensive tests of cross-reactivity with monospecific rabbit antisera to human γ and μ chains (19). The IgG of each of six mammalian species tested cross-reacted with anti-human IgG. Monkey IgG showed 100% cross-reactivity, horse IgG about 23%, and rat IgG, 15%. Chicken IgG did not cross-react. With anti-human μ chain antiserum the IgM of the monkey showed about 90% cross-reactivity; horse IgM exhibited 12–57% cross-reactivity with three different antisera, and that of the rat averaged 35%. Of considerable interest was the finding that chicken IgM cross-reacted to the extent of about 50% with human IgM, thus establishing the homology between the corresponding bird and mammalian proteins. The chicken immunoglobulin of low molecular weight showed no antigenic cross-reactivity with anti-human IgG; whether the chicken protein is homologous to mammalian IgG is uncertain (Chapter 7).

Immunological cross-reactivity of the IgA of various mammalian species with anti-human IgA is discussed in references 19a, 20, and 21. With respect to the four species under consideration here, all have been found to possess a protein which cross-reacts with antihuman IgA; classification of a protein as IgA is, however, also based on its localization in the body and on the presence of secretory piece and J chain.

For demonstrating serological cross-reactivity it is desirable to immunize a recipient animal which is not closely related to the two species whose immunoglobulins are to be compared. For example, Orlans and Feinstein immunized chickens with mammalian IgA proteins in order to demonstrate cross-reactivity (20). It is obvious that one should not use as recipient a species closely related to the donor since it may not recognize as foreign many of the determinants of the injected molecule.

Shared antigenic determinants in the IgE of mammalian species are discussed in the next section.

IV. HOMOCYTOTROPIC ANTIBODIES: IgE

The terms "reaginic" or "homocytotropic" antibody (HCA) are in general usage to denote antibodies capable of mediating passive cutaneous anaphylactic reactions within the autologous species (21a). In a number of species there is more than one class of molecule which has this property. When an immunoglobulin has the following characteristics it is generally considered to be homologous to human IgE: heat lability (56°C for 1 hour); persistence in skin with a long half-life (at least a few days); reactivity with anti-L chain antiserum; failure to react with antiserum specific for any other class of immunoglobulin; and a sedimentation coefficient of 8 S. Such antibody has been identified in primates, rats, guinea pigs, mice, rabbits, and other species. (For reviews, see references 19a, 22–24 and 24a.) Cross-reactivity with specific antiserum to human IgE, but not with antisera to other human immunoglobulin classes, is considered a definitive criterion for identification as IgE. Immunological cross-reactivity can also be shown by the capacity of anti-human IgE (prepared against a myeloma protein) to remove reaginic activity from a serum or to cause release of histamine from mast cells of the species under consideration. Such cross-reactivity was first demonstrated for proteins as disparate as monkey (24), dog (25), rat (26,27), and guinea pig (28) IgE (see also ref. 19a). Mouse IgE did not cross-react with anti-human IgE (29) and the cross-reaction of rabbit IgE is weak (30,31). Subsequently, a study of about 90 mammalian species was carried out by Neoh *et al.* (19a), who used antisera to human IgE prepared in a sheep or in several chickens. The plasma of nearly all primates contained a cross-reacting protein, presumably IgE. With a few exceptions, including the guinea pig, the plasma of most nonprimates failed to react with the antisera to human IgE used in this study.

The method of Vaz and Ovary (32), or an adaptation is frequently used in passive cutaneous anaphylactic tests for the presence of IgE antibody; 24–48 hours are allowed to elapse after injecting antibody before challenging with antigen (see also Section IX).

A second class of homocytotropic antibody, identified in a number of mammalian species, is relatively stable to heat, has a sedimentation coefficient of 7 S, and disappears from sensitized skin sites much more rapidly than IgE; in the mouse, for example, the half-life in skin is 3–4 hours (33). In the mouse (34–38) and guinea pig (39,40) the immunoglobulin is IgG1. [It has been suggested that guinea pigs may possess another heat-labile homocytotropic antibody, similar to IgG1 but of faster mobility (41).] In the rat, the molecule is designated IgGa (42). In the rabbit, the corresponding protein is IgG; it is present in both fast and slow electrophoretic fractions of purified IgG and its reactivity is complement dependent (43).

The relative amounts of the two types of homocytotropic antibodies produced may vary with the antigen and route of injection. For example, Levine and Vaz succeeded in producing a relatively high titer of reaginic (IgE) antibody in some inbred strains of mice by repeated injection of a low dose of antigen in aluminum hydroxide gel (44). Orr and Blair (45) and Bloch *et al.* (46) found that a reaginic response can be initiated in rats by injections of small doses of antigen incorporated in alum, followed by infection with *Nippostrongylus brasiliensis* larvae. Injection with certain parasites stimulates IgE production in experimental animals and in man (47). Numerous empirical procedures for the preferential induction of IgE antibodies have been reported.

V. RABBIT IMMUNOGLOBULINS

A. Light Chains

This section is complementary to the discussion of rabbit L chains presented with reference to allotypy (Chapter 9).

About 70 to 90% of L chains in rabbit serum are of the κ type; the remainder have the characteristics of λ chains (1,5,48,49). The λ chain population comprises those molecules which lack allotypic determinants controlled by the *b* locus (50). A partial subfractionation of L chains (8,48) can be accomplished if gel filtration (after cleavage of interchain disulfide bonds) is carried out in 6 M urea containing 0.05 M formic acid (51), rather than in 1 M propionic acid. Rejnek *et al.* utilized this chromatographic procedure after first breaking the interchain disulfide bonds of rabbit IgG with sulfite in the presence of cupric ion (49). Two well-defined peaks containing L chains were obtained. All the λ chains were found in the first fraction, together with part of the κ chain population. The second peak of L chains consisted entirely of κ chains. The κ chains in the two peaks were designated κ_A and κ_B, respectively. Allotypic markers controlled by the *b* locus are present in both κ_A and κ_B chains. (Lambda chains contain a different set of markers, controlled by the *c* locus.) κ_B molecules were found to differ structurally from κ_A; the former contain seven half-cystine residues, whereas κ_A molecules have five. This difference reflects the presence of an extra intrachain disulfide bond in κ_B, which spans the V_L and C_L domains, connecting half-cystines 80 and 171 (52,53). The slower migration through Sephadex of κ_B may reflect a more compact structure, related to the presence of the extra disulfide bond (49); this conformational difference would be of particular importance in the urea-formic acid solvent employed. The separation does not appear to be attributable to a significant difference in molecular weight (54). The weight ratio of κ_B to κ_A is a function of the allotype of the molecules, with b4 > b5 $\geq$ b6 > b9 (49). Interestingly, this is the same as the relative order of quantitative expression of these allotypes in heterozygous rabbits.

The isolation of rabbit λ chains is greatly facilitated by suppression of the production of κ chains with antiallotype antisera directed to specificities controlled by the *b* locus (3,55). (See Chapter 9.)

Allotype-related amino acid sequences are discussed in Chapter 9. Sequences of a number of κ chains from homogeneous rabbit antibodies are presented in Figs. 4.7 and 4.8.

B. Rabbit IgG

This class comprises well over 90% of the immunoglobulins in normal rabbit serum; IgM and IgA are present in very low concentration in serum and are difficult to isolate. A large proportion of antibody molecules elicited in response to many antigens upon hyperimmunization is of the IgG class. However, antibodies of the IgM class have been produced in significant titer in response to many bacteria, endotoxins, erythrocytes, and viruses.

Molecules of rabbit IgG are capable of fixing guinea pig complement, have the unique ability among the Ig classes to cross the placental barrier (56), and are capable of fixation to guinea pig skin to permit passive cutaneous anaphylaxis upon challenge with antigen (57,58). The half-life of rabbit IgG in the circulation is about 6 days (59,60). Rabbit IgG is readily prepared in good yield and in a high degree of purity from serum by precipitation with sodium or ammonium sulfate (61) followed by chromatography on DEAE-cellulose (62). Because of the considerable heterogeneity of IgG with respect to charge, some of the negatively charged IgG molecules can be eluted only under conditions which also release IgA or IgM (63); under appropriate conditions, however, the first peak contains only IgG. General structural features of rabbit IgG are very similar to those of human IgG (Figs. 1.1 and 1.2). In contrast to the human protein the γ chains of rabbit IgG comprise only one major subclass, although allotypic variants exist. The presence of a minor subclass has been reported (64). Subgroups of rabbit V_H regions are discussed in Chapter 9.

1. ENZYMATIC CLEAVAGE OF RABBIT IgG BY PAPAIN AND PEPSIN

Starting with the work of Parfentjev in 1936 (65), many investigators have treated immunoglobulins with enzymes and studied the properties of the larger fragments produced. We will not discuss the earlier literature, but will begin with a description of the work of Porter in the late 1950's (66,67), which represented a major advance in immunochemistry and formed a basis for subsequent structural work.

Treatment of rabbit IgG at 37°C and neutral pH with 0.1–1% by weight of crystalline papain, in the presence of reducing agent, cleaves the molecule into three fragments, each of approximate molecular weight 45,000–50,000 (Fig. 8.2; see also Fig. 1.1) (66,67). Two fragments, designated Fab (ab for antigen-binding), are univalent, and therefore lack the capacity to form the cross-linked network necessary for precipitation with an antigen. They can, however, preempt antigenic sites and prevent the precipitation (or agglutination) that would otherwise occur upon addition of untreated, bivalent antibody (66,67). As in the case of human IgG, papain cleaves the H chains in the hinge region. Each Fab fragment thus comprises a complete L chain and about half of an H chain (designated fragment Fd) (68). Fab fragments are very soluble and show no significant tendency to aggregate. The Fd fragment comprises the V_H and C_H1 domains of the H chain. It can be isolated by reductive cleavage of the Fab fragment followed by gel filtration in 1 M propionic acid; although L chains and Fd fragments have similar molecular weights they are separable because of the tendency of fragment Fd to aggregate (68).

A large amount of indirect evidence supports the view that the two Fab fragments of an individual molecule are identical. This identity has been demonstrated directly for myeloma proteins and certain homogeneous antibodies by amino acid sequence analysis. The net charge of an IgG molecule reflects that of its fragments; within a heterogeneous population the order of elution of Fab fragments from an ion-exchange resin parallels that of the parent IgG molecules (69). The two combining sites of an individual antibody molecule in a heterogeneous population were shown to have the same specificity (70).

The third fragment, Fc, is crystallizable and comprises the remainder of the two H chains (the C-terminal halves including part of the hinge region and all of the C_H2 and C_H3 domains). The two chain segments in fragment Fc are held together by noncovalent interactions (68) and by one interchain disulfide bond (71). The disulfide bond is cleaved if a high concentration of reducing agent is used during papain digestion; however, noncovalent interactions suffice to hold the two chain segments in fragment Fc together. If a very low concentration of reducing agent is employed, the interheavy chain disulfide bond remains intact in fragment Fc and serves as an additional link between the two H chain segments (72). Crystals of fragment Fc appear spontaneously in the cold, even when nonspecific immunoglobulin is the starting material (67); this suggested molecular homogeneity of fragment Fc, which was subsequently confirmed by amino acid sequence analysis (73,74). Preliminary crystallographic data on rabbit fragment Fc have been reported by Poljak *et al.,* who determined the space group and unit cell dimensions (75).

The enzyme pepsin also produces large fragments that retain an-

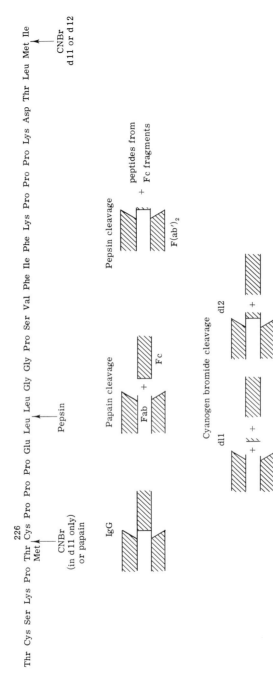

Fig. 8.2. Cleavage of rabbit IgG by papain, pepsin (pH 4.5), or cyanogen bromide (in HCl solution). Cleavage by papain is just N-terminal to the half-cystine which forms the interheavy chain disulfide bond [residue 226 by homology with the human γ_1 chain (protein Eu)]. Molecules of allotype d11 possess an extra methionine just N-terminal to the interheavy chain disulfide bond; this accounts for the difference in cleavage points between d11 and d12 molecules.

tibody activity (76,77) (Figs. 1.1 and 1.2). For this purpose proteolysis is carried out at pH 4.0–4.5, which is well above the optimal pH range of the enzyme. At a lower pH extensive degradation may occur, in part because the IgG molecule begins to unfold and is subject to attack at multiple positions in the polypeptide chains. In a typical reaction the amount of pepsin present is about 2% of the weight of antibody and digestion is allowed to proceed for 8 to 16 hours at 37°C. Although pepsin, like papain, cleaves the H chains in the hinge region, it produces a bivalent rather than a monovalent product, because it breaks a peptide bond on the C-terminal side of the interheavy chain disulfide bond. The locus of cleavage of rabbit IgG by pepsin is shown in Fig. 8.2. It is entirely analogous to the cleavage of human IgG. The product, designated $F(ab')_2$, has a molecular weight of approximately 95,000 and a sedimentation coefficient of 4.6 S. Being bivalent, it is about as effective as intact IgG in precipitation and agglutination (76,78). Fragment Fc is degraded by pepsin into heterogeneous peptides, whose size depends upon the conditions and length of the digestion. Some of these fragments have been partially characterized and localized (79–84); fragments with molecular weights as high as 27,000 have been isolated and antigenic determinants of fragments Fc were identified in fragments with molecular weight as low as 5,000 (79,80). The fragment of molecular weight 27,000 comprises a noncovalently bound dimer, corresponding approximately to the C_H3 domains of the molecule (81). This fragment is now designated pFc'. A closely related fragment (stFc) can be prepared by digestion with papain at pH 4.5 (84a).

In contrast to human IgG, only a single disulfide bond joins the two H chains of rabbit IgG. This, of course, is the bond that links the two univalent Fab' fragments after peptic digestion (71,85,86). This disulfide bond is extremely labile and can be reduced at neutral pH with 0.01 M 2-mercaptoethanol, thus allowing the two Fab' fragments to separate. The properties of fragment Fab' are practically indistinguishable from those of fragment Fab (76,77,87). When prepared from a human IgG1 myeloma protein, the two fragments give virtually identical X-ray diffraction patterns at 2.8 Å resolution (R. J. Poljak, personal communication).

If the reducing agent is removed under appropriate conditions, it is possible to reoxidize the sulfhydryl groups that were liberated upon reduction to reform fragment $F(ab')_2$ (87,88). When specifically purified antibody is used as starting material a substantial amount of precipitating activity is restored upon reoxidation. The possibility of separating and recombining Fab' fragments made it feasible to synthesize, *in vitro*, hybrid antibody molecules in which the two combining sites are of different specificity; such molecules are functionally monovalent and do not occur naturally. These preparations also contain some bivalent antibodies directed against each of the two antigens (89,90). If an equal amount of two specifically purified antibodies of different specificity (A-A and B-B) are treated with pepsin and then hybridized the theoretical ratio of $F(ab')_2$ products, AB, BB, and AA, is $2:1:1$. The experimental evidence indicates that the recombination is indeed random (90,91). The hybrid antibodies have been isolated by consecutive adsorption and elution from two immunoadsorbents, each containing one of the two antigens (92,93).

The initial evidence for the existence of hybrid molecules was the capacity of such preparations to precipitate a mixture of the two antigens (ovalbumin and bovine IgG) but neither individual antigen alone (89). A hybrid molecule would not be expected to form a continuous lattice with either antigen but should do so if both are present (see Fig. 6.4). The failure of molecules A-A or B-B in the mixture to precipitate the corresponding antigens was attributed to the blocking activity of A-B, which is univalent with respect to either antigen and is presumably present in twofold excess.

An experiment which provided a visual demonstration of the formation of antibodies of mixed specificity was carried out by Fudenberg *et al.* (94). It was based on the fact that chicken and human erythocytes can readily be distinguished under the microscope; the latter are disc-shaped and enucleate, whereas the former are oval, larger, and nucleated. The human red blood cells were coated with one antigen, ovalbumin, by the chromic chloride method (95); bovine γ-globulin was similarly attached to the chicken cells. When $F(ab')_2$ fragments from purified antiovalbumin were added to a mixture of the two types of coated cells, only the human cells were agglutinated (Fig. 8.3A). Similarly, the $F(ab')_2$ fragments of purified antibovine gamma globulin agglutinated only the chicken cells. A mixture of the two types of $F(ab')_2$ fragments agglutinated both types of cells, but individual clumps contained one cell type or the other. When a hybrid antibody was employed mixed agglutinates were seen (Fig. 8.3D). The blocking effect of the presence of an excess of either individual antigen (ovalbumin or bovine gamma globulin) on the nature of agglutinates formed was consistent also with the presence of molecules of mixed specificity (94).

Hybrid antibodies have found practical application in electron microscopy, where they have been used, for example, to localize surface antigens on cells. For such an experiment (96), mouse lymphocytes may first be coated with mouse antibodies to H-2 antigens present on the cell surface. Hybrid rabbit antibody is prepared with one combining site spe-

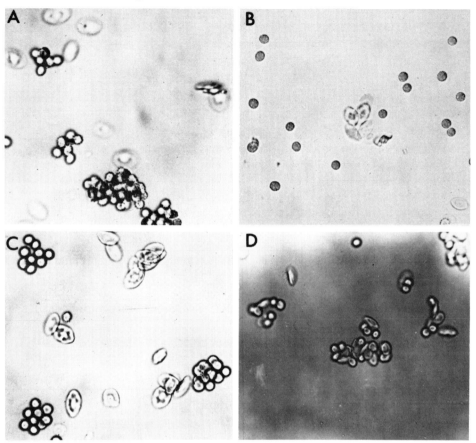

Fig. 8.3. Agglutination reactions of mixtures of chicken erythrocytes (oval and nucleated) and human erythrocytes (disc-shaped); the chicken cells were coated with bovine IgG (BGG) and the human cells with hen ovalbumin. The following rabbit F(ab′)$_2$ fragments were present in the mixtures: A, antiovalbumin; B, anti-BGG; C, mixture of antiovalbumin and anti-BGG; D, hybrid preparation of antiovalbumin and anti-BGG. From reference 94.

cific for mouse immunoglobulin and the other specific for ferritin which, by virtue of its high electron density, is readily visualized by electron microscopy. The hybrid antibody is attached to the mouse cells through one site, then treated with ferritin. This permits direct visualization of the distribution of H-2 antigens on the cell surface. Other markers that have been used in place of ferritin are southern bean mosaic virus or tobacco mosaic virus; antibody to the virus is used for preparation of the hybrid molecule (97).

2. LIMITED PROTEOLYSIS OF RABBIT IgG
   BY OTHER ENZYMES

It is possible to cleave rabbit IgG into discrete fragments with proteolytic enzymes other than papain and pepsin. For example, digestion
with ficin yields fragments which are identical by several criteria to
those obtained with papain (98)[3]. By tryptic digestion, Givol was able to
produce fragments very similar in properties to papain fragments Fab
and Fc, but only if the rabbit IgG was first mildly reduced and aminoeth-
ylated (99). (Aminoethylcysteine is positively charged and, like arginine
and lysine, provides a locus of attack for trypsin.) The bond cleaved is
Cys-Ser, evidently corresponding to positions 221–222 in Fig. 8.2. Untreated rabbit IgG is quite resistant to trypsin under the same conditions. It is evident from such results that peptide bonds in the hinge
region of the H chain are particularly susceptible to enzymatic attack at
neutral pH and that the Fab fragment is highly resistant. The degree of
degradation of fragment Fc is variable and dependent on the enzyme and
conditions of the reaction. Papain remains one of the most useful proteolytic enzymes because of the relative resistance of rabbit fragment Fc
to this enzyme.

Rabbit cathepsins D and E, obtained from spleen and bone marrow,
respectively, cleave rabbit IgG into fragments closely resembling the
$F(ab')_2$ fragments released by pepsin (100).

A fragment comprising all of the rabbit IgG molecule except the
two C_H3 domains was prepared by Connell and Porter (100a). Cleavage
is accomplished with rabbit or human plasmin at neutral pH but only
after exposure of the IgG to pH 2.5 for 1 hour. Cleavage occurs
between lysine 326 and alanine 327 (rabbit γ chain numbering system).
Thus, the C-terminal domain is removed from each H chain. The larger
fragment, designated Facb, retains the capacity to form specific precipitates and to fix complement.

Another interesting product is obtained in low yield after digestion
of rabbit IgG with very low concentrations of papain (100b) or for a
very short period of time (100c). It results from cleavage of only one of
the two H chains (in the hinge region) and comprises one complete Fab
segment and the Fc segment:

---

[3] In this investigation, Putnam *et al.* showed that a wide variety of proteolytic enzymes cleave human IgG into 3.5 S fragments. Proteolyses of porcine, equine, and bovine
IgG were also demonstrated (98).

A similar fragment, derived from human IgGl, has been denoted Fabc (100d).

3. CLEAVAGE OF RABBIT IgG BY CYANOGEN BROMIDE

Although the rabbit H chain has four or five methionine groups, each of which represents a potential site of attack by cyanogen bromide (101–104), cleavage occurs most readily next to a methionine located C-terminal to, and near the hinge region (105–107) (Fig. 8.2). This liberates a fragment, designated F(ab'')$_2$, which is slightly larger than F(ab')$_2$ and in which two Fab'' units are linked only by the disulfide bond which joins the H chains. Subsequent mild reduction releases univalent Fab'' fragments. Molecules of allotype d11 possess an additional methionine at position 215, just N-terminal to the interheavy chain disulfide bond (108). Cleavage by cyanogen bromide under mild conditions occurs also at this position, giving rise to univalent 3.5 S molecules instead of the bivalent 5 S product formed upon treatment of molecules of allotype d12 under the same mild conditions (109).

The selective cleavage at these two methionyl bonds occurs in dilute HCl solution, whereas concentrated formic acid is used for cleavage adjacent to all methionine groups. The susceptibility of these bonds to attack by cyanogen bromide is attributable to a relatively loosely folded structure in the hinge region. The antigen-binding sites in Fab'' and F(ab'')$_2$ remain active after exposure of the molecule to the low pH (required for cyanogen bromide cleavage) followed by neutralization (105).

C. Rabbit IgM

In its general properties, rabbit IgM is very similar to the corresponding human immunoglobulin. It is a decavalent molecule (109a,110) of approximate molecular weight 900,000–950,000 which comprises five 4-chain (IgMs) subunits (111) together with a J chain (112), and has a relatively high carbohydrate content. The IgMs subunits are linked to one another only by interheavy chain disulfide bonds which are readily reduced at neutral pH; i.e., without disruption of the secondary structure of the molecule. H and L chains can be isolated from IgMs by conventional methods (113).

Studies of human IgM have been greatly facilitated by the occurrence of large amounts of protein in sera of patients with Waldenström's macroglobulinemia; owing to its high concentration in such sera the IgM can readily be isolated. Monoclonal IgM has not been available in the rabbit, and the isolation of pure IgM from normal rabbit serum is a rather formidable task. As indicated earlier, certain types of antigen stimulate a fairly good IgM response. Such antibodies can be specifically purified and then fractionated by gel filtration to remove any IgG antibody that is present. Another property that facilitates separation from IgG is the somewhat greater average negative charge, as well as size, of IgM which permits partial separation from IgG on a DEAE-cellulose column at neutral pH; IgM is retained at low ionic strength while most of the IgG is eluted (62).

There has been some controversy as to the valence of rabbit IgM. Earlier reports, based on hapten-binding studies, suggested a valence of 5 for IgM (114–118). It appears, however, that about half of the combining sites in some populations are of low affinity and are therefore not readily detected (109a,110). It is uncertain whether this heterogeneity reflects differences in affinity of the combining sites of an individual molecule or heterogeneity of the population of IgM molecules. One would tend to favor the latter possibility on the basis that most antibody-producing cells synthesize a single species of L and H chain (119). It is conceivable, however, that some of the binding sites are subject to steric interference and therefore exhibit an artifically low binding affinity.

D. Rabbit IgA

IgA constitutes the major immunoglobulin of rabbit colostrum or milk, from which it can be isolated by gel filtration and ion-exchange chromatography (120). Since the isolation of IgA from serum is difficult, because of its low concentration, most studies of the physical and chemical properties of rabbit IgA have made use of the colostral protein, which is designated secretory IgA or sIgA. Rabbit colostral IgA has a molecular weight of 370,000 to 400,000 (121) and comprises two 7 S monomers (150,000 each), secretory component (∼ 70,000) (122,123), and a J chain (15,000) (123,124). As in other species, the J chain is disulfide-bonded to rabbit IgA through its Fc fragment. There are conflicting data as to whether or not disulfide bonds link all molecules of secretory component to rabbit IgA (120–123),[4] but there is general agreement that strong noncovalent forces are involved. The latter can be disrupted by concentrated guanidine hydrochloride; this permits separation of free secretory component by gel filtration.

---

[4] Dr. Katherine Knight has found that secretory component is disulfide bonded to all molecules bearing f-locus determinants, and that in some or all molecules with g-locus determinants it is linked only through noncovalent forces (personal communication).

Two major subclasses of rabbit sIgA, differing with respect to antigenic determinants in their H chains, have been described. These have not as yet been given designations (such as IgA1 and IgA2) but rather are defined through the existence of nonallelic allotypic markers controlled by the f and g loci (Chapter 9). Molecules of sIgA bearing f-locus determinants are much more resistant to the action of papain at neutral pH. Molecules with g-locus determinants are readily susceptible to digestion, yielding $Fab_{2\alpha}$ and $Fc_{2\alpha}$ fragments. This differential susceptibility provides a means of isolating Fc fragments bearing determinants controlled by the g locus; this in turn has made it possible to prepare monospecific antisera useful in the antigenic analysis of IgA (Chapter 9).

E. Rabbit IgE

Because of its very low serum concentration, rabbit IgE has not been isolated in a pure state. We have no precise estimate of its concentration in serum, but, from its general properties and by analogy with human IgE, its normal concentration is probably less than 1 μg per ml.

Despite its unavailability in a pure state, the evidence for the existence of a rabbit immunoglobulin corresponding to human IgE is quite strong (125–130). It appears to be the major homocytotropic antibody in the rabbit and, in common with the human protein, has a sedimentation coefficient of 8 S and a molecular weight of about 200,000. Approximations of molecular size are made by ultracentrifugation; fractions are assayed for the biological activity of the protein as a skin-sensitizing antibody. The molecule migrates in the fast gamma region upon immunoelectrophoresis. It loses reaginic activity upon heating to 60°C or upon mild reduction of disulfide bonds. Another important resemblance to human IgE is the long optimal latent period for skin sensitization (about 3 days) and the prolonged persistence of sensitization, for 2 to 3 weeks. The molecule is not subject to inactivation by treatment with antibody against rabbit IgG, IgM or IgA, but can be neutralized by an appropriately absorbed antiserum prepared against a fraction of serum enriched for reagin, or by antiserum to rabbit L chains.

The likelihood of elicitation of an IgE response to an antigen is enhanced by inoculation into the footpads (126–128). As indicated earlier, certain parasites induce the formation of relatively high titers of the homocytotropic antibody. Reports vary as to the possibility of elicitation of an anamnestic response.

A more complete discussion of the general biological properties of IgE, which applies to many species, is given in Chapter 3.

VI. GUINEA PIG IMMUNOGLOBULINS

A. Guinea Pig IgG

Guinea pig serum contains the major immunoglobulin classes found in many other mammalian species. As noted earlier, the nature of the subclasses of IgG varies markedly among species. In the guinea pig there are two major subclasses, IgG1 and IgG2 (Table 8.1). Each has a sedimentation coefficient of about 7 S and a low carbohydrate content (2–3%). The two subclasses, by definition, possess shared as well as unique antigenic determinants, present on H chains, and exhibit strong antigenic cross-reactivity (131–133). Peptide mapping indicates very close similarity of the Fab fragments of IgG1 and IgG2, but fewer than half of the spots in peptide maps of the Fc fragments of the two proteins appear in the same positions (134). The subclasses differ also with respect to average electrophoretic mobility, with IgG1 having the greater anodal mobility at slightly alkaline pH. Antibodies of the IgG1 subclass will sensitize guinea pigs for local and systemic anaphylaxis and fix complement only through the alternate pathway (135,136). A second heat-stable IgG subclass with anaphylactic activity has been described (41). It is distinct from IgG1 and IgG2, has a high average anodal electrophoretic mobility at neutral pH, and persists in the skin for long periods of time. IgG2 is incapable of mediating passive anaphylactic reactions but fixes complement by the conventional mechanism; it is involved in causing cell lysis or the Arthus reaction (135,137). IgG2 can be isolated free of IgG1, but the reverse is difficult to accomplish (138).

In general, IgG1 molecules are present in much lower concentration than IgG2 in the sera of nonimmunized animals, but the relative and total concentration of IgG1 may increase markedly upon challenge with certain antigens without the use of adjuvant; complete Freund's adjuvant tends to stimulate formation of IgG2 (133).

Digestion of guinea pig IgG with papain results in the formation of two fragments, designated S (slow) and F (fast anodal electrophoretic mobility) which can be separated by starch block electrophoresis, and which comprise fragments Fab and Fc, respectively (131,139). The Fc fragments of IgG1 (but apparently not IgG2) are readily crystallized (139). Peptic digestion and subsequent reduction proceed in a manner very similar to that of rabbit or human IgG (138). L and H chains from each subclass can be separated by conventional means (139); the two subclasses cannot be differentiated from one another or from other guinea pig immunoglobulins on the basis of their L chains.

B. Guinea Pig IgE

In the guinea pig, homocytotropic antibodies comprise molecules of IgE and of two subclasses of IgG (30,39,41). They can be elicited, for example, by immunization with polymerized *Ascaris suum* antigen followed by subsequent injection of the larvae of this parasite. As in the case of rabbit IgE a low serum concentration precludes the isolation in a pure state of guinea pig IgE. Thus IgE activity is determined by bioassay, in this case by the Prausnitz–Küstner (P–K) and passive cutaneous anaphylactic (PCA) reactions. Reaginic activity, measured as P–K activity present after a 6-day latent period following subcutaneous injection of antibody, was found in the 11 S and 8 S regions on sucrose density gradients and in the corresponding fractions of eluates from Sephadex G-200. Both the 11 S and 8 S reaginic activities could be absorbed by a rabbit antiserum active against guinea pig IgE or by monospecific rabbit antiserum to human IgE. It was proposed that the 11 S molecule is a dimer of the 8 S antibody (30).

C. Guinea Pig Secretory IgA

The properties of this class appear entirely analogous to those of human IgA. IgA is a very minor component in guinea pig serum and has not been studied in detail. Secretory IgA can be isolated from guinea pig milk by gel filtration, ion-exchange chromatography, and zone electrophoresis (140). The protein has the typical sedimentation coefficient of 11 S. In Ouchterlony analysis, antibody to sIgA reacts with a component of serum but sIgA forms a spur over the serum IgA; the spur is attributable to the presence of secretory component. Antigenic analysis revealed the presence of free (as well as bound) secretory component in guinea pig milk. As in many other mammals. the majority of antibody-producing cells in the intestinal mucosa of the guinea pig synthesize molecules of the IgA class (140).

VII. MOUSE IMMUNOGLOBULINS

A. Mouse IgG

Table 8.1 lists the subclasses of mouse IgG, which are defined on the basis of differences in their C_H regions. Additional discussion of their properties may be found in Chapter 9, which considers allotypy. As in the case of human immunoglobulins the availability of myeloma proteins has been an invaluable aid to structural studies, since such proteins are homogeneous and can be purified readily in good yield. For example, molecules of the IgG2a and IgG2b subclasses overlap to such an extent in their properties that it is virtually impossible to separate them from one another with normal serum as the source. Even normal IgG1, which has a somewhat greater average anodal electrophoretic mobility than IgG2, is difficult to isolate in a pure state. When molecules of these subclasses occur in high concentration as myeloma proteins they can, however, be separated with little difficulty. Antiserum monospecific for a particular class or subclass is generally prepared by using a myeloma protein as the immunogen and absorbing the antiserum with myeloma proteins of other classes and subclasses.

Multiple myeloma can be induced by intraperitoneal injection of mineral oil, certain other hydrocarbons, or solid plastics into BALB/c or NZB mice, or F_1 hybrids of these two strains, but rarely in any other strains (7,141–144).[5] An alternative, but less consistent method of eliciting high concentrations of apparently monoclonal protein is through the induction of leukemias with carcinogens (145–146); although this method may be applicable to a number of strains the associated serum proteins have not been extensively investigated.

An interesting method, devised by Potter and Lieberman, permits the induction of myeloma proteins corresponding in structure to the immunoglobulins of a variety of strains in addition to BALB/c and NZB (7,142). BALB/c mice are mated to a second strain (for example, C57BL), and the F_1 offspring are backcrossed to BALB/c mice. Those progeny which exhibit the allotypic (C_H region) determinants of C57BL are backcrossed to BALB/c. Again, offspring carrying the C57BL allotype are mated to BALB/c. After this is repeated for a number of generations, the resulting hybrid mice are mated and those which are homozygous for the C57BL allotype are selected. It is apparent that such congenic mice will have most characteristics of the BALB/c strain except for the allotype of their immunoglobulins and any closely linked traits. Multiple myeloma can be artificially induced in such mice, but the myeloma protein has H chains with C_H and probably V_H regions encoded by C57BL structural genes. (The linkage of V_H to C_H genes in the mouse is discussed in Chapter 11.)

Myeloma proteins have been used in the vast majority of structural studies. The incidence of immunoglobulin classes associated with tumors induced in BALB/c mice in several laboratories, as compiled by

---

[5] The genetic factors causing susceptibility are unknown.

Potter (147), is: IgA, 74%; IgG1, 10%; IgG2b, 8%; IgG2a, 7%; IgM, 0.5%; IgG3, 0.3%. These values do not include a small percentage of tumors producing only κ or λ chains, or a more substantial number (about one-fifth of all tumors) that are nonproducers of immunoglobulin. The high incidence of IgA tumors, which contrasts with the low serum concentration of IgA, may be related to the fact that tumors are induced within the peritoneum, where high concentrations of IgA-producing cells are localized on mucosal surfaces. It should be noted that the monoclonal IgA, found in serum or ascites fluid, does not contain secretory component and thus differs from secretory IgA. The monoclonal serum IgA may occur, however, as a variety of disulfide bonded polymers of 4-chain units, with sedimentation coefficients of 7S, 9S, 11S, or 13 S, corresponding to monomeric, dimeric, etc., forms of the basic 4-chain unit. As in human IgA, such polymers contain J chain (148). Evidence that the cells which become malignant may have already been stimulated by antigen includes the specific activity of certain myeloma proteins against antigens expected to be present in the mouse (Chapter 10), the idiotypic identity of certain of those myeloma proteins and induced antibodies of the same specificity (Chapter 11), and the low incidence of tumors in germ-free mice treated with mineral oil (149).

As in the human, a large proportion of mice with multiple myeloma excrete a urinary Bence Jones protein which, in an individual animal, is either κ or λ. The concentration is highly variable, ranging from a barely detectable level to a concentration as high as 50 mg/ml.

Most mouse myeloma and urinary Bence Jones proteins are of the κ type; the relatively low incidence of λ proteins is in accord with the low concentration of immunoglobulin of type λ in serum (3–5% of the total). The close similarity of the amino acid sequences of many λ chains, and sequences of κ chains and their subgroups, are discussed in Chapter 4.

Alternative nomenclatures are in use for the subclasses of mouse IgG; these are IgG2b (IgH), IgG2a (IgG), IgG1 (IgF). A more recently discovered class is IgG3 (150). The symbols in parentheses are the nomenclature of Potter and Lieberman (7). The other designations (IgG2b, etc.) are based on Fahey *et al.* (151,152).

IgG2a and IgG2b appear most closely related, sharing most but not all antigenic determinants, and overlapping greatly with respect to electrophoretic mobility (152). Both shared and unique allotypic determinants are associated with the two subclasses. In tryptic digests of fragment Fc, a number of peptides of IgG2a and IgG2b also are identical (142), but marked differences in amino acid sequences have been detected in the studies carried out so far (153).

Although very few IgG3 myeloma proteins have been detected, antiserum directed against unique, C_H region determinants of the IgG3 myeloma protein also reacts with a minor component of mouse serum, which is therefore assumed to be IgG3 (150).

All four subclasses of mouse IgG can be transported across the placenta; IgG3 is transported most rapidly (150,154). IgG2a and IgG2b fix guinea pig complement through the conventional pathway, whereas IgG1 and IgG3 do not (150,155,156). IgG1 molecules but not IgG2a, IgG2b or IgG3 are capable of mediating passive cutaneous anaphylactic (PCA) reactions in the mouse (150,157–159). Mouse IgG2a and IgG2b subclasses, but not IgG1, mediate the same reaction in the guinea pig (155,160–162).

Molecules of each IgG subclass are readily digested by papain to yield Fab and Fc fragments; the latter migrate more rapidly toward the anode than Fab during electrophoresis at neutral pH. Fc fragments of myeloma proteins of the IgA class can be crystallized (163), and the crystallized Fab fragments of an IgA myeloma protein are being studied by single-crystal X-ray diffraction methods (164). This work is of great interest because the myeloma protein has antibody-like activity directed toward the phosphorylcholine hapten group. Examination of diffraction patterns in the presence and absence of hapten has permitted localization of the active site in the three-dimensional structure. (See Chapter 5.)

Peptic digestion of mouse IgG has not provided large fragments in acceptable yields, possibly because mouse IgG unfolds at the low pH required for activity of the enzyme (165).

B. Mouse IgA

The structural properties of mouse secretory IgA are quite comparable to those of the human and guinea pig proteins in that both a secretory piece (mol. wt. 70,000) and a J chain (15,000) are present, as well as four H and four L chains (148,166–169).

The serum IgA, both normal and monoclonal, of BALB/c mice has an unusual disulfide bonded structure; the L chains are not disulfide bonded to H chains and, in most of the molecules, are disulfide bonded to one another (16,16a,17). At low pH, therefore, as the molecule dissociates into dimers of L chains and dimers of H chains as well as some monomers. In NZB mice, serum IgA has the typical disulfide bonded structure, with each L chain linked through a disulfide bond to an H chain (18). With respect to this structural feature NZB and BALB/c serum IgA proteins correspond to human IgA1 and to the $A_2m(1)$ allotype of human IgA2, respectively.

An interesting enzymatic cleavage of a mouse IgA myeloma protein (MOPC 315), having antibody activity against the Dnp hapten group, was reported by Inbar *et al.* (169a). Digestion with pepsin at pH 3.7 liberates a univalent fragment consisting only of the V_H and V_L domains, joined by noncovalent interactions. The active site remains intact and the fragment contains essentially all of the idiotypic determinants of the intact molecule (Chapter 11).

VIII. HORSE IMMUNOGLOBULINS

Historically, horse immunoglobulins have been of interest because of the use of horse antiserums, such as antitetanus toxin or antidiphtheria toxin, for therapeutic purposes. These are less widely employed now owing to the advent of antibiotics, the development of improved vaccines, and the hazards of serum sickness associated with inoculation of horse proteins into patients. Horse immunoglobulins are less thoroughly characterized, with respect to amino acid sequence, than mouse and human immunoglobulins, in part because equine myeloma proteins are not available.

The classes of immunoglobulins found in the horse are typical of most mammalian species; they include IgG, IgM, and IgA. To our knowledge, the presence in the horse of homocytropic antibodies, analogous to human IgE, has not been reported, but this may only reflect the difficulty in working with a large animal.

Horse IgG comprises several subclasses, designated IgGa, IgGb, IgGc, IgGl, and IgG(T) (170,171). For some time it was thought that IgG(T), which has the fastest average anodal electrophoretic mobility of the subclasses, corresponds to the IgA of other species. This view was based on its relatively high carbohydrate content (172), its electrophoretic mobility, and its existence as a 10 S dimer, which is dissociable into 7 S monomeric units upon reduction (170,173). It is now generally accepted that IgG(T) is a subclass of IgG. Evidence relating Ig(T) to IgG, rather than IgA, is the close similarity of the amino acid sequences of a C-terminal octadecapeptide of IgG (pool of subclasses) and IgG(T) (174). IgG(T) and IgG also show strong immunological cross-reactivity (175,176), sharing some but not all specificities present on the H chain. More recently, molecules with the characteristics of secretory IgA, and differing from IgG(T), have been isolated from horse secretions (177,178). This appears to disprove the hypothesis that IgG(T) corresponds to human IgA and indicates that IgG(T) should be considered a subclass of IgG.

Subclasses IgGa and IgGb have the slowest average anodal electrophoretic mobilities of the horse immunoglobulins. IgGc migrates in the γ_1-region, IgGa and IgGb in the γ_2-region. IgGa and/or IgGb are capable of fixing guinea pig complement by the conventional pathway[6] whereas IgGc and IgG(T) are not (170). IgG(T) is a major component of commercial antisera, suggesting that its concentration increases during prolonged immunization with many antigens (175).

IgG(T) exists in serum in the form of 7 S and 10 S molecules; the latter is a disulfide bonded dimer of the former. The disulfide bond may be formed by an extra half-cystine, present in the Fd fragment of IgG(T) but not the other subclasses of IgG (175). This extra disulfide bond may be responsible for the fact that digestion of IgG(T) with papain liberates 5 S bivalent fragments rather than the univalent 3.5 S product obtained from the other horse IgG subclasses (175,179).

Rockey (171) was able to identify eight antigenically distinguishable immunoglobulins in a purified horse antihapten antibody preparation (anti-*p*-azophenyl-β-lactoside). Under current terminology six of these would be designated IgGa, IgGb, IgGc, IgG(T), IgM, and IgG1 (10 S); an additional component with IgG(T) mobility and another migrating between IgGb and IgGc were noted.

An immunoglobulin with one or more unique antigenic determinants and a tendency to form aggregates had been observed earlier by Sandor *et al.* in certain horse antibacterial antisera, where it occurs in high concentration (180,181). The work of Zolla and Goodman (182) showed that such aggregated immunoglobulin can be dissociated without breaking covalent bonds (by urea, for example). They were also able to identify the component in all normal horse sera tested. On the basis of electrophoretic mobility, and its possession of some but not all antigenic determinants in common with IgG (176), the protein might be designated IgG1. It may correspond to Rockey's 10 S IgG1 immunoglobulin. The protein has been variously referred to as IgB (182a), "atypical macroglobulin," "aggregating immunoglobulin," or "γ_1-component."

Isolated IgGc, or a mixture or IgGa and IgGb, has a carbohydrate content of about 3%; that of IgG(T) is about twice as great. An unusual property of IgG(T) is the presence of about half of its carbohydrate in the Fd segment of the H chain (175).

Horse IgM has the typical pentameric structure, a high carbohydrate content and a molecular weight of 900,000 (173,183,184). The sIgA molecule closely resembles its counterpart in other mammalian species; it contains secretory component and J chain and has a sedimentation coefficient of 11 S (178).

---

[6] The assay for complement fixation was carried out with a mixture of IgGa and IgGb.

IX. PASSIVE CUTANEOUS ANAPHYLACTIC REACTIONS IN GUINEA PIGS MEDIATED BY HETEROLOGOUS IMMUNOGLOBULINS

Extensive studies have been carried out on passive cutaneous anaphylactic reactions (PCA) in guinea pigs. Much of this work has been done by Ovary and his collaborators (185,186). The technique generally employed consists of injection of antiserum, purified immunoglobulin, or its fragments intradermally into a nonimmune guinea pig. This is followed 4 hours later by intravenous inoculation of a saline solution containing specific antigen or an antiglobulin reagent and Evans Blue dye. The occurrence of an antigen-antibody reaction at the intradermal site results in vascular permeability and the appearance of a blue spot on the internal surface of the skin; its size provides a semiquantitative measure of the severity of the reaction. The test is very sensitive; it is capable of detecting as little as 0.02 μg of antibody. Immunoglobulins that can mediate PCA after intradermal injection are stated to be capable of "fixation" to the skin site. The cell type responsible is believed to be the mast cell, which liberates histamine and serotonin (187). As indicated above, two heat-stable classes of guinea pig immunoglobulin (IgG1 and a more negatively charged IgG subclass) and IgE, which is heat labile, are capable of mediating passive cutaneous anaphylactic reactions in guinea pigs.

The class of molecule from a heterologous species that mediates PCA in the guinea pig may differ from the class that causes the reaction in the autologous species. For example, mouse IgG2 (probably IgG2a) causes PCA in guinea pigs, but only mouse IgG1 causes PCA in mice (35). Human IgG1, IgG3, and IgG4, but not IgG2 (188) mediate PCA in guinea pigs but do not cause the Prausnitz–Küstner reaction in man. IgG of the monkey, rabbit, rat, or dog, but not of the horse, mediates PCA in guinea pigs (185). The portion of the IgG molecule that fixes to guinea pig skin is the Fc fragment; thus, intravenous inoculation of an anti-Fc reagent can cause PCA after intradermal inoculation of the Fc fragments of those IgG molecules that are capable of fixation to skin. The antiglobulin may be injected intravenously as whole serum, its IgG fraction, or as the F(ab')$_2$ fragments of the antiglobulin antibody; Fab fragments of the antiglobulin are inactive, indicating a requirement for bivalence. In contrast to fragment Fc, fragments Fab, Fab' and F(ab')$_2$ are incapable of "fixing" to guinea pig skin. The site on the Fc fragment of rabbit IgG that is involved in PCA differs from that responsible for complement fixation (189). The classes other than IgG from heterologous species have not been shown to be capable of fixation to guinea pig skin.

REFERENCES

1. Melcher, U., Vitetta, E.S., McWilliams, M., Lamm, M.E., Phillips-Quagliata, J.M., Uhr, J.W. (1974). *J. Exp. Med.* **140**, 1427.
1a. Hood, L.E., Gray, W.R., Sanders, B.G., and Dreyer, W.J. (1967). *Cold Spring Harbor Symp. Quant. Biol.* **32**, 133.
2. Nussenzweig, V., Lamm, M.E., and Benacerraf, B. (1966). *J. Exp. Med.* **124**, 787.
3. Appella, E., Mage, R.G., Dubiski, S., and Reisfeld, R.A. (1968). *Proc. Nat. Acad. Sci. U.S.* **60**, 975.
4. McIntire, K.R., Asofsky, R., Potter, M., and Kuff, E.L. (1965). *Science* **150**, 361.
5. Rude, E., and Givol, D. (1968). *Biochem. J.* **107**, 449.
6. Carbonara, A., and Mancini, G. (1968). *Atti Ass. Genet. Ital.* **13**, 229.
7. Potter, M., and Lieberman, R. (1967). *Advan. Immunol.* **7**, 91.
8. de Vries, G.M., Lanckman, M., and Hamers, R. (1969). *Eur. J. Biochem.* **11**, 370.
9. Nussenzweig, V., and Benacerraf, B. (1966). *J. Exp. Med.* **124**, 805.
10. Blomberg, B., Geckeler, W., and Weigert, M.G. (1972). *Science* **177**, 178.
10a. Parkhouse, R.M.E., Askonas, B.A., and Dourmashkin, R.R. (1970). *Immunology* **18**, 575.
11. Tomasi, T.B., and Grey, H.M. (1972). *Progr. Allergy* **16**, 83.
12. Vaerman, J.P. (1973). *In* "Research in Immunochemistry and Immunobiology" (J.B.G. Kwapinski and E.D. Day, eds.), pp. 99. University Park Press, Baltimore, Maryland.
13. Heremans, J.F., and Vaerman, J.P. (1971). *In* "Progress in Immunology"(D.B. Amos, ed.), p. 875. Academic Press, New York.
13a. Mestecky, J., and Lawton, A.R., III (eds.) (1973). *Advan. Exp. Med. Biol.* **45**, 1.
14. Grey, H.M., Abel, C.A., Yount, W.J., and Kunkel, H.G. (1968). *J. Exp. Med.* **128**, 1223.
15. Jerry, L.M., Kunkel, H.G., and Grey, H.M. (1970). *Proc. Nat. Acad. Sci. U.S.* **65**, 557.
16. Abel, C.A., and Grey, H.M. (1968). *Biochemistry* **7**, 2682.
16a. Seki, T.E., Appella, F., and Itano, H.A. (1968). *Proc. Nat. Acad. Sci. U.S.* **61**, 1071.
17. Grey, H.M., Sher, A., and Shalitin, N. (1970). *J. Immunol.* **105**, 75.
18. Warner, N.L., and Marchalonis, J.J. (1972). *J. Immunol.* **109**, 657.
19. Mehta, P.D., Reichlin, M., and Tomasi, T.B., Jr. (1972). *J. Immunol.* **109**, 1272.
19a. Neoh, S.N., Jahoda, D.M., Rowe, D.S., and Voller, A. (1973). *Immunochemistry* **10**, 805.
20. Orlans, E., and Feinstein, A. (1971). *Nature (London)* **223**, 45.
21. Vaerman, J.P., Querinjean, P., and Heremans, J.F. (1971). *Immunology* **21**, 443.
21a. Becker, E.L., and Austin, K.F. (1966). *J. Exp. Med.* **124**, 379.
22. Ishizaka, K., and Ishizaka, T. (1971). *Ann. N.Y. Acad. Sci.* **190**, 443.
23. Bennich, H., and Johansson, S.G.O. (1971). *Advan. Immunol.* **13**, 1.
24. Ishizaka, K., and Ishizaka, T. (1971). *In* "Progress in Immunology" (B. Amos, editor), Vol. I, p. 859. Academic Press, New York.
24a. Ishizaka, K. (1973). *In* "The Antigens" (M. Sela, ed.) Vol. 1, p. 479. Academic Press, New York.
25. Halliwell, R.E., Schwartzman, R.M., and Rockey, J.H. (1972). *Clin. Exp. Immunol.* **10**, 339.
26. Kanyerezi, B., Jaton, J-C., and Bloch, K.J. (1971). *J. Immunol.* **106**, 1411.

27. Liakopoulou, A., and Perelmutter, L. (1971). *J. Immunol.* **107**, 131.
28. Dobson, C., Rockey, J.H., and Soulsby, E.J.L. (1971). *J. Immunol.* **197**, 1431.
29. Schwartz, H.A., and Levine, B.B. (1973). *J. Immunol.* **110**, 1638
30. Zvaifler, N.J., and Robinson, J.O. (1969). *J. Exp. Med.* **130**, 907.
31. Levine, B.B., Chang, H., Jr., and Vaz, M.M. (1971). *J. Immunol.* **106**, 29.
32. Vaz, N.M., and Ovary, Z. (1968). *J. Immunol.* **100**, 169.
33. Levine, B.B., and Pfister, L. (1972). *J. Allergy* **49**, 92.
34. Nussenzweig, R.S., Merryman, C., and Benacerraf, B. (1964). *J. Exp. Med.* **120**, 315.
35. Ovary, Z., Vaz, N.M., and Warner, N.L. (1970). *Immunology* **19**, 715.
36. Ovary, Z., and Warner, N.L. (1972). *J. Immunol.* **108**, 1055.
37. Moto, I., Wong, D., and Sadum, E.H. (1968). *Life Sci.* **7**, 1289.
38. Barth, W.F., and Fahey, J.F. (1965). *Nature (London)* **206**, 730.
39. Ovary, Z., Benacerraf, B., and Bloch, K.J. (1963). *J. Exp. Med.* **117**, 951.
40. Nussenzweig, V., Benacerraf, B., and Ovary, Z. (1969). *J. Immunol.* **103**, 1152.
41. Parish, W.E. (1970). *J. Immunol.* **105**, 1296.
42. Bach, M.K., Bloch, K.J., and Austen, K.F. (1971). *J. Exp. Med.* **133**, 752.
43. Henson, P.M., and Cochrane, C.G. (1969). *J. Exp. Med.* **129**, 153.
44. Levine, B.B., and Vaz, N.M. (1970). *Int. Arch. Allergy Appl. Immunol.* **39**, 156.
45. Orr, T.S.C., and Blair, A.M.J.N. (1969). *Life Sci.* **8**, 1073.
46. Bloch, K.J., Ohman, J.L., Jr., Waltin, J., and Cygan, R.W. (1973). *J. Immunol.* **110**, 197.
47. Bloch, K.J. (1967). *Progr. Allergy* **10**, 84.
48. Rejnek, J., Mage, R.G., and Reisfeld, R.A. (1969). *J. Immunol.* **102**, 638.
49. Rejnek, J., Appella, E., Mage, R.G., and Reisfeld, R.A. (1969). *Biochemistry* **8**, 2712.
50. Dray, S., and Nisonoff, A. (1963). *Proc. Soc. Exp. Biol. Med.* **113**, 20.
51. Franek, F., and Nezlin, R.S. (1963). *Folia Microbiol.* **8**, 128.
52. Strosberg, A.D., Fraser, K.J., Margolies, M.N., and Haber, E. (1972). *Biochemistry* **11**, 4978.
53. Strosberg, A.D., Margolies, M.N., and Haber, E. (1974). *Fed. Amer. Soc. Exp. Biol. Proc.* **33**, 726.
54. Zikan, J., Skarova, B., and Rejnek, J. (1967). *Folia Microbiol.* **12**, 162.
55. Dubiski, S. (1967). *Nature (London)* **214**, 1365.
56. Brambell, F.W.R., Hemmings, W.A., Oakley, C.L., and Porter, R.R. (1960). *Proc. Roy. Soc. Ser.* **B.151**, 478.
57. Ovary, Z., and Karush, F. (1961). *J. Immunol.* **86**, 146.
58. Ishizaka, K., Ishizaka, T., and Sugahara, T. (1962). *J. Immunol.* **88**, 690.
59. Taliaferro, W.H., and Talmage, D.W. (1956). *J. Infect. Dis.* **99**, 21.
60. Weigle, W.O. (1958). *J. Immunol.* **81**, 204.
61. Kekwick, R.A. (1950). *Biochem. J.* **34**, 1248.
62. Levy, H.B., and Sober, H.A. (1960). *Proc. Soc. Exp. Med. Biol.* **103**, 250.
63. Onoue, K., Yagi, Y., and Pressman, D. (1964). *J. Immunol.* **92**, 173.
64. Rodkey, L.S., and Freeman, M.J. (1969). *J. Immunol.* **102**, 713.
65. Parfentjev, I.A. (1936). U.S. Patent 2,065,196.
66. Porter, R.R. (1958). *Nature (London)* **182**, 670.
67. Porter, R.R. (1959). *Biochem. J.* **73**, 119.
68. Fleischman, J.B., Porter, R.R., and Press, E.M. (1963). *Biochem. J.* **88**, 220.
69. Palmer, J.L., Mandy, W.J., and Nisonoff, A. (1962). *Proc. Nat. Acad. Sci. U.S.* **48**, 49.
70. Nisonoff, A., Winkler, M.H., and Pressman, D. (1959). *J. Immunol.* **82**, 201.

71. Palmer, J.L., and Nisonoff, A. (1964). *Biochemistry* **3**, 863.
72. Inman, F.P., and Nisonoff, A. (1966). *J. Biol. Chem.* **241**, 322.
73. Hill, R.L., Delaney, R., Fellows, R.E., and Lebovitz, H.E. (1966). *Proc. Nat. Acad. Sci. U.S.* **56**, 1765.
74. Hill, R.L., Delaney, R., Lebovitz, H.E., and Fellows, R.E. (1966). *Proc. Roy. Soc. Ser.* **B.166**, 159.
75. Poljak, R.J., Goldstein, D.J., Humphrey, R.L., and Dintzis, H.M. (1967). *Cold Spring Harbor Symp. Quant. Biol.* **32**, 95.
76. Nisonoff, A., Wissler, F.C., Lipman, L.N., and Woernley, D.L. (1960). *Arch. Biochem. Biophys.* **89**, 230.
77. Nisonoff, A., Wissler, F.C., and Lipman, L.N. (1960). *Science* **132**, 1770.
78. Fudenberg, H.H., Mandy, W.J., and Nisonoff, A. (1962). *J. Clin. Invest.* **41**, 2123.
79. Goodman, J.W. (1963). *Science* **139**, 1292.
80. Utsumi, S., and Karush, F. (1965). *Biochemistry* **4**, 1776.
81. Prahl, J.W. (1967). *Biochem. J.* **104**, 647.
82. Charlwood, P.A., and Utsumi, S. (1969). *Biochem. J.* **112**, 357.
83. Amiraian, K., and Ovary, Z. (1969). *J. Immunol.* **103**, 716.
84. Matthews, N., Stewart, G., and Stanworth, D.R. (1971). *Immunochemistry* **8**, 973.
84a. Utsumi, S. (1969) *Biochem. J.* **112**, 343.
85. Nisonoff, A., and Dixon, F. (1964). *Biochemistry* **3**, 1338.
86. Mole, L.E., Jackson, S.A., Porter, R.R., and Wilkinson, J.M. (1971). *Biochem. J.* **124**, 308.
87. Mandy, W.J., Rivers, M.M., and Nisonoff, A. (1961). *J. Biol. Chem.* **236**, 3221.
88. Nisonoff, A. (1960). *Biochem. Biophys. Res. Commun.* **3**, 466.
89. Nisonoff, A., and Rivers, M.M. (1961). *Arch. Biochem. Biophys.* **93**, 460.
90. Nisonoff, A., and Mandy, W.J. (1962). *Nature* (*London*) **194**, 355.
91. Nisonoff, A., and Palmer, J.L. (1964). *Science* **143**, 376.
92. Aoki, T., Boyse, E.A., Old, L.J., de Harven, E., Hämmerling, U., and Wood, H.A. (1970). *Proc. Nat. Acad. Sci. U.S.* **65**, 569.
93. Stackpole, C W., Aoki, T., Boyse, E.A., Old, L.J., Lumleyn, J., Frank, J., and de Harven, E. (1971). *Science* **172**, 472.
94. Fudenberg, H.H., Drews, G., and Nisonoff, A. (1964). *J. Exp. Med.* **119**, 151.
95. Jandl, J.H., and Simmons, R.L. (1957). *Brit. J. Haematol.* **3**, 19.
96. Hämmerling, U., Aoki, T., de Harven, E., Boyse, E.A., and Old, L.J. (1968). *J. Exp. Med.* **128**, 1461.
97. Aoki, T., Wood, H.A., Old, L.J., Boyse, E.A., de Harven, E., Lardis, M., and Stackpole, C.W. (1971). *Virology* **45**, 858.
98. Putnam, F.W., Easley, C.W., and Lynn, L.T. (1962). *Biochim. Biophys. Acta* **58**, 279.
99. Givol, D. (1967). *Biochem. J.* **104**, 39c.
100. Ghetie, V. and Mihaescu, S. (1973). *Immunochemistry* **10**, 251.
100a. Connell, G.E., and Porter, R.R. (1971). *Biochem. J.* **124**, 53P.
100b. Nelson, C.A. (1964). *J. Biol. Chem.* **239**, 3727.
100c. Goodman, J.W. (1965). *Biochemistry* **4**, 2350.
100d. Michaelsen, T.E., and Natvig, J.B. (1972). *Scand. J. Immunol.* **1**, 255.
101. Gross, E., and Winthrop, B. (1964). *J. Biol. Chem.* **237**, 1856.
102. Givol, D., and Porter, R.R. (1965). *Biochem. J.* **97**, 32c.
103. Cebra, J.J., Steiner, L.A., and Porter, R.R. (1968). *Biochem. J.* **107**, 79.
104. Hill, R.L., Lebovitz, H.E., Fellows, R.E., Jr., and Delaney, R. (1967). *3rd Nobel Symp.* p. 109. Wiley (Interscience), New York.
105. Cahnmann, H.J., Arnon, R., and Sela, M. (1965). *J. Biol. Chem.* **240**, 2762.

106. Lahav, M., Arnon, R., and Sela, M. (1967). *J. Exp. Med.* **125**, 787.
107. Givol, D., and De Lorenzo, F. (1968). *J. Biol. Chem.* **243**, 1886.
108. Prahl, J.W., Mandy, W.J., and Todd, C.W. (1969). *Biochemistry* **8**, 4935.
109. Kindt, T.J., Mandy, W.J., and Todd, C.W. (1970). *Immunochemistry* **7**, 467.
109a. Onoue, K., Grossberg, A.L., Yagi, Y., and Pressman, D. (1968). *Science* **162**, 574.
110. Kishimoto, T., and Onoue, K. (1971). *J. Immunol.* **106**, 341.
111. Lamm, M.E., and Small, P.A., Jr. (1966). *Biochemistry* **5**, 267.
112. Weinheimer, P.F., Mestecky, J., and Acton, R.T. (1971). *J. Immunol.* **107**, 1211.
113. Robbins, J.B., Kenny, K., and Suter, E. (1965). *J. Exp. Med.* **122**, 385.
114. Onoue, K., Yagi, Y., Grossberg, A., and Pressman, D. (1965). *Immunochemistry* **2**, 401.
115. Voss, E.W., Jr., and Eisen, H.N. (1968). *Fed. Proc. Fed. Amer. Soc. Exp. Biol.* **27**, 2631.
116. Clem, L.W., and Small, P.A., Jr. (1968). *Fed. Proc. Fed. Amer. Soc. Exp. Biol.* **27**, 2633.
117. Schrohenloher, R.E., and Barry, C.B. (1968). *J. Immunol.* **100**, 1006.
118. Lindqvist, K., and Baer, D.C. (1966). *Immunochemistry* **3**, 373.
119. Mäkelä, O., and Cross, A.M. (1970). *Progr. Allergy* **14**, 145.
120. Cebra, J.J., and Robbins, J.B. (1966). *J. Immunol.* **97**, 12.
121. Cebra, J.J., and Small, P.A., Jr. (1967). *Biochemistry* **6**, 503.
122. Tomasi, T.B. Jr., and Bienenstock, J. (1968). *Advan. Immunol.* **9**, 1.
123. Halpern, M.S., and Koshland, M.E. (1970). *Nature (London)* **228**, 1276.
124. O'Daly, J.A., and Cebra, J.J. (1971). *Biochemistry* **10**, 3843.
125. Zvaifler, N.J., and Becker, E.L. (1966). *J. Exp. Med.* **123**, 935.
126. Lindqvist, K. (1969). *Immunochemistry* **5**, 525.
127. Zvaifler, N.J., and Robinson, J.O. (1969). *J. Exp. Med.* **130**, 1969.
128. Henson, P.M., and Cochrane, C. G. (1969). *J. Exp. Med.* **129**, 153.
129. Richerson, H.B., Ching, H.F., and Seebohm, P.M. (1968). *J. Immunol.* **101**, 1291.
130. Ishizaka T., Ishizaka K., Bennich H., and Johanson, S.G.O. (1970). *J. Immunol.* **104**, 854.
131. Thorbecke, G.J., Benacerraf, B., and Ovary, Z. (1963). *J. Immunol.* **91**, 670.
132. White, R.G., Jenkins, G.C., and Wilkinson, P.C. (1963). *Int. Arch. Allergy Appl. Immuhol.* **22**, 156.
133. Benacerraf, B., Ovary, Z., Bloch, K.J., and Franklin, E.C. (1963). *J. Exp. Med.* **117**, 937.
134. Lamm, M.E., Lisowska-Bernstein, B., and Nussenzweig, V. (1967). *Biochemistry* **6**, 2819.
135. Ovary, Z., Benacerraf, B., and Bloch, J.J. (1963). *J. Exp. Med.* **117**, 951.
136. Sandberg, A.L., and Osler, A.G. (1971). *J. Immunol.* **107**, 1268.
137. Bloch, K.J., Kourilsky, F.M., Ovary, Z., and Benacerraf, B. (1963). *J. Exp. Med.* **117**, 965.
138. Nussenzweig, V., and Benacerraf, B. (1967). *3rd Nobel Symp. Gamma Globulins—Structure and Control of Biosynthesis*, p. 233. Interscience, New York.
139. Nussenzweig, V., and Benacerraf, B. (1964). *J. Immunol.* **93**, 1008.
140. Vaerman, J.P., and Heremans, J.F. (1972). *J. Immunol.* **108**, 637.
141. Merwin, R.M., and Redmon, L.W., (1963). *J. Nat. Cancer Inst.* **31**, 998.
142. Potter, M., and Lieberman, R. (1967). *Cold Spring Harbor Symp. Quant. Biol.* **32**, 187.
143. Herzenberg, L.A., and Warner, N.L. (1967). *In* "Regulation of the Immune Response" (B. Cinader, ed.), p. 322. Thomas, Springfield, Illinois.
144. Warner, N.L., (1967). *J. Immunol.* **107**, 937.

145. Rask-Nielsen, R., and Gormsen, H. (1956). *J. Nat. Cancer Inst.* **16,** 1137.
146. Rask-Nielsen, R., McIntire, K.R., and Ebbesen, P. (1968). *J. Nat. Cancer Inst.* **41,** 495.
147. Potter, M. (1972). *Physiol. Rev.* **52,** 631.
148. Halpern, M.S., and Coffman, R.L. (1972). *J. Immunol.* **109,** 674.
149. McIntire, H.R., and Princler, G.L. (1969). *Immunology* **17,** 481.
150. Grey, A.M., Hirst, J.W., and Cohn, M. (1971). *J. Exp. Med.* **133,** 289.
151. Fahey, J.L., Wunderlich, J., and Mishell, R. (1964). *J. Exp. Med.* **120,** 223.
152. Fahey, J.L., Wunderlich, J., and Mishell, R.J. (1964). *J. Exp. Med.* **120,** 243.
153. de Preval, C., Pink, J.R.L., and Milstein, C. (1970). *Nature (London)* **228,** 930.
154. Fahey, J.L., and Barth, J.L. (1965). *Proc. Soc. Exp. Biol. Med.* **111,** 596.
155. Nussenzweig, V. (1964). *J. Exp. Med.* **120,** 315.
156. Ovary, Z. (1966). *Ann. N.Y. Acad. Sci.* **129,** 776.
157. Ovary, Z. (1958). *Progr. Allergy* **5,** 459.
158. Ovary, Z. (1958). *J. Immunol.* **81,** 355.
159. Ovary, Z. (1960). *Immunology* **3,** 13.
160. Barth, W.S., and Fahey, J.L. (1965). *Nature (London)* **206,** 730.
161. Warner, N.L., Vaz, N.M., and Ovary, Z., (1968). *Immunology* **14,** 725.
162. Ovary, Z., Barth, W.F., and Fahey, J.L. (1965). *J. Immunol.* **94,** 410.
163. Fahey, J.L. (1963). *J. Immunol.* **90,** 576.
164. Rudikoff, S., Potter, M. Segal, D.M., Padlon, E.A., and Davies, D.R. (1972). *Proc. Nat. Acad. Sci. U.S.* **69,** 3689.
165. Gorini, G., Medgyesi, G.A., and Doria, G. (1969). *J. Immunol.* **103,** 1132.
166. Nash, D.R., Deckers, C., and Heremans, J.F. (1970). *Fed. Proc. Fed. Amer. Soc. Exp. Biol.* **29,** 704.
167. Benveniste, J., Lespinats, G., and Salomon, J.C. (1971). *J. Immunol.* **107,** 1656.
168. Parkhouse, R.M.E. (1972). *Nature New Biol.* **236,** 9.
169. D.H. Dayton, Jr., P.A. Small, Jr., R.M. Channock, H.E. Kaufman and T.B. Tomasi, Jr. (eds.) (1969). "The Secretory Immunologic System." U.S. Government Printing Office, Washington, D.C.
169a. Inbar, D., Hochman, J., and Givol, D. (1972). *Proc. Nat. Acad. Sci. U.S.* **69,** 2659.
170. Klinman, N.R., Rockey, J.H., Frauenberge, G., and Karush, F. (1966). *J. Immunol.* **96,** 587.
171. Rockey, J.H. (1967). *J. Exp. Med.* **125,** 249.
172. Heremans, J.F. (1959). *Clin. Chim. Acta* **4,** 96.
173. Rockey, J.H., Klinman, N.R., and Karush, F. (1964). *J. Exp. Med.* **120,** 589.
174. Weir, R.C., Porter, R.R., and Givol, D. (1966). *Nature (London)* **212,** 205.
175. Weir, R.C., and Porter, R.R. (1966). *Biochem. J.* **100,** 63.
176. Helms, C.M., and Allen, P.Z. (1970). *J. Immunol.* **105,** 1253.
177. Vaerman, J.P., Heremans, J.F., and Van Kerckhoven, G. (1969). *J. Immunol.* **103,** 1421.
178. Pahud, J.J., and Mach, J.P. (1972). *Int. Arch. Allergy Appl. Immunol.* **42,** 175.
179. Schultze, H.E., Haupt, H., Heide, K., Heimburger, N., and Schwick, H.G. (1965). *Immunochemistry* **2,** 273.
180. Sandor, G., Korach, S., and Mattern, P. (1964). *Nature (London)* **204,** 794.
181. Sandor, G., and Korach, S. (1966). *Ann. Inst. Pasteur Suppl. Paris* **111,** 7.
182. Zolla, S., and Goodman, J.W. (1968). *J. Immunol.* **100,** 880.
182a. Sandor, G., and Audibert, F. (1970). *C. R. Acad. Sci. Paris* **270,** 1538.
183. Helms, C.M., and Allen, P.Z. (1970). *J. Immunol.* **105,** 1253.
184. Kunkel, H.G. (1960). *In* "The Plasma Proteins" (F.W. Putnam, Ed.), Vol. 1, p. 229. Academic Press, New York.

185. Ovary Z. (1964). *In* "Immunological Methods" (J.F. Ackroyd, ed.), p. 259. Blackwell, Oxford.

186. Ovary, Z. (1966). *Ann. N.Y. Acad. Sci.* **129,** 776.

187. Prouvost-Danon, A., Peixoto, J.M., and Queiroz-Javierre M. (1966). *Life Sci.* **5,** 1867.

188. Ovary, Z., Kunkel, H.G., and Joslin, F.G. (1970). *J. Immunol.* **105,** 1103.

189. Amiraian, K., and Ovary, Z. (1969). *J. Immunol.* **103,** 716.

190. Waldmann, T.A., and Strober, W. (1969). *Progr. Allergy* **13,** 1.

191. Birshtein, B.K., Turner, K.J., and Cebra, J.J. (1971). *Biochemistry* **10,** 1.

192. Oliveira, B., and Lamm, M.E. (1971). *Biochemistry* **10,** 26.

193. LeFever, J.D., and Ishizaka, K. (1972). *J. Immunol.* **108,** 1698.

194. Pink, R., Wang, A.C., and Fudenberg, H.H. (1971). *Annu. Rev. Med.* **22,** 145.

195. Bloemmen, J., and Eyssen, H. (1973). *Eur J. Immunol.* **3,** 117.

196. Milstein, C., and Pink, J.R.L. (1970). *Progr. Biophys. Mol. Biol.* **21,** 209.

197. dePreval, C., and Fougereau, M. (1972). *Eur. J. Biochem.* **30,** 452.

9

Allotypes of Rabbit, Human, and Mouse Immunoglobulins

I. INTRODUCTION

In this chapter we will discuss the genetically controlled polymorphism of immunoglobulins, a property first discovered in 1956 by Grubb (1) and Oudin (2,3) through studies of antigenic determinants of human and rabbit immunoglobulins, respectively. (Definitive proof that the relevant antigens are present on immunoglobulins came from subsequent work of the original authors and of other investigators.) Oudin (2,3) coined the term "allotype" to denote a distinctive antigenic form of a serum protein found in some but not all individuals. A committee on terminology generalized the term to include any protein which exists in polymorphic forms in different members of an animal species (4). Thus, the IgG molecules of one rabbit may possess antigenic (allotypic) determinants differing from those of another rabbit. Since the differences in amino acid sequence associated with allotypy are small, rabbit IgG molecules of different allotype share most of their antigenic specificities. The discovery of allotypy thus required the production of antisera that would distinguish among closely related molecules. The term, allotype, would not be used to denote a protein that might be present in some members of a species and absent in others.

The IgG molecules of all rabbits share antigenic determinants which are absent, for example, from bovine IgG. These are the isotypic determinants. (The IgG molecules of the two species share other antigenic specificities.)

It is apparent that polymorphism can be defined more precisely in terms of molecular structure, when sufficient information is available, and in a number of instances the amino acid substitutions corresponding to allotypic differences are known. With one or two possible exceptions (e.g., human Isf groups), no allotypic differences have been ascribed to carbohydrate content.

Allotypy has been studied most extensively in the rabbit, man, and mouse. In each species allotypic variation is seen in both H and L chains. In the rabbit and in man, for which data are available, genes controlling allotypic determinants on H and L chains are unlinked. In the mouse, allotypic variability of L chains has been detected by peptide mapping but, so far, not through antigenic analysis.

In each species the inheritance of genes controlling allotypic determinants is strictly Mendelian and is not sex-linked. All genes studied so far are codominant; they are expressed phenotypically in a heterozygote. An individual antibody-producing cell, however, normally expresses only one of a pair of allelic genes (5,6). This is in accord with the fact that most, if not all normal antibody-forming cells can synthesize only a single species of L chain and a single species of H chain; i.e., a cell behaves with respect to antibody biosynthesis as if it were functionally haploid (7).

The results we will discuss are consistent with the hypothesis that the variable and constant portions of immunoglobulin H chains are under the control of separate genes. Indeed, the presence of identical V region allotypic markers in different rabbit H chain (C region) classes provides evidence for the separate genetic control of the two segments of the chain (8–11). Convenient genetic markers are not yet available for both the V and C regions of the L chains of any species; the control of a single polypeptide chain by two separate genes is, therefore, not as well substantiated for L as for H chains.

II. RABBIT ALLOTYPES

Oudin (2,3) found that the immunoglobulin of an individual rabbit, when injected as an immune precipitate, elicits antiimmunoglobulin antibodies detectable by precipitin reactions in agar gel, in some but not all other rabbits. Such antibodies react with immunoglobulins from certain other rabbits as well as the donor. Following the initial discovery of Oudin, investigations which unraveled the basic principles of the inheritance of rabbit allotypes were carried out in the laboratories of Oudin (12,13), Dray (14–16), Dubiski and Kelus (17–21), and others. Before summarizing their findings we will briefly describe some of the methodology employed.

A. Detection and Quantitation of Allotypic Determinants in Rabbit Immunoglobulins

Antiallotypic antibodies directed to rabbit immunoglobulins are generally elicited by immunization of a rabbit with immunoglobulin of a genetically nonidentical rabbit, although antisera can also be prepared in species other than the rabbit. The latter antisera must be absorbed with rabbit immunoglobulin which lacks the allotypic determinant in question. A rabbit lacking a given determinant will normally respond to that determinant with the production of antibodies. A rabbit is of course tolerant of determinants present in its own immunoglobulins. Prolonged immunization is frequently required to elicit antiallotypic antibodies.

Such antibodies were produced initially by immunization with immune precipitates, emulsified in Freund's adjuvant (2,3). Antibodies to the antigen present in the complex (and possibly to components of complement which adhere to the complex and which might exist in polymorphic forms) were formed by the recipient animal, along with antiallotypic antibodies directed to the antibody present in the precipitate. Alternatively, rabbits have been immunized with complexes of rabbit antibody with bacteria or simply with the whole IgG fraction of the donor's serum. (It is not necessary that the immunogen have known antibody activity.) The difficulty of producing an antiserum varies with the allotypic determinant. For example, it is easier to produce high titers of antibodies directed toward certain allotypic determinants on L chains than on H chains of rabbit IgG.

Early investigations employed precipitin tests in agar gel almost exclusively for the detection of allotypic specificities (2,3,12–21). As the antigen in such tests, whole serum or a purified immunoglobulin fraction can be used. The Oudin and Ouchterlony techniques (single and double diffusion, respectively, in agar gel) have been widely used; the former method has the advantage of quantifying the antigen, if a pure standard is available. Even in the absence of a standard Oudin's method provides relative concentrations, in different sera, of molecules bearing a given allotype. The Ouchterlony method can be adapted to the quantification of antigen by the method of Mancini et al. (22), but comparatively large amounts of antibody are needed for incorporation into the agar.

More recently, quantitative studies of percentages of immunoglobulin molecules bearing particular allotypic markers have been carried out by labeling IgG or Fab fragments with ^{125}I or [125]I-*p*-iodophenylsulfonyl groups, and precipitating with monospecific antiallotype antiserum (23–27). Exhaustive precipitation is accomplished by adding unlabeled carrier (antigen) and additional antiallotype antiserum to the supernatant. In some cases the number of antigenic determinants per molecule is too small to permit the formation of specific precipitates, or precipitation may be incomplete even with repeated additions of carrier and antiserum. In such circumstances soluble antigen–antibody complexes can be precipitated with an antiglobulin reagent (25). Consider, for example, a rabbit allotypic marker present on the Fab fragment of the molecule. Fab fragments are labeled with ^{125}I for the purpose of quantitation. The labeled fragments are then allowed to react with rabbit antiallotypic antiserum, followed by a precipitating antiserum specific for rabbit fragment Fc:

Step 1 — ^{125}I-Fab + excess rabbit antiallotypic antiserum; incubate.
Step 2 — Add goat anti-rabbit Fc.

The goat antibody is added in a quantity sufficient to precipitate all the rabbit IgG present. Any labeled Fab fragments bound to rabbit antibody of the IgG class will also be brought down. The percentage of total radioactivity in the specific precipitate is equivalent to the percentage of Fab fragments bearing the allotypic determinants in question. To prove precipitation is complete additional antiallotypic antiserum and anti-Fc antiserum are added to the supernatant and the percentage of radioactivity precipitated again determined (25).

Another type of radioimmunoassay (28–30) utilizes antiallotype antiserum rendered insoluble by polymerization with ethyl chloroformate. Such preparations bind ^{125}I-labeled IgG or its fragments bearing the appropriate allotypic markers. The concentration of molecules bearing the allotype in an unlabeled preparation can be estimated through its capacity to inhibit binding of the labeled ligand.

Passive hemagglutination has also been useful for identification of allotypes in nonprecipitating systems (e.g., 31). The immunoglobulin is coated onto the surface of erythrocytes, which are then subject to agglutination by antiallotypic antiserum. A single antigenic (allotypic) determinant per molecule of immunoglobulin suffices to permit agglutination since there is a multiplicity of molecules on each erythrocyte. This method can also be adapted to quantitation of the antigen in a complex mixture such as serum; free antigen (immunoglobulin bearing the allotypic marker), when present in sufficiently high concentration, will inhibit agglutination by preempting the combining sites of the antiallotype antibody. A standard inhibition curve can be set up with a known immunoglobulin preparation and used to quantify the same allotype in other sera. The method has been used to study certain rabbit and human allotypes.

B. Association of Allotypes with L Chain Types and H Chain Classes in the Rabbit

1. General Considerations and Nomenclature

We will not attempt to describe research on allotypes in its historical context but, rather, will summarize present information. Table 9.1 lists the allotypic markers of rabbit immunoglobulins and their associa-

TABLE 9.1

Allotypic Specificities in Rabbit Immunoglobulins

Chain or chain segment	Locus	Known specificities	Location	Allelism
C_γ	de^a	d11, d12	Hinge, position 215 (Met/Thr)	Yes
C_γ	de	e14, e15	Fc, position 309 (Thr/Ala)	Yes
C_γ	Unnamed	A8, A10	Fc	—
$C_{\alpha 1}{}^b$	f	f69, f70, f71, f72, f73	C_α	Yes
$C_{\alpha 2}{}^b$	g	g74, g75, g76, g77	Fc_α and Fab_α	Yes
C_μ	n	n81, n82		Yes
C_μ	Unnamed	Ms1, Ms2, Ms4,[c] Ms5, Ms6		Unknown
$V_H(\gamma, \alpha, \mu, \epsilon)^c$	a^d	a1, a2, a3		Yes
$V_H(\gamma, \alpha, \mu, \epsilon)$	x	x32		—
$V_H(\gamma, \alpha, \mu, \epsilon)$	y	y33		—
$\kappa(\kappa_A$ and $\kappa_B)$	b	b4, b5, b6, b9	$C_\kappa(V_\kappa?)$	Yes
λ	c	c7, c21		Probably pseudoalleles

[a] A single gene probably controls the d and e markers.

[b] α_1 and α_2 chains are in two subclasses of IgA.

[c] So far only the a locus markers have been demonstrated on ϵ chains; one would predict that ϵ chains utilize all V_H subgroups, i.e., have the x and y as well as group a markers.

[d] The a, x, and y loci control specificities on different V_H region subgroups, which are shared by the various H chain (C region) classes.

[e] It is uncertain whether Ms2 differs from Ms4 and Ms6 and whether the Ms markers are related to the n locus. The marker Ms1 is found only in association with a3. The possible explanations are that Ms 1 is a C_μ marker which requires an a3 V region for its expression or that it is a variant of a3 which is expressed only when it is part of a μ chain.

tion with H chain classes and L chain types. Allotypic determinants which behave as though controlled by allelic genes are listed as a group. The genes are italicized and the designation of allotypic markers (not italicized) corresponds to that of the controlling gene. When the locus is as yet unnamed the allotypic marker has the prefix A or, for certain μ chain markers, Ms. Markers with the same letter prefix behave as alleles, with the possible exception of those for which the controlling locus is uncertain.

The nomenclature currently in use is based on conventions established in 1962 (4). Originally, all markers were designated with the prefix A, e.g., Ab4. The prefix is now often omitted when the locus has been established. Some investigators use the prefix As without specifying the locus, e.g., As4. The present authors feel that use of the locus designation conveys useful information to the reader, particularly since markers controlled by a given locus may not be numbered sequentially (e.g., b4, b5, b6, b9; c7, c21).

As indicated in Table 9.1, genetic polymorphism or allotypy is observed in rabbit L chains of both the κ and λ types and in the C_H regions of IgG, IgM, and IgA. In addition a distinct set of allotypic markers is localized in the V_H regions; the same V_H region markers are present on all rabbit H chain classes studied [IgG (12,13,18), IgM (8), IgA (9,10), and IgE (11)], a finding consistent with sharing of the same pool of V_H genes by each class. All V_H and C_H genes studied so far have been found, through breeding studies, to be very closely linked, and certain combinations of V_H and C_H markers (designated phenogroups or haplogroups) are preferentially associated in the rabbit population (32–34a; Section II,G). (The existence of phenogroups is one type of evidence for the close linkage of all genes controlling the various classes of H chains.) That the number of phenogroups is limited may also reflect in part the fact that many studies are based on small laboratory populations or on colonies bred from a small number of rabbits.

Certain allotypic determinants in rabbit κ chains appear, on the basis of sequence analysis, to be present in the C_κ region (35,36,36a). There is also a suggestion (discussed below) that sequences controlling allotype may be present in V_κ regions (36–38). In contrast to genes controlling H chain markers on various classes of immunoglobulins, those associated with κ and λ chains are not linked to one another, or to genes coding for H chain markers (39,40).

When nonallelic markers are found on corresponding polypeptides (e.g., specificities a1 and x32 on V_H regions) it is thought that they are present on different subgroups (different subgroups of V_H regions in the example cited).

Markers controlled by the *b* and *c* loci were localized to L chains by demonstrating that they are present in Fab fragments and in isolated L chains but absent from highly purified H chains (41–44). Allotypic specificities under control of the *a* locus are localized to the V_H region by: (a) their presence in Fab fragments and absence from fragment Fc (41,42); (b) their presence in isolated H chains and absence in L chains (43–45); (c) the fact that amino acid sequences of H chains carrying different group a markers appear to be identical after residue 115 (46,47); this would localize differences to the V_H region; (d) finally, Mole and Koshland have isolated the V_H region of a rabbit IgG protein and demonstrated the presence of group a specificities (L.E. Mole, and M.E. Koshland, personal communication). Localization of other markers will be discussed as they are considered individually.

2. Allotypic Markers on Rabbit κ Chains

Four genes, b^4, b^5, b^6, and b^9 (4,48), control the biosynthesis of rabbit κ chains, which constitute 80–90% of a normal L chain population. The corresponding antigens are designated b4, b5, b6, and b9. The b5 and b6 markers are strongly cross-reactive; this problem can be eliminated by preparing anti-b5 in a b^6b^6 rabbit and vice versa. A single κ chain possesses only one of these four antigenic markers. The four genes behave in all respects as if they are allelic. The possibility cannot, however, be entirely ruled out that all individuals possess all four genes, whose expression is controlled by allelic regulatory genes.[1] Rabbit κ chains of each allotype are found in association with all H chain classes; the allotypic determinants of κ chains appear to be expressed identically in each class. Each allotypic marker is found in association with L chains of both the κ_A and κ_B subtypes (49) (Chapter 8). The ratio of κ_B to κ_A is highest in b^4 homozygotes and lowest in b^9 homozygotes ($b^4 > b^5 \geqslant b^6 > b^9$).

A phenotype, such as b4, defines a set of several antigenic deter-

[1] Dr. A.D. Strosberg (personal communication) has recently observed the presence of specificities a1, a2, a3, b4, b5, and b6 in each of two individual rabbits which were believed to be of genotype a^1a^2, b^4b^5. The a3 and b6 specificities appeared only after immunization with *Micrococcus lysodekticus,* and were transient. They were, however, present in substantial concentration. Further work is needed to elucidate the significance of this potentially most important observation. A possible explanation is that an individual rabbit possesses all of the six genes, but inherits regulatory genes which ordinarily permit the synthesis of molecules of only two allotypic specificities at a given locus. Alternatively, there may be multiple *V* genes in a rabbit, and a crossover occurred in Strosberg's colony which placed genes controlling two specificities on the same chromosome. Our discussion will be written as if the genes controlling allotypic specificities b4, b5, b6, and b9 are allelic. See also *Note added in proof,* p. 406.

minants on one κ chain. Light chains of allotype b4, b5, or b6 were found to possess a minimum of two to three determinants per chain (50); in other words, the symbol b4 in reality denotes a set of antigenic determinants.

Kindt *et al.* made the important observation that homogeneous rabbit antistreptococcal antibodies usually do not contain a full complement of antigenic determinants recognized by antiserum to a group a specificity, e.g., anti-a1 (51). Whereas nonspecific IgG from any rabbit of appropriate allotype tested, including that which provided the homogeneous antibody, caused essentially complete inhibition of binding of labeled IgG bearing the group a specificity, only partial inhibition was obtained with individual homogeneous antibody preparations. An explanation favored by the authors is that sequence changes responsible for the specificity of the antigen-binding site of the antistreptococcal antibody impose modifications on allotypic determinants; i.e., that the allotype-related sequence remains constant but that the combining region influences the expression of allotypic determinants. An alternative possibility might involve somatic mutations affecting allotype-related sequences. Heterogeneous antibody populations (even those directed to a single hapten) comprise all determinants controlled by a single allele at the *a* locus (52).

Each of a group of homogeneous antibodies tested was found to express the full range of allotypic specificities controlled by the *b* locus (53). The difference, as compared to the *a* locus, may reflect localization of most group b specificities to the C region of the L chain; group a specificities are apparently confined to the V_H region.

As already indicated, antiallotype antibody is elicited when rabbit IgG of a given allotype is inoculated into another rabbit which does not possess immunoglobulin of that allotype; e.g., b4 immunoglobulin will elicit anti-b4 antibody in a non-b^4 rabbit; a rabbit of allotype b^4 is tolerant of the antigen and will not produce anti-b4. The same principles apply to each allotypic marker. To obtain monospecific antiserum it is thus necessary to use a recipient rabbit which lacks only one marker (e.g., b4) present in the immunoglobulin of the donor. It is understood that a marker can comprise more than one antigenic determinant.

An individual rabbit possesses two genes, on separate chromosomes, which are controlled by the *b* locus and which determine allotypic markers on κ chains. Thus a rabbit may be homozygous (e.g., b^4b^4) or heterozygous (e.g., b^5b^6); the presence of three specificities, e.g., b4, b5, and b6 in an individual rabbit has, with the exceptions noted previously not been reported.[1]

The inheritance of allotypes follows the Mendelian law of indepen-

dent assortment and is not sex-linked. The offspring of parents which are
b^4b^4 and b^5b^5, respectively, are exclusively b^4b^5 heterozygotes. Such a
heterozygous rabbit expresses both phenotypes; i.e., its serum contains
molecules with κ chains of allotypes b4 and b5. A single IgG molecule,
however, will have either two b4 or two b5 κ chains (25), and an individual IgM molecule in a heterozygous rabbit has ten b4 or ten b5 polypeptide chains (54). Again, this reflects allelic exclusion in a single, antibody-producing cell.

In a heterozygous rabbit the ratio of the numbers of molecules
bearing κ chains of the two allotypes is not necessarily $1:1$. For example, in a nonimmunized rabbit of genotype b^4b^5, the number of serum
immunoglobulin molecules bearing the b4 antigen is frequently about
twice as great as the number of molecules of allotype b5 (26). The
frequency of occurrence in heterozygotes, in terms of quantitative expression of allotypes in normal immunoglobulin is b4 > b5 ≥ b6 > b9
(49).

A typical heterogeneous population of antibody molecules of a given
specificity from an individual rabbit also expresses both allelic allotypic
markers, although not necessarily in the same proportion as the total immunoglobulin fraction (55–59). Furthermore, antihapten and antibacterial antibodies of greatly restricted heterogeneity have been isolated
from heterozygous rabbits and found to express only a single phenotype
(60–64); this provides one important criterion for the homogeneity or
"monoclonal" nature of such an antibody preparation. Homogeneous
human and mouse proteins, including myeloma proteins, exhibit the
same characteristic of allelic exclusion.

Of the allelic genes controlling rabbit κ chains, b^4 is the most
common; a large percentage of random-bred rabbits in the United States
are b^4b^4 homozygotes; the b^5 gene is found occasionally, b^6 and b^9 only
rarely; allotype b9 was discovered more recently than the other markers
(48). The allotype b6 is more common in certain Western European
countries than in the United States. Rabbits homozygous for b^5, b^6, or b^9
are ordinarily obtained by breeding heterozygotes. The Jackson Laboratory, at Bar Harbor, Maine, has a partially inbred strain of rabbits which
are $a^3a^3b^5b^5$ and which are homozygous for b^5.

Allotypic specificities are, in all probability, determined by amino
acid sequences. Thus, there are characteristic and reproducible differences with respect to the average amino acid composition of normal L
chains of allotypes b4, b5, and b6. Light chains of allotypes b4 and b5
differ with respect to content of aspartic acid, threonine, arginine, serine,
proline, valine, and leucine; no differences are evident in the overall content of other amino acids. The average number of residue differences per

L chain, based on measurements of amino acid composition, are: b4 versus b5, 15; b4 versus b6, 28; b5 versus b6, 17 (65,66). These are average values since they are obtained with heterogeneous populations of L chains. However, it seems quite possible that differences not associated with allotype would be minimized in such heterogeneous populations. This is supported by the identity in average composition with respect to most amino acids.

Light chains of allotypes b4, b5, and b6 can also be distinguished by peptide mapping (67,68); despite the heterogeneity of the chains, attributable to their V regions, certain peptide spots are characteristic of each phenotype.

Light chains expressing specificities b4, b5, or b6 also have distinct C-terminal sequences (35,36a). (These are shown in Table 9.2 together with C-terminal sequences of human and mouse L chains, included for the sake of comparison.) In addition, Frangione and Lamm have isolated two small internal peptides, adjacent to half-cystine residues, with amino acid sequences that differentiate the b4 and b5 alleles (36). The same amino acids that are involved in the sequence differences identified so far were also implicated by data on overall amino acid composition.

Differences in the N-terminal sequences of rabbit κ chains have also been noted (37,38), but these data must be interpreted with caution since

TABLE 9.2

COMPARISON OF N- AND C-TERMINAL SEQUENCES OF HUMAN, MOUSE, AND RABBIT L CHAINS[a]

N-Terminal										
Rabbit b(−)	Glp	Thr	(Val,	Pro)	Leu					
Mouse λ	Glp	Ala	Val	Val	Thr	Gln	Gln	Ser	Ala	Leu
Human λ	Glp	Ser	Val	Leu	Thr	Glu	Pro	Pro	Ser	Ala
			Ala		Ala		Asx	Ala	Ala	Val
			Glu							
C-Terminal								
Rabbit b4	Ser	Phe	Asn	Arg	Gly	Asn	Cys	
Rabbit b5		Phe	Ser	Arg	Lys	Asn	Cys	
Rabbit b6			Ser	Arg	Lys	Ser	Cys	
Mouse κ	Ser	Phe	Asn	Arg	Asn	Glu	Cys	
Human κ	Ser	Phe	Asn	Arg	Gly	Glu	Cys	
Mouse λ	Lys	Ser	Leu	Ser	Arg	Ala	Asp	Cys	Ser
Human λ	Lys	Thr	Val	Ala	Pro	Thr	Glu	Cys	Ser
Rabbit b(−)	Ser	Leu	Ala	(Pro,	Ala,	Glu,	Cys)	Ser

[a] Data for the rabbit proteins are from references 35 and 73, which provide the original references for the partial sequences of human and mouse L chains.

the differences may reflect preferential association of particular V region subgroups with C regions corresponding to particular allotypes. (Subgroups, by definition, are nonallelic.) Whether there are allotype-related substitutions in the V region will have to be substantiated by studies of V region sequences in a number of homogeneous antibody preparations.

An interesting correlation between allotype and sequence in the V_L region was discovered by Thunberg *et al.* (38). They found that b9 L chains from each of three antistreptococcal antibody preparations of restricted heterogeneity have glutamic acid at position 16. Also glutamic acid is present at the same position in an appreciable percentage of pooled normal b9 L chains. It is apparently absent in L chains of other allotypes, and may therefore serve as the first genetic marker for the V_L region of rabbit κ chains. Since the antigenic determinants characteristic of most L chain allotypes appear to depend on C region sequences, linkage studies between V_L and C_L genes may be possible. (This assumes control of the chain by two genes, as in the case of H chains.)

3. Allotypic Markers on Rabbit λ Chains

The existence on rabbit L chains of antigenic determinants that are not under control of the *b* locus was indicated by the failure of antisera directed to group b specificities to precipitate all molecules of IgG from a rabbit homozygous at the *b* locus (24,69). Molecules bearing such determinants are present in all normal sera, and are under control of a second genetic locus, designated *c*, which also controls allotypic determinants on L chains. Genes at this locus are not linked to the *a* or *b* loci. They are autosomal, a characteristic held in common with other genes controlling allotypes. So far, two specificities, c7 and c21, have been identified (16,39). Recent investigations suggest that genes c^7 and c^{21} may be closely linked and pseudoallelic; i.e., they segregate as if they were allelic in some, but not all, breeding colonies. In other words, c^7 and c^{21} may be found on separate chromosomes or closely linked on the same chromosome. Since the c7 and c21 specificities are not present on the same molecule, the occurrence of the two genes on one chromosome reflects the presence of at least two separate cistrons coding for λ chains.

Light chains controlled by the *b* and *c* loci can be separated from one another, after cleavage of the interchain disulfide bonds of IgG, by gel filtration on Sephadex G-100 equilibrated with 6 *M* urea in 0.05 *M* formic acid. The first L chain peak consists largely of molecules bearing markers controlled by the *c* locus. Despite the exposure to urea at low pH, the chains are still able to react with antiallotype antiserum (70,71).

Isolation of such chains is greatly facilitated if the immunoglobulin is derived from rabbits in which the synthesis of molecules bearing *b* locus markers had been suppressed (Section V) by neonatal administration of antibodies directed to *b*-locus determinants.

Light chains controlled by the *c* locus appear, from a comparison with human and mouse L chains, to be of the λ type (71–73). The evidence includes the presence of a blocked N-terminal group (pyrrolidone-carboxylic acid), the C-terminal dipeptide, -Cys-Ser, characteristic of λ chains, and the sequence of eight amino acids at the C-terminus (Table 9.2).

4. INDEPENDENT ASSORTMENT OF GENES CONTROLLING ALLOTYPIC MARKERS ON RABBIT L CHAINS

Nearly all molecules of rabbit IgG, labeled with ^{125}I to permit quantitation, are precipitated by an appropriate combination of anti-b and anti-c antisera; this indicates that if loci other than *b* and *c* exist they must control the synthesis of a very small proportion of rabbit L chains in a normal population (74).

Genes, *b* and *c*, controlling the allotypic markers on rabbit κ and λ chains, assort independently and thus may be present on separate chromosomes (39). Moreover, genes controlling L chains are not linked to the genes controlling markers on rabbit H chains (12,16,19,40).

5. ALLOTYPIC MARKERS IN THE V_H REGIONS OF RABBIT IMMUNOGLOBULINS

As indicated earlier, genes at the *a* locus control determinants present on the H chains of each class of rabbit immunoglobulin. This is consistent with the fact that the *a* locus specifies determinants in the V_H region and that H chain classes are generally not distinguishable on the basis of their V_H sequences. (The latter point has been established for human immunoglobulins and probably applies to other species as well.) It is generally accepted that the same V_H genes contribute to the biosynthesis of all classes of immunoglobulin.

The three apparently allelic genes, a^1, a^2, and a^3, control the biosynthesis of 70 to 90% of rabbit H chains (26); the phenotypes are a1, a2, and a3, respectively. (Molecules lacking group a markers will be discussed later.) A rabbit inherits two allelic genes controlled by the *a* locus and may be homozygous or heterozygous. The inheritance is Mendelian and not sex-linked. Alleles are codominant; i.e., a heterozygous rabbit expresses both phenotypes. Both H chains of an individual molecule have the same allotypic markers (25), reflecting allelic exclusion at the cellular level. A rabbit can be induced to synthesize antibodies to any a-locus determinant which it lacks. In all these respects, characteristics of the a and b loci are similar.

Among rabbits surveyed in the United States, Canada, and Great Britain the a^1 allele is the most common. This information is based on relatively small, closed colonies. However, Dubiski and Good examined a large number of random-bred, unselected rabbits obtained from a number of small breeding colonies in Canada (33). The gene frequencies they observed were a^1, 0.57; a^2, 0.076; a^3, 0.35.

Allotypic determinants controlled by the a locus are present in the Fab fragment and, more specifically, in the V_H region. Thus, consistent differences are observed in average amino acid composition among Fab fragments (which include the V_H and C_H1 regions of the molecule) from normal IgG populations of different allotype (66,75,76). Fragments Fd of allotypes a1 and a2 differ by an average of approximately 6 amino acid residues; a1 and a3 by 11 or 12; and a2 and a3 by 9 or 10 residues. Also, differences among H chains of different allotype have been observed in the peptide maps of their Fd, but not their Fc fragments (77). Strong evidence that determinants controlled by the a locus are localized in the V_H region comes from sequence analyses of the constant portion of the Fd segment of the H chain (Section II,B,1); such analyses show no allotype-related sequence differences.

Identification of amino acid substitutions associated with differences at the a locus is complicated by the normal variability in the V_H region; also, some of the available sequences are those of nonspecific H chains (from rabbits homozygous at the a locus), from which it is difficult to obtain high yields of certain peptides, and which are probably contaminated with small proportions of a-negative molecules. Nevertheless, there is good correlation between much of the published data for V_H regions of nonspecific IgG and for homogeneous antibodies (outside of hypervariable regions). The data suggest that most allotype-related substitutions occur in the N-terminal 29 residues of the chain (46,77a–78a). Apparent differences between a1 and a3 at positions 80–85 (46) may not be allotype-related (78) since a homogeneous antibody of allotype a1 exhibited a sequence in that region that is closely related to that of the nonspecific a3 pool. On the basis of the existing data with homogeneous antibodies and nonspecific pools, and excluding hypervariable regions, likely candidates for allotype-related substitutions (numbering system of Jaton) are: a1 versus a2, positions 4,7,9,11,12,15,16; a1 versus a3, positions 1a,9,12,14,15,16,27,28; a2 versus a3, positions 1a,3,4,7,9,11,14,15,16,28. It should be noted that some allotype-related sequence differences may not affect antigenicity. Complete V_H sequences of homogeneous antipneumococcal antibodies of allotypes a1 and a2 suggest that there are no allotype-related substitutions between positions 36 and 67 or between positions 92 and 120 (J.-C. Jaton, personal communication). A few sequence differences between positions 68 and 84 may be associated with allotype, but this is uncertain. (Hypervariable regions are excluded from consideration in all of this discussion.)

The available evidence suggests that the group a allotypic determinants in different classes of immunoglobulin are very similar antigenically. IgG, IgA, and IgM give lines of identity in reacting with antisera to group a specificities (8–10), and the group a determinants on IgG and IgM of an individual rabbit appear to be the same according to quantitative tests (79). Average differences in amino acid composition, associated with differences in allotype, are quite similar in γ and μ chains (80).

Despite the inconclusive nature of the direct experimental evidence bearing on the question, it seems likely that H chains of various classes will prove to have the same allotype-related amino acid sequences. Thus, there is substantial indirect evidence, discussed at length in Chapter 12, that different genes encode the V and C regions of each H chain and that the various H chain classes share the same V genes. Since group a determinants are in V_H regions, one would predict that such determinants would be the same in the various classes.

It seems unlikely that carbohydrate can contribute significantly to either group a or b allotypic specificities. Fab fragments containing less than 0.25% carbohydrate after gel filtration fully expressed these specificities. This percentage corresponds to a molecular weight of 125, which is smaller than that of a pentose (81).

Oudin (12) and Dray *et al.* (16,82) noted the appearance of double precipitin lines in reactions of rabbit sera with antisera directed against allotypic markers a1, a2, b4, or b5. The corresponding phenotypic pairs are designated a2′, a2″, b4′, b4″, etc. Members of each pair of specificities are presumed to be encoded by closely linked genes since the phenotypic pair of specificities is always found together. As shown by Kakinuma (83) most if not all a2′ and a2″ determinants are present on separate immunoglobulin molecules and are not antigenically cross-reactive. He also found that the antigenic activity of a2′ molecules is much more sensitive than that of a2″ digestion by papain. The apparently greater sensitivity of the antigenic activity of a2′ molecules to papain is probably attributable to a smaller antigenic valence in the intact molecule, rather than to destruction of determinants. Evidence for this is that

Fab fragments of a2' IgG do not form precipitates with antiallotypic antiserum, but do inhibit the precipitation in agar gel of intact a2' molecules with anti-a2 antibodies. In contrast, Fab fragments of a2'' molecules are capable of forming precipitates with anti-a2 antibodies (83).

6. IgG MOLECULES LACKING GROUP a DETERMINANTS

When rabbit IgG is trace-labeled with radioactive iodine, then exhaustively precipitated with antiserum to group a determinants, 15–30% of the molecules remain in solution (25,26). Molecules which fail to precipitate are designated a-negative (25,26,69). It now appears that a-negative molecules have V_H regions belonging to one or more subgroups differing from those which carry the group a determinants. Knight et al. (84) suppressed the biosynthesis of a2 molecules in an a^2a^2 rabbit by induction of anti-a2 antibodies in the pregnant (non-a^2) mother, which had received a zygote transfer (Section V); the anti-a2 antibodies reached the zygote through the circulation. After birth, the serum of the offspring had no detectable IgG molecules with a2 determinants. The Fc fragments of the IgG of this suppressed rabbit and that of a normal a^2a^2 rabbit had identical peptide maps. There were, however, four or five peptide differences between the Fab fragments of the two rabbits; this suggested that the differences between a-positive and a-negative molecules reside in the Fd segment of the H chain.

An antiserum was produced by injecting the purified IgG of the suppressed (a-negative) rabbit into another, partially inbred rabbit of genotype a^1a^1 (84). This antiserum precipitated 80% of the IgG molecules of the a-negative donor but only 5% of their Fc fragments, indicating that the reactive determinants are in fragment Fab. Antisera to a-negative molecules were found to differentiate among the normal sera of different individual rabbits. They distinguished two antigenic determinants, initially designated A32 and A33 (32). (The use of the symbol A indicates that the allotypic locus is not defined.) Determinants A32 and A33 were shown in mating studies not to behave as alleles (32). For this reason it was concluded that the two determinants reside in different V_H subgroups and two new loci, designated x and y, were assigned; the determinants, then, are x32 and y33. Assignment to the V_H, rather than the C_H regions, was based on the presence of x32 and y33 in IgM and IgA, as well as IgG, and on the fact that these determinants appear in high, apparently compensatory concentration after suppression of allotypes controlled by the a locus, which is also associated with the V_H region. The x and y loci are closely linked to the a locus and to all other genes controlling rabbit H chains.

No two of the allotypic specificities, a2, x32, or y33 are located on the same molecule in a serum containing all three specificities (85). In some normal rabbits homozygous with respect to the *a* locus nearly all the molecules could be accounted for by summing those bearing the a, x, and y specificities, but a small additional percentage of molecules with unknown specificities were present in two rabbits; these molecules were postulated to contain specificities controlled by genes allelic to x^{32} and/or y^{33}; the postulated markers have not yet been identified serologically.

Tack *et al.* (85a), in agreement with Knight *et al.* (84), detected no differences among the Fc fragments of a-positive or a-negative molecules by serological techniques or peptide mapping; also, the C-terminal octadecapeptides were found to be identical. Prahl *et al.* (85b) found distinct compositional differences in the V_H regions of a-negative and a-positive IgG. The predominant N-terminal sequence in the a-negative H chains is PCA-Glu-Gln-; this is a minor sequence in pooled rabbit γ chains, where it probably reflects the presence of a-negative molecules.

C. Allotypic Determinants in the C_H Region of Rabbit IgG

The discovery of allotypic determinants in the C_H region of rabbit γ chains, which occurred subsequent to the description of determinants in the V_H region, has led to significant information concerning the genetic control of antibody biosynthesis. The rabbit H chain is thus far unique in that allotypic markers, identifiable by antisera, have been found in both the V and C regions of the chain. This makes it possible, through breeding experiments, to study the linkage of the two groups of markers. Such investigations permit genetic mapping and yield insight into the process of transcription. The sharing of *a* locus genes by the various immunoglobulin classes provides direct evidence for the "two genes-one polypeptide" hypothesis for the control of biosynthesis of the H chain.

1. The *de* Locus; Group d Determinants

The *de* locus controls allotypic determinants in the C_H region of rabbit IgG (31, 86–88). Determinants of groups d and e were discovered independently, group d by Mandy and Todd (31) and group e by Dubiski (87,88), and are located in different parts of the C_H region. The locus is designated *de* on the assumption that a single gene controls the C_H segment of the H chain. Antisera to group d determinants were prepared by conventional techniques, involving the immunization of a rabbit with the immunoglobulin of another rabbit, matched to the recipient with respect to genes at the a and b loci (31,86). The immunoglobulin was injected as IgG or in the form of an immune precipitate or agglutinate. Antiallotypic antibodies were assayed by the sensitive technique of hemagglutination inhibition. This method can detect antigens of low valence, including univalent antigens, since a single coated red blood cell carries many antigen molecules and is thus effectively multivalent. Rabbit erythrocytes, coated with IgG of the donor rabbit, are agglutinated by the antiallotypic antiserum; the agglutination is inhibited by the sera of rabbits carrying that allotypic marker. Two allelic genes, d^{11} and d^{12},[2] have been identified. The pattern of inheritance and phenotypic expression of the genes are as described for the a and b loci (86). In most colonies in the United States the d^{12} gene frequency is higher than that of d^{11}. The a and d loci, controlling determinants in the V_H and C_H regions, respectively, are closely linked (89). This is shown by the results of backcrosses of F_1 rabbits (e.g., a^1d^{12}/a^2d^{11})[3] to doubly homozygous rabbits of one parental genotype (e.g., a^1d^{12}/a^1d^{12}). One then examines the offspring for the presence of a chromosome bearing a^2 and d^{12}. So far one recombinant has been reported among hundreds of progeny investigated (89; W.J. Mandy, personal communication).

The amino acid substitution responsible for the d11-d12 phenotypic variation has been precisely identified (90). Heavy chains of allotype d11 have a methionine group in the hinge region at position 225 (numbering system of human γ_1 protein Eu), adjacent to a half-cystine which forms the interheavy chain disulfide bond. Molecules of allotype d12 have threonine in place of methionine at this position. The integrity of the interheavy chain disulfide bond is essential for the expression of group d antigenic determinants (86,91).

The presence of methionine on the N-terminal side of the interheavy chain disulfide bond was used as the basis of a procedure which permits isolation of molecules bearing the d12 marker. Cleavage of d11 molecules with cyanogen bromide, which attacks polypeptides specifically at bonds adjacent to methionine, yields Fab fragments of approximate molecular weight 47,000, as well as smaller fragments. In contrast, molecules of allotype d12, which lack the methionine at position 225, are cleaved at methionine 252, which is closer to the C-terminus. The interheavy chain disulfide bond therefore serves to link the

---

[2] It is understood that the same cistron also may control group e determinants.

[3] The symbol, a^1d^{12}/a^2d^{11}, indicates that the chromosome inherited from one parent carries the a^1 and d^{12} genes and that the other parental chromosome carries a^2 and d^{11}.

Fab fragments containing the two d12 chains, so that the major product of cyanogen bromide cleavage, designated $F(ab'')_2$, is bivalent and has a molecular weight of about 95,000, a value twice that of d11 fragments. The difference in molecular weight permits separation of d11 and d12 fragments by gel filtration (92,93).

This convenient chemical manipulation permitted the demonstration that the allotypic markers in the V_H and C_H regions of an individual IgG molecule are largely determined by the genes on a single chromosome (93). Thus, if a rabbit inherits parental chromosomes carrying the genes, a^1d^{12} and a^3d^{11}, respectively, its individual IgG molecules have the phenotype a1,d12, or a3,d11; few a1,d11, or a3,d12 molecules are produced. This was shown experimentally by cyanogen bromide cleavage of the IgG population, which yields Fab fragments (mol. wt. 47,000) from d11, and $F(ab'')_2$ fragments from d12 molecules. The Fab fragments were isolated by gel filtration and found to be almost exclusively a3; conversely, nearly all the isolated $F(ab'')_2$ fragments (mol. wt. 95,000) were a1. This experiment indicates that the information for the sequence of an H chain comes from the genes on a single parental chromosome. Subsequent studies, designed to detect low concentrations of molecules possessing markers controlled by genes on the two parental chromosomes, showed that such molecules do exist. The data are discussed in the next section.

2. GROUP e DETERMINANTS

The existence of another genetic locus, controlling allotypic determinants in the C_H region of rabbit IgG, was discovered by Dubiski in 1969 (87,88). The donor rabbit used in his initial immunization was of genotype a^1a^3, b^9b^9; the recipient was a^2a^3, b^6b^6. First, the donor was immunized with *Proteus mirabilis;* the resulting antiserum was used to prepare bacterial agglutinates containing antibody, which were injected into the recipient. The antiallotypic antiserum elicited contained anti-a1 and anti-b9 antibodies, but after these antibodies were removed by absorption with IgG of allotypes a1 and b9, antiallotypic activity was still detectable by the method of passive hemagglutination. The serum of the donor and of 45 of 211 other rabbits tested were inhibitory. The responsible allotypic determinant, which was localized to the Fc fragment of IgG, is now designated e14. An antiserum was subsequently prepared against an allelic determinant, e15, which is present in the sera of all rabbits lacking e14. Heterozygotes ($e^{14}e^{15}$) express both phenotypes; in other respects as well, the inheritance of e^{14} and e^{15} genes parallels that already described for the other allotypic loci (29,87,88). In a homozygous $e^{14}e^{14}$ or $e^{15}e^{15}$ rabbit about 90% of the IgG molecules can be removed by the corresponding antiallotypic antiserum. In the few heterozygous rabbits studied varying proportions of e14 and e15 molecules were present, but the sum was 85% or more in each case (29).

Family studies demonstrated a very close linkage of genes controlling group a and group e determinants. In a paper published in 1971, only one recombinant had been found after 150 relevant backcrosses (94). Direct studies of recombination involving group d and group e determinants have not been reported. The existence of fixed allogroups in populations of rabbits investigated (Section II,G; Table 9.3) argues, however, against frequent crossovers; for example, the combination $d^{11}e^{14}$ is very rare.

Quantitative investigations indicate a mechanism of transcription for the a and e loci analogous to that described for a and d; i.e., a single molecule is ordinarily encoded by the V_H and C_H genes on one chromosome. Thus, in a rabbit which had inherited chromosomes with gene pairs a^1e^{14} and a^2e^{15}, removal of a1 molecules by a specific immunoadsorbent simultaneously removed most e14 but few e15 molecules (29). The sensitivity of the experiments was not sufficient to exclude the presence of a small proportion of "recombinant" molecules (e.g., a1, e15). Further evidence that an individual molecule is encoded by genes on a single parental chromosome is the close similarity in percentages of a1 and e14, or of a2 and e15 molecules in a rabbit of genotype a^1e^{14}/a^2e^{15} (29).

Another experiment bearing on the same question was carried out by suppression, with antiallotypic antiserum, of allotypic specificities in

TABLE 9.3

ALLOGROUPS OF GENES CONTROLLING RABBIT H CHAINS[a,b]

$a^1x^-y^-$	n^{81}	$f^{73}g^{74}$	$de^{12,15}$
$a^1x^-y^{33}$	n^-	$f^{72}g^{74}$	$de^{11,15}$
$a^1x^{32}y^{33}$	n^-	$f^{71}g^{75}$	$de^{12,15}$
$a^1x^-y^{33}$	n^-	f^-g^{74}	$de^{12,14}$
$a^2x^{32}y^{33}$	n^{82}	f^-g^{74}	$de^{12,15}$
$a^2x^{32}y^{33}$	n^{82}	$f^{71}g^{75}$	$de^{12,15}$
$a^3x^{32}y^-$	n^-	$f^{72}g^{74}$	$de^{11,15}$
$a^3x^{32}y^-$	n^-	$f^{71}g^{75}$	$de^{12,15}$

[a] Possible allogroups of a, x, and y genes that were not detected are as follows: $a^1x^{32}y^-$, $a^2x^-y^{33}$, $a^2x^-y^-$, $a^2x^{32}y^-$, $a^3x^-y^{33}$, $a^3x^-y^-$, $a^3x^{32}y^{33}$.

[b] Colonies maintained by S. Dray, C.W. Todd, the Jackson laboratory, and the National Institutes of Health. The data are from references 34 and 34a.

a newborn rabbit. The rabbit was of genotype a^1e^{14}/a^2e^{15} and was suppressed through transfer of maternal anti-a1 antibody. This resulted in marked suppression of immunoglobulin bearing determinants a1 and e14 and enhancement of a2 and e15 (29). This finding can, again, readily be interpreted on the premise that in a single cell the biosynthesis of an IgG molecule is controlled by the V_H gene (*a* locus) and C_H gene (*de* locus) present on the same chromosome. It requires the further, and likely, assumption that the antiallotypic antibody acts by suppressing the activity of a cell.

More sensitive methods subsequently indicated the presence of a small proportion of molecules bearing markers encoded by genes on the two homologous parental chromosomes. The proportion of such molecules in doubly heterozygous rabbits was determined by Landucci-Tosi and Tosi, who utilized insolubilized antiallotype sera and ^{125}I-labeled IgG preparations to quantitate allotypic specificities on individual molecules of IgG (95). They found that in a rabbit of genotype a^1e^{14}/a^2e^{15}, 1.4% of the IgG molecules were phenotypically a1, e15 and 0.3% were a2, e14. A similar pattern of biosynthesis was observed in a rabbit of genotype a^1e^{15}/a^2e^{14}. The presence of molecules bearing markers from different parental chromosomes could reflect recombination within lymphoid cells or, perhaps less probably, a translocation of a V_H gene on one chromosome to link up with a C_H gene on the homologous chromosome. A somewhat higher percentage of "recombinant" molecules has also been identified in rabbit sIgA by Knight *et al.* (95a).

The existence of a small proportion of molecules encoded by genes on two chromosomes is supported by studies at the cellular level (96). Spleen cells containing antibody (mainly plasma cells) were successively stained, for example, with fluorescein or rhodamine conjugates of antibodies directed to allotypic specificities of groups a and e, or a and d, respectively. In most instances a single cell contained only allotypic specificities controlled by a single parental chromosome. However, a small percentage of the cells (0.4–2%) had specificities controlled by genes on both parental chromosomes. Similarly, a very small but significant percentage of cells contained allotypes of IgG and IgM controlled by both parental chromosomes; e.g., 2 cells of 1500 examined from a rabbit of genotype Ms^4 (neg), a^2/Ms^4 (pos), a^3 were doubly stained by reagents specific for a2 and Ms4, respectively.

Peptide mapping and partial sequence analysis were carried out on Fc fragments of e14 and e15 molecules by Appella *et al.* (97). In analyzing their data the previous sequence analyses of Hill *et al.* (98,99) and of Fruchter *et al.* (100) were useful. An amino acid substitution was identified at position 309, where the e14 H chain has a threonine residue and e15 has alanine. This was the only substitution detected, although the C_H sequence is not quite complete. On the basis of a single amino acid substitution one would expect either antigenic univalence, or bivalence if each chain expresses a determinant; this would account for the fact that anti-e14 and anti-e15 do not form specific precipitates in the standard tests. Passive hemagglutination is generally utilized to detect these antigens.

Subsequently, it was found (101) that the presence of specificities e14 or e15 can be demonstrated by direct precipitation, using the Ouchterlony method, if 2% polyethylene glycol (102) is incorporated in the agar. The authors suggested that the antigen is bivalent and that the linear complexes formed with bivalent antibody precipitate in the presence of polyethylene glycol; the mechanism is not clear.

3. THE A8 AND A10 MARKERS

Hamers and Hamers-Casterman have reported that some but not all rabbit IgG molecules with a1 determinants in the V_H region also possess linked antigenic determinants, A8 and A10, in the Fc segment (103,104). The relationship of A8 and A10 to determinants of groups d and e has not yet been elucidated.

D. Independent Assortment of Genes Controlling the *a*, *b* and *c* Loci

We have noted the close linkage between the *a* locus, which controls determinants in the V_H region of all Ig classes, and the *de* locus, associated with determinants in the C_H region of IgG. In contrast, the *a*, *b*, and *c* loci are unlinked (12,16,19,39,40). Thus, genes controlling different portions of the same polypeptide chain are in close proximity on the chromosome, whereas those controlling H and L chains, or different L chain types, are either on separate chromosomes or distally located on the same chromosome.

E. Allotypic Determinants on the Rabbit μ Chain

Kelus and Gell (105) and Sell (106) first described allotypic determinants present on rabbit IgM but not on IgG or IgA. Their exclusive presence on IgM molecules is presumptive evidence that the determinants are on μ chains rather than on L chains. Five markers have been described: Ms1, Ms2, Ms4, Ms5, and Ms6 (107,108); another marker, Ms3, appears to be associated with L chains in IgM rather than μ chains (108), and there is some uncertainty related to Ms1 since it occurs only in association with allotype a^3. Conceivably, it could be a C_μ marker which is expressed in association with an a3 V_H region or a V_H marker expressed only when C_μ is present. The nonidentity of Ms2 with Ms4 or Ms6 has not been established. Kelus and Gell (105) believe that Ms markers are controlled by at least three loci, although detailed genetic investigations have been hampered by the difficulty of isolating pure IgM, owing to its low concentration in normal rabbit serum.

Gilman-Sachs and Dray (109) identified two allotypic specificities (n81 and n82) in rabbit IgM; their relationship to determinants described by Kelus and his collaborators is not yet known. Determinants n81 and n82 are controlled by allelic genes at the *n* locus, which is closely linked to the *a* locus. It is very probable that these antigenic determinants are present in the C_H region of the μ chain, although this has not been demonstrated directly.

F. Allotypic Determinants of Rabbit IgA

In studying allotypes of rabbit IgA, immunizations are carried out with secretory IgA (sIgA) isolated from colostrum or milk (110–113). This is necessary because of the difficulty of isolating IgA from rabbit serum, where it is present in very low concentration. Localization of allotypic determinants has been approached by cleaving sIgA with papain into fragments designated $Fab_{2\alpha}$ and $Fc_{2\alpha}$, respectively (112). Some but not all of the $Fc_{2\alpha}$ fragments are still associated with secretory component after cleavage.

Our present information on allotypes of IgA is based almost entirely on investigations carried out with a limited breeding colony (10,110–113). It is quite likely that other combinations of genes, and perhaps other genes not yet identified, will be found among other groups of rabbits. Two genetic loci, *f* and *g*, have been identified. These are closely linked to the *a*, *x*, and *y* loci (34,114). Five allelic genes at the *f* locus, $f^{69}, f^{70}, f^{71}, f^{72}$, and f^{73}, control allotypic specificities f69, f70, etc. Specificities g74, g75, g76, and g77 are controlled by allelic genes at the *g* locus (111, 112, 112a). Nearly all molecules of IgA bear determinants specified by the *f* or *g* locus. These determinants are also found in serum IgA, which lacks both secretory component and J chain; this fact, and their absence from other classes of immunoglobulin, would localize the determinants to the C_α region. Since f and g determinants are not controlled by allelic genes, and are found on separate molecules, it was concluded that they are present on molecules belonging to two different subclasses of IgA. It is thought that f and g specificities are associated with amino acid sequence, although a possible contribution of carbohydrate has not been ruled out (111,112).

There is a pronounced difference among molecules bearing f or g determinants with respect to their susceptibility to digestion by papain; molecules with group f specificities are highly resistant, whereas molecules with group g specificities are readily cleaved into $Fab_{2\alpha}$ and $Fc_{2\alpha}$ fragments (112,115).

It appears that g74 and g75 each represent a set of allotypic determinants, present on both the Fab and Fc fragments. For example, in an Ouchterlony test with anti-g74 antiserum either fragment, Fab or Fc, forms a precipitin band which shows only partial identity with intact sIgA; i.e., each fragment reacts but is antigenically deficient as compared to the intact molecule. Also, the g74 specificities on Fab and Fc are antigenically distinct from one another.[4] Similar results were obtained with anti-g75 antisera. Specificities controlled by the *f* locus have not been localized to fragments Fab or Fc because of the resistance of such IgA molecules to papain (111,112).

In the populations of rabbits studied so far, only certain combinations of *f* and *g* alleles (allogroups or haplogroups) are present on a single chromosome. These are: $f^{71}g^{75}$; $f^{72}g^{74}$; or $f^{73}g^{74}$ (Table 9.3). Three of the six possible combinations have not yet been reported. The occurrence and persistence of allogroups is one kind of evidence for close linkage of the *f* and *g* loci (Section II,G).

The existence of allogroups complicates the preparation of certain monospecific antisera. Thus, anti-g74 antiserum normally contains antibodies to f72 or f73 as well. This problem can be circumvented by preadsorption of the IgA to be used as immunogen with an immunoadsorbent containing anti-f72 or anti-f73 antibodies.[4] A similar problem arises when one attempts to prepare monospecific anti-f71. In this instance g75 molecules, which are also present in an f71 preparation, can be digested with papain and removed by gel filtration, leaving undegraded f71 IgA for use as the immunogen.

1. LINKAGE OF *f* AND *g* TO OTHER LOCI CONTROLLING
   IMMUNOGLOBULIN POLYPEPTIDE CHAINS

As already indicated, the *f* and *g* loci are very closely linked to one another; no recombinants have thus far been observed (111). They are

---

[4] K.L. Knight and W. C. Hanly, personal communication.

also linked closely to the *a* locus which controls V_H regions of the several immunoglobulin classes (111). The pattern which emerges is one of very close linkage of all genes controlling the synthesis of both V_H and C_H regions. This is true in the mouse and man, as well as in the rabbit. Linkage of genes controlling L and H chains has thus far not been observed.

2. ALLOTYPIC SPECIFICITIES IN RABBIT SECRETORY COMPONENT

Two allotypic markers have so far been identified on secretory component (113). The markers are controlled by allelic genes. Immunizations are carried out with free secretory component isolated from the IgA of colostrum or tears. Genetic studies are complicated by the difficulty of obtaining pure sIgA from large numbers of individual rabbits, especially males, since the major source of sIgA is colostrum.

G. Linked Sets of Genes Controlling Rabbit Immunoglobulins

Dray *et al.* (34) and Mage *et al.* (34a) have delineated the linkage patterns of genes (allogroups) present on the same chromosome and controlling H chains (V_H and C_H regions) in the rabbits of four separate breeding colonies. Table 9.3 summarizes the allogroups which are present. It is evident that only a small fraction of all possible gene combinations is represented. Also, because of the extremely low crossover frequency, these linkage groups persist virtually unchanged within a population. Different allogroups are present in other colonies; for example, the specificity e14 is not even represented in three of the four breeding colonies that provided the data of Table 9.3.

H. Allotypic Markers in Other Lagomorphs

A number of investigators have used antisera specific for allotypic determinants in the domestic rabbit (*Oryctolagus cuniculus*) to test for the presence of the same markers in other lagomorphs (family, Leporidae), particularly in the hare (genus, *Lepus*) and the cottontail rabbit (genus, *Sylvilagus*). It is believed that the various genera, which have different chromosome numbers and will not interbreed, evolved from a common ancestor about 2×10^6 years ago. Kelus and Chambers (quoted in reference 40) showed that IgG of the hare reacts with some but not all preparations of anti-a2, anti-b4, or anti-b6 prepared against IgG of the domestic rabbit. Mandy and Rodkey (116), using a quantitative radioimmunoassay, showed the presence of substantial numbers of molecules bearing a2, a3, and b5 specificities but very few with the markers a1, b4, b6, or b9 in the IgG of individual hares. The markers a2, a3, and b5 were present in all twelve animals studied, suggesting the possibility that they are isotypic, rather than allotypic markers in hares.

Some if not all allotypic markers in lagomorphs are cross-reactive, rather than identical. For example, F(ab')$_2$ fragments from the cottontail (genus, *Sylvilagus*) were unable to displace radiolabeled F(ab')$_2$ fragments of the domestic rabbit from anti-b4 antibodies, although the same F(ab')$_2$ fragments were capable of direct binding to the antibodies (117).

The e15 marker was identified in the sera of all 35 cottontails tested and in 20 of 26 hares. The d11, d12, and e14 markers could not be detected in any of these sera (116). Mandy and Rodkey suggest that the e^{15} gene was present in the common ancestor of modern lagomorphs and that e^{14} and the d locus genes arose subsequently in *Oryctolagus* as a result of mutations.

By radioimmunoassay, Rodkey showed that the b5 marker in the hare is localized to L chains and that the IgM of the hare shares determinants a3 and b5 with its IgG (118). The L chains lack the a3 marker.

Studies of allotypy in hare immunoglobulins were also reported by Landucci-Tosi *et al.* (119) who used insolubilized antiallotype antisera, prepared against IgG of the domestic rabbit, and radiolabeled hare IgG. In addition to the b5 marker observed by Mandy and Rodkey, they detected b4 and b6 on 70–80% of the IgG molecules in a typical preparation; b5 was present on 55%. Since the sum exceeds 100%, two or three markers must be present on the same molecule. The markers were found in the IgG of all hares from a variety of geographical sources; this work suggests that the markers are isotypic rather than allotypic in hares. The difference in results obtained by the two laboratories may be attributable to differences in the cross-reactivity of the antisera employed.

III. HUMAN ALLOTYPES

Allotypic markers have been found on H chains of human IgG, IgM, and IgA and on κ chains, but not as yet on the H chains of IgD or IgE or in human λ chains. In each instance, antiserum has been used for the initial classification, but more recent studies have related a number of allotypic variations to differences in amino acid sequence. With one probable exception, allotypic differences attributable to carbohydrate have not been reported. All allotypic markers so far identified in human immunoglobulins are present in C_H and C_L regions.

Allotypy in human immunoglobulins was first demonstrated in 1956 by Grubb, and Grubb and Laurel (1,120), who noted that sera from certain patients with rheumatoid arthritis reacted with the anti-Rh (anti-D) antibodies of some individuals but not others. The test system they used is illustrated in Fig. 9.1. Rh+ erythrocytes are coated with nonagglutinating ("incomplete") anti-Rh antibodies, and the sera of rheumatoid patients are tested for their ability to agglutinate the coated cells; the agglutinating antibody is generally IgM. Some of these rheumatoid sera have proven useful for the detection of allotypic determinants. The sera of a large number of individuals can readily be tested for capacity to inhibit the agglutination. Sera which caused inhibition in Grubb's initial test system (by pre-empting the combining sites of antibodies reactive with the anti-Rh cell coat) were designated Gm(a+) and noninhibitory sera, Gm(a−) (Gm for genetic marker or gamma globulin.) Gm(a+) individuals constitute about 60% of the Caucasian and 100% of the Negro population (121). The number approaches 100% in nearly all non-European populations (122,123). Family studies indicated that Gm(a+) [now Gm(a)] is inherited according to the Mendelian law of indepen-

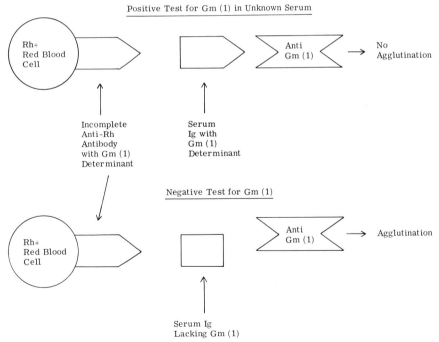

Fig. 9.1. Illustration of the test system initially used (and still widely employed) for the detection of Gm markers in human sera (1,120).

dent assortment and that the Gm^a gene is codominant and not sex-linked. The Gm(a) determinant is present exclusively on IgG1 molecules and was localized to the Fc region of the H chain (124). (Myeloma proteins are of great utility for the localization of allotypic determinants in immunoglobulin classes and subclasses and for identifying the related changes in amino acid sequence.) Following Grubb's initial discovery, the same technique and, in some instances, direct precipitation methods were used to identify a number of genetic markers on the H chains of

TABLE 9.4

ALLOTYPIC MARKERS ON THE H CHAINS OF HUMAN IgG MOLECULES
(Gm MARKERS)[a]

Subclass	Gm Designation	
	Current	Previous
IgG1	1	a
	−1	Non-a
	2	x
	4(3)	f(b^w, b^2)
	7	r
	17	z
	18	Rouen 2
	20	San Francisco 2
IgG2	23	n
IgG3	5(12)	b,b^1(b^γ)
	−5	Non-b,b^1
	6	c(c^3)
	11	b^β(b^0)
	−11	Non-b^β(non-b^0)
	13(10)	b^3(b^a)
	14	b^4
	15	s
	16	t
	21	g
	−21	Non-g
	24	c^5
	25	Bet
	Not assigned	b^5
IgG4		4a
		4b
Unclassified	19	Rouen 3

[a] Gm(8), Gm(9), and Gm(22) are omitted because there is some uncertainty as to whether they may actually be the same as Gm(−1) (127). It is probable that Gm(c^3) is the same as Gm(6) and that Gm(b^0) is the same as Gm(11). See text for a discussion of the nonmarkers.

human immunoglobulins and also on κ chains. Heavy chain markers on human IgG are designated Gm factors; those on κ chains are called Inv factors. A list of the most extensively investigated Gm factors is shown in Table 9.4 which also specifies the class of immunoglobulin with which the factor is associated. Two sets of terminology are included in the table. Letters of the alphabet were originally employed but replacement by numerals was recommended by a panel of the World Health Organization (125). Despite this recommendation, both sets of nomenclature are still in use. In some instances numerical designations have not yet been assigned and the letters are exclusively used. Either system would be easier to employ if it were organized with respect to distribution of the markers within subclasses of IgG.

Before a further discussion of the allotypic markers, some of the methodology used to identify them will be outlined briefly. For a more detailed description the reader is referred to the monograph by Grubb (123) and reviews by Fudenberg and Warner (126), Steinberg (122), and Natvig and Kunkel (127).

A. Methodology

The most widely used method for the detection of allotypic markers in human immunoglobulins is that of hemagglutination-inhibition, already described. Besides rheumatoid patients, multiply-transfused individuals and an occasional normal individual represent other important sources of agglutinating antibodies with specificity for Gm factors. The sera of very young children who are Gm-incompatible with their mothers also may express anti-Gm activity, owing to antigenic stimulation by maternal proteins transmitted across the placenta. Antisera which are useful for typing ideally should be specific for a single Gm factor. This occurs more frequently in normal sera with agglutinating activity than in rheumatoid sera. Multispecific antisera can be used if only one specificity matches that of the anti-Rh antibodies which are used to coat the red cells.

The problem of multispecificity of the anti-Gm serum is greatly reduced if the test erythrocytes are coated with a myeloma protein, which represents a single class of immunoglobulin, rather than with a heterogeneous anti-Rh antibody population. A myeloma protein possessing the desired Gm marker(s) can be linked to red blood cells for the agglutination test by using the bifunctional reagent, bisdiazotized benzidine (128) or by mixing the red blood cell suspension with the protein in the presence of a trivalent cation such as Cr^{3+} (129). Cells of blood

group O are generally used. The use of a myeloma protein may not completely solve the problem of multispecificity since more than one Gm
factor is frequently present on a single H chain. For example, in IgG1,
Gm(17), localized in the Fd region, is frequently associated with Gm(1)
in the Fc segment of the H chain; specificities 5,11,13,14, and 25 are
found on the same Fc fragment of IgG3 in some individuals (Table 9.5
and Section III,H,3).

Antibodies to Gm(1), (4), (5), (17), (21), (22), and (23) have been
produced by immunizing rabbits or primates with IgG, with the appropriate myeloma protein, or in the case of Gm(17), with the Fab fragment
of an IgG1 myeloma protein (130–137). The resulting antisera are ab-

TABLE 9.5

LOCALIZATION OF Gm FACTORS IN H CHAINS

Subclass	Domain		
	C_H1	C_H2	C_H3
IgG1	Gm(4) (Arg 214)		Gm(1) Arg Asp Glu Leu
			355 358
	Gm(17) (Lys 214)		Gm(−1) Arg Glu Glu Met[a]
			Gm(2)
IgG2		Gm(23)	
		Gm(−23)	
IgG3		Gm(5)	Gm(6)
		Gm(−5)	Gm(13)
		Gm(15)	Gm(11) (Phe 436)
			Gm(−11) (Tyr 436)
		Gm(16)	Gm(14)
		Gm(21) (Tyr 296)	Gm(b⁵)[b]
		Gm(−21) (Phe 296)	Gm(c³)[b]
IgG4		Gm(4a) Val Leu His	
		309	
		Gm(4b)[c] Val gap His	

[a] In IgG4 the corresponding sequence is Glu Glu Glu Met. In IgG2 and IgG3 the
Gm(−1) tetrapeptide is the same as that shown for IgG1; this accounts for the fact that
anti(−1) reacts with IgG2 and IgG3 but not IgG4.

[b] Letters are used where WHO numbers have not yet been assigned. However, there
is evidence that Gm(c³) is the same as Gm(6).

[c] Gm(4b) lacks the Leu present at position 309 in Gm(4a).

TABLE 9.6

COMMON GENE COMPLEXES PRESENT IN VARIOUS POPULATION GROUPS[a]

IgG1	IgG2	IgG3	IgG4	IgA2
Caucasians[b]				
4, −1[c]	23	5, 11, 13, 14, 25, −21[c]	4b	A2m(1)
4, −1	23−[c]	5, 11, 13, 14, 25, −21	4a	A2m(1)
1, 17	23−	21, −5	4a	A2m(1)
1, 2, 17	23−	21, −5	4a	A2m(1)
Melanesian				
1, 4		5, 13, 14		
1, 17		5, 13, 14		
1, 17		21		
1, 2, 17		21		
Negroes[d]				
1, 17	23−	5, 11, 13, 14		
1, 17	23−	5, 6, 11		
1, 17	23−	5, 6, 11, 14		
1, 17	23−	11, 13		

IgG1	IgG2	IgG3	IgG4	IgA2
Mongoloids				
1, 4	23	5, 11, 13, 14, 25	4a	A2m(1)
1, 17	23−	21	4a	A2m(1)
1, 17	23−	11, 13, 25		
Bushmen				
1, 17		5, 13, 14		
1, 17		21		
1, 17		5		
1, 2, 17		13		
Ainu				
1, 17		21		
1, 2, 17		21		
2, 17		21		
1, 17		13		

[a] Adapted from Grubb (123), Steinberg (122), and Natvig and Kunkel (127). Markers 7, 8, 9, 15, 16, 18, 19, 20, and 24 are not included because of incomplete data; Markers 11, 23, and 25 are tabulated where the data are available.

[b] The nonmarkers are indicated only for Caucasians.

[c] A minus sign preceding a number indicates a nonmarker; following a number it indicates the absence of that marker.

[d] Most Negroes carry the 4a marker in IgG4 and the A2m(1) marker in IgA2.

sorbed with serum or immunoglobulin lacking the genetic marker to be studied. Antibodies to Gm(17), Gm(22), and Gm(23) are obtained only from nonhuman sources (130–134). Although some of these antisera, in contrast to rheumatoid sera, form specific precipitates with the antigen, a more economical use of reagents is to test for activity by inhibition of passive hemagglutination of cells coated with a myeloma protein.

A major difficulty in typing is that two anti-Gm reagents which appear to separate a population of individuals into the same groups, i.e., which superficially appear identical, may actually be detecting different Gm factors. This can occur as a result of the presence of more than one allotypic marker on the same polypeptide chain in all members of the population studied; an antiserum to either marker would yield the same pattern of positive and negative reactions. In addition, genes controlling markers on different subclasses of IgG may occur as a gene complex which is the same in all members of a population under investigation; e.g., Caucasians whose IgG1 has the Gm(4) marker almost invariably have Gm(5) markers on their IgG3 molecules (Table 9.6). For this reason, the use of myeloma proteins of known class and subclass and of their Fab and Fc fragments has been of great value in the identification and localization of Gm specificities.

B. General Properties of the Gm System

Before discussing individual Gm factors a number of generalizations can be made:

1. Each subclass of IgG, with the exception of IgG4, has its own set of markers.

2. A single H chain may possess more than one Gm determinant; for example, IgG1 molecules of Caucasians frequently have three Gm markers: Gm(1) and Gm(2) on fragment Fc; and Gm(17) on fragment Fd (Table 9.5).

3. In a heterozygous individual, a single molecule possesses only one of two allelic determinants (123,127,138).

4. Amino acid substitutions associated with several of the Gm markers have been identified and others will undoubtedly be discovered.

5. Many important characteristics of the Gm system have been inferred through studies of myeloma proteins. It has nearly always been possible to extrapolate such conclusions to normal immunoglobulins.

6. Although Gm factors are associated only with H chains the expression of Gm(4) and Gm(17), localized in the Fd segment, requires the presence of L chains (139–141). This is probably attributable to a

conformational change which occurs in the H chain upon dissociation of the L chain. Gm markers localized in the Fc fragment are usually expressed in isolated H chains (140).

C. Presence of Different Gm Factors on the Same Polypeptide Chain

The location of various Gm markers within the H chain is listed in Table 9.5. Since some of the H chains exhibit more than one Gm specificity (all in C_H regions) it appears that a single gene can control more than one specificity.[5] (This is based on the assumption that one gene encodes the entire C_H segment.) The gene complexes observed vary among races. Thus, a gene, $Gm^{1,2,17}$ [encoding Gm(1,2, and 17)] is found in Caucasians but not in Mongoloids; the opposite is true of a gene, $Gm^{1,4}$. Other examples are presented in Table 9.6, which lists the common gene complexes in several population groups.

D. Gene Complexes Involving More than One Subclass of IgG

Since different genes control the C_H regions of the various sub-classes of IgG, it would seem possible that all combinations might occur in different individuals. In fact, this is not the case. Within a given population group only a few combinations of genes controlling the various subclasses are commonly observed. These are shown in Table 9.6. The gene complexes listed include an IgA marker. The stability of these complexes, which must reflect a very low recombination frequency, is consistent with the presence of a small number of C_H genes, located in very close proximity in the genome. This and other evidence has shown that all genes controlling the C_H regions of the various classes and subclasses of immunoglobulin are very closely linked. A few crossovers have been identified in population studies. These are described in Section III.K.

E. The Existence of "Nonmarkers"

There are certain determinants which are genetic variants in one subclass of IgG but which are present in all molecules of at least one other subclass. An example is the Gm(−1), determinant which is an allotypic marker for IgG1 but is present in all molecules of IgG2 or IgG3; it

---

[5] This also applies to mouse and rabbit C_H regions.

is absent in IgG4. In IgG1 the gene allelic to Gm^{-1} is Gm^1. Other examples are Gm(−21) which is an allotypic marker in IgG3 (allelic gene, Gm^{21}) but is present in all molecules of IgG2. Genes for two nonmarkers (−5) and (−11) are apparently allelic to Gm^5 and Gm^{11} in IgG3, but the nonmarkers are present in all IgG1 and IgG2 proteins (127,142,143). Two nonmarkers, designated 4a and 4b by Kunkel et al. (144), are apparently under the control of allelic genes in the IgG4 of Caucasians. Marker 4a is present in all IgG1 and IgG3 molecules, whereas 4b is present in all IgG2 molecules and absent from IgG1 and IgG3.

It is apparent that the study of the genetics of nonmarkers is most readily achieved through the use of myeloma proteins, since their presence on all molecules of one or more subclasses proscribes the use of whole serum. To study such a factor in normal serum the subclass of IgG in which it is a genetic marker must be isolated from the other subclasses in which the factor is present. In some instances this is best accomplished by treating with papain and isolating the desired Fc fragments (144,145). Perhaps the simplest genetic interpretation of nonmarkers is that they originally were encoded by DNA sequences controlling more than one subclass and that a mutation, creating the allele, occurred only in a gene controlling one subclass. (The genes for the individual subclasses of IgG probably arose through duplication followed by mutation.)

F. Possible Identity of Certain Markers with Different Designations

It has been suggested that certain markers listed separately in Table 9.4 are actually the same (123,127). This possibility arises because the amounts of reagents available are sometimes insufficient for adequate comparisons among different laboratories. Probable identities include Gm(3) and (4), Gm(10) and (13), and Gm(5) and (12).

G. Differentiation between Homoalleles and Heteroalleles

As already indicated a single gene may control more than one marker on a single polypeptide chain. Genes which behave as alleles and control markers that are located at the same position in two chains are referred to by Natvig and Kunkel as homoalleles (127); heteroalleles are genes that behave as alleles in genetic studies but which control markers at nonhomologous positions.

H. The Genetic Markers of IgG

Table 9.5 lists Gm markers identified in the four subclasses of IgG and their location, when known, in the H chain. The concentration of a given Gm marker in serum will, of course, reflect the concentration of the class or subclass to which it belongs. Table 9.6 shows major linkage groups found in various populations and includes the markers of IgA. Exceptions to the gene complexes listed in Table 9.6 are rare. We will discuss some of the more thoroughly studied Gm markers. The list of references, particularly of those to population studies, is necessarily abbreviated and the reader is referred to the reviews already cited for more detailed information. The monograph by Grubb (123) is an especially thorough description of the Gm and Inv markers.

1. IgG1 (1,120,146–149)

In Caucasians, the genes $Gm^{-1,4}$, $Gm^{1,17}$, and $Gm^{1,2,17}$ are allelic. If the entire C_H region is coded for by a single gene, then $Gm^{-1,4}$ is one gene coding for two different markers. In terms of the location of the markers on the chain, Gm(−1) and Gm(1) are related through a double amino acid substitution and Gm(4) and Gm(17) apparently through a single substitution (Table 9.5). The chemical basis for the Gm(2) marker is not known. $Gm^{-1,4}$ and $Gm^{1,2,17}$ are not found in African Negroes, nearly all of whom are homozygous for $Gm^{1,17}$. Gm(17) rarely occurs in the absence of Gm(1) in humans, although this has been observed in the chimpanzee (150). Mongoloids have a gene, $Gm^{1,4}$, which is not found in Caucasians or Negroes; such a gene could have arisen, for example, through a crossover involving $Gm^{-1,4}$ and $Gm^{1,17}$. A gene, $Gm^{2,17}$, is found among the Ainus of Northern Japan; in Caucasians the Gm(2) marker is nearly always present in association with Gm(1). The possibility that different gene combinations can arise through crossover events is supported by such findings as that of Natvig *et al.*, who identified the rare gene complex Gm(−1,2,4) controlling IgG1 in a few Caucasian families (150a).

Determinants 1 and 17, present in the IgG1 of all Negroes, are found in only 35–65% (depending on the ethnic group) of Caucasians. There is a marked geographical correlation of frequency of Gm(1) in European populations with the incidence increasing to the north and to the west. In nearly all non-European populations the incidence of Gm(1) approaches 100%; i.e., the Gm(−1) marker is found in IgG1 only of Europeans. Gm(1), the first Gm marker detected, has probably been the subject of the largest number of population studies.

2. IgG2 (128,133,151)

The genetic marker, Gm(23), is present in the IgG2 molecules of approximately 52% of Caucasians, 92% of Chinese, and 14% of Japanese, but is rarely seen in Negroes (133,152). An allelic gene must exist, but an antiserum that detects its product is not yet available.

3. IgG3

The marker Gm(21) (153) was present in about half the members of a Norwegian population studied. It is not found in African Negroes (152) but is present in a high percentage of Japanese (136). An allelic gene controls the nonmarker Gm(−21) (154). Gm(21) and Gm(−21) appear to be related by an amino acid interchange in the γ_3 chain: tyrosine versus phenylalanine at position 296 (155). A second important marker Gm(5) (156,157) is present in about 90% of Europeans and in all pure-bred Negroes. An antiserum has been prepared in baboons to the nonmarker Gm(−5); the marker was also identified by a rheumatoid factor (142). As indicated in Table 9.6, Gm^5 and Gm^{21} are not present on the same chromosome. They do not, however, encode markers present at homologous positions in the polypeptide chain. Gm(13) (157) which is probably equivalent to Gm(10) (121) is found in nearly all Caucasians who possess another IgG3 marker, Gm(5). It is present in 100% of African Negroes (157). Gm(6), another IgG3 marker, is found almost exclusively in Negroes (136,158–160). A recently discovered marker, Gm(25), is localized in the Fc fragment of IgG3 (161,162). Gm^{25} is closely linked to the gene complex $Gm^{5,10,11,14}$ in Caucasians and to $Gm^{5,10,11,14}$ or $Gm^{10,11}$ in Mongoloids, but the phenotype Gm(5,10,11,14,−25) is found in Negroes, in a frequency (up to 10%) varying with geographical location.

4. IgG4

The nonmarkers 4a and 4b behave as if under the control of allelic genes in Caucasians but only 4a is found in the IgG4 of Negroes or Mongoloids (127,144). The single amino acid deletion which provides a chemical basis for the difference between markers 4a and 4b (163) is shown in Table 9.5.

I. Localization of Gm Factors

Table 9.5 shows the location of Gm determinants within the H chains of each of the four subclasses of IgG and the sequences, when known, that correspond to the presence of the marker. (It should be noted that regions of the molecule in addition to that bearing the amino acid substitution may contribute to the formation of the antigenic determinant.) Each determinant, except Gm(4) and Gm(17), that has been localized is present in the Fc segment of the polypeptide chain. The nonmarker, Gm(−1), appears from sequence analysis to be localized in homologous positions in IgG1, IgG2, and IgG3; all molecules of IgG2 and IgG3 possess the determinant. (See footnote a, Table 9.5 for the sequence relationship in IgG4.) A single base change in a codon can account for each amino acid substitution observed in comparing markers with their corresponding nonmarkers. Only one or two substitutions are involved in each interchange. This is analogous to the small differences seen in allotypic interchanges in the C_H region of rabbit IgG, but differs from those in the rabbit V_H region, where multiple amino acid replacements distinguish markers controlled by the *a* locus.

J. Association of Genetic Markers Present in Different Subclasses (Allogroups)

The number of combinations of genes for the different subclasses present in any ethnic group is very limited and represents only a small fraction of the number of possible combinations (Table 9.6). Among Caucasians only four major gene complexes account for all populations studied; exceptions are quite rare. This is indicative of a low crossover frequency and is consistent with the presence of a small number of closely linked C_H genes. It is immediately apparent that different phenogroups characterize different populations. Markers that are very common in one population may not be found at all in another [e.g., Gm(4) and Gm(21) in Caucasians versus Negroes]. Genes controlling certain markers in different subclasses may always be together in the same gene complex in one ethnic group but always on separate chromosomes in another. An example is Gm^5 (IgG3) which is always associated with $Gm^{1,17}$ (IgG1) in African Negroes but only with $Gm^{-1,4}$ (IgG1) in Caucasians. Gm^{23} (IgG2) is present in the same gene complex as Gm^{-1} (IgG1) in Caucasians but is linked to Gm^1 in Mongoloids. A prominent example of a racial difference is the $Gm^{1,4}$ gene in Mongoloids and Melanesians, which is not found in Caucasians or Negroes; Gm^4 is not present in Negroes and is always associated with Gm^{-1} in Caucasians.

K. Unusual Combinations of Gm Factors in Family Groups

The occurrence of rare combinations of Gm factors in families is of significance since it permits an estimate of crossover frequency among the *Gm* loci, provides information relevant to the order on the chromosome of genetic loci controlling different subclasses, and suggests that most individuals have a single cistron for the C_H region of each subclass. The data on which these conclusions are based comes from studies of thousands of families by J.B. Natvig, H.G. Kunkel, A.G. Steinberg, E. van Loghem, and others.

1. DUPLICATION

Examples of duplications of genes, giving rise to two IgG1 genes on one chromosome, are described in references 127,164, and 165.[6] In two instances, members of a family group had the rare gene complex $Gm^{1,-1,4,17}$ on a single chromosome. (In Caucasians, Gm^4 and Gm^{17}, or Gm^4 and Gm^2, are normally not present on the same chromosome.) In addition, Gm(1) and (−1) were found, on separate molecules, in the same individual, as were Gm(4) and Gm(17). This again agrees with the concept that a total gene duplication had occurred, placing genes, $Gm^{1,17}$ and $Gm^{-1,4}$ on the same chromosome. Duplication can occur as a result of unequal crossing over.

2. HYBRIDIZATION

Of great interest was the observation in two individuals of an apparent hybridization of genes (164,166,167). This hybridization gave rise to molecules analogous to hemoglobin Lepore, in which different segments of the molecule are controlled by what are normally separate genes. (Hemoglobin Lepore is a hybrid of a β and a δ chain.) One individual was highly unusual in that his serum lacked all the following Gm markers: 1,2,4,5,11,13,15,16,21, and 23 (164,166,167); one or more of these markers is present in all normal Caucasians. The serum had normal amounts of IgG2 and IgG4, elevated amounts of the Fab segment of IgG3 (by antigenic analysis), and a complete absence of the Fc portion of IgG3 (166,167). Precisely the reverse was found for Fab and Fc antigens of IgG1. Addition to the serum of antibody to the Fab portion of IgG3 precipitated all IgG1 (Fc) antigens, as well as IgG3 (Fab) antigens; this indicated that the Fab portion of IgG3 and the Fc of IgG1 were on the same molecule. All these data can be explained by a mispairing of IgG1 and IgG3 cistrons at meiosis followed by a crossover which made contiguous the gene segments controlling the Fab of IgG3 and the Fc of IgG1 (Fig. 9.2). Another reported hybrid molecule was a myeloma protein from a Negro patient, in which the C_H1 and C_H2

---

[6] The interpretation of data presented here is that of Natvig *et al.* (127,165), who provide convincing evidence in support of their hypothesis.

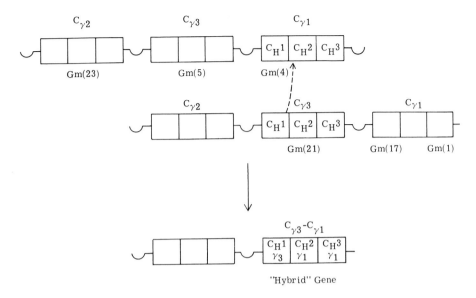

Fig. 9.2. Suggested crossover which yielded a gene coding the C_H1 domain (in the Fab fragment) of IgG3 and the C_H2 and C_H3 domains (Fc fragment) of IgG1. From references 127 and 166.

regions were those of IgG4, whereas the C_H3 region had antigenic properties of IgG2 (127); the authors state that such molecules have also been detected, on rare occasions, in the sera of normal Negroes.

These findings are of great importance since they suggest the presence of only a single cistron encoding the C_H region of a subclass of IgG. If more than one copy were present, it is difficult to see how a crossover event could result in the total loss of capacity to produce molecules of that subclass.

L. Ordering of Cistrons for the IgG Subclasses

Natvig and Kunkel (127) suggest the following order of genes in the chromosome: γ_4, γ_2, γ_3, γ_1, where γ_4 is the gene encoding the C_H region of IgG4, etc. The left end of the gene complex corresponds to the N-terminus of the polypeptide sequence. One line of evidence supporting this model comes from the individual, described above, whose IgG consisted in large part of hybrid molecules with H chains comprising the Fd segment of IgG3 and the Fc of IgG1. Since IgG2 and IgG4 levels were normal the genes for these two subclasses are presumably not located between those for IgG3 and IgG1; otherwise they would have been deleted during the crossover. The γ_3 gene is placed to the left of the γ_1

gene because the protein contained the Fd segment of IgG3 and the Fc segment of IgG1. The alignment of the γ_4 and γ_2 genes is based, by a similar line of reasoning, on the myeloma patient with hybrid IgG, who had molecules comprising the C_H1 and C_H2 regions of IgG4 and the C_H3 of IgG2. The somewhat weaker, but reasonable justification for placing the γ_4,γ_2 pair to the left of γ_3 and γ_1 is the close similarity of IgG2 and IgG3 molecules; this would suggest that the γ_2 and γ_3 genes may be related to one another through an early duplication, which placed one of the genes adjacent to the other.

M. Deletions of Genes

A number of examples of a gene deletion have been reported (152,164,168–170). This as well as duplication, can result from homologous but unequal crossing over. Deletions of the IgG3 cistron were found among members of several families and deletions of the IgG1 cistron in other families. In a few instances the defect was associated with an immune deficiency disease [reviewed in (127)]. Deletions of portions of an H chain (heavy chain disease) are discussed in Chapter 4, Section VII.

N. Other H Chain Determinants

In 1966, Ropartz *et al.* (171) described two antisera from healthy blood donors in San Francisco (sf), which reacted with a factor designated Isf(1). It is present on the Fd fragment of H chains of the IgG1 subclass in some individuals (172). They employed a hemagglutination system similar to that used to detect Gm factors. Two lines of evidence suggest that the Isf(1) antigen may be carbohydrate. First, the gene controlling Isf(1) is unlinked to that controlling Gm(1), Gm(2), or Gm(5), despite the presence of the Isf(1) determinant on IgG1 molecules. Second, Isf(1) frequency is age-dependent in Caucasians, occurring in 25% of infants, 40% of adults, and increasing to 60% in old age. This might be more readily interpreted in terms of regulation of attachment of carbohydrate than regulation of transcription of DNA. The Isf(1) phenotype is present in nearly all Negroes (92%) and is independent of age in that population group (173).

O. Allotypes of Human IgA

Human IgA has been differentiated into two subclasses, IgA1 and IgA2, on the basis of antigenic analysis (174–176). Certain IgA myeloma proteins show antigenic deficiency with respect to others when tested with rabbit anti-IgA antiserum. This permitted the development of antisera specific for the two subclasses. The antigenically deficient proteins, designated IgA2, comprise a minor proportion of serum IgA, which consists principally of IgA1.

Allotypy has so far been demonstrated only in the IgA2 subclass. It was discovered independently by Kunkel *et al.* (177) who now designate the first marker discovered as Am+ and by Vyas and Fudenberg (178,179) who called it Am(1). A useful designation currently employed is $A_2m(1)$ (180). The determinant was defined by using the sera of patients containing anti-IgA antibodies. The structure of IgA2 molecules bearing the $A_2m(1)$ marker is unique among human immunoglobulins in that the L and H chains are not joined by disulfide bonds; the chains are separable under denaturing conditions without prior reduction. (See sketch Table 3.1.) In addition, the L chains in $A_2m(1)$ molecules are linked to one another by disulfide bonds (181,182). By contrast, IgA molecules lacking $A_2m(1)$ determinants exhibit the normal disulfide bonded structure of L and H chains. The arrangement of interchain disulfide bonds in $A_2m(1)$ molecules is similar to that in IgA myeloma proteins of BALB/c mice.

The $A_2m(1)$ phenotype occurs in more than 98% of Caucasians, 30–50% of Negroes, 77% of Japanese, and 55–65% of Chinese (177,179). Simple Mendelian genetics apply to the inheritance of the allelic genes. The gene controlling $A_2m(1)$ is closely linked to genes encoding Gm antigens of the IgG3 subclass (177). In humans, as in mice, genes controlling H chains of all immunoglobulins are closely linked.

More recently, Wang *et al.* described a second marker, $A_2m(2)$, on IgA2 molecules (180). The reagent used was an antiserum from an IgA-deficient patient which reacted with IgA lacking $A_2m(1)$. The marker is present on the $F(ab')_2$ (presumably Fd) fragment of $A_2m(2)$ proteins. Family studies demonstrated that the A_2m^2 gene is closely linked to the *Gm* locus and behaves as an allele to A_2m^1. The geographical frequency of the A_2m^2 gene is in the order, Africa > Australia > Asia and Europe.

P. Allotypes of Human IgM

An allotypic marker on IgM, designated Mm1, was discovered by Wells *et al.* (183). The reagent used for typing was a human serum containing IgG antibodies directed to human IgM. Five of 23 monoclonal Waldenström IgM proteins, and the sera of some but not all individuals, interacted with the antibodies. The marker was found in 85% of Caucasians, 26% of Negroes, and 28% of Japanese tested. The gene controlling Mml is codominant and is inherited according to Mendelian laws. A reagent that detects the product of an allelic gene has not yet been described. The Mml determinant is not found on isolated μ chains; an intact molecule is required for its expression.

Q. Allotypic Markers on κ Chains (*Inv* Determinants)

These antigenic markers, initially described by Ropartz *et al.* (184,185) and Steinberg *et al.* (186), were first detected with sera from normal blood donors. The test system used is similar to that commonly employed in studying Gm factors; i.e., agglutination, by an appropriate serum, of Rh+ red blood cells coated with incomplete anti-Rh antibody, and tests of the inhibitory capacity of sera from various individuals. The known markers are Inv(1), (2), and (3). Inv(2) is always associated with Inv(1) but a small percentage of individuals are Inv(1,−2). The *Inv³* gene is allelic to genes encoding Inv(1,2) or Inv(1,−2). Agglutinating reagents useful for detecting Inv(2) and Inv(3) are rare. A κ Bence Jones protein which is positive for Inv(1) almost invariably lacks the Inv(3) marker and a protein which lacks Inv(1), with rare exceptions, carries the Inv(3) marker.

The Inv system can be described in terms of amino acid sequence. Kappa chains which are Inv(1,2,−3) have leucine at position 191, whereas chains which are Inv(−1,−2,3) have valine at this position (187–189). More recently, a Bence Jones protein which is Inv(1,−2,−3) was examined and found to have leucine at position 191 (189a). Unexpectedly, valine was found at position 153 in place of alanine. Valine had not previously been identified at position 153 because of the rarity of proteins which are Inv(1,−2,−3). The relationship between Inv type and sequence is:

	153	191
Inv(1, 2, -3)	Ala	Leu
Inv(-1, -2, 3)	Ala	Val
Inv(1, -2, -3)	Val	Leu

This means that anti-Inv(2) antibody recognizes the alanine-leucine combination; these residues are probably close enough to interact with a single antibody combining site.[7] For a positive reaction with anti-Inv(3) valine is required at position 191; whether it also involves alanine 153 is

---

[7] R.J. Poljak, personal communication.

uncertain. Anti-Inv(1) gives a positive reaction when leucine is present at position 191, with either alanine or valine at position 153.

The following observations indicate that the expression of Inv determinants is dependent on conformation (139,140,190): (a) L chains lose much of their Inv antigenicity when separated from H chains; (b) Inv determinants are expressed poorly when the L chains are combined with H chains of the IgG2 or IgG4 subclasses.

The Inv(1,2) marker is found in 10–20% of Caucasians, 30–60% of Negroes, and about 50% of the Japanese population. Inv(3) is present in more than 95% of Caucasians and about 90% of Negroes (122,123). These numbers are consistent with gene frequencies for Inv(3) of about 0.8 and 0.7, respectively, in Caucasians and Negroes.

R. Absence of Allotypic Markers on λ Chains

Allotypic markers have not been identified on human λ chains. Differences in amino acid sequences in the C regions of type λ Bence Jones proteins, once thought to reflect allotypy, have been shown in fact to be attributable to the presence of different isotypes of λ chains in most or all individuals (Chapter 3); this isotypy must reflect the presence of more than one C_λ gene.

S. Human Gm Markers in Nonhuman Primates

Many, although not all, of the Gm markers present in human IgG have been identified in nonhuman primates (150,191,192). Markers identified include several found in human IgG1 and IgG3 as well as Inv(1) and Inv(3); the association of markers with particular subclasses in primates has not as yet been established. The only marker for human IgG2, Gm(21) was not found in any of a variety of primate species tested. In some instances, a marker that is allotypic in humans appears to be isotypic in a primate species. For example, all gorillas, dwarf chimpanzees, and chimpanzees tested had the Gm(1), Gm(17), and b^5 markers.

Several human IgG3 markers are found in all gorillas but only in part of the chimpanzee population. Chimpanzees also appear to be polymorphic for Inv(1) and Inv(3). For each marker found in nonhuman primates there is a rather sharp cutoff on the evolutionary scale below which it can not be detected. It is somewhat difficult to generalize because various investigators have obtained different results with respect to certain markers. This is probably owing to the fact that the determinants in nonhuman primates are cross-reactive rather than identical with those in the human. The results might then vary with the antiserum.

From the patterns of Gm markers on the evolutionary scale and of isotypic markers characteristic of the four human subclasses, van Loghem and Litwin (192) conclude that molecules corresponding to human IgG2 appeared first, followed by IgG3 or IgG4, and that IgG1 evolved most recently (see also Chapter 7).

IV. MOUSE ALLOTYPES[8]

The immunoglobulins of the mouse comprise several classes, defined initially on the basis of antigenic determinants reflecting class-specific amino acid sequences in C_H regions. As is true in other species, the various classes are not distinguishable on the basis of their L chains (196), or, in all probability, on the basis of their V_H regions. Some of the properties of the major classes are discussed in Chapter 8.

Allotypic determinants have been detected in H chains of the IgG2a, IgG2b, IgG1, and IgA classes (34a,197,198), but not in IgG3 or IgM. Except for three specificities shared by IgG2a and IgG2b, and one shared by IgG1 and IgG2a, each class has a unique set of allotypic markers (197,198). An L chain marker is discussed in Section IV,E.

A. Methodology

Nearly all studies of allotypy in mice have been carried out with homologous antisera, prepared by injecting immune precipitates, immune agglutinates, or myeloma proteins from one strain into another inbred strain of mouse (34a,197,198). When normal (nonmyeloma) immunoglobulins are used the antiserum produced may react with allotypic determinants on more than one class of immunoglobulin. A thorough description of procedures used, and a list of strains that are efficient in the production of various antiallotype antibodies, are given by Mage et al. (34a). A few investigations with wild mice have been reported (199).

All individual mice of a given inbred strain share the same allotypic

[8] Early investigations of mouse allotypes were reported by Kelus and Moor-Jankowski (193), by Dubiski and Cinader (194), and by Lieberman and Dray (195). Much of the more recent work discussed here has been carried out in the laboratories of M. Potter, R. Lieberman, and L. Herzenberg.

specificities and are homozygous for each allelic gene (as well as for all other traits that are not sex-linked). Many isotypic specificities are shared by all strains and also by each of the IgG subclasses.

ANALYSIS OF DETERMINANTS DETECTED BY ANTIALLOTYPE ANTISERA

Antisera have been analyzed by qualitative and quantitative techniques; direct precipitation methods have been used in most investigations. More recently inhibition of passive hemagglutination (200) and radioimmunoassays (27,201) have been employed. Qualitative analysis is generally performed by the Ouchterlony method (double diffusion in agar gel). The quantitative procedure, used by Herzenberg and his collaborators (27,198) consists, first, in trace-labeling a purified mouse immunoglobulin preparation with radioactive iodine. Antiallotype antiserum is added and the percentage of radioactivity precipitated is determined. The presence of an allotypic determinant (present in the labeled immunoglobulin and recognized by that antiserum) in an unknown, unlabeled preparation is shown by its capacity to inhibit, partially or completely, the precipitation of radiolabeled antigen. Partial inhibition indicates that the inhibiting preparation shares some but not all of the allotypic specificities involved in the precipitation of the radiolabeled ligand.

It is informative to summarize some of the other rules employed by Herzenberg *et al.* in interpreting their data (198). (a) The recipient strain has none of the specificities recognized by the antiserum it produces. (b) The immunizing strain has all of the specificities detected. (c) The antiserum may not recognize all of the donor's allotypic specificities; first, because the recipient may have specificities in common with the donor and, second, because some potential determinants may not have induced antibody formation. (d) When the labeled antigen used in the test is from a strain (say, strain X) other than the donor, the only specificities detectable are those shared by the donor and strain X. (e) Two strains, each of which shows partial inhibition, may conceivably share no specificities. (f) The specificities detected always represent a minimum estimate of the true number.

B. Localization of Allotypic Determinants

Nearly all allotypic determinants studied in the mouse have been found on H chains (198,201–206). (A κ chain genetic marker will be described below.) With the exception of two specificities recently discovered in Fd fragments (201), all have been localized to fragment Fc. The mouse differs in important respects from the rabbit in that allotypic markers have not yet been identified in the V_H regions of mouse immunoglobulins, and no one has succeeded in preparing antiserum to allotypic determinants on mouse L chains.

The availability of inbred strains and the fact that the several H chain classes of mouse immunoglobulins are under control of separate genetic loci has permitted extensive investigation of genetic linkage. Through appropriate breeding studies it has been shown that genes encoding the C_H regions of IgG2a, IgG2b, IgG1, and IgA are all very closely linked. In a large number of matings, resulting in several thousand progeny, no crossovers have been seen (27,197,198,205,207).[9] A tentative conclusion as to the arrangement of these genes in the chromosome will be mentioned later.

Most investigations of allotypy in mice, in contrast to rabbits, have utilized highly inbred strains. Mouse myeloma proteins have been of great value in assigning allotypic markers to a particular subclass of immunoglobulin, primarily because it is difficult to isolate molecules of a given subclass in a pure state from normal mouse serum but relatively easy to purify myeloma proteins, owing to their high concentration. As a consequence, the association of an allotype with a particular subclass of immunoglobulin is often made by inference, based on data obtained with myeloma proteins of the BALB/c or NZB strains.[10] For example, if a given allotypic marker is associated only with IgG2a myeloma proteins from BALB/c mice, and the determinant is subsequently observed in another strain, the assumption is made that the determinant is present on IgG2a molecules in that strain as well (196–198).[10]

---

[9] Herzenberg and Warner (27) studied the specificities present on three myeloma proteins, GPC-5, GPC-7, and GPC-8, induced in F_1 hybrids (NZB × BALB/c). They found that the two IgG2a myeloma proteins, GPC-7 and GPC-8, both carry antigenic specificities determined by only one or the other of the *Ig-1* alleles inherited from its parents; i.e., GPC-7 carried only specificities of the *Ig-1[e]* locus (NZB) and GPC-8 carried the specificities of *Ig-1[a]* locus (BALB/c). However, GPC-5 carried one *Ig-3* specificity, 3.3 (IgG2b), and one Ig-*1* specificity, 1.5 (IgG2a), characteristic of the NZB strain. The rest of the *Ig-1* and *Ig-3* specificities of the NZB strain were missing. Since the *Ig-1* and *Ig-3* alleles are closely linked, Herzenberg and Warner proposed that the genetic information for this myeloma protein may have arisen from an intrachromosomal crossover between two sister chromatids, which resulted in the observed deletion. Information on the normal immunoglobulin of the donor mouse is not available.

[10] Potentially, myeloma proteins characteristic of other strains can be produced in congenic mice having the IgC_H locus (which controls Fc markers) of a second strain on a BALB/c or NZB background. Production of congenic mice is tedious and a limited amount of work with such mice has so far been reported, primarily with strains developed by Michael Potter (34a).

In considering mouse immunoglobulins it is necessary to separate clearly the concepts of allotype and allotypic specificity. A specificity represents an antigenic determinant recognized by an antiserum prepared in a mouse that was immunized with the immunoglobulin from another strain. (Such an antiserum can of course only be prepared in a mouse lacking that specificity.) Allotype is defined as a particular set of allotypic specificities, inherited as a group. For example, if one strain carries allotypic specificities 1, 2, and 3 of a particular class, e.g., IgA, whereas a second strain has specificities 1, 2, and 4, each set of specificities (or phenogroup) would represent a different allotype, despite the cross-reactions that would be observed with antisera directed to specificities 1 or 2. If mice from the two strains were mated, the immunoglobulins of each offspring would carry the specificities 1, 2, 3, and 4, but most individual IgA molecules would bear specificities 1, 2, and 3 or 1, 2, and 4. Tables 9.7 and 9.8 derived from the work of Herzenberg and co-workers (198) and of Potter, Lieberman and co-workers (34a, 197) list allotypes of the IgG2a, IgG2b, IgG1, and IgA classes. A different genetic locus controls the allotypic determinants on molecules of each class. For the IgG2a, IgG2b, IgG1, and IgA classes, the corresponding loci are designated by Herzenberg *et al.* (198) as *Ig-1*, *Ig-3*, *Ig-4*, and *Ig-2*, respectively.[11] Each allotypic specificity at a given locus is defined by two numerals separated by a decimal point; the first number identifies the locus. Thus, the antigenic specificities at the *Ig-1* locus (controlling the C_H region of IgG2a are 1.1, 1.2, 1.3, . . . , 1.12). Specificity 1.9 is now omitted because it has been found on both IgG2a and IgG2b molecules (208). For a similar reason specificities 3.5 and 3.6 are not listed.

As we have indicated, an allotype comprises a group of antigenic specificities (Table 9.7). Thus, molecules of the IgG2a class from

---

[11] Potter and Lieberman use the symbols IgF, IgG, and IgH for the three major subclasses of mouse IgG (equivalent to IgG1, IgG2a, and IgG2b, respectively). They are arranged here in decreasing order of average electrophoretic mobility toward the anode at neutral pH. Potter and Lieberman designate the antigenic markers detected on a molecule as superscripts to the right of the subclass designated; e.g., $G^{1,6,7,8}$ indicates the presence of allotypic determinants 1,6,7, and 8 on molecules of the IgG (or IgG2a) subclass (Table 9-8); the numerals bear no relation to those of Herzenberg. Superscripts to the left of the entire phenogroup designation indicate markers which have not been localized to a specific subclass; such markers are usually found in strains other than BALB/c, and hence no myeloma proteins containing these markers are available to help identify the subclass. It should be possible eventually to classify such determinants when myeloma proteins bearing them are raised in suitable congenic mice (See also footnote 10). Table 9.7 indicates those markers in the classifications of Herzenberg and of Potter, that are known to be identical.

BALB/c mice (allele *Ig-1ᵃ*) carry the antigenic specificities 1.1, 1.2, 1.6, 1.7, 1.8, 1.10, and 1.12. All these specificities are present on the same molecule. Mice of different inbred strains with different allelic genes may have some but not all of the same determinants in common; e.g., the allele *Ig-1ᶜ* controls specificities 1.2 and 1.7 in common with *Ig-1ᵃ*.

Tables 9.7 and 9.8 also list a prototype strain for each allele. In some cases many strains are allotypically identical to the prototype; for example, Herzenberg *et al.* (198) list 25 inbred strains of mice expressing the allele *Ig-1ᵃ* (prototype strain, BALB/c). The same reference gives an extensive tabulation of the allotypes of different strains of mice.

TABLE 9.7

HEAVY CHAIN LINKAGE GROUPS OF MICE[a]

Subclass	Locus	Allele	Specificities[b]	Prototype strain(s)
IgG2a	*Ig-1*	*Ig-1ᵃ*	1.1(G7),[c] 1.2(G8), 1.6, 1.7, 1.8, 1.10(G1), 1.12(G6)	BALB/cJ (+24 strains)[d]
		Ig-1ᵇ	1.4, 1.7	C57BL/10J (+17)
		Ig-1ᶜ	1.2(G8), 1.3(G3), 1.7	DBA/2J (+5)
		Ig-1ᵈ	1.1(G7), 1.2(G8), 1.5, 1.7, 1.12(G6)	AKR/J (+1)
		Ig-1ᵉ	1.1(G7), 1.2(G8), 1.5, 1.6, 1.7, 1.8, 1.12(G6)	A/J (+3)
		Ig-1ᶠ	1.1(G7), 1.2(G8), 1.8, 1.11(G5)	CE/J (+3)
		Ig-1ᵍ	1.2(G8), 1.3(G3)	RIII/J (+3)
		Ig-1ʰ	1.1(G7), 1.2(G8), 1.6, 1.7, 1.10(G1), 1.12(G6)	SEA/Gn (+4)
IgA	*Ig-2*	*Ig-2ᵃ,ʰ*	2.2(A12), 2.3(A13), 2.4(A14)	BALB/cJ, SEA/Gn
		Ig-2ᵇ		C57BL/10J
		Ig-2ᶜ,ᵍ	2.1	DBA/2J, RIII/J
		Ig-2ᵈ,ᵉ	2.3(A13)	AKR/J, A/J
		Ig-2ᶠ	2.4(A14)	CE/J
IgG2b	*Ig-3*	*Ig-3ᵃ,ᶜ,ʰ*	3.1, 3.2(H11), 3.4(H9) 3.7, 3.8	BALB/cJ, DBA/2J, SEA/Gn
		Ig-3ᵇ	3.4(H9), 3.7, 3.8, 3.9(H16)	C57BL/10J
		Ig-3ᵈ	3.1, 3.3, 3.7, 3.8	AKR/J
		Ig-3ᵉ	3.1, 3.3, 3.7	A/J
		Ig-3ᶠ	3.1, 3.2(H11), 3.3, 3.4(H9)	CE/J
		Ig-3ᵍ	3.1, 3.2(H11), 3.4(H9)	RIII/J
IgG1	*Ig-4*	*Ig-4ᵃ,ᶜ,ᵈ,ᵉ,ᶠ,ᵍ,ʰ*	Fast Fc (F8, 19)	BALB/cJ, DBA/2J, AKR/J, A/J, CE/J, RIII/J, SEA/Gn
		Ig-4ᵇ	Slow Fc	C57BL/10J

[a] From Herzenberg *et al.* (198) and Mage *et al.* (34a).

[b] There is no relationship (for example) between specificities 1.2, 2.2, or 3.2. The numeral before the decimal point refers to the locus; the numeral after the decimal point to the antigenic determinant. The letters F, G, H, and A refer to IgF, IgG, IgH, and IgA (designations of Potter *et al.*).

[c] The symbol in parentheses is the designation of Potter and Lieberman (Table 9.8) for the same specificity.

[d] The figure in parentheses is the number of other strains with the allele, listed by Herzenberg *et al.* (198).

TABLE 9.8

HEAVY CHAIN LINKAGE GROUPS OF INBRED AND WILD MICE[a]

Heavy chain phenogroup[b]	Prototype strain(s)
$G^{1,6,7,8}H^{9,11,22}F^{8,19}A^{12,13,14}$	BALB/c
$^{2}G^{-}H^{9,16,22}F^{-}A^{15}$	C57BL
$^{21}G^{3,8}H^{9,11}F^{8,19}A^{-}$	RIII
$^{20}G^{3,8}H^{9,11,22}F^{8,19}A^{-}$	DBA
$^{10}G^{4,6,7,8}H^{4,23}F^{8,19}A^{13,17}$	NZB, A
$^{10,18}G^{4,6,7,8}H^{4,23}F^{8,19}A^{13,17}$	AKR
$^{10,24}G^{4,6,7,8}H^{4,23}F^{8,19}A^{13,17}$	BL
$G^{5,7,8}H^{9,11}F^{8,19}A^{14}$	CE
$^{10}G^{1,6,7,8}H^{9,11,22}F^{8,19}A^{12,13,14}$	DD
$G^{3+5,7,8}H^{9,11}F^{8,19}A^{-}$	KH1[c]
$G^{3+5,8}H^{9,11}F^{8,19}A^{-}$	KH2[c]
$^{2}G^{1,6,7,8}H^{9,16}F^{-}A^{15}$	KY[c]

[a] Designation of Potter *et al.* (34a,197).

[b] Superscripts to the right of each letter indicate markers present on that subclass or class (IgG, IgH, IgF, or IgA = IgG2a, IgG2b, IgG1, or IgA, respectively). Superscripts to the left of the entire phenogroup designation, e.g. $^{10,18}G$, are markers for which the subclass of IgG is unknown. A dash indicates the absence of known markers.

[c] Wild mice (KH = Kitty Hawk, N.C.; KY = Kyushu, Japan). The determinant, G^{3+5} may involve a crossover of G^{3} and G^{5}, present in inbred strains.

It is of great interest that strains of each group listed as sharing allotypes controlled by the *Ig-1* locus also have the same allotypic markers controlled by each of the other loci (although the converse is not necessarily true).[12] Thus, all inbred strains for which SEA/Gn is the prototype at the *Ig-1* locus are allotypically identical to SEA/Gn at the *Ig-2* and *Ig-3* loci as well; this generality holds true for each strain and allele. Therefore, if two inbred strains have the same allotypic determinants on their IgG2a molecules they will also have the same markers on IgG2b, IgG1, and IgA. Herzenberg *et al.* have utilized this observation in designing a nomenclature of alleles at the three loci (27,198). For example, all strains carrying the *Ig-1ᵃ* or *Ig-1ʰ* alleles at the *Ig-1* locus have identical specificities at the *Ig-2* locus. The allele at the *Ig-2* locus is therefore designated *Ig-2ᵃ,ʰ*. The designation of alleles at the *Ig-2* and *Ig-3* loci is in this manner derived from that initially assigned on the basis of specificities controlled by the *Ig-1* locus.

The *Ig-4* locus which specifies the structure of IgG1 molecules has presented a special problem because of the difficulty of preparing anti-

[12] For example, BALB/c and SEA/Gn mice are identical at the *Ig-2* locus, which controls IgA, but are not identical at the *Ig-1* locus, which controls IgG2a.

allotype antisera. Mage *et al.* (34a) list two determinants, F8 and F19, present on the IgG1 of some but not all mice. Those mice whose IgG2a molecules are controlled by the *Ig-1*[b] allele (prototype strain C57BL) have IgG1 molecules which lack determinants F8 and F19; all other strains have IgG1 with these two determinants. Specificity F8 is probably identical with specificity G8 in the IgG2a (IgG) subclass (34a).

The same genetic polymorphism in IgG1 was demonstrated by Minna *et al.* through an entirely different approach (209). They discovered that inbred strains of mice can be divided into two groups on the basis of the electrophoretic mobility of the Fc fragments of their IgG1 molecules. Whole serum is digested with papain and subjected to immunoelectrophoresis; the pattern is developed with rabbit antiserum specific for mouse IgG1. The IgG1 of all strains carrying the F8(G8) = 1.2 specificity have Fc fragments of relatively fast (anodal) electrophoretic mobility at pH 8.2. The Fc fragments of all strains lacking F8 (prototype, C57BL) migrate more slowly. Thus one can determine the allotype of a strain at the *Ig-4* locus by physiochemical as well as immunological techniques.

C. Allotypes in Wild Mice

The linkage of genes controlling the various H chain classes has been explored in wild mice by Lieberman and Potter (199,210). Such mice almost always exhibit phenotypes that are found in individual inbred strains. However, in a survey of mice from various parts of North America and Japan, unusual combinations of allotypic specificities were detected in a few animals. In one location in North Carolina wild mice were found which had determinants G[3] and G[5] under control of a single gene. This was demonstrated by appropriate crosses with inbred mice. (Among all inbred strains tested the two markers are controlled by allelic genes.) Lieberman and Potter noted that the group of strains of which DBA/2 is the prototype possesses specificities 3 and 8, whereas another (prototype, CE/J) has specificities 5, 7, and 8. It is evident that an appropriate intragenic crossover could place all four of the specificities on a single chromosome and give rise to the observed gene, specifying G[3,5,7,8]. Similar suggestive evidence for crossing over was derived from the presence of an unusual heavy chain linkage group (allogroup) in a group of wild mice from Japan (Table 9.8).

On the basis of these apparent crossovers the following tentative order of loci on the chromosome was assigned (expressed in terms of the class or subclass under control of the genetic locus) IgG2a (IgG), IgG2b (IgH), IgG1 (IgF), IgA. Lieberman and Potter provide a detailed discussion of possible alternative mechanisms that could have produced the unusual phenogroups in wild mice (199). Homologous intragenic crossover was considered the most probable for the mice found in North Carolina. The possibility of a nonhomologous crossover was tentatively suggested to account for the unusual linkage of genes in the mice from Japan.

D. Allotypic Markers on the Fab Fragments of Mouse IgG

The allotypic markers discussed so far, all of which were identified by direct precipitation, are present in the Fc segments of mouse IgG or IgA (197,198). With more sensitive methods it is possible to identify markers in the Fd region of the H chain (201). Guinea pigs were immunized with polymerized Fab fragments of whole IgG from individual strains of mice. Tests for antibody activity were carried out by an indirect precipitation method using ^{125}I-labeled Fab of the donor IgG, the presumed guinea pig antiallotypic antiserum, and excess rabbit antiguinea pig IgG (to precipitate soluble complexes containing the radioactive label). This method should detect univalent antigen. The presence of a marker in various strains was determined by measuring the capacity of their sera to inhibit precipitation of the radioactive label. By these methods two different allotypic markers were identified on Fab fragments by two guinea pig antisera (201). One antiserum recognized determinant(s) present only in the IgG2a subclass. There was indirect evidence that the second antiserum also recognized markers on a single, unidentified subclass. Mice which fall into the same groupings on the basis of their reactivity with the anti-Fab antisera also belong to the same group when classified with conventional antiallotypic (anti-Fc) antisera. However, one antiserum divided a phenogroup based on Fc determinants (Herzenberg's *Ig-1^a* allele) into two subgroups. This, and the nonreactivity of L chains suggested that the markers detected are on the H chain (Fd segment) rather than on the L chain. Their restriction to one subclass would tend to localize the markers to the C_H1 segment since the V_H polypeptides are probably common to the various subclasses. Congenic mice, bearing the Fc allotypic marker of one strain on a second, background strain, possess the Fab allotypic marker of the first strain; this indicates close linkage or identity of the gene(s) controlling the Fab marker and the Fc segment of the chain.

E. Allotypic Specificity in the V Region of Mouse L Chains

By immunological techniques allotypic markers have so far not been identified in the L chains of mouse immunoglobulins. An alternative method appears, however, to differentiate the V regions of normal L chains of certain strains of mice (211). (Over 95% of the L chains in mice are κ.) The chains are first completely reduced, and the sulfhydryl groups liberated are alkylated with ^{14}C-iodoacetate. After tryptic digestion, peptide maps are prepared and radioactive peptides containing carboxymethylcysteine are identified by radioautography. The L chains of three strains of mice investigated were characterized by the presence of a unique peptide in the map; the maps of 14 other strains lacked this peptide, which encompasses residues 19–24 in the V region of the L chain population. If genetic polymorphism is discovered in the C_L region, linkage studies of genes controlling the two segments of polypeptide chain, similar to those carried out on the V_H and C_H genes in the rabbit, will be feasible.

F. Studies of Linkage of Immunoglobulin Genes

That the genes controlling the C_H regions of IgG2a, IgG2b, IgG1, and IgA subclasses are very closely linked to one another was demonstrated by Herzenberg (207) and by Lieberman and Potter (205). The latter investigators backcrossed F_1 (BALB/c × C57BL) to C57BL mice and examined 1054 progeny for allotypic determinants characteristic of BALB/c IgG2a and IgA. Both determinants were found in all of the same group of 539 mice and neither determinant in 515 mice; the absence of a crossover between genes controlling the C_H regions of IgG2a and IgA demonstrates very close linkage. Similar studies, involving fewer mice, indicate close linkage of IgG2a (IgG in Potter's nomenclature) with IgG2b (IgH), and of IgG2a with IgG1 (203,204). An obvious explanation for the infrequency or absence of crossovers is that a small number of genes, which are in very close proximity, control the synthesis of the C_γ and C_α polypeptides. Alternative possibilities, suggested by Potter and Lieberman, are that the H chain locus is close to a centromere or that the homologous chromosome regions in different strains are sufficiently different structurally to inhibit crossing over.

Further evidence for close linkage of the allotype-determining genes is the occurrence of only a few combinations of determinants (on IgG2a, IgG2b, and IgA) in a large number of inbred strains investigated (Table

9.7). The number of possible combinations of the major alleles at the four loci is 480 (198).[13] This great restriction of allelic combinations must be attributed, at least in part, to a very low recombination frequency. (In addition, it is possible that a relatively small number of mice gave rise to the domesticated mice from which most existing inbred strains arose. Wild mice are very difficult to breed.)

As already indicated, studies with wild mice are also consistent, in general, with maintenance of the same group of alleles as are found in inbred mice (199). Of 123 wild mice in one group studied, 75 were homozygous for linkage groups found in inbred mice and 46 had determinants consistent with heterozygosity. Only two mice in this study had groups of determinants which would not be found in the existent strains of inbred mice. They could have arisen through recombinations or independent mutations. The striking feature of these observations is the apparent maintenance of a limited number of linkage groups in wild mice.

G. Linkage of Genes Controlling Allotypic and Idiotypic Specificities

Using idiotypic specificity as a marker for V regions, very close linkage has been demonstrated among genes controlling V_H and C_H regions of mouse immunoglobulins (Chapter 11).

V. SUPPRESSION OF ALLOTYPIC SPECIFICITIES

Prenatal or early postnatal exposure to antiallotypic antibodies may suppress the appearance of the corresponding allotypic specificities. Such suppression has been accomplished in rabbits and in a particular strain of mice.

A. Suppression in Rabbits

The first experiments on suppression were reported by Dray and by Mage and Dray (212,213). Female rabbits of allotype b^4b^4 (κ chain locus), were mated with b^5b^5 bucks and were immunized during pregnancy with b5 immunoglobulin. The b^4b^5 offspring showed a greatly diminished serum concentration of b5, as compared to ordinary het-

---

[13] $8(Ig\text{-}1) \times 5(Ig\text{-}2) \times 6(Ig\text{-}3) \times 2(Ig\text{-}4)$.

erozygotes, and a compensatory increase of b4 immunoglobulin. The suppression was attributed to the production in the mother of anti-b5 antibodies, which were transmitted to the offspring *in utero.* Such suppression may last for as long as 1 to 3 years, and recovery is generally partial rather than complete; the concentration of the suppressed allotype often remains below 10% of the normal level. Suppression can be maintained indefinitely by the occasional administration of the appropriate antiallotype antiserum. Determinants specified by the *a,* as well as the *b* locus, can be suppressed by comparable methods (214). One can, alternatively, suppress an allotypic specificity by postnatal administration of antiallotypic antiserum. Several inoculations may be required for long-term suppression (213). Suppression of an allotype at the *b* locus (κ chains) does not affect the expression of allotypes controlled by the *a* locus (V_H regions).

There are technical difficulties in the suppression of an allotypic specificity for which an animal is homozygous. For example, neonatal suppression of the b4 allotype in homozygous offspring is complicated by the presence of maternal immunoglobulins which will bind any anti-b4 antibodies administered to the newborn rabbit. Dubiski (215) was able to achieve such suppression in a homozygote by breeding a b^4b^5 doe, which had itself been suppressed for allotype b5, to a b^5b^5 buck. In this situation molecules of allotype b5 were not transmitted to the progeny. Suppression of allotype b5 in b^5b^5 offspring could therefore be achieved by administration of anti-b5 antiserum.

Alternatively, the problem can be circumvented by a technique involving zygote transfer (216,217). For example, a fertilized egg of genotype b^5b^5 can be surgically transferred to a b^4b^4 surrogate mother (216). Obviously, there will be no maternal transfer of b5 molecules, and the progeny can be treated at birth with anti-b5 antiserum without difficulty. This results in almost complete suppression of group b markers. Typically, a rabbit will have recovered about 25% of its capacity to synthesize b5 within a month and 75% of its normal level will be attained within 6 months. Additional injections of anti-b5 antiserum can, however, prolong the suppression.

Alternatively (217), the doe into which the embryo is implanted can be immunized with immunoglobulin bearing the specificity (say a2) to be suppressed in a homozygous a^2a^2 embryo. Maternal anti-a2 antibodies are transmitted to the offspring, which then fails to synthesize a2 immunoglobulin. It is apparent that the foster mother must not possess an a^2 gene.

Suppression of allotype has proven to be a powerful tool in immunogenetic research. For example, suppression of rabbits homozygous at the b (κ chain) locus results in a compensatory increase of L chains bearing markers controlled by the c locus (73,218). This greatly facilitated the isolation and structural analysis of b-negative L chains, which were proven to be of the λ type. Similarly (32), the existence of V_H region subclasses in rabbit H chains was demonstrated through the suppression of molecules bearing allotypes controlled by the a locus (which encodes V_H genes). Molecules that are negative for all group a markers belong to a separate V_H subgroup.

Other studies of suppression have been carried out with rabbits of known genotype at both the a and e loci (which control V_H and C_H genes, respectively). When a rabbit of genotype a^1e^{14}/a^2e^{15} was suppressed with anti-a1 antiserum, there was a simultaneous, partial suppression of a1 and e14, and a compensatory increase in numbers of molecules bearing the a2 and e15 markers (29). One can explain this finding on the basis that only one chromosome of a homologous pair is expressed in a cell synthesizing immunoglobulin and that suppression occurs at the cellular level. When a doubly homozygous a^2e^{15}/a^2e^{15} rabbit was suppressed with anti-a2, the e15 marker was still found in the serum, but was associated with a-negative molecules, i.e., with molecules having V_H regions belonging to a different subgroup (219).

Harrison *et al.* showed that suppression of allotype b5 in homozygous b^5b^5 rabbits was accompanied by a complete absence of circulating lymphocytes having membrane-bound b5 immunoglobulins (220). During recovery from suppression the appearance of b5 molecules in the serum was preceded by the appearance of lymphocytes with membrane-bound b5 molecules. Determinants on the lymphocyte surface were detected with fluorescent or ^{125}I-labeled anti-b5 antibodies.

B. Suppression in Mice

Experiments analogous to those carried out in rabbits have been performed with inbred mice. For example, the offspring of a C57BL male (allele *Ig-1*^{b}), mated with a BALB/c female (allele *Ig-1*^{a}), which was then immunized during pregnancy against the paternal allotypic markers, exhibited an initial delay in the appearance of Ig-1^b immunoglobulin (221). Several months were required for the return to completely normal levels of immunoglobulins bearing Ig-1^b determinants. The degree of suppression was considerably less, however, than that observed in rabbits under similar circumstances.

More recently, Jacobson and Herzenberg showed that chronic suppression, similar to that observed in rabbits, can be induced in F_1 hybrid offspring of SJL and BALB/c mice (222). When males of the SJL strain (allele $Ig-1^b$) were mated with BALB/c females (allele $Ig-1^a$), which were then immunized against the paternal allotype, suppression of Ig-1^b markers persisted in about half the offspring for as long as 6 to 9 months; partial suppression was observed in most other F_1 offspring.

An important insight into the mechanism of suppression was obtained through adoptive transfer experiments (223). First, it was found that the repopulation of irradiated (600 R), chronically suppressed mice with spleen cells from nonsuppressed mice did not restore Ig-1^b production. This suggested that the chronic suppression was due to some active process which prevented the expression of the paternal ($Ig-1^b$) allele; this process is evidently resistant to irradiation. Next, it was shown that when cells from suppressed mice (SJL × BALB/c) are injected into irradiated syngeneic recipients, together with normal (nonsuppressed) syngeneic cells, the recipient mice failed to produce immunoglobulins controlled by the $Ig-1^b$ locus, despite the capacity of the normal cells to produce such molecules. (An initial burst of Ig-1^b production is frequently observed after the adoptive transfer.) Thus it appears likely that suppression is an active process involving members of the lymphocyte population. Present evidence suggests that the cell responsible for suppression is an activated T-cell which is present in a variety of lymphoid tissues.

REFERENCES

1. Grubb, R. (1956). *Acta Pathol. Microbiol. Scand.* **39**, 195.
2. Oudin, J. (1956). *C. R. Acad. Sci. (Paris)* **242**, 2489.
3. Oudin, J. (1956). *C. R. Acad. Sci. (Paris)* **242**, 2606.
4. Dray, S. Dubiski, S., Kelus, A.S., Lennox, E.S., and Oudin, J. (1962). *Nature (London)* **195**, 785.
5. Cebra, J.J., Colberg, J.E., and Dray, S. (1966). *J. Exp. Med.* **123**, 547.
6. Pernis, B., Chiappino, G., Kelus, A.S., and Gell, P.G.H. (1965). *J. Exp. Med.* **122**, 853.
7. Makela, O., and Cross, A.M. (1970). *Progr. Allergy* **14**, 145.
8. Todd, C.W. (1963). *Biochem. Biophys. Res. Commun.* **11**, 170.
9. Feinstein, A. (1963). *Nature (London)* **199**, 1197.
10. Lichter, E.A. (1967). *J. Immunol.* **98**, 139.
11. Kindt, T.J., and Todd, C.W. (1969). *J. Exp. Med.* **130**, 859.
12. Oudin, J. (1960). *J. Exp. Med.* **112**, 107.
13. Oudin, J. (1960). *J. Exp. Med.* **112**, 125.
14. Dray, S., and Young, G.O. (1958). *J. Immunol.* **81**, 142.
15. Dray, S., and Young, G.O. (1960). *Science* **131**, 738.
16. Dray, S., Young, G.O., and Gerald, L. (1963). *J. Immunol.* **91**, 403.

17. Dubiski, S., Skalba, D., Dubiska, A., and Kelus, A. (1959). *Nature (London)* **184,** 1811.
18. Dubiski, S., Dudziak, Z., Skalba, D., and Dubiska, A. (1959). *Immunology* **2,** 84.
19. Dubiski, S., Rapacz, J., and Dubiska, A. (1962). *Acta Genet.* **12,** 136.
20. Dubiski, S., and Kelus, A.S. (1961). *In* "Protides of the Biological Fluids" (H. Peeters, ed.), p. 172. Elsevier, Amsterdam.
21. Kelus, A.S., and Gell, P.G.H. (1963). *Proc. 11th Int. Congr. Genet.* Vol. 1, p. 194. Pergamon, New York.
22. Mancini, E., Tosi, R.M., Luzzati, A., and Carbonara, A. (1970). *Progr. Immunobiol. Stand.* **4,** 56.
23. Dray, S., Young, G.O., and Nisonoff, A. (1963). *Nature (London)* **199,** 52.
24. Dray, S., and Nisonoff, A, (1963). *Proc. Soc. Exp. Biol. Med.* **113,** 20.
25. Gilman, A.M., Nisonoff, A., and Dray, S. (1964). *Immunochemistry* **1,** 109.
26. Dray, S., and Nisonoff, A. (1965). *In* "Molecular and Cellular Basis of Antibody Formation" Proc. of Symposium Held in Prague, June, 1964, p. 175. Academic Press, New York.
27. Herzenberg, L.A., and Warner, N.L. (1967). *In* "Regulation of the Antibody Response" (B. Cinader, ed.), p. 322. Thomas, Springfield, Illinois.
28. Landucci-Tosi, S., and Mage, R.G. (1970). *J. Immunol.* **105,** 1046.
29. Landucci-Tosi, S., Mage, R.G., and Dubiski, S. (1970). *J. Immunol.* **104,** 641.
30. Tosi, R., and Landucci-Tosi, S. (1973). *Contemp. Topics Mol. Immunol.* **2,** 79.
31. Mandy, W.J., and Todd, C.W. (1968). *Vox. Sang.* **14,** 264.
32. Kim, B.S., and Dray, S. (1972). *Eur. J. Immunol.* **2,** 509.
33. Dubiski, S., and Good, P.W. (1972). *Proc. Soc. Exp. Biol. Med.* **141,** 486.
34. Dray, S., Kim, B.S., and Gilman-Sachs, A. (1974). *Ann. Immunol. (Paris)* 125C 41.
34a. Mage, R.G., Lieberman, R., Potter, M., and Terry, W.D. (1973). *In* "The Antigens" (M. Sela, ed.), Vol. 1, p. 299, Academic Press, New York.
35. Appella, E., Rejnek, J., and Reisfeld, R.A. (1969). *J. Mol. Biol.* **41,** 473.
36. Frangione, B., and Lamm, M.E. (1970). *FEBS Lett.* **11,** 339.
36a. Frangione, B. (1969). *FEBS Lett.* **3,** 341.
37. Waterfield, M.D., Morris, J.E., Hood, L.E., and Todd, C.W. (1973). *J. Immunol.* **110,** 227.
38. Thunberg, A.L., Lackland, H., and Kindt, T.J. (1973). *J. Immunol.* **111,** 1755.
39. Gilman-Sachs, A., Mage, R.G., Young, G.O., Alexander, C., and Dray, S. (1969). *J. Immunol.* **103,** 1159.
40. Kelus, A.S., and Gell, P.G.H. (1967). *Progr. Allergy* **11,** 141.
41. Kelus, A.S., Marrack, J.R., and Richards, C.B. (1961). *In* "Protides of the Biological Fluids" (H. Peeters, ed.), Vol. 9, p. 176. Elsevier, Amsterdam.
42. Marrack, J.R.M., Richards, C.B., and Kelus, A.S. (1961). *In* "Protides of the Biological Fluids" (H. Peeters, ed.), Vol. 9, p. 200. Elsevier, Amsterdam.
43. Stemke, G.W. (1964) *Science* **145,** 403.
44. Wilheim, E., and Lamm, M.E. (1966). *Nature (London)* **212,** 846.
45. Feinstein, A., Gell, P.G.H., and Kelus, A.S. (1963). *Nature (London)* **200,** 653.
46. Mole, L.E., Jackson, S.A., Porter, R.R., and Wilkinson, J.M. (1971). *Biochem. J.* **124,** 301.
47. Fleischman, J.B. (1973) *Immunochemistry* **10,** 401.
48. Dubiski, S., and Muller, P.J. (1967). *Nature (London)* **214,** 696.
49. Rejnek, J., Appella, E., Mage, R.G., and Reisfeld, R.A. (1969). *Biochemistry* **8,** 2712.
50. Mage, R.G., Reisfeld, R.A., and Dray, S. (1966). *Immunochemistry* **3,** 299.

51. Kindt, T.J., Seide, R.K., Tack, B., and Todd, C.W. (1973). *J. Exp. Med.* **138**, 33.
52. Spring, S.B., Nisonoff, A., and Dray, S. (1970). *J. Immunol.* **105**, 653.
53. Kindt, T.J., Seide, R.K., Lackland, H., and Thunberg, A.L. (1972). *J. Immunol.* **109**, 735.
54. Schenelle, J., Costea, N., Dray, S., Heller, P., and Yakulis, V. (1969). *Proc. Soc. Exp. Biol. Med.* **130**, 48.
55. Gell, P.G.H., and Kelus, A.S. (1962). *Nature (London)* **195**, 44.
56. Reider, R.F., and Oudin, J. (1963). *J. Exp. Med.* **118**, 627.
57. Lark, C.A., Eisen, H.N., and Dray, S. (1965). *J. Immunol.* **95**, 404.
58. Hoyer, L.W., and Mage, R.G. (1967). *J. Immunol.* **99**, 25.
59. Catty, D., Humphrey, J.H., and Gell, P.G.H. (1969). *Immunology* **16**, 409.
60. Nisonoff, A., Zappacosta, S., and Jureziz, R. (1967). *Cold Spring Harbor Symp. Quant. Biol.* **32**, 89.
61. Rodkey, L.S., Choi, T.K., and Nisonoff, A. (1969). *J. Immunol.* **104**, 63.
62. Jaton, J.C., Waterfield, M.D., Margolies, M., Bloch, K.J., and Haber, E. (1971). *Biochemistry* **10**, 1583.
63. Kindt, T.J., Todd, C.W., Eichmann, K., and Krause, R.M. (1970). *J. Exp. Med.* **131**, 343.
64. Strosberg, A.D., Jaton, J.C., Capra, J.D., and Haber, E. (1972). *Fed. Proc. Fed. Amer. Soc. Exp. Biol.* **31**, 771.
65. Reisfeld, R.A., Dray, S., and Nisonoff, A. (1965). *Immunochemistry* **2**, 155.
66. Reisfeld, R.A., and Inman, J.K. (1968). *Immunochemistry* **5**, 503.
67. Small, P.A., Reisfeld, R.A., and Dray, S. (1965). *J. Mol. Biol.* **11**, 713.
68. Frangione, B., Franklin, E.C., and Kelus, A.S. (1968). *Immunology* **15**, 599.
69. Bornstein, O., and Oudin, J. (1964). *J. Exp. Med.* **120**, 655.
70. DeVries, G.M., Lanckman, M., and Hamers, R. (1969). *Eur. J. Biochem.* **11**, 370.
71. Rejnek, J., Mage, R.G., and Reisfeld, R.A. (1969). *J. Immunol.* **102**, 638.
72. Mage, R.G., Young, G.O., and Reisfeld, R.A. (1968). *J. Immunol.* **101**, 617.
73. Appella, E., Mage, R.G., Dubiski, S., and Reisfeld, R.A. (1968). *Proc. Nat. Acad. Sci. U.S.* **60**, 975.
74. Vice, J.L., Hunt, W.L., and Dray, S. (1970). *J. Immunol.* **104**, 38.
75. Koshland, M.E. (1967). *Cold Spring Harbor Symp. Quant. Biol.* **32**, 119.
76. Prahl, J.W., and Porter, R.R. (1968). *Biochem. J.* **107**, 753.
77. Small, P.A., Reisfeld, R.A., and Dray, S. (1966). *J. Mol. Biol.* **16**, 328.
77a. Williamson, J.M. (1969). *Biochem. J.* **112**, 173.
78. Jaton, J.-C., Braun, D.G., Strosberg, A.D., Haber, E., and Morris, J.E. (1973). *J. Immunol.* **111**, 1838.
78a. Jaton, J.-C. and Haimovich, J. (1974). *Biochem. J.* **139**, 281.
79. Tosi, S.L., Mage, R.G., and Lawton, A.R. (1972). *Immunochemistry* **9**, 317.
80. Koshland, M.E., Davis, J.J., and Fujita, N.J. (1969). *Proc. Nat. Acad. Sci. U.S.* **63**, 1274.
81. Micheli, A., Mage, R.G., and Reisfeld, R.A. (1968). *J. Immunol.* **100**, 604.
82. Dray, S., and Young, G.O. (1961). *Fed. Proc. Fed. Amer. Soc. Exp. Biol.* **20**, 32.
83. Kakinuma, M. (1971) *J. Immunol.* **106**, 1095.
84. Knight, K.L., Gilman-Sachs, A., Fields, R., and Dray, S. (1971). *J. Immunol.* **106**, 761.
85. Kim, B.S., and Dray, S. (1973). *J. Immunol.* **111**, 750.
85a. Tack, B.F., Feintuch, K., Todd, C.W., and Prahl, J.W. (1973). *Biochemistry* **12**, 5172.

85b. Prahl, J.W., Tack, B.F., and Todd, C.W. (1973). *Biochemistry* **12**, 5181.
86. Mandy, W.J., and Todd, C.W. (1970). *Biochem. Genet.* **4**, 59.
87. Dubiski, S. (1969). *J. Immunol.* **103**, 120.
88. Dubiski, S. (1969). *In* "Protides of the Biological Fluids" (H. Peeters, ed.), Vol. 17, p. 117. Elsevier, Amsterdam.
89. Kindt, T.J., and Mandy, W.J. (1972). *J. Immunol.* **108**, 1110.
90. Prahl, J.W., Mandy, W.J., and Todd, C.W. (1969). *Biochemistry* **8**, 4935.
91. Mandy, W.J., and Todd, C.W. (1969). *Immunochemistry* **6**, 811.
92. Kindt, T.J., Mandy, W.J., and Todd, C.W. (1970). *Immunochemistry* **7**, 467.
93. Kindt, T.J., Mandy, W.J., and Todd, C.W. (1970). *Biochemistry* **9**, 2028.
94. Mage, R.G., Young-Cooper, G.O., and Alexander, C. (1971). *Nature New Biol.* **230**, 63.
95. Landucci-Tosi, S., and Tosi, R.M. (1973). *Immunochemistry* **10**, 65.
95a. Malek, T.R., Hanly, W.C., and Knight, K.L. (1974). *Eur. J. Immunol.* **4**, 692.
96. Pernis, B., Forni, L., Dubiski, S., Kelus, A.S., Mandy, W.J., and Todd, C.W. (1973). *Immunochemistry* **10**, 281.
97. Appella, E., Chersi, A., Mage, R.G., and Dubiski, S. (1971). *Proc. Nat. Acad. Sci. U.S.* **68**, 1341.
98. Hill, R.L., Delaney, R., Fellows, R.E., and Lebovitz, H.E. (1966). *Proc. Nat. Acad. Sci. U.S.* **56**, 1762.
99. Hill, R.L., Delaney, R., Lebovitz, H.E., and Fellows, R.E. (1966). *Proc. Roy. Soc.* **B166**, 159.
100. Fruchter, R.G., Jackson, S.A., Mole, L.E., and Porter, R.R. (1970). *Biochem. J.* **116**, 249.
101. Eby, W.C., Kim, B.S., Dray, S., Young-Cooper, G.O., and Mage, R.G. (1973). *Immunochemistry* **10**, 417.
102. Harrington, J.C., Fenton, J.W., II, and Pert, J.H. (1971). *Immunochemistry* **8**, 413.
103. Hamers, R., and Hamers-Casterman, C. (1965). *J. Mol. Biol.* **14**, 288.
104. Hamers, R., and Hamers-Casterman, C. (1967). *Cold Spring Harbor Symp. Quant. Biol.* **32**, 129.
105. Kelus, A.S., and Gell, P.G.H. (1965). *Nature (London)* **206**, 313.
106. Sell, S. (1966). *Science* **153**, 641.
107. Kelus, A.S. (1967). *In* "Nobel Symposium on the Gamma-Globulins" (J. Killander, ed.), p. 329. Interscience, New York.
108. Kelus, A.S., and Pernis, B. (1971). *Eur. J. Immunol.* **1**, 123.
109. Gilman-Sachs, A., and Dray, S. (1973). *Eur. J. Immunol.* **2**, 505.
110. Conway, T.P., Dray, S., and Lichter, E.A. (1969). *J. Immunol.* **102**, 544.
111. Hanly, W.C., Knight, K.L., Gilman-Sachs, A., Dray, S., and Lichter, E.A. (1972). *J. Immunol.* **108**, 723.
112. Hanly, W.C., Lichter, E.A., Dray, S., and Knight, K.L. (1973). *Biochemistry* **12**, 733.
112a. Lammert, J.M., Hanly, W.C., Knight, K.L., Lichter, E.A., and Dray, S. (1974). *Fed. Proc. Fed. Amer. Soc. Exp. Biol.* **33**, 737.
113. Knight, K.L., Rosenweig, M., Lichter, E.A., and Hanly, W.C. (1974). *J. Immunol.* **112**, 877.
114. Kim, B.S. (1973) *Fed. Proc. Fed. Amer. Soc. Exp. Biol.* **32**, 990.
115. Hanly, W.C., Lichter, E.A., and Knight, K.L. (1973). *Fed. Proc. Fed. Amer. Soc. Exp. Biol.* **32**, 1003.
116. Mandy, W.J., and Rodkey, L.S. (1974). *Immunochemistry* **11**, 29.
117. Rodkey, L.S., and Conrat, A.H. (1972). *J. Immunol.* **109**, 342.

118. Rodkey, L.S. (1973). *Immunochemistry* **10**, 661.
119. Landucci-Tosi, S., Tosi, R., and Perramon, A. (1973). *J. Immunol.* **110**, 286.
120. Grubb, R., and Laurell, A.B. (1956). *Acta Pathol. Microbiol. Scand.* **39**, 390.
121. Ropartz, C., Rivat, L., Rousseau, P.Y., Baitsch, H., and van Loghem, J. (1963). *Acta Genet. (Basel)* **13**, 109.
122. Steinberg, A.G. (1969). *Annu. Rev. Genet.* **3**, 25.
123. Grubb, R. (1970). "The Genetic Markers of Human Immunoglobulins." Springer-Verlag, New York.
124. Harboe, M., Osterland, C.K., and Kunkel, H.G. (1962). *Science* **136**, 979.
125. *Bull. WHO* (1965). **33**, 721.
126. Fudenberg, H.H., and Warner, N.L. (1970). *Advan. Human Genet.* **1**, 131.
127. Natvig, J.B., and Kunkel, H.G. (1973). *Advan. Immunol.* **16**, 1.
128. Natvig, J.B., and Kunkel, H.G. (1967). *Nature (London)* **215**, 68.
129. Vyas, G.N., Fudenberg, H.H., Pretty, H.M., and Gold, E.R. (1968). *J. Immunol.* **100**, 274.
130. Hess, M., and Butler, R. (1962). *Vox. Sang.* **7**, 93.
131. Alepa, F.P., and Steinberg, A.G. (1964). *Vox. Sang.* **9**, 333.
132. Litwin, S.D., and Kunkel, H.G. (1967). *J. Exp. Med.* **125**, 847.
133. Kunkel, H.G., Yount, W.J., and Litwin, S.D. (1966). *Science* **154**, 1041.
134. Litwin, S.D., and Camp, F.R., Jr. (1969). *Vox. Sang.* **17**, 194.
135. Litwin, S.D., and Kunkel, H.G. (1966). *Transfusion* **6**, 140.
136. van Loghem, E., and Martensson, L. (1967). *Vox. Sang.* **13**, 369.
137. Yount, W.J., Kunkel, H.G., and Litwin, S.D. (1967). *J. Exp. Med.* **125**, 177.
138. Martensson, L. (1961). *Acta Med. Scand.* **170** (Suppl. 367), 87.
139. Polmar, S.H., and Steinberg, A.G. (1964). *Science* **145**, 928.
140. Polmar, S.H., and Steinberg, A.G. (1967). *Biochem. Genet.* **1**, 117.
141. Steinberg, A.G. (1964). *Cold Spring Harbor Symp. Quant. Biol.* **29**, 449.
142. Gaarder, P.I., and Natvig, J.B. (1972). *J. Immunol.* **108**, 617.
143. van Loghem, E., and de Lange, A. (1972). *Vox. Sang.* **22**, 193.
144. Kunkel, H.G., Joslin, F.G., Penn, G.M., and Natvig, J.B. (1970). *J. Exp. Med.* **132**, 508.
145. Michaelsen, T.E., and Natvig, J.B. (1971). *Immunochemistry* **8**, 235.
146. Harboe, M., and Lundevall, J. (1959). *Acta Pathol. Microbiol. Scand.* **45**, 357.
147. Gold, E.R., Martensson, L., Ropartz, C., Rivat, L., and Rousseau, P.Y. (1965). *Vox. Sang.* **10**, 299.
148. Gold, E.R., Mandy, W.J., and Fudenberg, H.H. (1965). *Nature (London)* **207**, 1099.
149. Litwin, S.D., and Kunkel, H.G. (1966). *Nature (London)* **210**, 866.
150. van Loghem, E., Shuster, J., and Fudenberg, H.H. (1968). *Vox. Sang.* **14**, 81.
150a. Natvig, J.B., Michaelsen, T.E., and Nielsen, J.C. (1974). *Scand. J. Immunol.* **3**, 127.
151. Natvig, J.B., Kunkel, H.G., and Gedde-Dahl, T. (1967). *Nobel Symp.* **3**, 313.
152. Natvig, J.B., Kunkel, H.G., Yount, W.J., and Nielsen, J.C. (1968). *J. Exp. Med.* **128**, 763.
153. Natvig, J.B. (1966) *Nature (London)* **211**, 318.
154. Natvig, J.B., Kunkel, H.G., and Joslin, F.G. (1969). *J. Immunol.* **102**, 611.
155. Grey, H.M., and Abel, C.A. (1970). *Protides Biol. Fluids Proc. Colloq.* **17**, 229.
156. Harboe, M. (1959). *Acta Pathol. Microbiol. Scand.* **47**, 191.
157. Steinberg, A.G., and Goldblum, R. (1965). *Amer. J. Human Genet.* **17**, 133.
158. Steinberg, A.G., Giles, B.D., and Stauffer, R. (1960). *Amer. J. Human Genet.* **12**, 44.
159. Steinberg, A.G., and Wilson, J.A. (1963). *Amer. J. Human Genet.* **15**, 96.
160. Ropartz, C., Rousseau, P.Y., and Rivat, L. (1963). *Rev. Fr. Etud. Clin. Biol.* **8**, 465.

161. Blanc, M., Ducos, J., and Ruffie, J. (1970). *C. R. Acad. Sci. (Paris)* **271**, 145.
162. Rivat, L., Blanc, M., Rivat, C., Ropartz, C., and Ruffie, J. (1971). *Humangenetik* **13**, 108.
163. Abel, C.A. (1972). *Fed. Proc. Fed. Amer. Soc. Exp. Biol.* **31**, 742.
164. Steinberg, A.G., Muir, W.A., and McIntire, S.A. (1968). *Amer. J. Human Genet.* **20**, 258.
165. Natvig, J.B., Michaelsen, T.E., and Kunkel, H.G. (1971). *J. Exp. Med.* **133**, 1004.
166. Kunkel, H.G., Natvig, J.B., and Joslin, F.G. (1969) *Proc. Nat. Acad. Sci. U.S.* **62**, 144.
167. Steinberg, A.G., Terry, W.D., and Morell, A.R. (1970). *In* "Protides of the Biological Fluids" (H. Peeters, ed.), Vol. 17, p. 111. Elsevier, Amsterdam.
168. van Loghem, E., and Natvig, J.B. (1970). *Vox. Sang.* **18**, 421.
169. Litwin, S.D., Yount, W.J., Kunkel, H.G., Martensson, L., van Loghem, E., and Natvig, J.B. (1973). Quoted in Ref. 127.
170. Yount, W.J., Hong, R., Seligmann, M., Good, R., and Kunkel, H.G. (1970). *J. Clin. Invest.* **49**, 1957.
171. Ropartz, C., Rivat, L., Rousseau, P.Y., Fudenberg, H.H., Molter, R., and Salmon, C. (1966). *Vox. Sang.* **11**, 99.
172. Ropartz, C., Rivat, L., Rivat, C., and Rousseau, P.Y. (1968). *Vox. Sang.* **14**, 458.
173. Ropartz, C., Fudenberg, H.H., Rivat, L., Rousseau, P.Y., and Lebreton, J.P. (1967). *Rev. Fr. Etud. Clin. Biol.* **12**, 267.
174. Feinstein, D., and Franklin, E.C. (1966). *Nature (London)* **212**, 1496.
175. Kunkel, H.G., and Prendergast, R.A. (1966). *Proc. Soc. Exp. Biol. Med.* **122**, 910.
176. Vaerman, J.P., and Heremans, J.F. (1966). *Science* **153**, 647.
177. Kunkel, H.G., Smith, W.K., Joslin, F.G., Natvig, J.B., and Litwin, S.D. (1969). *Nature (London)* **223**, 1247.
178. Vyas, G.N., and Fudenberg, H.H. (1969). *Clin. Res.* **17**, 469.
179. Vyas, G.N., and Fudenberg, H.H. (1969). *Proc. Nat. Acad. Sci. U.S.* **64**, 1211.
180. Wang, A.C., van Loghem, E., and Shuster, J. (1973). *Fed. Proc. Fed. Amer. Soc. Exp. Biol.* **32**, 1003.
181. Grey, H.M., Abel, C.A., Yount, W.J., and Kunkel, H.G. (1969). *J. Exp. Med.* **128**, 1223.
182. Jerry, L.M., Kunkel, H.G., and Grey, H.M. (1970). *Proc. Nat. Acad. Sci. U.S.* **65**, 557.
183. Wells, J.V., Bleumers, J.F., and Fudenberg, H.H. (1973). *Proc. Nat. Acad. Sci. U.S.* **70**, 827.
184. Ropartz, C., Rivat, L., and Rousseau, P.Y. (1964). *Proc. 9th Congr. Int. Soc. Blood Transfusion, Mexico, 1962,* **9**, 455.
185. Ropartz, C., Lenoir, J., and Rivat, L. (1961). *Nature (London)* **189**, 586.
186. Steinberg, A.G., Wilson, J., and Lanset, S. (1962). *Vox. Sang.* **7**, 151.
187. Hilschmann, N., and Craig, L.C. (1965). *Proc. Nat. Acad. Sci. U.S.* **53**, 1403.
188. Milstein, C. (1966). *Nature (London)* **209**, 370.
189. Baglioni, C., Alescio Zonta, L., Cioli, D., and Carbonara, A. (1966). *Science* **152**, 1519.
189a. Milstein, C.P., Steinberg, A.G., McLaughlin, C.L., and Solomon, A. (1974). *Nature (London)* **248**, 160.
190. Litwin, S.D., and Kunkel, H.G. (1967). *J. Immunol.* **99**, 603.
191. Goldsmith, E.I., and Moor-Jankowski, J. (eds.) (1969). *Ann. N.Y. Acad. Sci.* **162.**
192. van Loghem, E., and Litwin, S.D. (1972). *Transplant. Proc.* **4**, 129.
193. Kelus, A.S., and Moor-Jankowski, J.K. (1961). *Nature (London)* **191**, 1405.

194. Dubiski, S., and Cinader, B. (1963). *Nature (London)* **197**, 705.
195. Lieberman, R., and Dray, S. (1964). *J. Immunol.* **93**, 584.
196. Potter, M., and Lieberman, R. (1967). *Cold Spring Harbor Symp. Quant. Biol.* **32**, 187.
197. Potter, M., and Lieberman, R. (1967). *Advan. Immunol.* **7**, 91.
198. Herzenberg, L.A., McDevitt, H.O., and Herzenberg, L.A. (1968). *Annu. Rev. Genet.* **2**, 209.
199. Lieberman, R., and Potter, M. (1969). *J. Exp. Med.* **130**, 519.
200. Lieberman, R., Paul, W.E., Humphrey, W., Jr., and Stimpfling, J.H. (1972). *J. Exp. Med.* **136**, 1231.
201. Spring, S.B., and Nisonoff, A. (1974). *J. Immunol.* **113**, 470.
202. Mishell, R., and Fahey, J.L. (1964). *Science* **143**, 1440.
203. Dray, S., Potter, M., and Lieberman, R. (1965). *J. Immunol.* **95**, 823.
204. Lieberman, R., Dray, S., and Potter, M. (1965). *Science* **148**, 640.
205. Lieberman, R., and Potter, M. (1966). *J. Mol. Biol.* **18**, 516.
206. Potter, M., Lieberman, R., and Dray, S. (1966). *J. Mol. Biol.* **16**, 334.
207. Herzenberg, L.A. (1964). *Cold Spring Harbor Symp. Quant. Biol.* **29**, 455.
208. Warner, N.L., and Herzenberg, L.A. (1967). *J. Immunol.* **99**, 675.
209. Minna, J.D., Iverson, G.M., and Herzenberg, L.A. (1967). *Proc. Nat. Acad. Sci. U.S.* **58**, 188.
210. Lieberman, R., and Potter, M. (1966). *Science* **154**, 535.
211. Edelman, G.M., and Gottlieb, P.D. (1970). *Proc. Nat. Acad. Sci. U.S.* **67**, 1192.
212. Dray, S. (1962). *Nature (London)* **195**, 677.
213. Mage, R.G., and Dray, S. (1965). *J. Immunol.* **95**, 525.
214. Mage, R.G., Young, G.O., and Dray, S. (1967). *J. Immunol.* **98**, 502.
215. Dubiski, S. (1967). *Nature (London)* **214**, 1365.
216. Vice, J.L., Hunt, W.L., and Dray, S. (1969). *Proc. Soc. Exp. Biol. Med.* **130**, 730.
217. David, G.S., and Todd, C.W. (1969). *Proc. Nat. Acad. Sci. U.S.* **62**, 860.
218. Vice, J.L., Hunt, W.L., and Dray, S. (1969). *J. Immunol.* **103**, 629.
219. Landucci-Tosi, S., Mage, R.G., Gilman-Sachs, A., Dray, S., and Knight, K.L. (1972). *J. Immunol.* **108**, 264.
220. Harrison, M.R., Mage, R.G., and Davie, J.M. (1973). *J. Exp. Med.* **137**, 254.
221. Herzenberg, L.A., Herzenberg, L.A., Goodlin, R.C., and Rivera, E.C. (1967). *J. Exp. Med.* **126**, 701.
222. Jacobson, E.B., and Herzenberg, L.A. (1972). *J. Exp. Med.* **135**, 1151.
223. Jacobson, E.B., Herzenberg, L.A., Riblet, R.J., and Herzenberg, L.A. (1972). *J. Exp. Med.* **135**, 1163.

Note added in proof: T.J. Kindt (personal communication) has found that group a determinants other than the major gene products are often detectable in very low concentration (1 to 35 µg/ml) in normal, preimmune rabbit sera; about 30% of rabbits tested possess such determinants. The concentration of such "latent" allotypes may increase markedly upon immunization with streptococci. Two interpretations of these findings are (a) all genes controlling rabbit allotypes are present in each animal, and regulatory genes, which behave predominantly (but not entirely) as alleles control their expression; (b) the array of *V* genes in one chromosome comprises mainly a single allotype but may also include a small number of genes of another allotype; this could reflect crossover events. Immunization may expand the population bearing the "latent" allotype if products of the relevant *V* genes react with the antigen.

10

Homogeneous Antibodies and Myeloma Proteins with Antibody Activity

I. INTRODUCTION

During the past few years it has become evident that antibody populations in individual animals often contain substantial amounts of homogeneous antibodies; i.e., molecules with identical structure. It seems logical to discuss such antibody populations together with myeloma proteins having antibody activity since both represent homogeneous groups of molecules with the capacity to interact specifically with antigens. Homogeneous proteins with antibody activity have a major practical use in the study of the relationship of amino acid sequence and 3-dimensional structure of an antibody to its specificity. In rabbits, which do not develop multiple myeloma, homogeneous antibodies are also being used to localize amino acid sequences that determine the allotypic markers in V regions and to identify residues responsible for antigen-binding specificity and idiotypic variability; this work is in its early stages. Investigation of the structure and biosynthesis of homogeneous antibodies and myeloma proteins has also provided much of our current insight into the genetic control of antibody diversity. More recently, homogeneous antibodies with a number of different specificities have been elicited in inbred mice. These have been studied rather extensively with respect to idiotypic specificities and for this reason are discussed mainly in the next chapter. In some instances antibodies elicited in BALB/c mice have proved to be closely related structurally to artificially induced myeloma proteins with antibody activity directed toward the same antigen.

It is generally accepted that homogeneous antibody populations and myeloma proteins are synthesized by individual clones of cells which have undergone extensive proliferation, frequently at the expense of the biosynthesis of other immunoglobulins. In the case of antibodies to bacterial vaccines induced in experimental animals, the antibody concentration in serum often exceeds the total concentration of immunoglobulin in normal, nonimmunized animals. This concentration relationship, of course, also applies to myeloma proteins. Homogeneous subpopulations of heterogeneous antibody may be identified, however, even when present at a concentration as low as 1 mg/ml, which might represent only 10% of the total serum immunoglobulin concentration.

Continuous immunization is necessary to maintain a high concentration of homogeneous antibody; and, in the face of repeated challenge by antigen, clones producing homogeneous antibody may on occasion diminish and be replaced by other clones of cells manufacturing antibody differing in structure but having specificity for the same antigen. In contrast, clones of cells manufacturing a myeloma protein undergo virtually uncontrolled proliferation, apparently without antigenic stimulus.

Animals producing very high titers of antibody may do so without overt symptoms of disease, although antigen–antibody complexes may accumulate in the kidney and antiglobulins may appear in rather high concentration in the serum. This again is in contrast to multiple myeloma, which is accompanied by bone destruction, infections, and other systemic complications. It has been observed that in animals producing high concentrations of antipneumococcal antibody, the architecture and histological appearance of the spleen appears normal, although it may be considerably enlarged (1,2).

In many instances, plasma cells associated with multiple myeloma can be maintained in continuous tissue culture; the capacity to maintain cells in culture is generally associated with chromosomal aberrations.

The induction of antibodies of restricted heterogeneity should be considered in the context of the clonal selection theory of antibody formation, which has gained universal acceptance. Cells of bone marrow origin which have not been processed by the thymus (B cells) are known to possess receptors for antigen which have the properties of immunoglobulin. These receptor molecules are present prior to contact with antigen and are representative of the antibody that will later be produced by descendants of the cell, after the antigenic stimulation which triggers proliferation. The heterogeneity of antibody produced in response to a given antigen or hapten thus reflects the heterogeneity of lymphocyte receptors, and the presence of a homogeneous subpopulation must be based on extensive proliferation of a clone, which in all probability is descended from one or a small number of precursor cells, each bearing a single molecular species of receptor.

The factors leading to production of large amounts of homogeneous antibody are not well understood. It is probably advantageous if the antigen itself does not possess a large spectrum of different determinants, and this may account for the lesser degree of heterogeneity of antibodies produced in response to bacterial polysaccharides, which have repeating determinants, as compared to protein antigens. Homogeneity with respect to antigenic determinants of antigen is not, however, a strict requirement. Homogeneous subpopulations of antibodies are also present in many antihapten antisera, despite the fact that protein–hapten conjugates used for immunization must present the hapten to the host in many different conformations (3).

A portion of this chapter will be concerned with antibodies to bacterial vaccines, particularly killed streptococci and pneumococci. Such antigens are of unique value for the production of homogeneous antibodies because of the very high concentrations of precipitable antibody which can be induced in experimental animals, as well as the frequent appearance of uniform subpopulations. Serum concentrations exceeding 15 mg/ml are common and values as high as 60 mg/ml have been reported (e.g., 4). Not all such sera possess a readily demonstrable homogeneous component; when the latter is present it may account for a small or a large fraction of the antibody.

The most commonly used screening method for demonstrating the presence of homogeneous antibody is zone electrophoresis. Examples, reproduced from the studies of Eichmann *et al.* (4) and Pincus *et al.* (5) are shown in Figs. 10.1 and 10.2. Figure 10.1 shows examples of "monoclonal," "restricted," and "heterogeneous" responses to carbohydrate antigens of streptococcal cell walls. In Fig. 10.2a the sharp band on the left contrasts with the diffuse, broad pattern which results after electrophoresis of normal IgG or of IgG from most hyperimmune antisera. The band is eliminated upon absorption with the pneumococcal antigen (Fig. 10.2b).

The very high concentrations of antibody resulting from immunization with bacterial vaccines have been of particular importance for the isolation of homogeneous antibody in amounts sufficient for physicochemical studies and determinations of amino acid sequence. In addition, the high titers facilitate the detection of homogeneous subpopulations.

The reasons underlying the extensive proliferation of a clone of cells, leading to the production of a large homogeneous subpopulation of molecules, are poorly understood. The investigations of Eichmann, Braun, Kindt, and Krause with rabbit antistreptococcal antibodies have clearly implicated genetic factors, since rabbits can be bred for the production of high or low titers of antibody. On the other hand, immunizations with various bacterial vaccines, if sufficiently frequent and prolonged, may induce at some time reasonably high concentrations of antibody with homogeneous components in nearly all randomly selected recipient rabbits (see below).

More recently, rabbit antihapten antisera have become a significant source of homogeneous antibody, despite the moderate concentrations

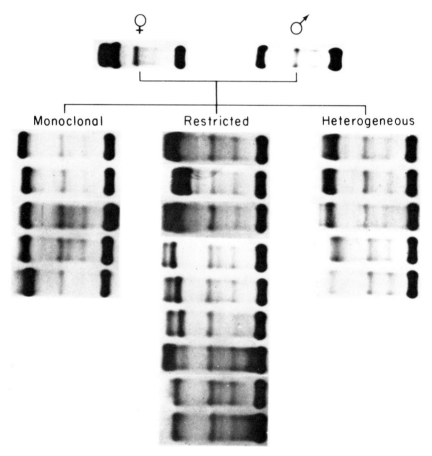

Fig. 10.1 Microzone electrophoretic patterns of antisera obtained after secondary immunization of a pair of breeding rabbits (top) and of their 19 offspring with Group C streptococcal vaccine. The anode is at the right and the sharp band at the right of each pattern is albumin. The IgG region at the left is pale and diffuse in normal rabbit serum. Reprinted by permission from Eichmann *et al.* (4).

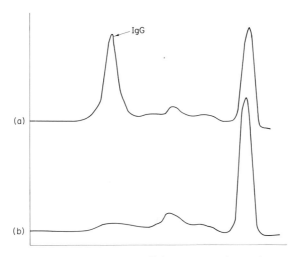

Fig. 10.2 Densitometric tracing of a cellulose acetate electrophoretogram of a rabbit anti-type VIII pneumococcal antiserum, before (a) and after (b) precipitation at equivalence with Type S8 polysaccharide. In normal rabbit serum the major peak at the left in the upper tracing is replaced by a broad, shallow peak corresponding to IgG. Reprinted by permission from Pincus *et al.* (5).

of antibody which they normally contain. Such antibodies will be discussed after considering the homogeneous antibacterial antibodies. Other examples of the appearance of homogeneous antibody components will then be briefly described. This will be followed by a discussion of the monoclonal proteins which appear in serum in association with lymphoproliferative diseases without external immunization.

II. HOMOGENEOUS ANTISTREPTOCOCCAL ANTIBODIES

Krause and his collaborators, beginning in 1966, have reported on an extensive series of investigations in which antibodies of restricted heterogeneity were elicited in rabbits by immunization with heat-killed, pepsin-digested streptococci (6–8). Such treatment removes the hyaluronic acid capsule and protein antigens of the cell wall, leaving the group-specific carbohydrate exposed. Despite the fact that the carbohydrate of the cell wall constitutes less than 10% of the dry weight of the bacteria, more than 95% of the antibodies produced upon immunization are directed to this component. The isolated carbohydrate is a very poor immunogen but precipitates strongly with antisera to the treated bacte-

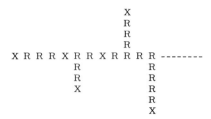

Fig. 10.3 General structure of streptococcal cell wall carbohydrate X, *N*-acetylglucosamine for Group A and *N*-acetylgalactosamine for Group C. Rhamnose (R) itself is the immunodominant grouping in Group A-variant streptococci. The average molecular weight is about 10,000. From Krause (7).

ria. Homogeneous antibodies can frequently be isolated from the antibody populations of restricted heterogeneity.

Most of the investigations in Krause's laboratory have utilized Group A, Group A-variant, or Group C streptococci. The chemical structure of the cell wall carbohydrate of each of these organisms is illustrated in Fig. 10.3, in which the "immunodominant" determinant is also shown. An antigenic grouping, or hapten, is designated as immunodominant on the basis of its capacity to inhibit strongly the precipitation of the isolated polysaccharide with the antibacterial antibodies. The reactions of antibodies to the different groups are quite specific; for example, *N*-acetylglucosamine strongly inhibits anti-Group A antibodies but has no demonstrable effect on antibodies to bacteria of Group C.

High titers of antibodies can be elicited in rabbits to each of these heat-killed bacterial vaccines, which are generally administered intravenously. A typical course of immunization comprises several injections per week, over a period of 4 weeks, followed by a resting period of a few months, after which intravenous inoculations are resumed. Applied to a random group of New Zealand rabbits, this schedule elicits homogeneous components, readily detectable by zone electrophoresis, in a substantial fraction of the recipients. Many of the immunized rabbits acquire antibody concentrations exceeding 20 mg/ml (9).

Methods used to isolate the homogeneous component include preparative zone electrophoresis on agarose and affinity chromatography on Sepharose to which an appropriate hapten or, in the case of Group C streptococci, a large oligosaccharide of the cell wall, is covalently bound (9,10). Isoelectric focusing has also been successfully employed. In each instance, the antibody is first purified specifically by precipitating with cell wall carbohydrate and separating the antibody from the antigen; the purified antibody is then fractionated further. During affinity chromatography it is eluted from the column by applying a concentration gradient of an appropriate hapten, i.e., a compound related or identical to the immunodominant group (Fig. 10.3), or by means of a pH and salt gradient (10). More than one homogeneous component can sometimes be isolated from the serum of an individual rabbit. Examples of antisera containing two such components are illustrated in Fig. 10.1.

Various criteria, in addition to zone electrophoresis, are used to prove molecular uniformity of the major product obtained after subfractionation. These include the electrophoretic homogeneity of L chains isolated from the antibody; the presence of only one of two allelic allotypic specificities in the antibody of a heterozygous rabbit; and, most significantly, the presence of a single amino acid at each position in the variable region of a polypeptide chain of the molecule. A number of sequences of homogeneous rabbit antibodies are presented in Chapter 4. (The ability to obtain a meaningful sequence is in itself evidence for restricted heterogeneity.) The criterion of uniformity with respect to allotype (11–13) of the isolated subpopulation is impressive because antibodies directed to a single antigen or hapten, derived from an individual heterozygous rabbit, normally express both allelic allotypic specificities.

An additional criterion of homogeneity, that has been applied to antipneumococcal and antihapten antibodies (discussed below), is uniformity with respect to binding affinity, as evidenced by agreement of the binding curve, relating concentration of hapten bound by antibody to the free hapten concentration at equilibrium, with that predicted for a homogeneous population of binding sites. Such binding measurements have generally been made by the method of equilibrium dialysis.

III. HOMOGENEOUS ANTIBODIES TO PNEUMOCOCCAL POLYSACCHARIDES

The work of Haber, Pappenheimer, and their colleagues (1,2,5,14) has established the feasibility of producing large amounts of homogeneous rabbit antibodies to formalin-treated pneumococci, particularly of types III or VIII. The specificity of such antibodies is directed toward the carbohydrate of the cell wall. The chemical structures of the type III and type VIII cell wall carbohydrates are (14):

SIII:$[\rightarrow 3]$-β-D-glcA-$(1\rightarrow 4)$-β-D-glc-$(1]\rightarrow_n$

SVIII:$[\rightarrow 4]$-β-D-glcA-$(1\rightarrow 4)$-β-D-glc-$(1\rightarrow 4)$-β-glc-$(1\rightarrow 4)$-α-D-gal-$(1]\rightarrow_n$

where glc represents glucose, glcA is glucosamine, and gal is galactose.

The pneumococcal antigens elicit, at some time during immunization, antisera containing homogeneous subpopulations of antibody in nearly all recipient rabbits, when an appropriate regimen of inoculation is used. The rabbits are challenged with antigen two or three times a week over a period of months. In some rabbits homogeneous subpopulations appear after a few weeks; in others many months are required (2,5,15). The antibodies of restricted heterogeneity are identified by zone electrophoresis and are specifically purified with an immunoadsorbent. One adsorbent used in Haber's laboratory consists of an octasaccharide, derived from the pneumococcal cell wall, covalently linked to bovine serum albumin, which in turn is coupled to bromacetyl cellulose. The antibodies are adsorbed onto this matrix and eluted with the homologous or a cross-reacting oligosaccharide (16). It is sometimes possible by this method to subfractionate the antipneumococcal antibodies so as to isolate a homogeneous subpopulation. Furthermore, some antisera contain such a large proportion of homogeneous antibody that such subfractionation is hardly necessary, and the total specifically purified antibody fraction can be used for amino acid sequence analysis of both H and L chains. The validity of such sequence analysis is shown by the presence of only a single major amino acid constituent at each position in the sequence (Fig. 4.8).

IV. HOMOGENEOUS ANTIHAPTEN ANTIBODIES

Pressman and his collaborators have shown that antihapten antibodies from individual rabbits frequently contain identifiable homogeneous subpopulations (17–19). They inoculated rabbits repeatedly over an extended period of time with the *p*-azobenzoate hapten conjugated to bovine γ-globulin. Fourteen of 21 antisera examined contained antibodies of restricted heterogeneity, as shown by the limited number of protein bands observed upon isoelectric focusing of the specifically purified antibenzoate antibody. By the same technique, L chains from each of five of the antibody populations gave only a single band. Four of these five antibody preparations also showed evidence of homogeneity when hapten-binding studies were carried out by the method of equilibrium dialysis; a plot of reciprocals of bound versus free hapten concentration gave a straight line. Several types of evidence indicated that the homogeneous subpopulations persisted in rabbits over a prolonged period of time; this persistence is undoubtedly mediated through memory cells since the half-life of an antibody, or of most antibody-producing cells, is relatively brief.

The complete amino acid sequence of the L chain of a homogeneous anti-*p*-azobenzoate antibody from an individual rabbit (19) is presented in Chapter 4 (Fig. 4.7).

An early example of a homogeneous antibenzoate antibody was a preparation from an individual rabbit that crystallized spontaneously in the cold after specific purification and concentration to 60 mg/ml (11). Subsequently, crystallization occurred at much lower antibody concentrations. Other evidence for homogeneity was the linearity of the hapten-binding curve, a restricted electrophoretic mobility, and the presence of but a single allotype at the a (V_H) locus, despite the heterozygosity of the rabbit. The X-ray diffraction pattern of the crystals proved to be inadequate for analysis.

Restricted heterogeneity has also been demonstrated in some antisera from individual rabbits immunized against the *p*-azotrimethylammonium group (20,21). In some instances apparently homogeneous subpopulations could be isolated from the purified antibody by preparative isoelectric focusing. Criteria of homogeneity included: the isoelectric focusing profile; the hapten-binding curve; disc electrophoretic patterns of isolated L chains; the presence of a single amino acid at the N-terminus; and homozygosity with respect to allotype in antibodies derived from heterozygous rabbits.

In another study (22) anti-*p*-azobenzenearsonate and anti-*p*-azophenyltrimethylammonium antibodies of restricted heterogeneity were isolated from serums collected from rabbits over a long period of time. Antibodies were specifically purified from the pooled antiserum of an individual rabbit, and were subfractionated by isoelectric focusing in liquid medium. L chains isolated from individual fractions showed marked restriction of heterogeneity with respect to amino acid sequence up to the first hypervariable region, which begins near residue 30. Surprisingly, each fraction was heterogeneous with respect to sequence within the hypervariable segment. These interesting data indicate that antihapten antibodies with similar isoelectric points may be heterogeneous but may still have L chains with similar properties, i.e., belonging to the same subtype and with similar sequences in at least a portion of the V_L region.

Another example of antihapten antibodies of restricted heterogeneity are anti-Dnp antibodies, elicited by Montgomery and Pincus upon immunization of rabbits with ϵ-Dnp-lysine conjugated to type III pneumococci (22a). The isoelectric focusing spectrum was the criterion for restricted heterogeneity.

A number of other instances of the production of rabbit antibodies of restricted heterogeneity has been reported (e.g., 23–27). So far none of these antibodies has been subjected to detailed amino acid sequence analysis. In some cases attempts were made to elicit homogeneous rabbit antibodies by immunization with antigens of restricted heterogeneity. For example, Brenneman and Singer (24) prepared a derivative of papain containing a single Dnp-lysine group attached to the sulfhydryl group in the active site of the enzyme. Rabbit anti-Dnp antibodies produced early in the response to this antigen were of restricted heterogeneity but of low titer. As immunization continued the antibodies became more heterogeneous. Richards *et al.* (28) immunized rabbits with a synthetic polymer of L-lysine containing Dnp groups at equally spaced intervals. Antihapten antibodies of restricted heterogeneity were elicited in some rabbits but, again, at relatively low concentration.

One of the most successful efforts to elicit antibodies of restricted heterogeneity by using a homogeneous carrier of low molecular weight was reported by Montgomery *et al.;* they utilized a Dnp conjugate of gramicidin, which is a cyclic decapeptide (28a). Each of several immunized rabbits produced antibodies of restricted heterogeneity, as indicated by their hapten-binding curves and isoelectric focusing patterns. Moderate concentrations of antibody, up to 0.3 mg/ml, were elicited.

V. RELATIONSHIP OF STRUCTURE OF ANTIGEN TO THE DEGREE OF HETEROGENEITY OF ANTIBODY

The frequency of appearance of antibodies of restricted heterogeneity in response to polysaccharide antigens has often been attributed, at least in part, to the presence of repetitive antigenic structures on the antigen. The finding that antihapten antibodies frequently contain homogeneous subpopulations is, however, not readily interpretable on this basis. It is well established that antibodies directed to a small hapten, such as benzoate or the dinitrophenyl group recognize a portion of the protein carrier as well as the hapten, and the carrier surface would necessarily introduce structural heterogeneity (3). The potential heterogeneity of antihapten antibodies is also reflected in the wide range of association constants that can generally be observed in the antihapten antibodies of a given specificity in an individual animal, and by the fact that antihapten antibodies produced in different rabbits rarely share idiotypic specificities.

To account for the frequent appearance of subpopulations of antihapten antibodies of limited heterogeneity, Roholt *et al.* suggest that it is attributable to selective stimulation of only a few of many cells capable of producing antibody to the hapten (17). Thus, once a clone is established it may compete effectively against other precursor cells for the antigen subsequently injected, owing to the relatively large number of memory cells in the clone.

A related point concerns the interpretation of hapten-binding data. The results have frequently been analyzed on the basis of an assumed Gaussian distribution of binding energies (29,30). Hapten-binding curves can, however, be interpreted mathematically as well, and in many instances more adequately (30a), on the assumption of a discrete number of homogeneous populations of antibodies with appropriately assigned associations constants (Chapter 2, Section VI). The discovery of homogeneous subpopulations in many antihapten antisera indicates that the latter interpretation is more realistic. [That antihapten antibodies from an individual animal are frequently of limited heterogeneity has also been inferred from studies of idiotypic specificities (Chapter 11).]

VI. RESTRICTED HETEROGENEITY OF HUMAN ANTIBODIES TO POLYSACCHARIDE ANTIGENS

Extensive studies of the degree of heterogeneity of purified human antibodies directed to dextran, levan, blood group A substance, and teichoic acid have been reported by Yount *et al.* (31). Although no sub-

TABLE 10.1

NONRANDOM DISTRIBUTION OF HEAVY CHAIN CLASS AND LIGHT CHAIN TYPE AMONG HUMAN ANTIBODIES TO DEXTRAN AND LEVAN[a]

			Percentage of total population								
				Ig class			IgG subclass (heavy chain)				L chain type	
Subject	Antibody specificity	Serum conc. (mg/ml)	IgG	IgA	IgM	γ_1	γ_2	γ_3	γ_4	κ	λ
1[b]	Dextran	0.41	100	0	0	0	100	0	0	97	3
1	Levan	0.32	100	0	0	0	100	0	0	100	0
20	Dextran	0.31	92	8	0	0	100	0	0	30	70
J.Ge	Dextran	0.62	100	0	0	(3)	97	0	0	79	21
Fo.	Dextran	0.27	68	32	0	50	50	0	0	75	25

[a] Data are from Yount *et al.* (31).
[b] Number assigned to subject.

populations of proved homogeneity were isolated there was considerable evidence for restricted heterogeneity. Some of their data are shown in Table 10.1. Six of eight purified antidextran antibodies from different individuals were predominantly IgG2; in some instances, 100% of the isolated molecules belonged to this subclass. (It should be recalled that IgG2 represents only about 20% of normal IgG.) In general, both κ and λ chains were represented in the isolated antibody. One antibody population was fractionated to give subpopulations that were predominantly either IgG2(κ) or IgG2(λ). These individual subfractions were also greatly restricted with respect to allotype on IgG2 molecules despite the fact that the donor was heterozygous (n^+n^-).

Electrophoretic analysis substantiated the conclusion that many of these antibodies are of restricted heterogeneity. However, none seemed to be monoclonal; the degree of heterogeneity appeared, upon electrophoresis of whole molecules or of H and L chains, to be greater than might have been expected from the antigenic analysis. It seems possible, nevertheless, that some of these antibodies were nearly homogeneous and that the electrophoretic heterogeneity arose in part from degradative changes occurring in serum (31,32).

VII. INFLUENCE OF GENETIC FACTORS ON THE MAGNITUDE OF THE RESPONSE OF RABBITS TO STREPTOCOCCAL ANTIGENS

We have already discussed the work of Krause and his collaborators which led to the isolation of homogeneous antistreptococcal cell wall antibodies. Breeding studies were carried out in that laboratory to ascertain whether genetic factors influence the magnitude of the immune response and, second, the incidence of homogeneous subpopulations. Positive correlations were obtained in both instances, and antibodies of restricted heterogeneity were observed in both high and low responders. The initial studies were done with Group C streptococci as antigen (4). When high responders (> 15 mg/ml of serum antibody) were bred for two generations, all of the offspring were high responders. In an unselected population the incidence of high responders is approximately 10% (9). The mean titer among the third generation of high responders was two to three times as great as that in a random population of rabbits. (A controlled schedule of immunization was employed.)

A similar study was carried out by mating low responders (< 10 mg/ml of serum antibody). Within two generations the sera of nearly all the offspring fell into the low range. Thus two or three generations of selective breeding is sufficient to segregate high and low responding populations from a random group.

VIII. INFLUENCE OF GENETIC FACTORS ON THE HETEROGENEITY OF RABBIT ANTIBODIES PRODUCED AGAINST STREPTOCOCCAL ANTIGENS

Eichmann *et al.* (4) also investigated the inheritance in rabbits of the capacity to produce antistreptococcal antibody of restricted heterogeneity. Antisera obtained after a secondary response were subjected to zone electrophoretic analysis and classified as "heterogeneous," "restricted," or "monoclonal" according to the patterns that resulted. Examples of these electrophoretic patterns are shown in Fig. 10.1. The term "monoclonal" was applied to antisera in which more than 60% of the IgG was present in a single narrow band. When 30–60% was localized to one band the antiserum was classified as "restricted."

The results of mating studies of rabbits immunized with Group C streptococci may be summarized as follows. Thirty-six of 37 offspring of matings of "heterogeneous" rabbits produced heterogeneous antibodies. When "restricted" rabbits were mated, 50% of the offspring produced restricted antibodies and, in addition, 20% produced "monoclonal" antibodies; only 7 of 24 offspring formed heterogeneous antibodies. When one parent was of the "monoclonal" type, 33% of the offspring exhibited a monoclonal response and only 6 of the 33 offspring formed heterogeneous antibodies. Comparable results were obtained when rabbits were immunized with Group A rather than Group C streptococci. Investigations of this type were extended by using Group A-variant streptococci as the antigen, with very similar results (32a).

These data demonstrate that powerful genetic factors control the type of response, with respect to heterogeneity and titer, exhibited by a rabbit upon challenge with streptococcal antigens.

Relationship between the Structures of Monoclonal Antistreptococcal Antibodies Produced by Members of a Family Group

Since the capacity to produce monoclonal antibodies is inherited, one may ask the following question: When a parent and its offspring possess monoclonal antibodies, are these antibodies identical in structure? This question was approached by Eichmann and Kindt through studies of idiotypic determinants in antistreptococcal antibodies (33). They found a high incidence of idiotypic cross-reactions, suggestive of structural identity or close similarity of antibodies, in an inbred family group in which the initial brother–sister mating pair was selected on the basis of capacity to produce antistreptococcal antibodies of limited heterogeneity. Inheritance of idiotype, in inbred mice as well as rabbits, is discussed in some detail in Chapter 11.

IX. AMINO ACID SEQUENCES OF HOMOGENEOUS RABBIT ANTIBODIES

Most sequence analyses of rabbit L chains have been carried out on κ chains, which occur with greater frequency than λ chains, and which have the advantage of possessing an unblocked N-terminal group. Figure 4.8 summarizes some of the data reported so far. A more complete listing of sequences was compiled by Braun and Jaton (34), who identified the six subgroups shown in Fig. 4.8. It seems probable that, as in the case of mouse κ chains, the number of subgroups may eventually prove to be quite large.

The studies of Braun and Jaton (34) also indicated that rabbits belonging to the same inbred family group frequently produce antistreptococcal antibodies with κ chains of the same subgroup and with remarkably similar N-terminal sequences. In some instances such antibodies also exhibit cross-idiotypic specificity (defined in Chapter 11, Section II,A).

The amino acid sequence of the H chains of a homogeneous rabbit antistreptococcal antibody (allotype a2) was investigated by Fleischman (35,36), who reported the sequence of the N-terminal 70 amino acid residues, and of positions 127–179 in the C_H region. Again, the presence of a single sequence is proof of restricted heterogeneity.

X. COLD AGGLUTININS FROM PATIENTS WITH CHRONIC COLD HEMAGGLUTININ SYNDROME (CHS)

Chronic cold agglutinin disease is a term applied to a group of disorders which have in common, as the name implies, the presence of serum agglutinins which are autoreactive with the patient's erythrocytes (37). The agglutinins are nearly always of the IgM class. Clinically, these patients have a hemolytic anemia which is variable in degree but rarely severe. They often exhibit acrocyanosis (Raynaud-like phenomenon) upon exposure to the cold. Frequently, the patients are found to have or to develop subsequently a lymphoproliferative disorder analogous to Waldenström's macroglobulinemia.

The sera of such patients contain a high titer of antibodies which agglutinate erythrocytes, including those of the patient. The antibodies are active at low temperature, but inactive at 37°C, and are directed toward the blood group specificities i, I, or Pr; the most frequently occurring cold agglutinins are anti-I.[1] Anti-Pr cold agglutinins are quite rare. The i and I antigens appear to be carbohydrates (38); the chemical nature of Pr antigens has not yet been determined. Cold agglutinins are nearly always IgM(κ). For example, Harboe *et al.,* examined 87 patients with CHS, all of whom had IgM(κ) cold agglutinins (39). A few cases in which the agglutinin was IgM(λ) were reported by Feizi and Schumacher (40). Occasional reports of IgG or IgA cold agglutinins have also appeared.

Cold agglutinins can readily be isolated by taking advantage of their thermal properties. They are adsorbed to red cells or stroma at low temperature (0°–20°C); after centrifugation to separate the cells from plasma, the agglutinins can be eluted by raising the temperature to 37°C. The purified agglutinins retain antibody activity and are capable of agglutinating red cells at low temperature or of lysing the cells in the presence of complement.

Strong evidence for the restricted heterogeneity of cold agglutinins is provided by the work of Cooper, who studied the IgM proteins from 16 patients (41). In each case the isolated cold agglutinin migrated, upon electrophoresis on cellulose acetate, as a single, narrow band with the mobility of a β- or γ-globulin. Light chains isolated from the protein gave three or four bands, with two usually predominating, when subjected to starch gel electrophoresis at alkaline pH. In contrast, nonspecific L chains formed ten bands, four or five of which were relatively strong. By this criterion, the L chains of cold agglutinins were not much more heterogeneous than several Bence Jones proteins that were tested.

Another type of evidence for the restricted heterogeneity of cold agglutinins was provided by the investigations of Cooper and Steinberg (42), who worked with the same panel of sixteen proteins. Six of these came from patients heterozygous at the *Inv* locus, which controls allo-

---

[1] The I antigen is found on normal adult erythrocytes, the i antigen on those of the fetus or the newborn. The transformation from i to I takes place during infancy, but adult cells normally contain small amounts of the i antigen. The description of I, i, and Pr specificities is oversimplified since there are subdivisions of each specificity.

typic determinants on κ chains. Light chains isolated from the cold agglutinins of each of these patients bore only one of the two allelic markers present in the patient's immunoglobulin. This finding is consistent with a monoclonal derivation of cold agglutinins. (It is relevant that type κ cold agglutinins may bear either of the two major allelic Inv markers; i.e., the κ chain may have either leucine or valine at position 191.) The strongest evidence for molecular homogeneity of cold agglutinins comes from amino acid sequence analyses (so far largely restricted to the N-terminal region of the L chain), which frequently show the presence of a single type of amino acid at each position (43–45a). There is a high incidence of κ chains belonging to the $V_{\kappa III}$ subgroup. (Subgroup designation of L. Hood.) The frequency of $V_{\kappa III}$ proteins, within the limited number of cold agglutinins studied so far, is about 70% as compared to 35% in the general population of κ chains (45).

Of considerable interest are the studies by Gergely *et al.* of amino acid sequences in the L chains ($V_{\kappa III}$) of the IgM anti-I cold agglutinins from two patients (45a). In determining amino acid sequences through residue 35 they observed identity throughout the first hypervariable region (positions 27–33), with an uncertainty at one position. The two L chains differed only at position 19, which is not in a hypervariable segment. Identity in hypervariable regions could account for the cross-idiotypic specificities observed by others.

Wang *et al.* studied N-terminal amino acid sequences of the L chains of two cold agglutinins with anti-Pr specificity (45b). Each L chain was of restricted heterogeneity, as evidenced by the presence of a single type of amino acid at each position in the sequence, which was determined through residue 22. The two L chains were identical except for position 4. They differed, however, from the prototype $V_{\kappa II}$ or $V_{\kappa III}$ sequences by a minimum of 7 of the first 22 positions, a surprisingly high value. On this basis the authors suggested that the two L chains derived from anti-Pr cold agglutinins represent a separate V_κ subgroup.

Cooper *et al.* (46) noted that 13 of 14 monoclonal IgM anti-I cold agglutinins studied had H chains belonging to a minor subdivision of μ chains. [Two species of μ chain are distinguishable by antigenic analysis or peptide mapping (47,48).[2]] Thus, these proteins show a special restriction both with respect to V_κ and, probably, V_H subgroup. In this regard it is of interest that each of four IgM cold agglutinins with anti-I specificity was found to belong to the V_{HI} subgroup (45a,45b).

Another important observation made by Cooper *et al.* was that L

---

[2] Natvig and Kunkel suggest that these may actually reflect V_H region subgroups present in different IgM proteins (49).

chains of different cold agglutinins vary markedly with respect to electrophoretic mobility. This indicated nonidentity of cold agglutinins from different individuals, despite their shared antibody specificity and, frequently, shared cross-idiotypic specificity. It seems possible that some of these proteins may show a greater degree of similarity in hypervariable regions than in other segments of the polypeptide chain. Further sequence analyses will be of great interest.

XI. RHEUMATOID FACTORS AND CRYOGLOBULINS

A. Monoclonal Rheumatoid Factors

A general discussion of rheumatoid factors was presented in Chapter 3. In this section we will consider monoclonal rheumatoid factors which occur in about 1% of patients with rheumatoid arthritis (50). In 1971, Potter (51) cited 24 such cases in the literature and numerous additional examples have been reported since then. Many more have undoubtedly been unreported, particularly as special conditions, such as low pH, are sometimes necessary to demonstrate RF activity in monoclonal proteins.

The first unequivocal demonstration of monoclonal IgM with anti-IgG activity appears to be that of Kritzman *et al.* (52). The serum of their patient had an extremely high level of IgM with restricted electrophoretic heterogeneity. The protein precipitated strongly with aggregated IgG from pooled human serum; the optimal pH for the reaction, however, was 5.5 and no precipitation occurred at pH 8. Similarly, the serum, or its isolated IgM, agglutinated erythrocytes or latex particles coated with aggregated human IgG, again only at reduced pH. (In contrast, a typical RF is effective at neutral pH.) With coated red cells the agglutination titer of the patient's serum was 32,000 at pH 5.2 and 128 at pH 8. Aggregated IgG, conjugated with fluorescein isothiocyanate, was seen to stain many plasma cells and atypical lymphocytes in the bone marrow of the patient, thus providing further evidence that the active anti-IgG component was an IgM paraprotein and not an ordinary RF. The patient exhibited no symptoms of the joint disease characteristic of rheumatoid arthritis. This is a typical observation and is evidence suggesting that anti-IgG is not a primary causative factor in rheumatoid arthritis.

Detailed investigations of a Waldenström's macroglobulin with anti-IgG activity were reported by Stone and Metzger (53,54). Quantitative studies of the binding of IgG or its fragments to the purified macroglobulin or its subunits were carried out by methods involving ultracentrifugation or "molecular sieving." Major goals were to determine the number of combining sites, or valence, of the anti-IgG macroglobulin and the equilibrium constant for its association with IgG. The most striking result was that nearly all Fabμ fragments, obtained from the macroglobulin by tryptic digestion, were capable of binding IgG. This indicates that the IgM, which possesses ten Fab fragments, has a valence of 10. There is evidence that rabbit IgM is also decavalent (55).

Because of its tendency to form precipitates with IgG, intact IgM was not studied by Stone and Metzger. However, IgMs, the 7 S, 4-chain subunit of IgM obtained by mild reduction, was tested for its capacity to bind the Fc fragment of IgG. Surprisingly, despite the presence of two Fabμ fragments in an IgMs subunit, a maximum of one Fc fragment could be bound by IgMs. The authors attributed this to close proximity of the two binding sites, with consequent steric interference.

The affinity of the macroglobulin for IgG was quite low; the average association constant was approximately $3 \times 10^4 \ M^{-1}$. The binding curve was consistent with homogeneity of the binding sites of the IgM molecule and also of the antigenic determinant on IgG with which it combined. This was further evidence for the monoclonal nature of the IgM molecule.

A related investigation was carried out by Chavin and Franklin (56), who utilized IgM RF isolated from the serum of a patient with mixed cryoglobulinemia. The cryoglobulin precipitate contained the patient's IgG and the IgM RF. Each Fabμ fragment of the RF was capable of binding human or rabbit fragment Fc on a 1:1 molar basis. The effective valence of the 7 S (IgMs) monomer of the IgM was, however, only 1, despite the presence of two Fabμ fragments in each IgMs molecule. This, again, was attributed to steric interference, occurring when the first binding site is occupied.

In contrast, an IgA rheumatoid factor was found to bind two moles of the Fc fragment of IgG per mole of IgA (57). This would suggest a lesser degree of steric interference between the two combining sites of IgA, as compared with the IgMs subunit. This interpretation is uncertain, however, since various rheumatoid factors may combine with different regions of the Fc fragment, with consequent differences in the degree of steric hindrance associated with occupancy of the first binding site.

A major difference between a monoclonal anti-IgG and polyclonal rheumatoid factor is that the former would be expected to recognize only one kind of antigenic determinant on the IgG molecule. Stone and

Metzger found that one molecule of IgG, acting as the antigen, was capable of binding only one Fab fragment of the anti-IgG. Actually this result was somewhat unexpected since, in view of the symmetrical structure of the IgG antigen, one might predict that each antigenic determinant would be repeated twice. Possible explanations put forth by the authors were: (a) that combination with one Fab fragment of anti-IgG sterically prevented access of the second Fab fragment; or, (b) that the single antigenic determinant comprised portions of two H chains. (Light chains are not implicated because the determinant was localized to the Fc fragment.)

Although monoclonal anti-IgG appears to be monospecific, anti-IgG from different patients may have different specificities. This is shown, for example, by differences in their relative strengths of interaction with human, as compared to rabbit IgG. The ratios of the two titers vary from one anti-IgG to the next and an occasional monoclonal IgM protein reacts more strongly with rabbit than with human IgG (58). Anti-IgG from one individual reacted with human IgG only after treatment of the latter with neuraminidase to remove sialic acid (59). We have not found a report of a monoclonal IgM reactive with a Gm factor on IgG, although there are, of course, numerous instances of polyclonal rheumatoid factors with such reactivity.

Many monoclonal IgM proteins which have anti-IgG activity are cryoglobulins; that is, they fail to precipitate with IgG at 37°C but do form precipitates at lower temperatures. The IgM antiglobulin can be dissociated from the IgG in the precipitate by gel filtration at low pH. Such IgM proteins are often structurally related and have been studied extensively from the standpoint of idiotypic specificity and amino acid sequence (Chapter 11, Section II).

B. Hypergammaglobulinemic Purpura

A rare disease, first described by Waldenström in 1943 (60), is characterized by recurrent purpura (capillary hemorrhage) of the lower extremities, increased erythrocyte sedimentation rate, and elevated levels of an immunoglobulin which is nearly always IgG. The condition is benign but there are reports of subsequent development of multiple myeloma. The disease generally occurs in females and is frequently associated with the presence of other antibodies, such as antinuclear factors or, less frequently, an IgM rheumatoid factor. An IgG fraction present in high concentration in the serum of these patients has anti-IgG activity; this results in the formation of circulating immune complexes which are often associated with hyperviscosity. It is possible that deposition of these complexes results in microinfarction of small blood vessels. Interference with platelet function by immune complexes coated nonspecifically on the cell surface may also be a factor in the development of purpura.

Electrophoresis of sera from most patients fails to reveal an immunoglobulin component with restricted heterogeneity, although some such cases have been reported. Nevertheless, it now appears that the anti-IgG is often homogeneous and that the apparent heterogeneity is attributable to circulating IgG–anti-IgG complexes. Capra *et al.* (61) isolated the anti-IgG components from 16 patients by repeated adsorption and elution from cross-linked insoluble normal IgG. Eleven of 12 proteins that were classified belonged to the IgG1 subclass, and one was IgG2. Eight of these proteins were subjected to further study. Six gave zone electrophoretic patterns indicative of restricted heterogeneity, which was reflected also in the electrophoretic patterns of their isolated L chains. The L chains of several proteins exhibiting restricted electrophoretic heterogeneity have been subjected to partial amino acid sequence analysis (62). The presence of a single amino acid at each position provides the strongest evidence for homogeneity of some of these anti-IgG proteins. It appears, then, that many but not all sera associated with hypergammaglobulinemic purpura contain a homogeneous anti-IgG component.

Striking resemblances are observed among the sequences of some of these homogeneous anti-IgG proteins, and homologies with monoclonal IgM cryoglobulins having anti-IgG activity were also observed (62). For example, the L chains of two IgG antiglobulins were sequenced up to residue 40 and found to be identical at each position. Another L chain (from an IgM–anti-IgG) belonging to the same subgroup ($V_{\kappa I}$), was not identical to the first two but possessed in common with them an unusual asparagine at position 30. Similarly, several of the κ chains had serine at position 31 in the first hypervariable region, where it is rarely found in other κ chains. Sequence analysis of the N-terminal regions of H chains indicates very close resemblances among certain of these proteins (63,64). In some instances similarities are found in hypervariable regions. These data as well as idiotypic specificities of IgM antiglobulins are discussed in the next chapter.

C. Cryoglobulins

A syndrome in which proteins reversibly precipitate from blood upon cooling was described by Wintrobe and Buell in 1933 (65) and was later termed "cryoglobulinemia" (66). The term "cryoimmunoglobulin" (67) would be accurate for the purpose of the present discussion since we will not consider other plasma proteins which sometimes precipitate in the cold; for convenience, however, we shall use the abbreviated term. A thorough review of this topic has been provided by Grey and Kohler (67).

The presence of a cryoglobulin is often associated with Raynaud's syndrome, which is characterized by vasoconstriction of skin capillaries triggered by deposition of immunoglobulin, particularly in cold weather, and also by serum hyperviscosity which is increased by exposure to low temperature. The hyperviscosity is caused by aggregation of immunoglobulin. Cryoglobulinemia is frequently caused by a lymphoproliferative disorder, such as multiple myeloma or Waldenström's macroglobulinemia, with the concomitant presence of a monoclonal immunoglobulin. It is sometimes observed as well in other connective tissue disorders, such as systemic lupus erythematosus.

The two major categories of cryoglobulin are monoclonal immunoglobulins (IgG, IgM or, rarely, IgA), which are generally associated with malignancy, or immunoglobulin complexes (68) produced by antiglobulin in the patient's serum. The complexes may comprise one class (e.g., IgG-anti-IgG) or, more frequently, are mixed, consisting of IgG complexed with anti-IgG of another class, i.e., with a rheumatoid factor. The anti-IgG is generally IgM but may also occur as IgA; the antiglobulin is sometimes monoclonal. When the antiglobulin is polyclonal the amount of cryoglobulin that precipitates in the cold is generally low (69). A large preponderance (>90%) of monoclonal IgM cryoglobulins have κ chains; this disproportion, whose basis is not understood, does not apply to monoclonal IgG cryoglobulins (67). In cryoglobulins comprising an immunoglobulin complex the molecule acting as the antigen is invariably IgG.

Meltzer and Franklin examined 29 patients with cryoglobulinemia and found that more than half possessed monoclonal serum proteins, and that 12 had mixed cryoglobulins (70). Of the latter, 11 comprised IgM–anti-IgG complexes and 1 was IgG–anti-IgG. In all but 2 of the patients with mixed cryoglobulinemia the disease was benign, whereas it was malignant in most of the group having a monoclonal protein. A large proportion of polyclonal cryoglobulins was observed in an extensive study by Brouet *et al.* (69), who used sensitive methods capable of detecting small amounts of cryoprecipitate.

Grey *et al.* examined a group of patients with the relatively rare IgG–anti-IgG complex (71). Four of five cryoglobulins with anti-IgG activity proved to be of the IgG3 subclass; this may be compared with a value of about 5 to 10% for the frequency of occurrence of IgG3 myeloma proteins. As a possible explanation for the high incidence of anti-IgG cryoglobulins of the IgG3 subclass, Grey *et al.* cited the tendency of IgG3 to form aggregates.

The reason for the decreased solubility of monoclonal cryoglobulins at low temperature is not understood. It appears, however, to reflect the structure of the Fab fragment. Working with an IgG1 cryoglobulin, Saha *et al.* (72,73) showed that its $F(ab')_2$ fragments formed cryoprecipitates and that Fab fragments dimerized at low temperatures. One might have predicted that the Fab region would be responsible for the unique properties of monoclonal cryoglobulins in view of the constancy of structure of the Fc segment. The noncovalent bonds causing cryoprecipitation are usually quite weak; in general, they are quickly dissociated by lowering the pH to 5 or below. At 37°C, the immune complexes of a cryoglobulin ordinarily dissociate completely; this is in contrast to complexes formed by most rheumatoid factors, which are stable at 37°C.

If a mixed cryoglobulin consists of IgG and an IgM antiglobulin the two components can be separated by gel filtration at low pH. The IgM thus isolated will react with IgG from other sources (74). An interesting situation can exist in the case of an IgG–anti-IgG cryoglobulin, in which the same molecule may act as antigen or antibody. Pope *et al.* present evidence that an IgG antiglobulin may form a more stable complex, with the same molecule acting as the antigen and as the antibody, than with normal IgG as the antigen (75).

XII. HUMAN MONOCLONAL PROTEINS WITH ANTIBODY ACTIVITY TOWARD ANTIGENS OTHER THAN IgG

A. General Considerations

Ever since the close structural relationship between monoclonal proteins and normal immunoglobulins was established in the early 1960's, it was suspected that many and possibly all myeloma proteins might have the capability of reacting with some unknown antigen. Although many myeloma proteins have now been shown to have antibody activity, this problem is still not resolved. A more fundamental question is whether the immunoglobulin which acts as a receptor on the surface of a lymphocyte is necessarily an antibody with activity against some antigen. However, even if many such receptors should lack a useful antigen-binding site, it would still be possible that all myeloma proteins possess a functional site. This would be true if the transformation to malignancy always occurs after antigenic stimulation. We do not know whether this is the case, although there is suggestive supporting evidence, based on the antigen-binding specificity of certain myeloma proteins. Later in this chapter that evidence will be summarized.

Another complex question concerns the criteria to be used in classifying a myeloma protein as having antibody activity to a given antigen. At a minimum the molecule should have one antigen-binding site in each Fab fragment, should combine with a reasonably high affinity ($K > 10^4$ M^{-1}), and should show specificity comparable to that of an induced antibody. Even when each of these criteria is fulfilled there is no guarantee that an antigen identified as being reactive with the myeloma protein is the "correct" one; i.e., that the protein might not combine much more strongly with a different antigen. In the case of a myeloma protein with antihapten activity, the binding affinity for a variety of related haptens can provide some evidence bearing on this question, but cannot give a conclusive answer. A criterion that is very useful but difficult to apply is that the antigen should make contact with one or more hypervariable regions of the myeloma protein. In a few cases this has been shown to be true by affinity labeling or by X-ray crystallography.

There are instances, however, in which the "true" specificity of a myeloma protein is known with some certainty. Certain myeloma proteins from BALB/c mice which combine with phosphorylcholine (76–78) or with $\alpha(1 \rightarrow 3)$dextran (79), appear to be structurally identical to some of the normal antibodies induced in the same mouse strain by immunization with those antigens. This provides perhaps the strongest evidence we have that there is no essential difference between a myeloma protein and an antibody molecule.

B. Monoclonal Proteins Reactive with the 2,4-Dinitrophenyl (Dnp) Hapten Group

One obvious but tedious method for determining whether a myeloma protein has antibody activity is to screen a large number of myeloma proteins for activity against a particular antigen. This method was first applied successfully by Eisen *et al.* (80). These investigators took advantage of a spectral shift, which occurs when 2,4-dinitrophenyl (Dnp) derivatives combine with antibody, to screen 88 human myeloma sera for anti-Dnp activity. One serum of the 88 tested gave a positive result and its activity was shown to reside in the myeloma protein [IgG1(λ)]. The binding of Dnp-lysine by the isolated myeloma protein was measured by equilibrium dialysis and fluorescence quenching. When

TABLE 10.2

<small>SPECIFICITY OF A HUMAN MYELOMA PROTEIN WITH ANTI-DNP ACTIVITY</small>

Ligand[a]	r/c $(M^{-1} \times 10^{-4})$[b]
ϵ-Dnp-L-lysine	2.36
ϵ-2,4,6-Tnp-L-lysine	0.26
ϵ-Dnp-6-aminocaproate	1.0
2,4-Dinitroaniline	0.21
p-Mononitroaniline	0.06

[a] Dnp = 2,4-dinitrophenyl; Tnp = 2,4,6-trinitrophenyl.

[b] r, Moles hapten bound/mole antibody; c, free hapten concentration. Data obtained by equilibrium dialysis. The free hapten concentration varied over a relatively small range. From Eisen *et al.* (80).

the amount of hapten bound was measured as a function of the free hapten concentration, the quantitative relationship was characteristic of a homogeneous antibody. The association constant determined by this method was $2.3 \times 10^4 \ M^{-1}$ and the valence, 2.0 ± 0.1. Each Fab fragment possessed one of the two binding sites, and the Fc fragment had no activity. Data relating to the specificity of the myeloma protein are shown in Table 10.2. ϵ-Dnp-6-aminocaproate combined with an affinity almost equal to that of ϵ-Dnp-L-lysine; this is consistent with the structural similarity of the two molecules. The presence of the additional nitro group in ϵ-trinitrophenyllysine was associated with a large decrease in affinity. Dinitro- and mononitroaniline also interacted very weakly with the myeloma protein, indicating the importance of the lysine side chain. The specificity of this protein is quite reminiscent of that of induced antibody.

The observed K value of $2.3 \times 10^4 \ M^{-1}$ is, however, low as compared to that of a typical, induced anti-Dnp antibody, except for those antibodies that appear very early in the immune response. Furthermore, the myeloma protein failed to form precipitates with Dnp-protein conjugates or to fix complement. While it seems likely that the myeloma protein has a typical antigen-binding site, it is doubtful that Dnp is an optimal antigenic determinant.

A Waldenström's macroglobulin with anti-Dnp activity was discovered by Ashman and Metzger (81). Despite its affinity for ϵ-Dnp-6-aminocaproate the protein differed markedly in specificity from that investigated by Eisen *et al.*, since it had very low affinity for ϵ-Dnp-L-lysine. Investigations by equilibrium dialysis indicated a valence of 10 for the IgM and a binding affinity for ϵ-Dnp-6-aminocaproate of

$3.8 \times 10^4\ M^{-1}$. The shape of the hapten-binding curve was characteristic of a protein containing homogeneous binding sites (see Fig. 2.7). Each IgMs (7 S) subunit possessed two binding sites and each Fab fragment had one. Dnp derivatives of highest affinity were able to quench the fluorescence of the molecule. Over 60 different ligands were tested; only analogs of ϵ-Dnp-6-aminocaproate were active. Actually, 4-nitrophenyl-ϵ-Dnp-6-aminocaproate had a slightly higher binding affinity than the corresponding dinitro derivative.

Two large-scale screening programs for myeloma proteins with anti-Dnp and other activities were reported by Terry *et al.* (82) and by Yoo and Franklin (83). Quite different results were obtained by the two groups; neither, however, found any proteins with high binding affinity for the ligands tested. Terry *et al.* investigated more than 500 human sera containing monoclonal proteins and 60 normal sera. They screened each serum for activity against ϵ-Dnp-L-lysine and ϵ-Dnp-6-amino-caproate by using tritiated haptens and a modified Farr technique; this method makes use of the fact that hapten bound to immunoglobulin, but not free hapten, is precipitated by ammonium sulfate. Nine of the sera showed hapten-binding activity against one, or in some instances both of the haptens. Binding affinities were not reported in this paper but the lowest association constant that would permit positive results was calculated to be approximately $10^3\ M^{-1}$. In a subsequent study (84) one of the proteins $[\mathrm{IgA}(\lambda)]$ was found to have an association constant for ϵ-Dnp-lysine of $2.6 \times 10^4\ M^{-1}$; the monomeric form of the protein had a valence of 2. Terry *et al.* (82) also screened their proteins by precipitin analysis, using Dnp or Tnp (2,4,6-trinitrophenyl) groups conjugated to bovine serum albumin as the test antigen. About 10% of the sera tested gave positive results by double diffusion in agar gel; however, 12% of normal sera similarly gave precipitin lines. Oddly, none of the sera that were positive by precipitation showed binding by the Farr technique, and the converse was also true. The authors concluded that double diffusion in agar gel is an unreliable screening procedure for detecting monoclonal proteins with antibody activity for nitrophenyl ligands.

A large-scale and careful investigation with uniformly negative results was reported by Yoo and Franklin (83), who tested 275 human myeloma proteins. Their data contrast with those of Terry *et al.*, since no activity against the Dnp group was detected in any serum by precipitin analysis or by fluorescence quenching.

Nineteen additional antigens also failed to react with any of their myeloma sera. Antigens tested included thirteen different haptens, pneumococcal polysaccharide, and four mycoplasma antigens. The authors contrasted their results with those obtained with mouse myeloma pro-

TABLE 10.3

ANTIGENS REACTIVE WITH HUMAN MYELOMA PROTEINS[a]

Antigen	Ig class
Blood group antigens	
I, i	IgM, IgA
Sp$_1$	IgM
A$_1$	IgM
Streptolysin O	IgG
Staphylolysin	IgG
Klebsiella	IgM
Brucella	IgG
Rubella	IgG
IgG	IgM, IgG, IgA
Immune complexes	IgM
Fibrin monomer	IgG
Lipoproteins	IgG
Transferrin	IgG
Serum albumin	IgM
α_2-Macroglobulin	IgG
Dnp	IgM, IgG, IgA
Cardiolipids	IgM
Phosphorylcholine	IgM

[a] Adapted from Seligmann and Brouet (85). Antigens included are those for which the evidence of specificity is strongest. The original sources of data may be found in reference 85.

teins, in which antibody activity against DNP, nucleic acids or polysaccharides is observed quite frequently. It is uncertain whether the distinction lies in the species from which the myeloma protein is derived or some factor involving the method of testing. In addition, the reason for the differences in the results of Terry *et al.* and of Yoo and Franklin, with human myeloma proteins, is unclear. A number of examples of human myeloma proteins with antibody-like activity, compiled by Seligmann and Brouet (85), is shown in Table 10.3

XIII. MOUSE MYELOMA PROTEINS WITH ANTIBODY ACTIVITY

There has been a rather large number of reports of monoclonal mouse proteins with antibody activity to a variety of antigens. Most of these proteins have been derived from sera of BALB/c mice with plasmacytomas induced by the method of M. Potter. A partial list of some of the activities reported is given in Table 10.4 (86). The myeloma proteins listed are those for which the corresponding antigen is one to which it seems likely that the mouse may have been exposed. As indicated earlier, however, the formation of precipitin bands does not provide very strong evidence for true antibody-like activity; it is very useful if, in addition, an association constant can be measured.

Rather extensive studies have been carried out on mouse (BALB/c) myeloma proteins with specificity for the Dnp group, phosphorylcholine or $\alpha(1 \to 3)$dextran. One protein with anti-Dnp activity, designated MOPC 315, was elicited by M. Potter and its properties were described by Eisen *et al.* (87). The activity was discovered by screening a large number of BALB/c myeloma proteins for their reaction with the Dnp hapten by the method of spectral shift analysis that had already been applied to screen human myeloma sera. Protein 315 has a binding affinity for ϵ-Dnp-L-lysine of approximately 10^7 M^{-1} and a very similar affinity for ϵ-Dnp-6-aminocaproate. The H chains are of the IgA class but the L chains have an unusual amino acid sequence which resembles that of normal λ chains, but differs with respect to approximately 27 residues in the C-terminal half (C_L domain). On the basis of this comparison, Schulenburg *et al.* (88) concluded that there are at least two subtypes of

TABLE 10.4

MOUSE MYELOMA PROTEINS WITH ANTIBODY ACTIVITY AGAINST ANTIGENS
IN THE ENVIRONMENT OF THE MOUSE[a]

Antigenic activity	Suspected natural antigenic source
Mima antigen	*Mima polymorpha*
Phosphorylcholine	*Lactobacillus-A*
	Trichoderma
$\beta(1 \to 6)$-D-Galactan	Wheat
	Hardwood bedding
$\alpha(1 \to 3)$Dextran	Various possible bacterial sources
Fructosan	*Bacillus circulans*
α-Methyl-D-galactoside	*Proteus mirabilis* sp-2
α-Methyl-D-mannoside	*Proteus mirabilis* sp-2
Common trypsin-sensitive *Salmonella* antigen	*Pasteurella pneumotropica*
Pronase-sensitive antigen in wheat extract	Wheat extract

[a] The known antigenic activity and suspected natural antigenic source are given. For some antigens, e.g., phosphorylcholine, $\alpha(1 \to 3)$dextran, and $\beta(1 \to 6)$-D-galactan a number of myeloma proteins with the same specific antibody activity have been identified. Table adapted from Potter (86).

mouse λ chains, which they designated λ1 and λ2; MOPC 315 belongs to the λ2 subtype. Despite the relatively high affinity of this protein for Dnp derivatives, it proved quite difficult to establish its valence. Initially it appeared to have one combining site per molecule of approximate molecular weight 120,000. Subsequent studies, however, revealed the presence of an additional combining site, which is active only at high protein concentration (89). This phenomenon is not well understood. The complete amino acid sequence of the V_α region of this protein has recently been reported (90).

Interestingly, only eight differences were observed between the amino acid sequences of the variable regions of the λ chains of MOPC 315 and MOPC 104 (88); the latter myeloma protein combines specifically with a different ligand, $\alpha(1 \rightarrow 3)$dextran. About half of these differences fall in the hypervariable regions. The binding curves for the haptens, ε-Dnp-L-lysine and ε-Dnp-6-aminocaproate, reacting with protein 315, are characteristic of a homogeneous group of combining sites, as would be predicted for a myeloma protein.

Another mouse myeloma protein with high affinity for a hapten is MOPC 460 [IgA(κ)], which also has been extensively investigated by Eisen and his collaborators (91). This protein binds ε-Dnp-L-lysine with an association constant of $3 \times 10^5\ M^{-1}$ and Dnp-naphthol with an affinity of $5 \times 10^6\ M^{-1}$. Both proteins, 315 and 460, have specificity patterns characteristic of an antibody. They combine much more weakly or not at all with a large number of compounds which are unrelated to Dnp.

A number of different mouse myeloma proteins [IgA(κ)] have the capacity to bind phosphorylcholine (77,92–94). There is evidence that some of these proteins, which arose independently in different mice, may be very similar or identical in structure. This evidence includes idiotypic specificity and partial sequence analyses (Chapter 11). These proteins also react with pneumococcal type C polysaccharide, which contains haptenic determinants resembling phosphorylcholine. There exist other mouse myeloma proteins which are also reactive with phosphorylcholine but which differ in structure, as shown by differences in their idiotypic determinants, affinities for various haptens related to phosphorylcholine, and partial amino acid sequences. Leon and Young (92) recognized three classes of myeloma proteins with antiphosphorylcholine activity. Class 1 is characterized by a fairly high affinity for choline as well as phosphorylcholine; the other two classes do not combine well with choline. Classes 2 and 3 are distinguished by differences in affinity for phosphonocholine. Leon and Young identified four proteins in class 3; all of these had previously been shown by Potter and Liebermann (77) or by Cohn *et al.* (76) to have identical idiotypic specificities. The single proteins identified in classes 1 and 2 differ idiotypically from the proteins in class 3. Sher and Tarikas (95) studied quantitatively the capacity of one of these proteins to bind phosphorylcholine. They obtained an association constant of 9.5×10^5 M^{-1}, a valence of two for the purified monomer, and binding curves characteristic of homogeneous antibody. Very similar binding properties and shared idiotype were noted for two different myeloma proteins with antiphosphorylcholine activity.

The Fab' fragment of a mouse myeloma protein (number 603) with antiphosphorylcholine activity has been subjected to X-ray crystallography at high resolution (Chapter 5).

The frequency of appearance of myeloma proteins with antiphosphorylcholine activity poses interesting questions concerning their origin. A possible explanation (96,97) is that the induction of the myeloma occurs in cells that have already been committed to an antigen. On this basis one might propose that a substantial number of such normal cells, activated by bacterial antigens that cross-react with phosphorylcholine, exist in the intestinal tract of the normal BALB/c mouse prior to the treatment with mineral oil to induce a myeloma tumor. In support of this view, Potter and Liebermann (77) demonstrated that a polysaccharide derived from *Lactobacillus acidophilus,* a common inhabitant of the intestinal tract of BALB/c mice, cross-reacts antigenically with phosphorylcholine. In addition, myeloma proteins have been found to form precipitates with polysaccharides extracted from other bacterial flora of the mouse. Potter (97) also showed that certain myeloma proteins react with carbohydrate extracts of the wood shavings used as bedding for mice or with extracts of mouse food. Table 10.4 presents other examples of myeloma proteins with activity against antigens that may be present in the mouse.

That the antigen-binding specificity of a myeloma protein may be related to antigenic stimulation is also suggested by studies of Seligmann and his collaborators (98,99). One human patient, whose $\alpha_2 M$ myeloma protein had antibody activity against horse $\alpha_2 M$ serum protein, had received two inoculations of unpurified horse antitetanus serum about 35 years before the onset of multiple myeloma. Another patient, with an IgG myeloma protein possessing strong antistreptolysin 0 activity, had suffered from recurrent attacks of rheumatic fever.

A number of myeloma proteins induced in BALB/c mice have been found to bind $\alpha(1 \rightarrow 3)$dextran. They have been studied extensively by Cohn, Weigert, and their associates (79,100). Many of these proteins share idiotypic determinants, and when this is the case they have λ

chains with identical or nearly identical amino acid sequences. The molecules with shared idiotypic specificity include an IgM as well as IgA proteins (Chapter 11).

Fairly extensive studies of cross-reactions of one of these proteins [MOPC 104; IgM(λ)] with a variety of oligosaccharides were reported by Leon *et al.* (101). The specificity characteristics of the protein are quite similar to those of induced anticarbohydrate antibodies.

Cisar *et al.* investigated the specificity of mouse myeloma proteins [mainly IgA(κ)] reactive with dextrans, fructosans, and levans (102). The proteins varied with respect to their specificity for glycosidic linkages. Three proteins showed specificity for $\alpha(1 \rightarrow 6)$dextrans similar to that previously observed in induced human antidextran antibodies. The number of monosaccharide units in a polymer required for optimal binding ranged from three to six. Another investigation (103) demonstrated that myeloma proteins with anticarbohydrate activity and shared idiotypic specificity have very similar hapten-binding specificity, although (as in the case of myeloma proteins with antiphosphorylcholine activity) the converse is not always true.

Weigert *et al.* (100) have considered possible explanations for the relatively high incidence of myeloma proteins having anti-$\alpha(1 \rightarrow 3)$dextran activity and λ chains that are apparently identical in structure. They conclude that in the BALB/c mouse the prototype λ chain (λ_0) is controlled by a germ line gene, which is expressed in a relatively large number of precursor lymphocytes. These are stimulated to proliferate by $\alpha(1 \rightarrow 3)$dextran, or closely related molecules, present in the intestinal tract of the mouse. The frequency of appearance of the corresponding myeloma protein is then assumed to be related to the abundance of these clones of cells.

XIV. SUMMARY OF EVIDENCE RELATING MYELOMA PROTEINS WITH SPECIFIC BINDING ACTIVITY TO INDUCED ANTIBODIES

1. Amino acid sequence analysis has not revealed fundamental structural differences among myeloma proteins and antibodies.

2. Myeloma proteins with antibody activity generally possess one combining site per Fab fragment.

3. The specificities and affinities of myeloma proteins sometimes resemble those of induced antibodies.

4. Myeloma proteins have been affinity labeled (Chapter 2). As is

true of antibodies, either the H or L chain or both can be labeled. When localized, the label has been found in or near hypervariable regions.

5. Myeloma proteins with antibody activity have in some instances been found to share idiotypic specificity and amino acid sequence with induced antibodies reactive against the same antigen. This is perhaps the strongest evidence for the essential identity of myeloma proteins and antibodies.

XV. UNUSUAL IMMUNOLOGICAL CROSS-REACTIONS

A number of interesting and unexpected cross-reactions have been discovered in studies of the specificity of myeloma proteins and of certain induced antibodies. Schubert *et al.* (104) found that about 10% of a large number of mouse myeloma proteins tested had antibody activity against one of a panel of five haptens, comprising Dnp, 2,4,6-Tnp, 5-acetyluracil, purine, and adenosine monophosphate. Surprisingly, several of the myeloma proteins showed activity against more than one hapten, apparently unrelated in structure, such as Dnp and 5-acetyluracil. When such unusual cross-reactions occurred they took place via the same hapten-binding sites, as shown by cross-inhibition experiments. All their tests were carried out by precipitin analyses, using conjugates of the haptens to protein carriers, and specificity was tested by measuring hapten inhibition of precipitation. As a consequence, data were not obtained in this study as to the affinities of the reactions.

Related findings were reported by Eisen and his collaborators, who showed that mouse myeloma protein, MOPC 315, which has anti-Dnp activity, also combines weakly with 5-acetyluracil, caffeine, and riboflavin, and somewhat more strongly with menadione (2-methyl-1,4-naphthaquinone) (105). None of these compounds is closely related structurally to the dinitrophenyl group. Cross-reactions with 5-acetyluracil of anti-Dnp antibodies induced in some but not all rabbits and guinea pigs were also observed (106).

Evidence that certain naturally occurring antibodies of the nurse shark may be multispecific was presented by Rudikoff *et al.* (107). Antibody specifically purified by absorption to, and elution from a Dnp-conjugate, agglutinated sheep and pigeon erythrocytes and bound guanosine monophosphate.

Another unexpected cross-reaction was observed by Hannestad, who discovered a Waldenström macroglobulin with activity against IgG and also toward the Dnp group (108,109). The affinity, K_0, for ϵ-Dnp-L-lysine was low (10^4 M^{-1} or less). A possible explanation for this type of result is that a hydrophobic binding site which is large enough to accommodate the Dnp group may have sufficient complementarity to permit a weak interaction with Dnp even though the fine specificity of the antibody is directed toward a quite unrelated determinant. This view is supported by the finding of Terry, already discussed, that about 10% of normal human sera and an equivalent percentage of human myeloma proteins have measurable antibody-like activity directed to the Dnp group. In addition, weak anti-Dnp activity has been demonstrated in normal rabbit sera. There perhaps has been too much stress on studies of proteins with weak anti-Dnp activity. The observation of weak, unusual cross-reactions with low affinity may simply reflect the fact that extensive screening studies have been carried out with this hapten.

Rosenstein *et al.* (110) observed an unusual cross-reaction which they interpret as indicating that an antibody combining site can be polyfunctional; i.e., can accommodate structurally unrelated haptens in different segments of the active site. They noted that the mouse myeloma protein, MOPC 460, binds ϵ-Dnp-L-lysine or 2-methyl-1,4-naphthaquinone thioglycollate within the same active site, as shown by competitive binding. Further, they were able to carry out certain chemical modifications which eliminated the capacity of the protein to combine with one hapten but not the other. They concluded that there is spatial separation between the contact regions for the two haptens in the active site of protein 460 and concluded that multispecificity may be a general property of antibody combining sites. Evidence that the two haptens, ϵ-Dnp-lysine and menadione thioglycollate, (MenTG) are not bound in precisely identical positions was obtained by chemically substituting a sulfhydryl group in or near the active site with a bulky (Dnp-S) group. This resulted in loss of affinity for MenTG but not for ϵ-Dnp-lysine.

That the phenomenon of multiple binding specificity may have biological significance is strongly suggested by a subsequent report from the same laboratory (111). Rabbit antibody binding two diverse haptens–A (the immunogen), and an unrelated hapten, B–was identified in a serum by isoelectric focusing; also present were other antibodies reactive only with A. Upon secondary challenge with a protein conjugated to hapten B, only those species of antibody binding both A and B were evoked.

If combining sites are indeed multispecific, this could greatly reduce the number of structural genes needed to encode the library of specificities available to an individual animal. A clearer picture of the nature of the active site, and in particular as to its size, is emerging from X-ray crystallographic investigations. This should indicate whether this type of multispecificity is possible. It is already apparent that the surface area comprising amino acids from hypervariable regions is much larger than a typical hapten group and would thus have the potential for multi-specificity (Chapter 5).

It seems probable that unusual cross-reactions will be detected more frequently in myeloma proteins than in induced antibodies. Since the latter are heterogeneous, each subset of a given population might cross-react with a different set of antigenic determinants, and only a very small fraction of the population might cross-react with any particular "unrelated" antigen. In a homogeneous myeloma protein, any unusual cross-reaction would apply to all the protein molecules. The concept of multispecificity of antibodies was introduced by Talmage in 1959 (111a), but only gained wide acceptance as a result of recent investigations.

XVI. ANTIBODY ACTIVITY IN CRYSTALLIZED Fab′ FRAGMENTS

In Chapter 5, we discussed X-ray crystallographic models of the Fab′ fragments of a human myeloma protein (protein New, IgG1-λ) and of a mouse myeloma protein [McPc 603; IgA(κ)], as well as human Bence Jones proteins. The mouse protein was found to bind one mole of radiolabeled phosphorylcholine per mole of Fab′, either in the form of crystals or in free solution (112). The binding curve obtained in solution was indicative of homogeneity of the protein, and yielded a K value of $1.7 \times 10^5 \ M^{-1}$. The K value for the protein in the crystals was estimated as $3.9 \times 10^3 \ M^{-1}$. The difference might be due to the presence of a high concentration of ammonium sulfate in the mother liquor surrounding the crystals. The Fab′ fragments of protein New were found to bind vitamin K_1OH with an affinity of about $10^5 \ M^{-1}$ (113). This specificity was discovered by an empirical screening procedure. The ability to bind haptens with reasonably high affinity has permitted the unequivocal localization of the antibody combining site in X-ray crystallographic models.

XVII. INDUCTION OF HOMOGENEOUS ANTIBODY AFTER ADOPTIVE TRANSFER OF LIMITED NUMBERS OF CELLS

One approach to the production of homogeneous antibody involves adoptive transfers of limited numbers of cells into irradiated syngeneic mice.

Klinman immunized BALB/c mice to the Dnp hapten, then trans-ferred $\sim 10^6$ immune spleen cells into irradiated recipients (114). After 1 day, small fragments (~ 1 mm) were prepared from the spleens of the recipients and cultured in the presence of Dnp-protein conjugate. Such culture fluids eventually contain up to 2 μg of homogeneous antibody which can be isolated by immunoadsorption. Evidence for homogeneity included the linearity of the hapten-binding curve (r/c versus r, Chapter 2), the electrophoretic pattern of radiolabeled antibody, and the isoelec-tric focusing pattern (115). K values for antibodies from individual foci varied from 4.9×10^6 to 1.3×10^8 M^{-1}. Nearly all hapten-binding activ-ity was recovered when the H and L chains of two such preparations were separated and then recombined. In contrast, ordinary specifically purified anti-Dnp antibody showed about a tenfold decrease in its associ-ation constant when similarly treated. These data were taken as further evidence for the homogeneity of the antibodies produced in the culture fluids.

A somewhat different approach was taken by Askonas *et al.* (116). They selected a CBA mouse which had produced anti-Dnp antibodies of restricted heterogeneity and transferred portions of its spleen (4 to 5×10^6 cells) into a number of different irradiated syngeneic recipients, together with the antigen, bovine IgG-Dnp. A number of recipients produced antibody of limited heterogeneity, as evidenced by the isoelec-tric focusing spectrum. Antibody with identical properties was produced by irradiated recipients in up to seven serial transfers, starting with a mouse which had produced anti-Dnp antibodies of very restricted heter-ogeneity. The maximum serum concentration of homogeneous antibody rapidly declined, from a peak value of 2 to 3 mg/ml, after the fourth gen-eration (117).

Briles and Krause carried out adoptive transfers using 10^7 spleen cells from SWR/J mice that had produced antibody of restricted hetero-geneity to group A streptococcal carbohydrate (118). Recipient mice produced antibodies that were identical to those of the donor by the cri-teria of electrophoretic mobility and idiotype.

REFERENCES

1. Pincus, J.H., Jaton, J.C., Bloch, K.J., and Haber, E. (1970). *J. Immunol.* **104,** 1149.
2. Kimball, J.W., Pappenheimer, A.M., Jr., and Jaton, J.C. (1971). *J. Immunol.* **106,** 1177.
3. Singer, S.J. (1964). *Immunochemistry* **1,** 15.
4. Eichmann, K., Braun, D.G., and Krause, R.M. (1971). *J. Exp. Med.* **134,** 48.
5. Pincus, J.H., Jaton, J.C., Bloch, K.J., and Haber, E. (1970). *J. Immunol.* **104,** 1143.

6. Osterland, C.K., Miller, E.J., Karakawa, W.W., and Krause, R.M. (1966). *J. Exp. Med.* **123**, 599.

7. Krause, R.M. (1970). *Fed. Proc. Fed. Amer. Soc. Exp. Biol.* **29**, 59.

8. Krause, R.M. (1970). *Advan. Immunol.* **12**, 1.

9. Braun, D.G., Eichmann, K., and Krause, R.M. (1969). *J. Exp. Med.* **129**, 809.

10. Eichmann, K. and Greenblatt, J. (1971). *J. Exp. Med.* **133**, 424.

11. Nisonoff, A., Zappacosta, S., and Jureziz, R. (1967). *Cold Spring Harbor Symp. Quant. Biol.* **32**, 89.

12. Kindt, T.J., Todd, C.W., Eichmann, K., and Krause, R.M. (1970). *J. Exp. Med.* **131**, 343.

13. Rodkey, L.S., Choi, T.K., and Nisonoff, A. (1970). *J. Immunol.* **104**, 63.

14. Haber, E. (1970). *Fed. Proc. Fed. Amer. Soc. Exp. Biol.* **29**, 66.

15. Chen, F.W., Strosberg, A.D., and Haber, E. (1973). *J. Immunol.* **110**, 98.

16. Jaton, J.C., Waterfield, M.D., Margolies, M.N., and Haber, E. (1970). *Proc. Nat. Acad. Sci. U.S.* **66**, 959.

17. Roholt, O.A., Seon, B.K., and Pressman, D. (1970). *Immunochemistry* **7**, 329.

18. Hoffman, D.R., Grossberg, A.L., and Pressman, D. (1971). *J. Immunol.* **107**, 325.

19. Appella, E., Roholt, O.A., Chersi, A., Radzimski, G., and Pressman, D. (1973). *Biochem. Biophys. Res. Commun.* **53**, 1122.

20. Freedman, M.H. and Painter, R.H. (1971). *J. Biol. Chem.* **246**, 4340.

21. Painter, R.H. and Freedman, M.H. (1971). *J. Biol. Chem.* **246**, 6692.

22. Freedman, M.H., Guyer, R.B., and Terry, W.D. (1972). *J. Biol. Chem.* **247**, 7051.

22a. Montgomery, P.C. and Pincus, J.H. (1973). *J. Immunol.* **111**, 42.

23. Haber, E., Richards, F.F., Spragg, J., Austen, K.F., Vallotton, M., and Page, L.B. (1967). *Cold Spring Harbor Symp. Quant. Biol.* **32**, 299.

24. Brenneman, L. and Singer, S.J. (1968). *Proc. Nat. Acad. Sci. U.S.* **60**, 258.

25. Wu, W-H. and Rockey, J.H. (1969). *Biochemistry* **8**, 2719.

26. Trump, G.N. and Singer, S.J. (1970). *Proc. Nat. Acad. Sci. U.S.* **66**, 411.

27. Givas, S.J., Centeno, E.R., Manning, M., and Sehon, A.H. (1968). *Immunochemistry* **5**, 314.

28. Richards, F.F., Pincus, J.H., Bloch, K.J., Barnes, W.T., and Haber, E. (1969). *Biochemistry* **8**, 1377.

28a. Montgomery, P.C., Rockey, J.H., and Williamson, A.R. (1972). *Proc. Nat. Acad. Sci. U.S.* **69**, 228.

29. Karush, F. (1962). *Advan. Immunol.* **2**, 1.

30. Nisonoff, A. and Pressman, D. (1958). *J. Immunol.* **80**, 417.

30a. Werblin, T.P. and Siskind, G.W. (1972). *Immunochemistry* **9**, 987.

31. Yount, W.J., Dorner, M.M., Kunkel, H.G., and Kabat, E.A. (1968). *J. Exp. Med.* **127**, 633.

32. Dorner, M.M., Yount, W.J., and Kabat, E.A. (1969). *J. Immunol.* **102**, 273.

32a. Braun, D.G., Kjems, E., and Cramer, M. (1973). *J. Exp. Med.* **138**, 645.

33. Eichmann, K. and Kindt, T.J. (1971). *J. Exp. Med.* **134**, 532.

34. Braun, D.G. and Jaton, J.C. (1973). *Immunochemistry* **10**, 387.

35. Fleischman, J.B. (1971). *Biochemistry* **10**, 2753.

36. Fleischman, J.B. (1973). *Immunochemistry* **10**, 401.

37. Schubothe, H. (1966). *Sem. Hematol.* **3**, 27.

38. Feizi, T., Kabat, E.A., Vicari, G., Anderson, B., and Marsh, W.L. (1971). *J. Exp. Med.* **133**, 39.

39. Harboe, M., van Furth, R., Schubothe, H., Lind, K., and Evans, R.S. (1965). *Scand. J. Haematol.* **2**, 259.

40. Feizi, T. and Schumacher, M. (1968). *Clin. Exp. Immunol.* **3**, 923.

41. Cooper, A.G. (1968). *Clin. Exp. Immunol.* **3**, 691.
42. Cooper, A.G. and Steinberg, A.G. (1970). *J. Immunol.* **104**, 1108.
43. Edman, P. and Cooper, A.G. (1968). *FEBS Lett.* **2**, 33.
44. Cohen, S. and Cooper, A.G. (1968). *Immunology* **15**, 93.
45. Capra, J.D., Kehoe, J.M., Williams, R.C., Jr., Feizi, T., and Kunkel, H.G. (1972). *Proc. Nat. Acad. Sci. U.S.* **69**, 40.
45a. Gergely, J., Wang, A-C., and Fudenberg, H.H. (1973). *Vox. Sang.* **24**, 432.
45b. Wang, A-C., Fudenberg, H.H., Wells, J.V., and Roelcke, D. (1973). *Nature New Biol.* **243**, 126.
46. Cooper, A.G., Chavin, S.I., and Franklin, E.C. (1970). *Immunochemistry* **7**, 479.
47. Franklin, E.C. and Frangione, B. (1967). *J. Immunol.* **99**, 810
48. Franklin, E.C. and Frangione, B. (1968). *Biochemistry* **7**, 4203.
49. Natvig, J.B. and Kunkel, H.G. (1973). *Advan. Immunol.* **16**, 1.
50. Migliore, P.J. and Alexanian, R. (1968) *Cancer* **21**, 1127.
51. Potter, M. (1971). *New Engl. J. Med.* **284**, 831.
52. Kritzman, J., Kunkel, H.G., McCarthy, J., and Mellors, R.C. (1961). *J. Lab. Clin. Med.* **57**, 905.
53. Stone, M.J. and Metzger, H. (1967). *Cold Spring Harbor Symp. Quant. Biol.* **32**, 83.
54. Stone, M.J. and Metzger, H. (1968). *J. Biol. Chem.* **243**, 5977.
55. Onoue, K., Grossberg, A.L., Yagi, Y., and Pressman, D. (1968). *Science* **162**, 574.
56. Chavin, S.I. and Franklin, E.C. (1969). *J. Biol. Chem.* **244**, 1345.
57. Abraham, G.N., Clark, R.A., and Vaughan, J.H. (1972). *Immunochemistry* **9**, 301.
58. MacKenzie, M.R., Goldberg, L.S., Barnett, E.V., and Fudenberg, H.H. (1968) *Clin. Exp. Immunol.* **3**, 931.
59. Zinneman, H.H., Levi, D., and Seal, U.S. (1968). *J. Immunol.* **100**, 594.
60. Waldenström, J. (1943). *Nord. Med.* **20**, 2288.
61. Capra, J.D., Winchester, R.J., and Kunkel, H.G. (1971). *Medicine* **50**, 125.
62. Capra, J.D., Kehoe, J.M., Winchester, R.J., and Kunkel, H.G. (1971). *Ann. N.Y. Acad. Sci.* **190**, 371.
63. Capra, J.D., Kehoe, M.J., Winchester, R.J. and Kunkel, H.G. (1973). *Fed. Proc. Fed. Amer. Soc. Exp. Biol.* **32**, 989.
64. Capra, J.D. and Kehoe, M.J. (1975). *Advan. Immunol.* , in press.
65. Wintrobe, M.M. and Buell, M.V. (1933). *Bull. Johns Hopkins Hosp.* **52**, 156.
66. Lerner, A.B. and Watson, C.J. (1947). *Amer. J. Med. Sci.* **214**, 410.
67. Grey, H.M. and Kohler, P.F. (1973). *Semin. Hematol.* **10**, 87.
68. Lo Spalutto, F., Durward, B., Miller, W., and Ziff, M. (1962). *Amer. J. Med.* **32**, 142.
69. Brouet, J.C., Clarrel, J.P., Danon, F., Klein, M., and Seligmann, M. (1972). *In* "Actualities Hematologiques" (J. Bernard, ed.), p. 42. Masson, Paris.
70. Meltzer, M. and Franklin, E.C. (1966). *Amer. J. Med.* **40**, 828.
71. Grey, A.M., Kohler, A.F., Terry, W.D., and Franklin, E.C. (1968). *J. Clin. Invest.* **47**, 1875.
72. Saha, A. (1968). *Immunochemistry* **5**, 341.
73. Saha, A., Sambury, S., Smart, K., Heiner, D.C., Sargent, A.U., and Rose, B. (1969). *J. Immunol.* **102**, 476.
74. Meltzer, M., Franklin, E.C., Elias, K., McCluskey, R.T., and Cooper, N. (1966). *Amer. J. Med.* **40**, 837.
75. Pope, R.M., Tiller, D.C., and Mannik, M. (1974). *Proc. Nat. Acad. Sci. U.S.* **71**, 517.
76. Cohn, M., Notani, G., and Rice, S.A. (1969). *Immunochemistry* **6**, 111.
77. Potter, M. and Lieberman, R. (1970). *J. Exp. Med.* **132**, 737.
78. Cosenza, H. and Köhler, H. (1972). *Proc. Nat. Acad. Sci. U.S.* **69**, 2701.
79. Carson, D. and Weigert, M. (1973). *Proc. Nat. Acad. Sci. U.S.* **70**, 235.

80. Eisen, H.N., Little, J.R., Osterland, C.K., and Simms, E.S. (1967). *Cold Spring Harbor Symp. Quant. Biol.* **32**, 75.

81. Ashman, R.F. and Metzger, H. (1969). *J. Biol. Chem.* **244**, 3405.

82. Terry, W.D., Boyd, M.M., Rea, J.S., and Stein, R. (1970). *J. Immunol.* **104**, 256.

83. Yoo, T.J. and Franklin, E.C. (1971). *J. Immunol.* **107**, 365.

84. Terry, W.D., Ashman, R.F., and Metzger, H. (1970). *Immunochemistry,* **7**, 257.

85. Seligmann, M. and Brouet, J.C. (1973). *Semin. Hematol.* **10**, 163.

86. Potter, M. (1973). *Semin. Hematol.* **10**, 19.

87. Eisen, H.N., Simms, E.S., and Potter, M. (1968). *Biochemistry,* **7**, 4126.

88. Schulenburg, E.P., Simms, E.S., Lynch, R.G., Bradshaw, R.A., and Eisen, H.N. (1971). *Proc. Nat. Acad. Sci. U.S.* **68**, 2623.

89. Underdown, B.J., Simms, E.S., and Eisen, H.N. (1971). *Biochemistry* **10**, 4359.

90. Francis, S.H., Leslie, R.G.Q., Hood, L., and Eisen, H.N. (1974). *Proc. Nat. Acad. Sci. U.S.* **71**, 1123.

91. Jaffe, B.M., Simms, E.S., and Eisen, H.N. (1971). *Biochemistry* **10**, 1693.

92. Leon, M.A. and Young, N.M. (1971). *Biochemistry* **10**, 1424.

93. Hood, L.E., Potter, M., and McKean, D. (1970). *Science* **170**, 1207.

94. Sher, A., Lord, E., and Cohn, M. (1971). *J. Immunol.* **107**, 1226.

95. Sher, A. and Tarikas, H. (1971). *J. Immunol.* **106**, 1227.

96. Lennox, E.S. and Cohn, M. (1967). *Annu. Rev. Biochem.* **36**, 365.

97. Potter, M. (1971). *Ann. N.Y. Acad. Sci.* **190**, 306.

98. Seligmann, M., Danon, F., Basch, A., and Bernard, J. (1968). *Nature (London)* **220**, 711.

99. Seligmann, M., Sassy, C., and Chevalier, A. (1973). *J. Immunol.* **110**, 85.

100. Weigert, M.G., Cesari, I.M., Yonkovich, S.J., and Cohn, M. (1970). *Nature (London)* **228**, 1045.

101. Leon, M.A., Young, N.M., and McIntire, K.R. (1970). *Biochemistry* **9**, 1023.

102. Cisar, J., Kabat, E.A., Liao, J., and Potter, M. (1973). *J. Exp. Med.* **139**, 159.

103. Weigert, M., Raschke, W.C., Carson, D., and Cohn, M. (1974). *J. Exp. Med.* **139**, 137.

104. Schubert, D., Jobe, A., and Cohn, M. (1968). *Nature (London)* **220**, 882.

105. Eisen, H.N., Michaelides, M.C., Underdown, B.J., Schulenberg, E.P., and Simms, E.S. (1970). *Fed. Proc. Fed. Amer. Soc. Exp. Biol.* **29**, 78.

106. Underdown, B.J. and Eisen H.N. (1971). *J. Immunol.* **106**, 1431.

107. Rudikoff, S., Voss, E.W., and Siegel, M.M. (1970). *J. Immunol.* **105**, 1344.

108. Hannestad, K. (1969). *Clin. Exp. Immunol.* **4**, 555.

109. Hannestad, K. (1969). *Ann. N.Y. Acad. Sci.* **168**, 63.

110. Rosenstein, R.W., Musson, R.A., Armstrong, M.Y.K., Konigsberg, W.H., and Richards, F.F. (1972). *Proc. Nat. Acad. Sci. U.S.* **69**, 877.

111. Varga, J.M., Konigsberg, W.H., and Richards, F.F. (1973). *Proc. Nat. Acad. Sci. U.S.* **70**, 3269.

111a. Talmage, D.W. (1959). *Science* **129**, 1643.

112. Rudikoff, S., Potter, M., Segal, D.M., Padlan, E.A., and Davies, D.R. (1972). *Proc. Nat. Acad. Sci. U.S.* **69**, 3689.

113. Amzel, L.M., Poljak, R., Saul, F., Varga, J.M., and Richards, F.F. (1974). *Proc. Nat. Acad. Sci. U.S.* **71**, 1427.

114. Klinman, N.R. (1971). *J. Immunol.* **106**, 1345.

115. Klinman, N.R. (1972). *J. Exp. Med.* **136**, 241.

116. Askonas, B.A., Williamson, A.R., and Wright, B.E.G. (1970). *Proc. Nat. Acad. Sci. U.S.* **67**, 1389.

117. Askonas, B.A. and Williamson, A.R. (1972). *Nature (London)* **238**, 337.

118. Briles, D.E. and Krause, R.M. (1972). *J. Immunol.* **109**, 1311.

11

Idiotypic Specificities of Immunoglobulins[1]

I. INTRODUCTION

Monotypic immunoglobulins, such as myeloma and Bence Jones proteins, and antibody populations from individual animals possess individually specific antigenic determinants (1–4). For example, one can prepare an antiserum in a rabbit which when appropriately absorbed will react with the human myeloma protein used as immunogen but, with rare exceptions, not with any other myeloma protein or immunoglobulin (1). Alternatively, one can immunize a rabbit with antibody from an individual human or rabbit and elicit specific anti-antibodies (2,3,4). Oudin (5) has proposed the term, "idiotypic determinants," to designate those antigenic determinants in a population of antibody molecules which are not observed in other immunoglobulins of the donor animal or in antibody directed to the same antigen from other animals of that species. The restriction of idiotypic determinants to antibodies of a single specificity from an individual donor clearly differentiates idiotypy from allotypy, since allotypic determinants are shared by various antibodies of an individual.

As defined by Oudin, "idiotypy" applies to determinants recognized by an antiserum prepared in the same species, and the term, "individually specific antigenic determinant," has been utilized in reference to determinants defined by an antiserum prepared in a heterologous species, such as a rabbit antiserum directed to a purified human antibody or

---

[1] This chapter is an expanded and updated version of an earlier review by two of the authors, which appeared in *Advan. Immunol.* **13,** 57 (1971).

myeloma protein (6). In recent publications, however, idiotypic specificity has come into usage in referring to determinants recognized by heterologous as well as homologous antisera. For convenience, this terminology will be adopted here. As an abbreviation for antiidiotypic antibody, the term "anti-D-antibody" will frequently be used [D for donor (7)].

There may be no essential difference between idiotypic and individually specific antigenic determinants since either must reflect one or more unique amino acid sequences, characteristic of a given myeloma protein or antibody, and therefore present in the variable regions of polypeptide chains. It is possible that heterologous and homologous antisera may tend to recognize different idiotypic determinants on the same molecule. This is not always the case, however, since the region of the antigen-binding site of certain antibodies, or of myeloma proteins with antibody activity, has been recognized as an important idiotypic determinant by both homologous and heterologous antisera.

A contribution of the constant region of a polypeptide chain to an idiotypic determinant is conceivable, but idiotypic differences among proteins must reflect differences in the variable regions. Isotypic and allotypic antigenic determinants similarly reflect particular amino acid sequences, which in many instances have been defined.

It is noteworthy that antiidiotypic antibodies can be prepared against antibodies from an individual donor, despite the heterogeneity of the immunogen. It is apparent therefore that an anti-D antiserum may recognize several specificities present in the donor population. The frequent appearance of multiple lines in double-diffusion experiments in agar gel supports this view. In a sense this is also true of a homogeneous myeloma protein, since unrelated determinants may be present on the same molecule. [This is probably the case since precipitates are sometimes (not always) formed in the reactions of Fab fragments of myeloma proteins with anti-D antisera, indicating multivalency of the antigen; however, as would be expected, only a single line is ordinarily observed in a double-diffusion experiment, since all the determinants are on one molecule.]

It seems quite certain that immunoglobulin molecules synthesized by a single clone of cells share idiotypic specificity. It does not follow, however, that all molecules which share idiotype are identical in structure. For example, molecules of different classes (e.g., IgG and IgM) can have common idiotypic specificities. In such molecules the V regions must be very similar or identical although the C_H regions obviously are not. In addition, there can be microheterogeneity within V regions of molecules of the same class; i.e., differences in amino acid sequence that are sufficiently small so that the nonidentical molecules share idiotypic specificity. An interesting example of shared idiotypy among molecules differing in structure was recently reported by Kindt *et al.*, who observed an idiotypic cross-reaction between two populations of rabbit antibodies directed to the same antigen, Group C streptococcal carbohydrate; the antibodies were isolated from the same rabbit but differed with respect to group a allotype (7a). One antibody was of allotype a3 and the other was a-negative. Since markers controlled by the *a* locus are localized in the V_H regions this demonstrates that identity of variable regions is not required for the expression of the same idiotype. It is noteworthy, however, that the L chains of the two antibodies were structurally similar or identical. This might account in large part for the shared idiotypy. Examples of shared idiotype among molecules that are very similar but not identical in amino acid sequence will be discussed in Sections II and V.

In this context, a concept whose significance has only recently become widely appreciated is that of "cross-idiotypic" specificity (6). For example, many IgM cold agglutinins share antigenic specificities that are not found in other immunoglobulins, including other IgM proteins. Nonetheless, if significantly sensitive techniques are used, each cold agglutinin can be shown to possess at least one unique idiotypic specificity, not present on other cold agglutinins (nor on other immunoglobulins). The shared, or cross-specificity is demonstrable with antiserum absorbed with normal immunoglobulins; further absorption with heterologous cold agglutinins leaves antiidiotypic antibody which recognizes only the cold agglutinin used as immunogen. This work, by Kunkel, Capra, and co-workers, as well as related studies on "cross-idiotypic" specificity, is discussed in more detail in Section II.

Within an animal more than one precursor cell may express the same genetic information. Evidence for this is the fact that a relatively small number of cells taken from an inbred mouse may sometimes express idiotypes characteristic of that strain, either in culture or after adoptive transfer. Thus, *in vivo,* there may be more than one clone synthesizing molecules of the same idiotype. It is probable, however, that only closely related structural genes encode molecules with shared idiotype, and the number of such genes may be small for a given idiotype. In humans and rabbits, in which adoptive transfer experiments are not feasible, there is no direct evidence on this point.

Oudin and Michel (8) have pointed out that idiotypy in proteins may be restricted to the immunoglobulins; i.e., that other proteins do not have structures that differ extensively among individuals of a species. If, however, all antibody sequences are encoded by germ line genes, the variations observed could reflect the expression of different genes in different individuals, each possessing essentially the same genetic capabilities. On the other hand, if antibody diversity is based on somatic mutation the number of potential sequences may be so large that the capacity of an individual to produce a unique antibody molecule may be a valid concept.

Idiotypic cross-reactions are much more frequent among mice of an inbred strain than among outbred animals. Even in inbred mice, however, the frequency of cross-reactions varies greatly, depending on the antigen and on the strain of mouse. All mice of a given strain may produce antibodies, some of which cross-react idiotypically, in response to a particular antigen, whereas antibodies to the same antigen may show very weak and infrequent *intra*strain idiotypic cross-reactions among the individual mice of another strain. *Inter*strain cross-reactions are also quite unpredictable at present; a pattern should emerge as more data become available (Section V).

The original definition of idiotype did not consider cross-reactions among different individuals. The term is, however, now used even when such cross-reactions are frequent, for example, with certain antigens in inbred mice. Although no formal revision of the definition has been proposed, in practice the term now applies to determinants which are found only on antibodies of a given specificity and which are not represented in detectable quantity in antibodies of other specificities from the same animal. The possibility has been considered that an idiotypic specificity is characteristic of a minor V region subgroup rather than a particular antibody; but this can practically be ruled out by demonstrating quantitatively that the specificity is not detectable by sensitive techniques in other immunoglobulins. For example, it has been shown by radioimmunoassay that the proportion of molecules bearing certain specificities in a preimmune immunoglobulin population is less than 1 in 50,000 (9). In addition, the region of the antibody combining site has been shown to be an important idiotypic determinant, and X-ray crystallography has demonstrated that amino acids in hypervariable regions are concentrated in the active site (Chapter 5). Amino acids in hypervariable regions do not appear to be subgroup-specific.

The existence of idiotypic determinants has proven very useful in pursuing a number of lines of investigation relating to the structure and biosynthesis of antibodies. These include the following: (a) Idiotypy has been used as a marker in probing the onset, persistence, and replacement of antibody molecules of a given structure during the course of prolonged immunization. These data have been interpreted as reflecting the persistence and replacement of clones of antibody-forming cells. (b)

Evidence has been adduced for the biosynthesis of IgG and IgM by a single clone of cells, and a relationship between the primary structures of molecules of the two classes produced by a single clone has been proposed. (c) The region of the combining site of an antibody molecule has been found to be an important idiotypic determinant. (d) The role of H and L chains in idiotypy has been explored. (e) Evidence has been secured for the existence of homogeneous subpopulations in the heterogeneous antibody of a single specificity from an individual donor. (f) The broad range of idiotypic specificities of antibodies directed to a single antigen or hapten has provided additional insight into the great diversity of antibody molecules. (g) The sharing of idiotypic determinants on antibodies of certain specificities in all mice of a given strain, and their absence from other strains, permits the use of idiotypic specificity as a phenotypic marker for genes encoding V regions (or, less probably, for regulatory genes). (h) The biosynthesis of molecules bearing particular idiotypic specificities can be suppressed, *in vivo* or *in vitro,* by the administration of antiidiotypic antibody. This should permit an investigation of the mechanism of the eventual escape from suppression, through recovery of suppressed cells or via the emergence of new precursor cells. Suppression *in vitro* provides a useful approach to the study of cell receptors, since it is probable that suppression is mediated by the direct interaction of antiidiotypic antibody with immunoglobulin receptors on B cells. Also, K. Eichmann (personal communication) has been able to demonstrate the presence of suppressor T cells, after administration of antiidiotypic antibody under appropriate conditions.

II. IDIOTYPIC SPECIFICITIES IN HUMAN MONOCLONAL PROTEINS

Before the discovery of individual antigenic specificities of myeloma proteins it had been known for some time that such proteins are deficient in antigenic determinants as compared with nonspecific immunoglobulin preparations. This was taken generally as evidence for the abnormality of these monotypic proteins. The present interpretation would be that a myeloma protein has H and L chains belonging to just one subclass or type and would therefore react with only part of the antibodies produced against pooled nonspecific immunoglobulin of the same class. Also, in some of the earlier work, the myeloma proteins studied may have been of the IgA class but were tested against antiserum prepared against a mixture of IgG and IgA.

Early experiments of Wuhrmann *et al.* (11) and von Habich (12) suggested the presence of individually specific antigenic determinants in myeloma proteins and Waldenström macroglobulins (see also reference 10). Conclusive evidence was obtained in 1955 by Slater *et al.* (1) who studied myeloma proteins from 21 patients. The proteins were classified as γ- or β-globulins according to electrophoretic mobility; from their properties these proteins may have been IgG and IgA, respectively. Antisera to individual myeloma proteins gave maximal precipitation at equivalence with the protein used as immunogen; γ-myeloma proteins cross-reacted with other γ-proteins more strongly than with β-myeloma proteins and vice versa. Absorption experiments showed that each of several myeloma proteins tested possessed individual antigenic specificities. Thus, rabbit antiserum to a given myeloma protein failed to precipitate with any myeloma protein after absorption with the immunogen; however, precipitin reactions with the immunogen persisted after absorption with nonspecific γ-globulin or with any of the 20 heterologous myeloma proteins. In the Ouchterlony test, with the homologous and a heterologous protein placed in adjacent cells, the homologous protein formed a spur in the reaction with its unabsorbed antiserum.

These results were confirmed by Korngold and Lipari (13) who prepared antibodies in rabbits against three human myeloma proteins, migrating in the slow γ, fast γ, and β-globulin regions, respectively. Tests of specificity were carried out by precipitin tests with 24 myeloma globulins. Each of the three immunogens possessed individually specific determinants. All of the 24 proteins had determinants in common with nonspecific γ-globulin.

Korngold and Van Leeuwen (14,15), and Boerma and Mandema (16) extended these findings to include human macroglobulins isolated from sera of patients with Waldenström's disease. With appropriately absorbed rabbit antisera it was shown by the Ouchterlony method that each macroglobulin possessed determinants not present in any of the several other macroglobulins tested. Similar investigations were carried out with human Bence Jones proteins (L chains) of the κ and λ types by Stein *et al.* (17), who also utilized rabbit antisera. Numerous subsequent studies have amply confirmed these findings. It appears that each myeloma or Bence Jones protein possesses unique, individually specific antigenic determinants, demonstrable with antisera prepared in a heterologous species and suitably absorbed. Cross-reactions, which have been observed among certain myeloma proteins, will be considered later.

Idiotypic determinants in monotypic IgG or IgM are present in the Fab fragment produced by proteolysis of these proteins (18,19). This is as expected, since fragment Fc is common to immunoglobulins of a given class and would not be expected to express idiotypy. More recently idiotypic determinants have been localized to fragment Fv, which comprises only the V regions of L and H chains (20). Localization of idiotypic determinants is considered in detail in Section IX.

Mehrotra (21) observed that cold agglutinins of patients with acquired hemolytic anemia possess idiotypic specificities; by analogy with subsequent findings these proteins were probably all of the IgM class. The methods he used were similar to those employed in the investigations already summarized. Absorbed rabbit antisera and a panel of seven cold agglutinins were utilized and individual specificity was found in each protein by the precipitin test. The presence of idiotypic specificity in 19 S cold agglutinins was confirmed in the studies of Harboe and Deverill (22), who utilized rabbit antisera prepared against cold agglutinins from six patients.

A. Cross-Idiotypic Specificities

Idiotypic specificities were detected by Williams *et al.* (23) in each of ten human cold agglutinins of the IgM class investigated by precipitin techniques with rabbit antisera. In addition, however, they showed that these proteins possessed other antigenic specificities common to cold agglutinins from many individuals but not present in any of 50 Waldenström macroglobulins tested. The common specificities were demonstrated with partially absorbed antisera. Individual antigenic specificity was identified by spur formation in the Ouchterlony test, showing unique determinants on the immunogen not present in other cold agglutinins. Only one of the cross-reacting cold agglutinins had λ chains; the remainder were κ. Hypotheses put forth to explain these results were: (a) the combining site of the cold agglutinin is an antigenic determinant, and thus cold agglutinins may have similar combining sites; (b) the cold agglutinins belong to a minor subgroup of IgM.

The findings of Williams *et al.* define a unique category of antigenic specificities, present in a group of molecules with similar function—in this case the capacity to agglutinate erythrocytes at low temperature. This type of idiotypic cross-reaction is referred to by Kunkel as "cross-idiotypic" specificity (6). It is advisable in attempting to distinguish "true" from "cross-idiotypic" specificity, to use a test (such as passive hemagglutination or the indirect precipitation of soluble complexes of labeled D and anti-D with an antiglobulin reagent) that will detect an antigen of low valence, since the "true" idiotypic specificity may sometimes comprise only one determinant per Fab fragment.

Apparently related observations were made by Hannestad *et al.* (24) who investigated two IgM monotypic proteins with different electrophoretic mobilities, isolated from the serum of a single patient. Both proteins reacted specifically with a trinitrophenyl derivative of hemocyanin. The IgM proteins were not, however, identical in specificity since only one of them reacted with a *Klebsiella* polysaccharide. Each protein had individual, unrelated idiotypic determinants but also held in common other antigenic determinants that were not found in 99 other serums from patients with Waldenström's macroglobulinemia or rheumatoid arthritis. This appears, then, to be another example of cross-idiotypic specificity.

Subsequent investigations in two laboratories indicated that cross-idiotypic specificity also exists among human IgM proteins with antibody activity toward human IgG (25–27). Such IgM antibodies can be isolated from immune complexes, which precipitate at low temperature from serum of patients with the "mixed cryoglobulin" syndrome. Kunkel *et al.* found that the IgM antiglobulins can be separated into two groups (prototype proteins Wa and Po) on the basis of cross-idiotypic specificity; proteins in a group cross-react with one another but not with proteins of the other group (27). A few IgM antiglobulins did not belong to either major group. The antiserum used to demonstrate cross-specificity was prepared in a rabbit against an individual IgM antiglobulin and was absorbed with nonspecific immunoglobulin and with IgM lacking antiglobulin activity. (Absorption with a heterologous antiglobulin of the same group would leave antibody reactive only with the immunogen and hence not useful for demonstrating cross-specificity.) Passive hemagglutination tests were used to evaluate cross-reactions, since the tendency of the antiglobulins to form precipitates with rabbit immunoglobulin would complicate the interpretation of precipitin reactions. A useful technique is to coat the red cells with an antiglobulin exhibiting the cross-idiotype, rather than with the immunogen itself; this greatly increases the sensitivity of tests for cross-idiotypic specificities.

Franklin and Frangione (25) made the interesting observation that one patient with mixed cryoglobulinemia, possessing IgM with anti-IgG activity, also had multiple myeloma. Associated with the disease was an IgA myeloma protein which lacked anti-IgG activity but, nevertheless, shared idiotypic specificity with the IgM antiglobulin present in the same serum. Other examples of individuals having two different monoclonal proteins with shared idiotypic specificity are discussed in Section VIII,

B. Whether the proteins studied by Franklin and Frangione possessed true or cross-idiotypic specificity is uncertain since the anti-D antisera were absorbed with various immunoglobulins but not with heterologous anti-IgG cryoglobulins.

B. Chemical Basis of Cross-Idiotypic Specificity

Progress toward elucidating the molecular basis of cross-idiotypic specificity is being made with respect to the antiglobulins and cold agglutinins. Capra *et al.* (27a,27b) found striking resemblances in the V_H sequences of two IgM antiglobulins (Lay and Pom; group Po) which show cross-idiotypic specificity (27). Remarkably, these two proteins have nearly identical sequences in all four hypervariable (V_H) regions, exhibiting only three differences in sequence out of 41 potentially hypervariable positions. Outside the hypervariable regions, five differences were noted; this degree of variation is typical of two randomly selected V_{HIII} sequences. The L chains of proteins Lay and Pom show no particular relationship and actually belong to different V_κ subgroups (27a). Thus in antiglobulins of group Po the H chains may account for cross-idiotypic specificity.

In the Wa group the L chains, and possibly the H chains, are similar. In each protein studied the L chain belonged to the $V_{\kappa III}$ subgroup[2] (subsubgroup $V_{\kappa IIIb}$) (27c). The sequences of two of these L chains were determined to position 40 and exhibited only one difference, at position 22, which precedes the first hypervariable region (27b). Limited data available on the H chains of the Wa group indicate that they all belong to the V_{HII} subgroup.

Gergely *et al.* found that the first hypervariable regions of the L chains of cold agglutinins with anti-I specificity of 2 patients were identical (27d). (There was an uncertainty in the sequence at one position.) Through residue 35 there was only one difference in the sequence; this occurred at position 19 which is not in a hypervariable segment. Studies from the same laboratory indicated that L chains of two other cold agglutinins (with anti-Pr specificity) were identical, with one exception, up to position 22 and furthermore contained seven unusual substitutions as compared to other typical V_κ sequences (27e). Idiotype was not studied, but the strong possibility of cross-idiotypy may be inferred from the investigations already discussed.

From the studies reported so far it seems likely that proteins exhibiting cross-idiotypic specificity have L chains, H chains, or both

---

[2] Some investigators reverse the subgroup designations of $V_{\kappa II}$ and $V_{\kappa III}$ (Chapter 4).

belonging to the same V_L or V_H subgroup and that striking similarities exist in hypervariable regions.

III. IDIOTYPIC SPECIFICITIES IN RABBIT AND HUMAN ANTIBODY POPULATIONS

A. Qualitative Investigations

Induced antibody populations as well as myeloma proteins possess unique antigenic specificities (2–4). Oudin and Michel elicited anti-*Salmonella typhi* antibodies in individual rabbits, coated bacteria with these antibodies, and immunized individual recipient rabbits with the antibody–bacteria complexes. After prolonged immunization, antibodies were produced in recipients which reacted, in precipitation or passive cutaneous anaphylaxis tests, with the hyperimmune serum of the donor rabbit, but not with the preimmune serum of the donor, or with hyperimmune (antisalmonella) serums of 17 other rabbits. By immunoelectrophoresis, the antigenic reactivity was shown to reside in the γ-globulin fraction of the donor's serum; this reactivity was almost completely removed by adsorption of that serum with *Salmonella typhi*. The reactivity of the donor serum disappeared after 11 months without challenge by salmonella (Fig. 11.1). Thus, the reactivity of the donor serum was attributable to the presence of antisalmonella antibodies and was not observed in antisalmonella antibodies of other rabbits. Although the allotypes of the donor and recipient animals were not specified, allotypy did not appear to play a significant role in these experiments since pre- and postimmune donor sera were not reactive with the anti-antibodies.

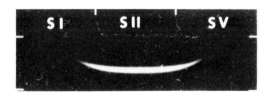

Fig. 11.1. Double-diffusion reactions in agar gel of antiidiotypic antiserum directed to anti-*Salmonella* antibody from a donor rabbit. The antiidiotypic antiserum was placed in a trough across the lower edge of the figure. A trough comprising three sections (SI, SII, and SV) was present across the upper edge. SI, Preimmune serum from the donor rabbit; SII, hyperimmune anti-*Salmonella* antiserum; SV, serum taken from the same rabbit 11 months later, with no intervening inoculations. Reprinted, by permission, from Oudin and Michel (2).

Kunkel *et al.* (3) demonstrated idiotypy in human immunoglobulins by utilizing rabbit antisera prepared against isolated human antibodies. For example, specifically purified human anti-A substance from an individual donor was used to immunize a rabbit, and the resulting antiserum was absorbed with normal human serum and γ-globulin. Two of seven anti-A preparations tested elicited antibodies to individually specific antigenic determinants; the absorbed rabbit antibodies reacted only with the immunogen, and not with anti-A antibodies from seven other individuals, or with a variety of other antibodies or normal sera. An immunoelectrophoretic pattern demonstrating reactions of absorbed and unabsorbed rabbit antiserum to purified anti-A antibody is shown in Fig. 11.2. The anti-A antibodies were shown to be 7 S γ-globulins and their individually specific antigenic determinants were localized to the Fab or Fab' fragment. Subsequently, Kunkel *et al.* prepared rabbit antibodies against a third human anti-A preparation; a panel of 28 human anti-A antibodies was used to test the absorbed rabbit antisera. Positive precipitin reactions were noted only with the homologous preparation (28).

Idiotypic specificity was also demonstrated in human antidextran and human antilevan antibodies (3). Of considerable interest was the finding that two antibodies, anti-A substance and antilevan, isolated

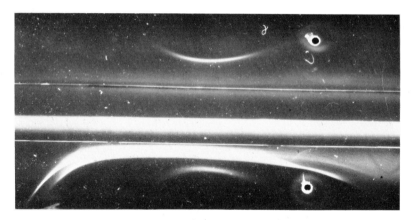

Fig. 11.2. Immunoelectrophoretic patterns showing the reaction of a serum containing human anti-A substance with a rabbit antiserum to anti-A antibodies specifically purified from that human serum. In each case the human anti-A antiserum was first subjected to electrophoresis. In the lower section the unabsorbed rabbit antiserum was placed in the trough; in the upper section the rabbit antiserum had been absorbed with normal human serum. The arc in the upper section which has its counterpart also in the lower section, represents the reaction with individually specific antigenic determinants in the human anti-A antibody. Reprinted, by permission, from Kunkel *et al.* (3). Copyright 1963 by the American Association for the Advancement of Science.

from the serum of one individual, possessed unrelated idiotypic specificities.

Extensive studies of idiotypic specificities in rabbit anti-*Proteus vulgaris* antibodies were carried out by Kelus and Gell (7), who immunized rabbits with complexes of proteus with antiproteus antibody from an individual donor rabbit. The allotypes of the donor and recipient were matched with respect to several major specificities to minimize the possibility of eliciting antiallotype antibodies. Rabbits were immunized against antiproteus antibodies from ten different donors and a panel of serums from 60 rabbits hyperimmunized to proteus was used in testing for cross-reactions. In each instance the reactive antigen in the donor population was antiproteus antibody of the IgG class. Each antiidiotypic antiserum formed a precipitate only with antiproteus antibody of the donor and not with the donor's preimmune serum, or with antiproteus antibodies from the large panel of hyperimmunized rabbits, which in some cases included members of the family group of the donor. Absorption of antiproteus antibody from a donor's serum invariably eliminated its reactivity with the antiidiotypic antiserum. No precipitation reactions were observed with the normal sera of 80 relatives and progeny of one of the donors. Autoimmunization of rabbits was attempted with their own antiproteus antibody, complexed to bacteria; no antibodies were produced that reacted with antiserum of high titer against proteus, collected earlier from the same rabbit. The idiotypic determinants of the donor antibody were localized to the Fab fragment. Kelus and Gell were successful in eliciting antiidiotypic antibodies in nearly every attempt, when immunization was sufficiently prolonged.

Although purified antibodies or antigen–antibody complexes have generally been used as the immunogen to elicit anti-D antibodies, this may not be essential. An IgG fraction of hyperimmune donor serum has also been used successfully; tests of antiidiotypic specificity were carried out with the purified donor antibodies (29).

Antiidiotypic antibodies directed against rabbit antibenzoate antibody have been induced in recipient rabbits actively producing high titers of antibenzoate antibodies (30). This supports the view that rabbits are capable of producing a wide variety of antibodies directed to that hapten group; one would expect a recipient rabbit to be tolerant of idiotypic structures already present in the animal at a significant concentration. [Recent data, however, indicate the feasibility of producing antiidiotypic antibodies after disappearance from the animal's serum of the antibodies to be used subsequently as the immunogen (Section XIII).]

The research we have summarized established the presence of idiotypic determinants in myeloma proteins, macroglobulins, and Bence

Jones proteins as well as in human and rabbit antibodies directed to a variety of antigens. Although not all immunizations were successful in eliciting antiidiotypic antibodies, there appears to be no strong evidence against the possibility that essentially all monoclonal proteins and antibody populations possess idiotypic specificities. The infrequency of idiotypic cross-reactions is consistent with the great heterogeneity of the variable regions of H and L chains of immunoglobulin molecules.

B. Quantitative Investigations

The studies described so far utilized qualitative techniques, principally double diffusion in agar gel. A question of interest is the percentage of molecules in a donor myeloma or antibody population reactive with its antiidiotypic antiserum. In the case of myeloma proteins one might expect that this fraction would approach 100%; evidence that this is the case is presented below. However, for antibody populations, which are heterogeneous, the answer to this question is not necessarily predictable.

1. Precipitating Antibody Systems

Quantitative investigations of the fractions of antibody populations reactive with antiidiotypic antisera were undertaken by using specifically purified rabbit anti-p-azobenzoate antibody as the immunogen (31,32). Each recipient rabbit was matched to the donor with respect to nine allotypic specificities. A high percentage of positive responses was obtained when the donor antibody was polymerized with glutaraldehyde prior to inoculation. Quantitative precipitin tests were carried out with monomeric ^{125}I-labeled antibenzoate (donor) antibodies. Fractions of donor populations precipitated varied from 2 to 74%. Positive tests were obtained by the Ouchterlony procedure when as little as 2 to 4% of the antigen molecules were precipitable. With antiidiotypic antisera prepared against purified antibenzoate antibodies from seven donors, no cross-reactions were observed by direct precipitation; antibenzoate antibodies from a panel of 14 rabbits were used for the tests. These antibodies comprised all the major allotypic specificities of the donor rabbits. Removal of antibenzoate antibodies from donor sera eliminated the capacity to precipitate with antiidiotypic antisera. A sensitive quantitative test for cross-reactivity, based on coprecipitation of heterologous ^{125}I-labeled antibenzoate antibodies, similarly failed to reveal any cross-reactions.

2. Nonprecipitating Antibody Populations

It was found that idiotypic specificities are present on molecules which are not directly precipitable by antiidiotypic antisera (32). This observation came from experiments based on an indirect method of precipitation, utilizing ^{125}I-labeled $F(ab')_2$ fragments of the purified donor (rabbit antibenzoate) antibody, antiidiotypic rabbit antiserum, and goat

TABLE 11.1

Comparison of Percentages of Donor Antibody (Antibenzoate) Precipitable by Antiidiotypic Antisera by the Direct and Indirect Methods[a]

Donor rabbit	Recipient rabbit	Allotype of donor and recipient	Ouchterlony test	Percentage precipitable[f]	
				Direct precipitation	Indirect precipitation
AZ5[b]	RD5	1, 3, 4, 7, 21	+	2	23
AZ5[c]	9Y		+	33	70
AZ11	2X	1, 3, 4, 21	+	7	13
AZ1[d]	1I	1, 3, 4, 7, 21	0	1	34
AZ1[d]	RD8		0	1	42
AZ1[e]	9N		+	22	51
A5	7A	1, 3, 4, 7, 21	+	4	29
A5	7C		+	10	43
A5	7D		+	11	43
A6A	7O	1, 3, 4, 7	+	14	58
A6A	7E		+	13	41
A6B	7I	1, 4, 7	0	4	28
A6B	7K		0	4	32
A7	7B	1, 4, 7, 21	+	56	69
A7	7M		+	41	74
V15	E1	1, 4, 7	+	32	35
V15	E2		+	29	31

[a] Data compiled from references 32 and 41.

[b] Antibenzoate antibodies isolated approximately 2 months after the start of immunization of rabbit AZ5.

[c] Antibenzoate antibodies isolated approximately 8 months after the start of immunization of rabbit AZ5.

[d] Antibenzoate antibodies isolated approximately 2 months after the start of immunization of rabbit AZ1.

[e] Antibenzoate antibodies isolated approximately 8 months after the start of immunization of rabbit AZ1.

[f] ^{125}I-Labeled, specifically purified, anti-*p*-azobenzoate antibody from the donor rabbit was used as antigen in the direct precipitations; ^{125}I-labeled $F(ab')_2$ fragments were used in the indirect method.

anti-rabbit Fc. The latter reagent, present in excess, precipitates all rabbit IgG in the antiidiotypic antiserum as well as soluble complexes of labeled $F(ab')_2$ fragments with antiidiotypic antibody. A comparison of results obtained by direct and indirect precipitation is shown in Table 11.1. In nearly all instances a higher percentage of the donor population is precipitable by the indirect method; in some cases, substantial amounts of donor antibody fragments were precipated by antisera that had failed to react in the Ouchterlony test with the donor (antibenzoate) population. It appears, therefore, that direct precipitation may fail to reveal the presence of some or all molecules bearing idiotypic determinants. The greater sensitivity of the indirect method was attributed to a low antigenic valence of molecules in the donor population; the indirect test should detect even univalent antigens, but at least three antigenic determinants per molecule may be minimal for direct precipitation (33).

Additional evidence for the importance of antigenic valence is the finding of Potter *et al.* (34) and Potter and Lieberman (35) that Fab fragments of mouse myeloma proteins often fail to precipitate with antiidiotypic antibodies which form precipitates with the intact myeloma protein. Also, Harboe *et al.* (36) reported inhibition of the precipitation of monoclonal IgM by its antiidiotypic antiserum in the presence of the 7 S subunit of the IgM; the latter would necessarily have a lower antigenic valence. Increased precipitability by the indirect method has also been observed in quantitative studies of certain rabbit allotypic specificities (37). The fact that Fab fragments sometimes form precipitates with antiidiotypic antibodies and sometimes inhibit precipitation is attributable to variation in the number of idiotypic determinants recognized by different antisera.

IV. IDIOTYPIC CROSS-REACTIONS AMONG RABBIT ANTIBODIES

A. Antibodies from Different Donors

The indirect precipitation test provided a sensitive means for investigation of idiotypic cross-reactions among antibenzoate antibodies from different donor rabbits (32). Such tests were carried out by utilizing unlabeled antibenzoate antibody, or whole serum containing such antibody, in large excess as inhibitor of the indirect precipitation of ^{125}I-$F(ab')_2$ fragments by homologous antiidiotypic antiserum. As expected, the unlabeled immunogen was a potent inhibitor in each system. However, in a large number of tests the degree of inhibition by a 60-fold excess of unlabeled heterologous antibenzoate antibodies did not exceed 21%. Significant inhibition (greater than 10%) was noted in 13 of the 138 tests of cross-reactivity.

Cross-reactions were also investigated, in a smaller number of systems, by testing the capacity of heterologous antiidiotypic antisera to react, by the indirect procedure, with ^{125}I-F(ab')$_2$ fragments of antibenzoate antibodies. One strong cross-reaction occurred in these tests.

One may conclude that direct precipitation may fail to reveal cross-reactions that are detectable by the more sensitive methods of indirect precipitation or inhibition of indirect precipitation. Such cross-reactions are, however, infrequent among antibodies from different, unrelated rabbits and usually involve a small proportion of the idiotypic antibody population.

Cross-reactions have been demonstrated by direct precipitation methods (ring tests or double diffusion in agar gel) by Oudin and Bordenave (38), who prepared rabbit antiidiotypic antisera against anti-*Salmonella abortus equi* (anti-SAE) antibodies from individual donor rabbits. In contrast to the anti-*Salmonella typhi* system (2,8) discussed earlier, a considerable number of cross-reactions was observed when anti-SAE antisera from individual rabbits were tested against heterologous antiidiotypic antisera. In 132 such tests, utilizing six different antiidiotypic antisera, 23 positive results were obtained by the ring test; 9 of these reactions were also visible in agar gel. Ten of the 22 anti-SAE antisera tested exhibited no cross-reactions. Frequently the homologous idiotypic reaction gave several lines in agar gel, none of which could be completely abolished by absorption of the antiidiotypic antiserum with a cross-reacting (heterologous) anti-SAE serum. On this basis the authors concluded that the anti-SAE antibodies in cross-reacting antisera were similar but not identical in structure. Since whole sera were used for absorption the amounts were necessarily limited because of dilution effects, so that the presence of small concentrations of identical molecules does not appear to be completely ruled out. Nevertheless, this appears to be a case of cross-idiotypic specificity (Section II,A).

A similar example is provided by the work of Braun and Krause (39). Goat antiserum was prepared against a relatively homogeneous preparation of specifically purified antistreptococcal (Group C) antibody from an individual rabbit. Absorption of the antiserum with nonspecific rabbit γ-globulin eliminated the precipitability of the goat serum with purified antistreptococcal antibodies from several other rabbits, but not with the immunogen. The absorbed goat antiserum did precipitate with antistreptococcal antibody from one other rabbit, but the homologous precipitin line formed in agar gel spurred over the line due to the heterologous reaction. Presumably, further absorption of the goat antiserum with the cross-reacting rabbit antibody would have rendered it specific for "true" idiotypic determinants on the rabbit antistreptococcal antibody used as the immunogen.

B. Antistreptococcal Antibodies from Partially Inbred Rabbits

Strong idiotypic cross-reactions were demonstrated by Eichmann and Kindt (40) within a partially inbred family of rabbits. The group studied comprised the parents, 25 F_1, and 15 F_2 offspring. The initial mating pair and the F_1 rabbits selected for further breeding had all produced high titers of antistreptococcal antibodies of restricted electrophoretic heterogeneity. Antiidiotypic antisera were prepared in guinea pigs against the purified antibodies of 3 of the 42 rabbits. Each absorbed antiserum cross-reacted with at least three and as many as seven antisera from the 42 rabbits in the group. Antistreptococcal antibodies from 48 unrelated rabbits showed no such cross-reactivity. A subsequent investigation demonstrated that the nature of the cross-reactions is consistent with sharing of cross-idiotypic rather than true idiotypic specificity; i.e., the antibody used as immunogen possesses at least one determinant not present on the idiotypically cross-reactive molecules (40a). Idiotypic cross-reactions within a family group of rabbits, immunized with Group A-variant streptococci, were also detected by Braun and Kelus (40b).

These results, together with data on idiotypic specificities in inbred mice, indicate that idiotype can be transmitted genetically. It should be noted, however, that studies of rabbit antiproteus (7), antisalmonella (8) and antipneumococcal (40c) antibodies have not revealed any pattern of cross-reactivity within a family. Why rabbits producing high titers of antistreptococcal antibodies tend to produce antibodies with shared idiotype remains to be elucidated. A similar question arises with respect to inbred mice; the occurrence of strong intrastrain idiotypic cross-reactions varies with the antigen and the strain.

C. Unrelatedness of Idiotypic Determinants in Antibodies of Different Specificity from the Same Individual

As indicated earlier Kunkel *et al.* (3) observed that anti-A substance and antilevan, specifically purified from the serum of a single human donor, possessed unrelated idiotypic specificities. Similarly, Oudin and Michel (2) found that a rabbit antiserum directed to idiotypic determinants in rabbit antisalmonella antibody failed to react with antipneumococcal antibody from the same donor rabbit. In a subsequent experiment antibodies from a single donor, specific for *Salmonella typhi* and *Salmonella tranoroa*, respectively, were found to have unrelated idiotypic specificities (8). Kelus and Gell (7) studied this question by immunizing a rabbit with *Proteus vulgaris*, allowing the titer to disappear, and then injecting human IgG. Antiidiotypic antibodies directed to the antiproteus did not react with the antiserum, taken subsequently, which contained anti-IgG. Daugharty *et al.* (31) and MacDonald and Nisonoff (41) utilized rabbit antiidiotypic antisera directed to specificity purified rabbit antibenzoate antibodies. Such antisera reacted with the serum of the donor rabbit, but the reaction was eliminated by absorption of antibenzoate antibodies from the serum. Each donor rabbit had been immunized with bovine γ-globulin conjugated with *p*-azobenzoate groups and possessed a high titer of antibodies against the protein carrier. The failure of antiidiotypic antiserum to react with the donor serum after removal of antibenzoate antibodies indicates that the antibovine γ-globulin and antibenzoate antibodies do not share idiotypic determinants. Thus, different determinants present on the same immunogen molecule, bovine γ-globulin-azobenzoate, elicited antibodies with unrelated idiotypic specificities.

A related question is whether antibodies derived from an individual animal, and directed to a particular antigen, possess more than one set of idiotypic specificities. In view of the known heterogeneity of antibodies reactive with a single antigen or hapten, one might predict that multiple idiotypic specificities would be present, and there is good evidence that such is the case. Thus, multiple precipitin lines are frequently observed when the donor antibody and antiidiotypic antiserum are allowed to react by double diffusion in agar gel (2,7,8). Also, Braun and Krause (39) and Eichmann *et al.* (42) were able to isolate subfractions of purified anti-streptococcal cell wall antibodies from an individual rabbit by taking advantage of differences in electrophoretic mobility. Goat antisera prepared against each subfraction and absorbed with nonspecific rabbit IgG identified different idiotypic determinants in the two populations of anti-streptococcal antibodies, although some evidence for partial cross-reactivity (cross-idiotypic specificity) was also obtained in one instance. Another approach to this question was made by Hopper *et al.* (32), who immunized different recipient rabbits with specifically purified anti-*p*-azobenzoate antibody from one rabbit. Frequently, antiidiotypic antisera from two recipients reacted with overlapping but nonidentical subfractions of the molecules in the donor (antibenzoate) population. Since an indirect method of precipitation was used, only a single antigenic determinant would have sufficed for precipitation; the differences therefore cannot be attributed to recognition of additional idiotypic determinants on the same molecule by that antiserum which precipitated the larger percentage of donor molecules. The results indicate the presence in a rabbit of antibenzoate antibodies bearing different idiotypic specificities, as well as subpopulations of antibenzoate antibodies lacking specificities detectable by the antiidiotypic antisera employed (since the antiidiotypic antibodies did not precipitate 100% of the radioactive ligand).

D. Unusual Idiotypic Cross-Reactions among Immunoglobulins of Different Specificity

Unusual idiotypic cross-reactions in rabbit antiovalbumin populations have been reported by Oudin and Cazenave (43). Antiidiotypic antibodies were prepared in rabbits against specifically purified rabbit anti-hen ovalbumin from individual rabbits. Antiovalbumin preparations from different donor rabbits did not cross-react idiotypically, nor did antiidiotypic antisera react with preimmune donor sera. The anti-antibodies thus satisfied these two criteria for antiidiotypic specificity. The surprising finding was that specific immune absorption of all antiovalbumin antibodies did not remove the capacity of the adsorbed serum to react with antiidiotypic antisera. (In other studies removal of specific antibody from donor serum has also removed the capacity to react with antiidiotypic antiserum.) The remaining, idiotypically reactive component contained immunoglobulin, but the percentage of nonimmunoglobulin components was not determined. Shared idiotypic specificities were also observed in different subfractions of the anti-hen ovalbumin population from an individual donor; for example, a fraction that cross-reacted with duck ovalbumin shared idiotype with another fraction of the same antiserum that failed to cross-react with duck ovalbumin. Further work is needed to elucidate the significance of these interesting observations, in particular, the unique finding of shared idiotypic specificity in a population of molecules that lacked specificity for ovalbumin.

V. IDIOTYPIC CROSS-REACTIONS AMONG ANTIBODIES AND MYELOMA PROTEINS OF INBRED MICE

A. Examples of Strong Idiotypic Cross-Reactions; Chemical Basis of Cross-Reactions

It is clear that idiotypic cross-reactions among rabbit or human antibodies of a given specificity, or among human myeloma proteins, are infrequent. They are much more prevalent, although by no means universal, among mice of the same inbred strain.[3] Also, a number of mouse myeloma proteins, appearing in different BALB/c mice with induced plasmacytomas, share idiotype and are apparently identical in structure. Of particular interest are mouse myeloma proteins which have antibody activity and which share idiotype with one another and with normally induced antibodies of the same specificity. In this section we discuss such myeloma proteins, as well as idiotypically cross-reactive mouse antibodies. The terms, "intrastrain" and "interstrain," are used to indicate idiotypic cross-reactivity among antibodies of a given specificity produced in mice of the same strain, or of different strains, respectively.

Cohn *et al.* (44) investigated an IgA myeloma protein from a BALB/c mouse which reacted specifically with pneumococcal C-carbohydrate. Antiidiotypic antibodies to the myeloma protein precipitated with the immunogen, but with only 1 of 160 other BALB/c myeloma proteins tested. Of great import was the finding that this single cross-reacting IgA protein also combined with pneumococcal C-carbohydrate. Antisera from normal BALB/c mice immunized with pneumococci were then tested with the same antiidiotypic antiserum. Positive reactions were obtained in the Ouchterlony test with 6 of 10 hyperimmune sera. Thus, the myeloma protein with anti-C-carbohydrate activity shared idiotypic determinants with normal antibodies of the same specificity. Also implied by this work was the possibility that normal antibodies of a given specificity produced in inbred mice might in general show a much greater frequency of idiotypic cross-reactions than antibodies elicited in humans or outbred rabbits.

This work was confirmed and extended by Potter and Lieberman (35) who isolated six additional IgA myeloma proteins, from BALB/c mice bearing induced tumors, which precipitated with pneumococcal C-carbohydrate. Antiidiotypic antisera were prepared in other strains of inbred mice against all eight of the available myeloma proteins with activity against this antigen. Three of the eight proteins possessed idiotypic specificities unrelated to one another or to any of 120 myeloma proteins tested by precipitin analysis. However, the remaining five myeloma proteins with anti-C-carbohydrate activity had idiotypic specificities that were indistinguishable from one another in precipitin tests in agar gel. The latter group included the two cross-reacting proteins with anti-C carbohydrate activity that were discovered by Cohn *et al.* It was later

---

[3] Much of the literature on inbred mice concerns antigens and strains in which strong intrastrain idiotypic cross-reactions occur, since conclusions of considerable interest have resulted from such studies. There are numerous instances, however, in which intrastrain idiotypic cross-reactions are weak; some of these are mentioned in Section V,B.

shown that each of the myeloma proteins with shared idiotype reacts, in addition, with phosphorylcholine (45,46) which is, or closely resembles, a constituent of the pneumococcal cell wall, and also with an extract of *Lactobaccilus acidophilus*. Since the latter organism is prevalent in the gastrointestinal tract of BALB/c mice, it was suggested that the cell which underwent malignant transformation belonged to a clone which had been stimulated by the *Lactobacillus* organism.

The chemical basis for these observations was elucidated by Barstad *et al.* (46a), who showed that three myeloma proteins (TEPC 15 group) which bind phosphorylcholine and share idiotype have identical N-terminal amino acid sequences up to position 36, both in their L and H chains. This includes the first hypervariable region of either chain. The possibility of complete identity is suggested. Of further interest was their discovery that two other myeloma proteins which bind phosphorylcholine but do not share idiotype with the first group have different N-terminal L chain sequences. The N-terminal H chain sequences (to position 36) of the five proteins are, however, identical. Thus, specificity for phosphorylcholine is associated with a particular H chain sequence, but the L chain sequence can vary. Shared idiotype is associated with identical N-terminal sequences, both in L and H chains, at least in this system. Barstad *et al.* propose that the corresponding structural genes are in the germ line, since they considered it unlikely that identical genes could be generated repeatedly in different mice by a random somatic process.

Amino acid sequence studies were carried out by Rudikoff *et al.* on six BALB/c IgA myeloma proteins, each of which binds $\beta(1 \rightarrow 6)$-D-galactan (46b); several of the proteins exhibited cross-idiotypic specificity but each had at least one unique determinant. The L chains (type κ) were sequenced from the N-terminus through position 23 and found to be identical. Among the six H chains, four were identical to position 30, and the other two chains each exhibited only one substitution as compared to the four identical proteins.

Cosenza and Kohler (47,48) and Sher and Cohn (49) found that antiidiotypic antibodies to the myeloma proteins, TEPC 15 or S107, which have antipneumococcal (antiphosphorylcholine) activity, almost completely inhibit plaque formation by spleen cells from BALB/c mice immunized with heat-killed strain R36A pneumococci. Erythrocytes used in the plaque-forming tests could be coated either with pneumococcal C-polysaccharide or with phosphorylcholine, with similar results. These significant experiments indicated that nearly all the antibodies produced by BALB/c mice in the primary *in vitro* response to the pneumococcal polysaccharide share idiotype with a group of mouse myeloma proteins having antibody activity to the polysaccharide or, more precisely, to the determinant group, phosphorylcholine. This is convincing evidence for the close similarity or identity of the combining sites of certain myeloma proteins, having antibody activity against a particular antigen, with those of naturally occurring antibodies to the same antigen. It is of interest that both myeloma proteins used in these studies are IgA whereas the antibodies produced by the immunized mice, or by spleen cells *in vitro,* are IgM. Shared idiotype among molecules of different classes and its rationalization on the basis of a translocation of *V* genes are discussed elsewhere (Section VIII). In the context of the present discussion it is germane that the antipneumococcal antibodies of all mice tested shared idiotype with the two myeloma proteins and therefore with one another. A related finding is that the sera of conventionally raised, but not germ-free, BALB/c mice, raised at the National Institutes of Health, contained 8 to 64 μg/ml of a protein which binds phosphorylcholine and shares idiotype with the TEPC 15 group of proteins (49a). The idiotype appeared in germ-free mice when they were exposed to conventional conditions. The implication is that the anti-phosphorylcholine antibody appears in response to microbial antigens. The occurrence of the idiotype in normal mice appears to vary among different colonies.

The anti-*p*-azophenylarsonate (anti-Ar) antibodies of A/J mice provide another example of strong intrastrain idiotypic cross-reactions (50,51). All A/J mice immunized with that hapten conjugated to keyhole limpet hemocyanin produce anti-Ar antibodies with cross-reacting idiotype, detectable with any of several rabbit antisera prepared against the specifically purified anti-Ar antibody of individual A/J mice. Many of these cross-reactions probably involve "true," rather than cross-idiotype since antiserum from any A/J mouse can almost completely displace radiolabeled donor antibody (the immunogen) from its antiidiotypic antibodies, and the weight of unlabeled antibody required is frequently not much greater than that of the donor mouse. A typical antiidiotypic antiserum will bind 20–80% of the labeled immunogen. The absence of the cross-reacting anti-Ar idiotype from many other strains of mice provided a basis for genetic studies, to be discussed below.

Strong intrastrain idiotypic cross-reactions were observed among antibodies to Group A streptococcal carbohydrate synthesized by A/J mice (52). An antiidiotypic antiserum was prepared against a monoclonal antibody synthesized by several irradiated mice, each of which had been reconstituted with lymphoid cells from a single A/J mouse producing a high titer of antibody of restricted heterogeneity. Four other A/J mice produced antistreptococcal antibody having the cross-reactive idiotype; in one mouse the antibody was only partially cross-reactive. Adoptive transfer of idiotype has also been demonstrated by Briles and Krause (53) for antistreptococcal antibodies of SWR/J mice. This idiotypic specificity may also prove useful for genetic studies since 5 of 14 SWR/J mice, but none of the A/J mice tested, shared the SWR idiotypic specificity under investigation.

Another example of idiotypic cross-reactivity between myeloma proteins and induced antibodies was reported by Weigert and his collaborators (54,55). They found that a small but significant percentage of myeloma proteins induced in BALB/c mice have antibody activity against $\alpha(1 \rightarrow 3)$dextran and share idiotypic specificity. These include an IgM as well as a number of IgA proteins; all are of type λ. The same idiotypic specificity was found in anti-$\alpha(1 \rightarrow 3)$dextran antibodies of all immunized, normal BALB/c mice.

Amino acid sequences of a number of λ chains from myeloma or Bence Jones proteins were determined and several, designated λ_0, were found to be identical (56). [They were also identical in sequence with two λ chains that had been sequenced earlier by Appella and Perham (57,58).] Three other λ chains differed from this basic sequence by $1(\lambda_1)$, $2(\lambda_2)$, or $3(\lambda_3)$ residues, with the substitutions restricted to hypervariable regions. When the H chains of one protein having λ_0 chains were reconstituted with the λ_0 chains from another protein, the idiotypic specificity and capacity to bind $\alpha(1 \rightarrow 3)$dextran were restored (55). Reconstitution with a λ_1 (one substitution) or a λ_2 chain fully restored the idiotypic specificity. Partial restoration of idiotypic occurred when a λ_3 chain was used. These important findings indicate that small differences in amino acid sequence, even in the hypervariable regions, are not necessarily reflected as changes in idiotypic specificity. They indicate that there may be microheterogeneity among antibody molecules of an individual animal which have the same apparent idiotypic specificity.

In the same investigation (55) it was found that an IgM myeloma protein with λ_0 chains and anti-$\alpha(1 \rightarrow 3)$dextran activity had all the idiotypic determinants of an IgA (λ_0) protein with the same activity, but that relatively high concentrations of the IgM protein were required to inhibit binding of the IgA protein to its antiidiotypic antibodies. This result suggested that the V_H regions of the proteins may be similar but not identical.

B. Examples of Absence of Intrastrain Idiotypic Cross-Reactions in Inbred Mice

The amount of published data on this subject is quite limited. In the case of anti-Ar antibodies, strong *intra*strain cross-reactions have been observed in strains A/J, AL/N, and A/He, but they are weak or nonexistent in C57BL/6J, DBA/2J, SWR/J, RF/J, AKR, and C57BR/cdj (59); e.g., antiidiotypic antibodies prepared against the anti-Ar antibodies of an individual DBA mouse do not cross-react strongly with the anti-Ar antibodies of another DBA mouse. This statement requires qualification in that a limited number of antiidiotypic antisera (2–4) have been tested in each system. One cannot rule out the possibility that cross-reactions might be observed with other antisera.

C. Interstrain Idiotypic Cross-Reactions; Idiotype as a Genetic Marker

When antibodies cross-react idiotypically within all or nearly all members of one inbred strain of mice but not with antibodies of the same specificity from another strain, the idiotype is potentially useful as a genetic marker, presumably for genes encoding V regions or, less probably, for some type of regulatory gene. A number of such systems has now been identified. One, mentioned above, involves the anti-Ar antibodies of A/J mice. All members of the A/J strain or of the closely related strains, A/He, AL/N, and A/WySn produced anti-Ar antibodies, some of which cross-react idiotypically (60,60a). A large number of unrelated strains produce anti-Ar antibodies which do not share idiotype with those of the A strains; one of these nonproducing strains (NZB) belongs to the same H chain allotype group as A/J. Congenic mice, having a different *H-2* gene on an A/J background, are quantitatively equivalent to A/J in the expression of the idiotype (60). Antibodies to the *p*-azobenzoate group produced in BALB/c and A/J mice share idiotypic specificity with one another but not with DBA or C57BL/6 antibodies of the same specificity (50). Antibodies to Group A streptococcal carbohydrate produced in a number of A/J mice were found to share idiotypic specificities with one another but not with antibodies of the same specificity from eight other strains tested (52,60b). The idiotype of antiphosphorylcholine antibodies of BALB/c mice (prototype myeloma protein, S107) was present in antibodies of that specificity produced in eight strains tested, but was absent in four other strains (49); mice producing the cross-reactive idiotype included strains which differ from BALB/c with respect to H chain allotype or H-2 type. Qualitative methods were used in the latter investigation. Another antiphosphorylcholine marker, differing in strain distribution from the one above, is described by Lieberman *et al.* (49a). A very useful marker involves anti-$\alpha(1 \rightarrow 3)$dextran antibodies of BALB/c mice, which share idiotype with the corresponding antibodies of several strains, but not with a number of other strains (54,55). The strains with shared idiotype

belong to the same H chain linkage group as BALB/c (i.e., share allotypic specificity); at least one strain in the same linkage group does not,
however, produce the idiotype. The same idiotype is also present on
BALB/c myeloma proteins (type λ) with antibody activity against
$\alpha(1 \rightarrow 3)$dextran.

A different type of genetic marker was discovered by Imanishi and
Makela (60c), who observed differences among strains with respect to
titers of antibody produced in response to the 4-hydroxy-5-iodo-3-
nitrophenylacetyl hapten group (NIP). There is a direct correlation with
H chain allotype. All strains tested that belong to the Ig-1^b allele group
are high responders, whereas strains in the Ig-1^a group produce low
titers of the antibody. F_1 offspring of high and low responders
(C57BL/6 × CBA) are high responders. The authors did not report on
the idiotypes of these antibodies.

D. Linkage of Genes Controlling Idiotype and Heavy Chain Allotype in Inbred Mice

In at least three systems, idiotype has been found to be closely
linked genetically to H chain allotype controlled by the IgC_H locus and
localized in C_H regions. The basis of each investigation is the existence
of strong idiotypic cross-reactions among antibodies of a particular
specificity produced in most or all members of an inbred mouse strain; in
each case, mice of another strain produce antibodies lacking the cross-
reactive idiotype. Idiotypic specificity then provides a genetic marker
and linkage studies are possible.

Very close linkage of idiotype to allotype was observed in studies of
anti-p-azophenylarsonate (anti-Ar) antibodies in A/J mice (51,61,62).
The idiotype characteristic of all A/J mice is not present in the anti-Ar
antibodies of BALB/c mice but is found in all immunized mice of the
AL/N strain, which is closely related to A/J. Congenic mice, bearing the
H chain allotype of the AL/N strain on a BALB/c background, all
expressed the A/J idiotype. Quantitative studies indicated that the concentration of the idiotypic marker in the anti-Ar antibodies of the
congenic strain was, on the average, about the same as is found in immunized A/J mice. The congenic mice used had been bred by Dr.
Michael Potter, starting with F_1 (BALB/c × AL/N) mice, backcrossing
to pure BALB/c for 9 to 20 generations, and selecting offspring for the
AL/N H chain allotype at each stage; further breeding was then carried
out to make the congenic strain homozygous for the AL/N allotypic
marker. The association of idiotype with allotype in the congenic mice
suggests very close linkage of genes controlling the anti-Ar idiotype of
the A strain and the allotype of the C_H region.

In F_1 (A/J × BALB/c or A/J × C57BL/6J) mice, about 9 out of 10 animals immunized with KLH-Ar produced the cross-reactive idiotype (62). This indicates that the absence of the idiotypic marker in BALB/c or C57BL antibodies is not due to the presence of a dominant gene which suppresses its expression; F_1 mice would carry this gene and lack the idiotype.

In other studies of the linkage of idiotype and allotype, Blomberg *et al.* used $\alpha(1 \rightarrow 3)$dextran as the immunogen (54). As already mentioned, BALB/c mice produce antidextran antibodies with a common idiotype, which is also shared by certain BALB/c myeloma proteins having antibody activity to $\alpha(1 \rightarrow 3)$dextran. C57BL/6 mice produce anti-$\alpha(1 \rightarrow 3)$dextran antibodies which do not cross-react idiotypically with the BALB/c antibodies. Members of the F_2 generation (BALB/c × C57BL/6) were inbred to obtain strains homozygous for *H-2* allele or H chain allotype (63). These are referred to as recombinant inbred strains. All combinations of *H-2* locus and allotype (characteristic of BALB/c or C57BL/6) can be obtained. Blomberg *et al.* found that only those recombinant inbred strains having the H chain allotype of BALB/c mice exhibited the BALB/c idiotype when immunized with $\alpha(1 \rightarrow 3)$dextran. The response was independent of the *H-2* allele. Their results indicate close linkage between loci controlling the H chain allotype and anti-$\alpha(1 \rightarrow 3)$dextran idiotype, and an absence of linkage to the *H-2* locus.

A different type of result was obtained upon immunizing a strain of congenic mice carrying the C57BL/6 allotype marker on a BALB/c background (54). These mice produced antidextran antibodies having the characteristic BALB/c idiotype. It was concluded that a crossover must have occurred during the backcrossing to produce the congenic mice, and that this brought together on the same chromosome genes controlling V_H regions characteristic of BALB/c and C_H regions of C57BL/6.

Evidence for linkage of idiotype and H chain allotype was also obtained by Sher and Cohn (49), who studied antibodies to type C pneumococci [IgM(κ)] produced in BALB/c mice.

The simplest interpretation of the linkage of idiotype and H chain allotype is that genes controlling V_H and C_H regions are in close proximity on the same chromosome; but the possibility that there is, instead, a regulatory gene closely linked to the IgC_H locus cannot be ruled out.

Since the idiotypes of antidextran, antiphosphorylcholine, and anti-Ar antibodies all depend on specific H and L chain interaction the question remains as to the genetic control of L chain biosynthesis in congenic or recombinant inbred mice. Blomberg *et al.* (54) suggest the possibility that the genetic locus controlling the biosynthesis of the V regions of λ

chains is closely linked to the H chain locus. Such linkage between L and H chains is not observed in rabbits or humans. An alternative possibility (61,62) is that the two strains of mice used in each breeding experiment are capable of synthesizing the same kind of L chains. Then, congenic mice carrying the AL/N allotype on a BALB/c background could have synthesized molecules carrying H chains of AL/N derivation and L chains encoded by BALB/c genes. This possibility does not seem remote since no one has succeeded in preparing antiallotype antiserum to mouse L chains [although differences among strains, attributable to V_L sequences, have been identified by peptide mapping (64)].

Eichmann (65) found that in a backcross of F_1 (A/J × BALB/c) to BALB/c, individual molecules of antistreptococcal antibody which carry the idiotype characteristic of A/J mice also are of the A/J allotype (present in the C_H region). These results are not proof of close linkage but do not indicate that individual molecules are in general encoded by V_H and C_H genes on the same chromosome. A similar finding was made in studies of rabbit V and C region allotypes (Chapter 9).

An example of an apparent crossover involving genes controlling two idiotypic markers was reported by Eichmann *et al.* (65a). Since genes controlling both markers had been shown to be linked to the locus controlling C_H regions it is assumed that the genes specifying the two idiotypes are V_H genes. The idiotypes concerned are present on anti-Ar and antistreptococcal antibodies of A/J mice and are absent in BALB/c mice. The apparent crossover was detected by backcrossing F_1 (A/J × BALB/c) to BALB/c mice. One of the progeny exclusively possessed the allotype (C_H marker) of the BALB/c strain but also expressed the antistreptococcal idiotype characteristic of A/J mice; the anti-Ar idiotype was absent. It was assumed that the crossover took place between V_H genes controlling the two idiotypes and that the gene for the antistreptococcal idiotype is located in closer proximity to the C_H gene. This type of investigation may permit mapping of V_H genes, since a number of markers are now available.

Results obtained with congenic (60–62) and recombinant inbred (54) mice indicate the absence of close linkage between genes controlling idiotype and the *H-2* locus.

VI. EVIDENCE BASED ON IDIOTYPIC SPECIFICITY FOR LIMITED HETEROGENEITY OF NORMAL ANTIBODY POPULATIONS

Most if not all myeloma proteins possess idiotypic specificity. In addition, such specificities are observed in relatively homogeneous rabbit antibody populations. However, most populations of antibody of a given specificity from an individual animal are quite heterogeneous. Investigations of idiotypic specificities to be considered here suggest that this heterogeneity is limited in the sense that homogeneous subpopulations are generally present in substantial concentration in specifically purified antibodies from an individual donor. One would anticipate that such homogeneous subfractions might be more prevalent in antibodies directed to haptens, or to antigens with repeating determinants, such as erythrocytes or bacterial cell walls, than in antiprotein antibodies.

One type of evidence suggestive of limited heterogeneity is the small number of bands generally observed in idiotypic precipitin reactions carried out by double diffusion in agar gel. Although several bands are sometimes seen, one or two often predominate (7,8,31).

Quantitative measurements of percentages of antibenzoate molecules from an individual donor reactive with antiidiotypic antisera from two or more recipients led to a similar conclusion (32). Often, two different antisera reacted with the same subpopulation of molecules in the donor antibody preparation. When one antiserum reacted with a larger fraction than the other, the larger subpopulation invariably included the smaller. It was proposed that the reactive fraction of the donor molecules comprises a discrete number of homogeneous (i.e., monoclonal) subpopulations. The remainder is so heterogeneous that it is nonimmunogenic in any recipient. That different recipient rabbits often produce antisera reacting with the same donor antibody molecules was shown qualitatively by Kelus and Gell (7), who utilized the Ouchterlony method.

Finally, it seems reasonable that elicitation of antiidiotypic antibody would require the presence of a significant amount of homogeneous antibody in the population of molecules used as the immunogen. Identification of homogeneous subpopulations by other methods is discussed in Chapter 10.

VII. PERSISTENCE AND CHANGES OF ANTIBODY POPULATIONS DURING PROLONGED IMMUNIZATION

A. Evidence Based on Idiotypic Specificities

Since the half-life of an antibody molecule or of most antibody-producing cells is of the order of a few days, one may ask whether antibody molecules isolated at various times during the course of immunization are structurally related.

Roholt *et al.* (66) have shown that the activity of H chains of a rabbit antihapten antibody is not appreciably enhanced upon recombination with L chains isolated from antibody of the same specificity, but from another rabbit, whereas a substantial fraction of the original antibody activity is recovered if the autologous L chains are utilized in preparing the recombinant. With this general approach it was found that structurally related antibody molecules are present in the serum of an immunized rabbit for a long period of time (67). Anti-*p*-azobenzoate antibodies were purified from sera of individual hyperimmunized rabbits at intervals of about 6 months. Recombinants of H (or L) chains from the earlier bleeding of a rabbit with L (or H) chains from the later bleeding of the same rabbit had specific activities 60–100% as great as the activities of the autologous recombinants. It was proposed that memory cells give rise upon subsequent challenge by antigen to antibody molecules identical to those synthesized initially by that cell line; i.e., that a long-lived clone of cells continues to synthesize molecules of a particular structure.

The study of idiotypic specificities provides a much more convenient tool for following the persistence of structurally similar or identical antibody molecules during prolonged immunization. A fundamental experimental variable in this type of investigation is the frequency of challenge by antigen; i.e., whether the animal is allowed to rest for a long period of time between inoculations or is repeatedly stimulated. One might, for example, predict that frequent exposure to antigen would tend to stimulate new clones of cells and thus lead to a more rapid replacement of idiotypic specificities than would be observed if the antigen were given infrequently. Experiments were therefore carried out in which the antigen (bovine IgG-*p*-azobenzoate) was administered to rabbits at weekly or biweekly intervals (68,41). Antiidiotypic antibodies were prepared in rabbits against specifically purified anti-*p*-azobenzoate antibodies isolated from the donor rabbit after 2 months or 8 months of immunization. Quantitative measurements of the persistence of idiotypic antibodies were carried out by an indirect precipitation method which utilizes ^{125}I-F(ab')$_2$ fragments of antibenzoate antibody (the immunogen) and its homologous antiidiotypic antiserum. Unlabeled antibenzoate antibodies from the same rabbit, isolated at intervals from 2 to 17 months after the start of immunization, were tested as inhibitors. Results obtained with one donor rabbit are shown in Figs. 11.3 and 11.4. In Fig. 11.3 the antiidiotypic antibody was prepared against antibenzoate antibody from the "month 2" bleedings. The homologous unlabeled antibody inhibited the indirect precipitation almost completely when present in excess. It is evident that antibodies having the same individ-

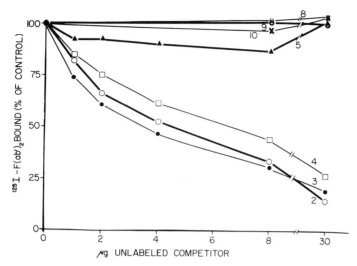

Fig. 11.3. Inhibition of binding of labeled F(ab')$_2$ fragments of anti-*p*-azobenzoate anti-bodies from rabbit AZ1 to homologous antiidiotypic antiserum. The antibenzoate antibodies used as immunogen were isolated from sera taken approximately 2 months after the start of immunization of rabbit AZI. Competitors are unlabeled, specifically purified antiben-zoate antibodies prepared from sera of rabbit AZ1 at various times after the start of im-munization; the approximate number of months is indicated by the numeral on each curve. Reprinted, by permission, from MacDonald and Nisonoff (41).

ual specificities were still present in comparable concentrations 2 months later. After month 4, however, there was a rapid transition and new, unrelated individual specificities emerged. The transition occurring after month 4 was confirmed with antiidiotypic antibodies prepared against antibenzoate antibodies from the month 8 bleeding (Fig. 11.4). The anti-idiotypic antibodies were not inhibited by antibodies from bleedings taken at months 2, 3, or 4. Idiotypic specificities present at month 8 were first identified at month 5 and then persisted through month 17, although gradual changes in the concentration of idiotypic specificities occurred. The most effective inhibitor was the immunogen, i.e., the anti-body isolated during month 8. The change in idiotype after month 4 was noted in two other rabbits, similarly immunized, although the transi-tion was more gradual in one of these animals. Prolonged persistence of idiotype for at least a year was observed also in the rabbits which sur-vived for that period of time. Similar results have since been obtained with other schedules of immunization (69,70).

Oudin and Michel (8), utilizing double diffusion in agar gel, inves-tigated the persistence of idiotype in antisalmonella antibodies of four rabbits. In one rabbit, molecules of the same or related idiotype were

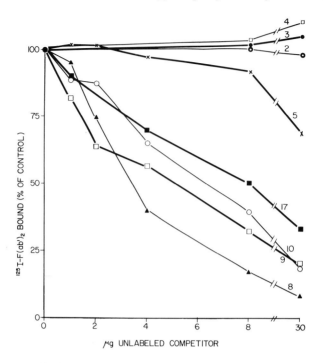

Fig. 11.4. Inhibition of binding of labeled F(ab′)$_2$ fragments of anti-*p*-azobenzoate anti-bodies from rabbit AZ1 to antiidiotype antiserum prepared in a recipient rabbit. The anti-benzoate antibodies were isolated from sera taken approximately 8 months after the start of immunization of rabbit AZ1. Competitors are unlabeled specifically purified antiben-zoate antibodies prepared from the sera of rabbit AZ1 at various times after the start of im-munization; the approximate number of months is indicated by the numeral on each curve. Reprinted, by permission, from MacDonald and Nisonoff (41).

present over a period of 29 months. The rabbit was allowed to rest for 17 months before the final set of injections and bleedings. In another rabbit they observed a loss of one set of idiotypic specificities but per-sistence of another set during the first few weeks of immunization. Idio-typic specificities persisted in two other rabbits during a period between 2 and 5 weeks after the start of immunization.

Persistence of idiotype has also been demonstrated in antibody pop-ulations of limited heterogeneity elicited in certain rabbits by bacterial antigens. Eichmann *et al.* (42) were able to separate from the serum of individual rabbits antistreptococcal antibody populations having distinct electrophoretic mobilities. Two examples are shown in Fig. 11.5. Goat antisera were prepared against each of the two major components which had been separated by preparative electrophoresis. Individual antigenic specificity was indicated by formation of a spur in an Ouchterlony test when the immunogen was placed in a well adjacent to nonspecific rabbit

IgG, with the goat antiserum in the center well. In an individual rabbit, the antibodies of slow and fast mobility were shown to have different idiotypic specificities. In two rabbits, the individual specificity present in a particular electrophoretic component after a primary course of immunization was observed in a component of the same mobility after a secondary course, 7 months later. It was not detected during an interval between courses of immunization when the serum did not contain anti-

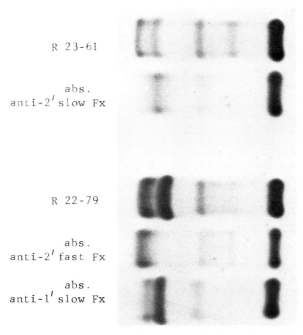

R 23-61

abs.
anti-2′ slow Fx

R 22-79

abs.
anti-2′ fast Fx

abs.
anti-1′ slow Fx

Fig. 11.5. Microzone electrophoretic patterns of antisera directed to streptococcal (Group A) cell walls, before and after absorption with antiidiotypic antisera. The uppermost pattern is that of immune serum from rabbit R23-61 after secondary immunization. The two major IgG components (bands on the left) were isolated, and goat antiserum was prepared against the slower moving fraction and rendered specific for idiotypic determinants by absorption with nonspecific rabbit γ-globulin. The antiidiotypic antiserum was then insolubilized by polymerization with glutaraldehyde. The antistreptococcal antiserum was absorbed with this polymer; the electrophoretic pattern subsequent to absorption is shown in the second diagram from the top. The lower three patterns show the results of similar experiments with the hyperimmune antistreptococcal antiserum of another rabbit (R22-79) after secondary immunization. However, in this case, the last pattern was obtained by absorbing the antistreptococcal antiserum with polymerized goat antiidiotypic antiserum directed to the slow electrophoretic component present in an earlier bleeding of the rabbit. The symbols 1′ and 2′ refer to primary and secondary immunizations. This experiment shows that the slow and fast components (labeled S and F) have different idiotypic specificities and that, for rabbit R22-79, the slow component after primary immunization showed some of the idiotypic specificity of the corresponding component observed after secondary immunization. Reprinted, by permission, from Eichmann *et al.* (42).

streptococcal antibody. These interesting experiments illustrate another means of following the persistence of molecules of a particular idiotype, namely through their characteristic electrophoretic mobility.

The effect of several parameters on the persistence of idiotypic specificites was investigated in several rabbits immunized against the *p*-azobenzoate group (41,69,70). Idiotypic specificites present in the earliest bleedings were completely replaced after a few months; subsequent changes occurred much more slowly. On a quantitative basis the population of molecules used as immunogen always reacted most effectively with the homologous antiidiotypic antiserum. Little effect of increased antigen dosage on the rate of change of idiotype was observed. Even large amounts of antigen administered every 2 weeks caused only gradual changes in idiotypic specifities. This was attributed either to more effective capture of antigen by relatively large numbers of memory cells, as compared to precursor cells, or to the induction of tolerance in those clones that were not expressed. In two of three rabbits on a monthly injection schedule, the idiotypic specificities identified underwent very slow changes over a period as long as 17 months. Changes occurred more rapidly when antigen was administered every 2 weeks. All idiotypic specificities identified before a 5-month rest period were still present afterward, indicating the survival of essentially all clones of antibody-producing cells during that interval. Quantitative inhibition data indicated that some new clones were initiated during the rest period, or as a consequence of the injection that terminated the period.

B. Evidence Based on Amino Acid Sequence Analysis for Persistence of Similar or Identical Molecules in Serum

A third, and most definitive method for observing persistence is the analysis of amino acid sequence; the idiotype of a molecule must be defined by sequences in the variable portions of its H and L chains. Amino acid sequence analysis has been used to observe the persistence of molecules of related or identical structure during repeated immunizations with type VIII pneumococcal vaccine (71). A rabbit received three 1-month courses of immunization with a rest period of 1 month after each course. Antibodies isolated after successive courses are referred to as Ab-1, Ab-2, and Ab-3. Specifically purified Ab-2 was homogeneous by the criterion of electrophoresis. Antiidiotypic antiserum specific for this purified antibody also reacted, although not as strongly, with Ab-1 and Ab-3. Light chains of Ab-2 were found to have a unique sequence for the first N-terminal 21 residues. This contrasts with nonspecific L chains of the same allotype (b4) which have multiple residues at many positions (72). The unique sequence observed in the L chains of Ab-2 also predominated in the L chains isolated from Ab-1 and Ab-3; the latter two preparations, however, were not homogeneous by the criterion of sequence since more than one amino acid was found at many positions. There was a good quantitative correlation between the percentage of molecules bearing the idiotypic determinants of Ab-2 and the percentage of L chains having the same partial sequence of amino acids as the L chains of Ab-2. Slightly less than half of the L chains of Ab-1 and Ab-3 shared the unique sequence found at the N-terminus of the L chains of Ab-2.

VIII. SHARED IDIOTYPIC DETERMINANTS IN RABBIT ANTIBODIES OR HUMAN MYELOMA PROTEINS BELONGING TO DIFFERENT CLASSES

Shared idiotypy among mouse myeloma proteins of different classes, or among BALB/c myeloma proteins having antibody activity and normally induced BALB/c antibodies, has been discussed in Section V. Here we shall consider data on rabbit antibodies and human myeloma proteins.

A. Shared Determinants in Antisalmonella Antibodies

Oudin and Michel (73) isolated IgG and IgM fractions of antisera prepared in two rabbits against *Salmonella typhi*. In each case the IgM and IgG gave lines of identity in their reaction in agar gel with antiidiotypic antiserum directed to the total antisalmonella antibody population. This important finding strongly suggested that IgG and IgM are synthesized by cells of the same clone, i.e., by cells derived from the same precursor. Since both IgG and IgM molecules with the same idiotype were present at widely spaced intervals during the course of immunization, the work of Oudin and Michel also indicated that there is constant regeneration, within a clone, of cells capable of synthesizing IgM as well as IgG.

B. Structural Relationship between Myeloma Proteins of Different Classes Produced by the Same Individual

Investigations of the serum of a single patient with multiple myeloma having two monoclonal proteins, IgG and IgM, provided insight into a possible switching mechanism which permits the biosynthesis of IgG and IgM by a single clone of cells.

The patient (Til), having two monotypic serum proteins [IgG2(κ) and IgM(κ)], was studied by Wang *et al.* (74). The L chains of the two proteins were isolated and found to be identical by several criteria, including the peptide map, amino acid composition, and optical rotatory dispersion. Upon electrophoresis in starch gel at pH 3 or 8 the L chains derived from the two proteins had identical electrophoretic mobilities. Subsequently, a sequence of 38 amino acids starting at the N-terminus was shown to be identical in the L chains (75).

Antisera were prepared in rabbits against the isolated monoclonal IgG and IgM and rendered specific for idiotypic determinants by appropriate absorptions (76). No cross-reactions were observed in tests with over 30 sera from other patients with multiple myeloma. Antiidiotypic antiserum to Til IgG gave a line of identity in its reaction with Til IgG and IgM. The antiidiotypic serum to Til IgM formed two lines in reacting with Til IgM, one of which showed identity with Til IgG.

In quantitative studies, about 90% of ^{125}I-labeled F(ab')$_2$ or Fab fragments of Til IgG or IgM were precipitable by the antiglobulin technique. Either unlabeled Til IgG or IgM was capable of completely displacing labeled F(ab')$_2$ fragments of Til IgG or Til IgM from antiidiotypic antibodies to Til IgG; the IgG was somewhat more effective on a molar basis. In the converse experiment, utilizing labeled Fab fragments from Til IgM, unlabeled IgM completely displaced the fragments from antiidiotypic antibody directed to Til IgM, but the IgG gave a maximum of 45% displacement. Thus, Til IgG and IgM share individually specific determinants but quantitative analysis demonstrated that they are not identical (76). Of particular interest was the finding that Til L chains did not precipitate with antiidiotypic antiserum to either Til IgG or IgM and was incapable of inhibiting the reaction of labeled Fab fragments of the Til proteins with antiidiotypic antisera. A recombinant of Til L chains with Til γ chains reacted with the antisera but a recombinant of Til L chains with H chains from another myeloma protein was completely inactive. These findings indicated that the H chains of the IgG and IgM contribute to the shared individual antigenic specificity.

A structural relationship between the V_H regions of Til IgM and Til IgG was then established by amino acid sequence analysis; so far no differences have been seen (76,77). The regions sequenced comprise residues 1–34 and 83–108; these include amino acids in each of three hypervariable regions. It seems quite possible, therefore, that the entire V_H regions will prove to be identical. Both of the H chains have an unblocked N-terminus (glutamic acid) and belong to the V_{HIII} subgroup.

Thus, Til IgG and IgM share identical or nearly identical V_H regions as well as identical L chains. The quantitative differences observed between Til IgG and IgM in reactions with antiidiotypic antisera might be due to steric hindrance or to a contribution of the C_H region to idiotypic determinants.

Related observations were reported by Penn *et al.* (78). Monotypic IgG and IgM from the same patient were found to share individually specific determinants which were not present on isolated L chains. These findings were later extended to several other patients who were found to have double myelomas of various immunoglobulin classes with shared idiotypic determinants (79). Other examples of shared idiotype in the monoclonal proteins of an individual include an IgA(κ) and IgM(κ) pair (79a), and IgG2(λ) and IgA(λ) (79b,79c). In both instances there is evidence that the shared idiotype may be based on very similar or identical L chains and V_H regions.

To account for the data obtained with Til proteins it was proposed that a clone of malignant cells originally synthesized either Til IgG or IgM and that a switching mechanism occurred in one or more cells which repressed the gene controlling, say, C_μ and simultaneously derepressed the gene controlling C_γ (76). That at least two genes control the biosynthesis of a single L or H chain had been proposed by a number of investigators (80–83). The data obtained with the proteins of patient Til provide direct evidence in support of this hypothesis.

On the basis of these data, and the shared idiotypic determinants in IgG and IgM discovered by Oudin and Michel (73), it was further proposed (76) that a similar switching event occurs during normal immunoglobulin biosynthesis; i.e., that different cells of a single normal clone synthesize IgG and IgM (and perhaps other classes as well) and, in particular, that the L chains as well as V_H regions of the molecules synthesized within that clone are identical. A corollary of this proposal is that molecules of different classes made by the same clone of cells may have identical antigen-binding sites. The fact that the binding site appears to be part of a major idiotypic determinant (84) lends additional weight to this hypothesis. It is not known whether switching occurs in a small or a large percentage of normal precursor cells.

Although the nature of the switching mechanism is obscure, it would appear that it involves only the C_H gene and does not affect the expression of the genes controlling the C_L, V_L, or V_H regions. The structural relationship between Til IgG and IgM and, hypothetically, between normal IgG and IgM from a single clone of cells is illustrated in Fig. 11.6.

Some of these findings were supported by studies carried out at the

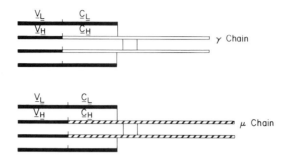

Fig. 11.6. Shared amino sequences (shaded areas) in the H and L chains of the monoclonal IgG and IgM of patient Til, and, hypothetically, in normal IgG and IgM antibodies produced by a single clone of cells. It is assumed that three of four genes controlling the four chain segments are the same for the two classes of molecule.

cellular level. Individual plasma cells derived from the bone marrow of patient Til were shown, with class-specific fluorescent antisera, to synthesize either IgG or IgM, but no individual cells producing both classes were identified (85). However, all plasma cells that were stained by anti-D antibodies to Til IgG also reacted with anti-D antibodies prepared against Til IgM. Nearly all of the plasma cells in the patient's bone marrow were stained by the fluorescent antiidiotypic reagents.

That IgG and IgM may be synthesized by a single clone of cells had been suggested earlier by the investigations of Nossal *et al.* (86). Their data indicated that a single cell is capable of synthesizing both IgG and IgM molecules when tested *in vitro* approximately 4 days after the start of immunization. Prior to this time single cells manufactured only IgM, and a week or more later, only IgG. Identification as IgM or IgG was based on sensitivity or resistance to mercaptoethanol. More recently, Nossal and associates (87), using a plaque technique, confirmed the synthesis of IgG and IgM by a single cell. Also Pernis *et al.* have shown that up to 15% of IgG-containing rabbit lymphoid cells have IgM of the same allotype on the cell surface; this finding is consistent with biosynthesis of IgG and IgM by members of the same cell line (88).

Studies of Cooper, Asofsky, Lawton, and their collaborators (89–91) as well as those of other investigators, have indicated that treatment of immunologically immature animals with anti-μ chain antiserum can suppress the subsequent production of IgG and IgA, as well as IgM. The precise mechanisms involved remain to be elucidated, but the results are consistent with a switch or transformation within a clone from the biosynthesis of one class of immunoglobulin to another class.

In the examples cited above, the idiotypically related paraproteins of different immunoglobulin class, derived from individual sera have contained L chains of the same type (κ or λ). More recently, Hopper reported on two paraproteins in the same human serum, which comprised light chains of different types; the proteins were IgM(λ) and IgG(κ). The two proteins shared idiotypic determinants localized in the V_H regions of the μ and γ chains (91a). In addition, the IgG(κ) protein possessed idiotypic determinants specific to the κ chain that were not found on the IgM(λ) protein. N-terminal sequence analysis of the two H chains revealed V_H regions belonging to separate V_H subgroups. The μ chain belonged to the V_{HIII} subgroup, the γ chain to V_{HI}, with an unusual unblocked N-terminal group (91b). The hypervariable regions have not yet been sequenced so that the structural basis for the shared idiotype has not as yet been ascertained. The possibility of separate genetic control of hypervariable and nonhypervariable (framework) regions is suggested by the author.

IX. LOCALIZATION OF IDIOTYPIC DETERMINANTS

A. Localization to V Region Sequences

One would predict that idiotypic determinants must be largely, if not entirely, determined by variable sequences in immunoglobulin molecules. Evidence has already been presented that such determinants are confined to the Fab fragment, which includes all of the variable sequence of each chain as well as invariant regions. More recently, Wells *et al.* demonstrated that the Fv fragment of a mouse IgA myeloma protein (MOPC 315), which comprises only the V regions of the L and H chains, is quantitatively equivalent to the complete myeloma protein in its reaction with antiidiotypic antibodies in the intact molecule (20).

Idiotypic specificities on free L chains have been localized to the variable half of the polypeptide chain by Tan and Epstein, who isolated such fragments from the urine of a patient with multiple myeloma (92). The corresponding, intact Bence Jones protein was also purified and used to prepare antibodies in rabbits which, after appropriate absorption, reacted with idiotypic determinants of the immunogen. A line of identity was obtained in the reaction of these anti-D antibodies with the Bence Jones protein and the fragment comprising the variable region. Thus, all the individually specific determinants appeared to be represented in the variable segment.

This work was extended by Solomon and McLaughlin (93), who utilized the urine of a patient with multiple myeloma, which contained Bence Jones protein as well as fragments corresponding to the V_L and

C_L regions. Anti-D antibodies to the Bence Jones protein failed to react with C_L but gave a line of identity in their reaction with V_L and the Bence Jones protein.

Solomon and McLaughlin were also able to cleave the Bence Jones protein, or L chains isolated from the serum myeloma protein, with proteolytic enzymes and in this way to produce artifically the V_L and C_L segments.[4] Enzymes that were effective included trypsin, pepsin, subtilisin, and papain, as well as an enzyme present in normal or pathological urine. In each of three patients the undegraded Bence Jones protein gave a line of identity with the V_L fragment in reacting with anti-D antiserum to the Bence Jones protein; the C_L fragment did not react.

Investigations of the monoclonal proteins of patient Til also showed that the V_H region contributes to the individual antigenic specificity; i.e., Til IgG and IgM, which have different C_H regions, share idiotypic specificity which requires participation of the H chain.

B. Localization of a Major Idiotypic Determinant to the Region of the Combining Site of an Antibody Molecule

Quantitative studies of antiidiotypic antibodies directed to specifically purified rabbit anti-p-azobenzoate antibody indicated that the combining site of the antibenzoate antibody is part of, or close to a major idiotypic determinant (84). The reaction of ^{125}I-labeled F(ab')$_2$ fragments of antibenzoate antibody with each of six antiidiotypic antisera tested was significantly inhibited by a large number of homologous haptens, i.e., by benzoate derivatives. There was a close correlation between the affinity of a hapten for the antibody and its capacity to prevent the combination of antibenzoate antibody with antiidiotypic antibody. Compounds unrelated to benzoate were not inhibitory. As much as 69% inhibition was observed when the hapten of highest affinity, p-(p'-hydroxy)phenylazobenzoate, was tested at a concentration of 1.6×10^{-3} M.

Alternative interpretations of these data are (a) The combining site of antibenzoate antibody is part of a major idiotypic determinant and the hapten interferes sterically with the interaction; (b) the hapten causes a

---

[4] The capacity of various enzymes to cleave the L chain in the same general region indicated that the V_L and C_L segments are compact and relatively resistant to proteolysis, but are joined by an exposed sequence of amino acids which is susceptible to enzymatic attack. This was confirmed by X-ray crystallographic data. Upon prolonged digestion the C_L region was degraded whereas the V_L segment was relatively resistant; this could explain the more frequent detection of V_L, as compared to C_L fragments in the urine of patients with multiple myeloma.

conformational change in antibenzoate antibody which results in an alteration of one or more idiotypic determinants in a region removed from the combining site. If the second hypothesis is correct, the conformational change must be limited in scope since haptens were shown to have little effect on the reaction of F(ab′)$_2$ fragments of antibenzoate antibodies with goat anti-rabbit Fab, and no detectable effect on the reaction of the same fragments with rabbit antiallotype antisera directed to determinants on either H or L chains (84). Thus, if conformational changes which affect antigenic determinants do occur they are probably restricted to the region of the hapten-binding site of the antibody molecule.

Approximately the same results were obtained whether the hapten was added to the F(ab′)$_2$ prior or subsequent to the anti-D antiserum. Thus, the hapten is capable of displacing antiidiotypic antibody.

Subsequently, the region of the antibody-combining site was found to be a significant idiotypic determinant in a number of immunoglobulins, including myeloma proteins with activity against Dnp (94,95), phosphorylcholine (96) or dextran (55).

It should be emphasized that the region of the active site is not necessarily the only idiotypic determinant on an antibody molecule. This is clearly demonstrated by the capacity of Fab fragments to form precipitates with antiidiotypic antibody in some (but not all) systems; precipitation implies antigenic multivalence. Also, antiidiotypic antibodies prepared against soluble complexes of rabbit antibenzoate antibody with excess antigen did not react with the active site of the antibenzoate antibody; i.e., when the active site of the donor antibody is blocked the immunogenicity of other idiotypic determinants becomes clearly evident (96a). Sirisinha and Eisen (95) found, however, that BALB/c antiidiotypic antibodies to a BALB/c myeloma protein having anti-Dnp activity were almost entirely inhibitable by Dnp derivatives; this suggests that the region of the active site may be the only important determinant recognized by an isologous mouse.

C. Idiotypic Determinants in Isolated Heavy and Light Chains and in Reconstructed Molecules; Determinants Dependent on Native Conformation

In a number of investigations H and L chains have been isolated and tested for their reactivity with anti-D antibody directed against the parent immunoglobulin. Some of this work will be described below. To summarize, variable results have been obtained, but, with some notable exceptions, the isolated polypeptide chains have reacted less strongly and sometimes not at all with such anti-D antibodies. When poor reactivity of isolated chains is observed, it may be attributable either to a change in conformation upon isolation of the chain or to the dependence of idiotypic determinants on a structure resulting from the combination of H and L chains. Indeed, in many instances idiotypic determinants are restored only when the homologous H and L chains are allowed to recombine, and are not found in heterologous recombinants, consisting of the L (or H) chain of the immunogen and an H (or L) chain from a different molecule. This indicates the dependence of idiotypic determinants on the integrity of the native structure in such molecules, but does not necessarily prove that a determinant comprises amino acids of both the H and L chain. For example, a determinant might be localized exclusively on the L chain, but might only be expressed when the L chain is combined with its autologous H chain. The data generally do not permit a distinction to be made between these two possibilities. Since the combining site of an antibody molecule appears to comprise portions of both the H and L chain, it is possible that those idiotypic determinants of an antihapten antibody which are blocked in the presence of small hapten molecules sometimes comprise amino acids from both chains.

Grey *et al.* (18) examined the L and H chains from 11 human IgG myeloma proteins for their capacity to react with rabbit anti-D antisera directed to the intact protein. (In three instances insolubility of the H chains prevented antigenic analysis.) In the five proteins with λ chains idiotypic determinants were localized only in the L chain of three proteins and only in the H chain of the other two. In each instance a line of identity formed when the isolated polypeptide chain bearing the idiotypic specificity was compared by double diffusion in agar gel with the intact protein; this suggested that all the specificity was restricted to one or the other chain. A finding that is difficult to interpret was the absence of idiotypic determinants from molecules prepared by recombining the homologous L and H chains of each of the five proteins of type λ, despite their presence in either the isolated L or H chain.

Quite different results were obtained with the six proteins having κ chains. The isolated L chains did not form precipitates with anti-D antiserum directed to the intact myeloma protein. In two cases the isolated H chains did react, giving a line of partial identity in agar gel with the myeloma protein. Recombination of the H and L chains was required for restoration of idiotypic determinants of the other four proteins. There was no obvious correlation between the retention of idiotype in the isolated chains and the subclass of IgG to which the myeloma protein belonged (18).

Comparable, although not identical results with respect to L chain type were obtained by Hurez *et al.* (97), who investigated two human myeloma proteins of the IgG class. Rabbit anti-D antiserum to one of these proteins [IgG(κ)] failed to precipitate with isolated H or L chains in agar gel, but a recombinant of the chains gave a line of identity with the native myeloma protein. In contrast, the isolated L chains of the second protein (type λ) did react in agar gel with anti-D antiserum against the native protein, but were antigenically deficient with respect to the intact myeloma protein.

Somewhat similar data were obtained with two monoclonal IgM proteins, one κ and one λ, from patients with Waldenström's disease (98). Rabbit antibodies directed to each macroglobulin, and absorbed so as to render them specific for idiotypic determinants, formed precipitates with the Fab subunit of IgM and also with the 7 S subunit, IgMs, prepared by reduction. Isolated L chains of the type κ protein failed to precipitate with anti-D antibodies; a weak reaction was obtained with H chains. In contrast, L chains of the type λ protein reacted with anti-D antibodies to the macroglobulin, although they proved to be antigenically deficient when compared with the Fab fragment. The H chains of this protein showed no reaction.

Thus, monoclonal IgG and IgM are similar in that L chains of the κ type have consistently failed to react with idiotypic antiserum directed to the corresponding native protein whereas, in several instances, λ chains reacted. The IgM differed in that the λ chains gave a reaction of only partial, rather than complete, identity with the intact protein.

Caution is required in interpreting reactivity of H chains with anti-D antisera; when the H chains are isolated by gel filtration of reduced immunoglobulin in acetic or propionic acid, they are frequently contaminated with L chains.

Data described so far were based on qualitative precipitin tests in agar gel. Quantitative studies were carried out to assess the capacity of isolated H and L chains to react with rabbit anti-D antibodies directed to a human IgG myeloma protein having L chains of the κ type (76). Substantial inhibitory activity was observed in an autologous recombinant, comprising H and L chains of the immunogen, but not in isolated L chains or in recombinants in which only one of the chains was derived from the immunogen. Very similar results were obtained with rabbit anti-D antibodies to two other monotypic proteins of the κ type, one IgG and one IgM (99).

In summary, results obtained with human myeloma proteins indicate that the native structure is generally essential for the expression of idiotypic determinants on proteins of the κ type, whereas isolated L or H chains of type λ proteins frequently have activity. The existing data do not rule out the possible presence on λ proteins of additional determinants that require the interaction of H and L chains since the λ chains were sometimes antigenically deficient; also, a line of identity in Ouchterlony analysis does not exclude the possible presence of an additional antigenic determinant. In view of the limited sample of λ myeloma proteins investigated, it is premature to draw general conclusions.

The presence of idiotypic determinants on isolated L and H chains of rabbit antibodies was investigated by Bordenave (100), who utilized rabbit anti-D antisera directed against rabbit anti-*Salmonella abortus equi* (anti-SAE) antibodies. In each case isolated H chains gave a positive ring test in liquid medium when tested with the antiidiotypic antiserum. The L chains of one donor antibody failed to react with each of the three homologous antiidiotypic antisera. However, a recombinant of the same L chains with nonspecific H chains reacted weakly with two of the antisera. In another system isolated L chains did react weakly with two anti-D antisera directed to the intact molecule but only after prolonged immunization; anti-D antibodies with strong reactivity against the native anti-SAE antibody, but with no activity directed to isolated L chains, appeared early in the course of immunization. It is evident that the major idiotypic determinants in these rabbit antibodies require the interaction of H and L chains but that reactions can sometimes be obtained with the isolated chains. Tests, by double diffusion, for antigenic similarity between the isolated chains and the native protein were not reported.

Studies of mouse myeloma proteins with antibody specificity for phosphorylcholine (101) or $\alpha(1 \rightarrow 3)$dextran (55) demonstrated that the expression of idiotypic determinants requires the participation of both H and L chains. It is of interest that the latter proteins are of type λ.

X. CROSS-REACTIONS OF ANTIIDIOTYPIC ANTIBODIES WITH NONSPECIFIC IMMUNOGLOBULINS

Data to be summarized here suggest that there are two kinds of idiotypic determinants in myeloma proteins. The first type cannot be detected in nonspecific immunoglobulin, even with extremely sensitive techniques. The second is apparently present in the nonspecific population; however, it is not certain whether the cross-reacting determinants are identical or only related in structure.

The most convincing evidence that certain determinants of human myeloma proteins are absent from nonspecific immunoglobulin was presented by Kunkel (6). Antiidiotypic antisera were prepared in monkeys or rabbits and were tested by passive hemagglutination, using erythrocytes to which the immunogen (IgG myeloma protein) was covalently conjugated. In a typical test system, 8×10^{-6} mg/ml of the homologous myeloma protein significantly inhibited passive hemagglutination whereas 60 mg/ml of nonspecific human Fraction II was not inhibitory; the ratio of the two numbers is 7.5×10^6. In the twelve systems studied no inhibitory capacity was detected in pooled nonspecific immunoglobulin. Minimum ratios reported for the inhibitory capacities of the immunogen, as compared to nonspecific IgG, ranged from 6×10^5 to 3×10^7. In other words, less than one molecule in 3×10^7 of nonspecific IgG, in the latter instance, shared the individual antigenic specificity of the myeloma protein.

The same methods were applied to four Bence Jones proteins (6). Again, no inhibition of the passive hemagglutination with antiidiotypic antisera was observed with high concentrations of nonspecific human IgG or its L chains. The ratio of the inhibitory capacity of the homologous Bence Jones protein to that of nonspecific L chains exceeded 7×10^4 in each system.

Similar results were obtained with a different but less sensitive test system (76,102), utilizing 0.5 μg of ^{125}I-labeled F(ab')$_2$ fragments of IgG myeloma protein and rabbit antiidiotypic antiserum. Complexes were precipitated by goat anti-rabbit Fc. The ratio of the inhibitory capacity of homologous protein to nonspecific IgG exceeded 3×10^4 to 1 (102).

The presence of unique idiotypic determinants that are not detectable in other immunoglobulins is characteristic of induced antibodies as well as myeloma proteins. Idiotypic determinants characteristic of anti-*p*-azophenylarsonate antibodies of A/J mice were not detectable in nonspecific A/J IgG or in A/J antibodies of different specificity; the ratio of the inhibitory capacity of the anti-*p*-azophenylarsonate antibody used as immunogen to that of the other immunoglobulins was in excess of $5 \times 10^4 : 1$ (9).

Quite different results have been obtained when cross-reactions were investigated by inhibition of specific precipitation. In several systems nonspecific IgG inhibited, partially or completely, the precipitation in liquid medium of human IgG myeloma proteins by rabbit anti-D antisera; classical precipitin tests were utilized (18,97).

When both precipitin and binding tests were carried out with the same system, it was found that nonspecific IgG had no effect on the binding of labeled F(ab')$_2$ fragments of an IgG myeloma protein by anti-D antibodies but, when present at high concentration, the IgG completely inhibited precipitation of the myeloma IgG by the anti-D antiserum (102). Other myeloma proteins tested had no effect on either precipitation or binding.

Possible explanations for these results are (a) Precipitation requires the participation of multiple idiotypic determinants, only some of which are present, in similar or identical form, in nonspecific immunoglobulin. At least one determinant in the myeloma protein must be completely unique to account for the data; the region of the combining site is a likely candidate. (b) A high concentration of normal immunoglobulin nonspecifically inhibits precipitation. This seems unlikely since concentrations as low as 20 mg/ml of nonspecific IgG are inhibitory in some cases; this value does not greatly exceed the concentration in normal serum. The fact that other myeloma proteins failed to inhibit precipitation also argues against this hypothesis. (A myeloma protein would not possess the spectrum of determinants of nonspecific IgG.) (c) A third possibility would invoke the difference in conditions of the precipitin and binding tests. The latter were carried out with much lower concentrations of antiidiotypic antibodies. If the determinants shared by nonspecific IgG are cross-reacting and combine with low affinity, they might conceivably not be effective in inhibiting binding reactions but could be active at the higher concentrations used in preciptin tests.

XI. SUPPRESSION OF IDIOTYPIC SPECIFICITIES

A. Suppression of Humoral Responses

The existence of strong idiotypic cross-reactions among different mice of the same strain, with respect to certain antigens, made it feasible to attempt suppression of a particular idiotype with antiidiotypic antiserum. This could be analogous to suppression of an allotype in heterozygous animals with antiallotypic antiserum (Chapter 9). The appearance of an idiotype, characteristic of anti-p-azophenylarsonate (anti-Ar) antibodies of A/J mice was suppressed for periods up to 5 months, in neonatal or adult A/J mice, by intraperitoneal administration of a saline solution of 2 or 4 mg of an IgG fraction of rabbit anti-D antiserum (103). It was shown that suppression is not caused by simple absorption of anti-Ar antibodies by the antiidiotypic antibodies injected. There was no concomitant suppression of the total antihapten response or of production of antibody to the protein carrier.

The suppressed mice produced anti-Ar antibodies in titers comparable to those of controls. Interestingly, the idiotypic specificities of the anti-Ar antibodies arising in different, suppressed A/J mice were not cross-reactive with one another (104). This result indicates that A/J mice are capable of synthesizing a large variety of antibody molecules specific for the azophenylarsonate group but that expansion of one or a few identical clones occurs in all nonsuppressed mice of that strain.

Immunological memory, for the production of the cross-reactive idiotype, can also be suppressed after primary immunization with the phenylarsonate–protein conjugate (104a). This observation indicates that memory cells are subject to inactivation by heterologous antiidiotype antibodies and, also, that they are accessible *in vivo*.

Suppression was attributed to the reaction of antiidiotypic antibodies with receptors (antibodies) present on the surface of B lymphocytes. Whether it is due to reversible inactivation or to destruction of cells is uncertain, although the latter explanation seems more plausible in view of the long-term nature of the suppression. Fab' and F(ab')$_2$ fragments of the rabbit anti-D antibodies were ineffective (105); this might be attributable either to rapid clearance of the fragments from the mouse or to their inability to fix mouse complement.

Studies carried out by Cosenza and Köhler (48) and by Sher and Cohn (49) demonstrated that mouse antiidiotypic antibodies can suppress the production *in vitro* of BALB/c antipneumococcal C-polysaccharide antibodies. This was shown by a plaque assay using, as the target, red cells coated with phosphorylcholine or with the antigenically cross-reacting pneumococcal C-polysaccharide. These experiments suggest that nearly all antibodies to the polysaccharide, produced in a primary response in BALB/c mice, share idiotypic specificity. The antibodies are of the IgM class, but cross-react idiotypically with certain IgA myeloma proteins having antiphosphorylcholine activity. Actually, the anti-D antisera used by the two groups of investigators were prepared against such IgA myeloma proteins.

Eichmann exploited intrastrain idiotypic cross-reactions, observed in nearly all A/J mice immunized with Group A streptococci, to study suppression of a particular idiotype by guinea pig antiidiotypic antisera (106). Suppression was mediated by guinea pig IgG2 antibodies but not by IgG1; the former but not the latter are capable of fixing complement and binding to macrophages. Cells adoptively transferred from suppressed A/J mice to irradiated syngeneic recipients failed to produce the cross-reactive idiotype, in contrast to nonsuppressed cells from normal controls; this proved that suppression is attributable to elimination of the relevant clone of cells.

B. Suppression of Cell-Mediated Responses

Since the antigen receptors on B lymphocytes are immunoglobulins, the suppression of B-cell mediated responses by antiidiotypic antibodies can readily be attributed to antireceptor activity. More recent observations, starting with work of Ramseier and Lindenmann (107–108a), suggest that cell-mediated responses can also be inhibited by such antisera, possibly indicating an interaction of antiidiotypic antibody with T cells. The rationale of their experiments, carried out with inbred rats, mice, and hamsters, is as follows: If lymphoid cells from inbred strain A are injected into $(A \times B)F_1$ rats, the host may respond by producing antibodies against receptors in the donor (A) lymphocytes that are specific for antigens of strain B. The F_1 recipients possess essentially all antigens of strain A, but, being tolerant of B antigens, should lack anti-B receptors; they are therefore capable of producing anti-anti-B. Anti-antibodies of the same specificity can in theory be produced by injecting anti-B antibodies, produced by challenging A recipients with B antigens, into $(A \times B)F_1$ recipients. Their data are in accord with these premises. Anti-anti-B was formed as a result of either procedure. The assay consists of testing the resulting antiserum for its ability to prevent a mixed lymphocyte reaction involving A and B lymphoid cells. Their unique assay for the occurrence of a mixed lymphocyte reaction is described in detail in reference 108a.

McKearn (109) elicited antiidiotypic antibodies against antibodies from inbred Lewis rats having activity toward histocompatibility antigens of the BN rat strain. The latter antibodies were purified, then injected into F_1(Lewis × BN) (LBN) rats, which produced the antiidiotypic antibody. Of great interest was the observation that when the immunized LBN hosts were challenged with Lewis spleen cells the graft versus host reaction, as evidenced by increase in weight of local lymph nodes, was diminished as compared with nonimmunized controls. Whether this was caused by an interaction of antiidiotypic antibodies with receptors on T cells remains to be established.

XII. PRODUCTION OF ANTIIDIOTYPIC ANTIBODIES WITHIN THE SAME STRAIN OF MOUSE; ANTITUMOR ACTIVITY OF ANTIMYELOMA PROTEIN ANTIBODIES

Although it is sometimes difficult to accomplish, antiidiotypic antibodies have been produced in certain instances by immunization of mice of the same strain as that which produced the immunoglobulin. Sirisinha and Eisen (95) succeeded in producing antiidiotypic antibodies in BALB/c mice against two BALB/c myeloma proteins (Nos. 315 and 460) having antibody activity specific for the 2,4-dinitrophenyl (Dnp) group. The antiidiotypic antibodies were almost entirely inhibitable by free Dnp derivatives, suggesting that the region of the antibody-combining site is the most important idiotypic determinant for isoimmunization. Of particular interest was the finding that BALB/c mice immunized with a BALB/c myeloma protein rejected doses of the corresponding tumor cells which became established in control BALB/c mice (109a). Rejection was attributed to the presence of antiidiotypic antibodies or to cellular immunity mediated by lymphocytes with antiidiotypic specificity. Upon challenge with cells from the MOPC 315 tumor, some mice that had been immunized with protein 315 developed variant tumors that secreted only the L chains of that protein. (Free L chains lack the idiotypic determinants of the complete molecule.) It was subsequently found (110) that the MOPC 315 tumor ordinarily contains about 5 to 10% of cells which secrete only L chains. Thus, antiidiotypic antibodies (or lymphocytes) evidently suppress cells synthesizing complete molecules and permit the multiplication of cells producing free L chains.

Another example of autoimmunization is afforded by the work of Eichmann (52), who succeeded in eliciting anti-D antibodies to A/J antistreptococcal carbohydrate antibodies by attaching the antibodies to streptococci and immunizing A/J mice with the complex.

Yakulis *et al.* (111) were able to produce anti-D antibodies specific for two BALB/c myeloma proteins, MOPC 195 and LPC 1, by immunization of BALB/c mice with proteins polymerized with glutaraldehyde. The anti-D was detected by passive hemagglutination. The enhancement of immunogenicity through polymerization may be explained in terms of the earlier work of Iverson (112), who was unable to produce anti-D against a BALB/c myeloma protein in a second strain of mouse that shared H chain allotype with BALB/c, but was successful in eliciting anti-D antibodies if the protein was first modified with Dnp groups prior to inoculation.

The work of Janeway and Paul (113) indicates that the mechanism of enhancement by the attached Dnp groups involves the production of anti-Dnp antibodies in the recipient mouse; these antibodies evidently form complexes with the immunogen which are capable of eliciting antiidiotypic antibodies reactive with the native myeloma protein.

An alternative method for enhancing the immunogenicity of a BALB/c myeloma protein in BALB/c mice is to copolymerize the protein with homologous (C57BL) or heterologous (rabbit) IgG (114). Such copolymers proved to be much more immunogenic than the self-polymerized myeloma protein.

XIII. PRODUCTION OF ANTIIDIOTYPIC ANTIBODIES BY AN ANIMAL AGAINST ITS OWN ANTIBODIES

This subject is provocative since it introduces the possibility that antiidiotypic antibodies are regularly produced against one's own antibodies and that this provides a regulatory mechanism for antibody production. The data so far are limited.

Rodkey (115) immunized rabbits with protein conjugated to *p*-azophenyl-*N*-trimethylammonium groups, collected and purified the antibodies, and prepared $F(ab')_2$ fragments. The latter were polymerized and injected into the same rabbit after a rest period of 14 months. Antiidiotypic antibodies were synthesized as a consequence of this procedure.

McKearn (109) states that Lewis rats injected with fibrosarcoma cells from strain BN rats develop not only antibodies to the antigen but also, on prolonged immunization, antiidiotypic antibodies to the anti-BN antibodies.

REFERENCES

1. Slater, R.J., Ward, S.M., and Kunkel, H.G. (1955). *J. Exp. Med.* **101,** 85.
2. Oudin, J. and Michel, M. (1963). *C. R. Acad. Sci. (Paris)* **257,** 805.
3. Kunkel, H.G., Mannik, M., and Williams, R.C. (1963). *Science* **140,** 1218.
4. Gell, P.G.H. and Kelus, A.S. (1964). *Nature (London)* **201,** 687.
5. Oudin, J. (1966). *Proc. Roy. Soc. Ser.* **B166,** 207.
6. Kunkel, H.G. (1970). *Fed. Proc. Fed. Amer. Soc. Exp. Biol.* **29,** 55.
7. Kelus, A.S. and Gell, P.G.H. (1968). *J. Exp. Med.* **127,** 215.
7a. Kindt, T.J., Klapper, D.G., and Waterfield, M.D. (1973). *J. Exp. Med.* **137,** 636.
8. Oudin, J. and Michel, M. (1969). *J. Exp. Med.* **130,** 595.
9. Pawlak, L.L., Wang, A.L., and Nisonoff, A. (1973). *J. Immunol.* **11,** 587.
10. Hopper, J.E. and Nisonoff, A. (1971). *Advan. Immunol.* **13,** 57.
11. Wuhrmann, F.H., Wunderly, C.H., and Hassig, A. (1950). *Brit. J. Exp. Pathol.* **31,** 507.
12. Von Habich, H. (1953). *Schweiz. Med. Wochenschr.* **52,** 1253.
13. Korngold, L. and Lipari, R. (1956). *Cancer* **9,** 183.
14. Korngold, L. and Van Leeuwen, G. (1957). *J. Exp. Med.* **106,** 467.
15. Korngold, L. and Van Leeuwen, G. (1957). *J. Exp. Med.* **106,** 477.
16. Boerma, F.W. and Mandema, E. (1957). *J. Lab. Clin. Med.* **49,** 358.
17. Stein, S., Nachman, R.L., and Engle, R.L., Jr. (1963). *Nature (London)* **200,** 1180.
18. Grey, H.M., Mannik, M., and Kunkel, H.G. (1965). *J. Exp. Med.* **121,** 561.

19. Seligmann, M., Meshaka, G., Hurez, D., and Mihaesco, C. (1965). *4th Int. Symp. Immunopathol.*, p. 229. Schwabe and Co., Basel.
20. Wells, J.V., Fudenberg, H.H., and Givol, D. (1973). *Proc. Nat. Acad. Sci. U.S.* **70,** 1585.
21. Mehrotra, T.N. (1960). *Nature (London)* **185,** 323.
22. Harboe, M. and Deverill, J. (1964). *Scand. J. Haematol.* **1,** 223.
23. Williams, R.C. Jr., Kunkel, H.G., and Capra, J.D. (1968). *Science* **161,** 379.
24. Hannestad, K., Eriksen, J., Christensen, T., and Harboe, M. (1970). *Immunochemistry* **7,** 899.
25. Franklin, E.C. and Frangione, B. (1971). *J. Immunol.* **107,** 1527.
26. Agnello, V., Joslin, F.G., and Kunkel, H.G. (1972). *Scand. J. Immunol.* **1,** 283.
27. Kunkel, H.G., Agnello, V., Joslin, F.G., Winchester, R.J., and Capra, J.D. (1973). *J. Exp. Med.* **137,** 331.
27a. Capra, J.D., Kehoe, J.M., Winchester, R.J., and Kunkel, H.G. (1971). *Ann. N.Y. Acad. Sci.* **190,** 371.
27b. Capra, J.D. and Kehoe, J.M. (1975). *Advan. Immunol.,* in press.
27c. Kunkel, H.G., Winchester, R.J., Joslin, F.G., and Capra, J.D. (1974). *J. Exp. Med.* **139,** 128.
27d. Gergely, J., Wang, A.C., and Fudenberg, H.H. (1973). *Vox. Sang.* **24,** 432.
27e. Wang, A.C., Fudenberg, H.H., Wells, J.V., and Roelcke, D. (1973). *Nature New Biol.* **243,** 126.
28. Kunkel, H.G., Killander, J., and Mannik, M. (1966). *Acta Med. Scand.* **445,** 63.
29. Schade, S.Z. and Nisonoff, A. (1972). *J. Immunol.* **108,** 1295.
30. Spring-Stewart, S., Brient, B.W., and Nisonoff, A. (1972). *J. Immunol.* **108,** 1288.
31. Daugharty, H., Hopper, J.E., MacDonald, A.B., and Nisonoff, A. (1969). *J. Exp. Med.* **130,** 1047.
32. Hopper, J.E., MacDonald, A.B., and Nisonoff, A. (1970). *J. Exp. Med.* **131,** 41.
33. Valentine, R.C. and Green, N.M. (1967). *J. Mol. Biol.* **27,** 615.
34. Potter, M., Lieberman, R., and Dray, S. (1966). *J. Mol. Biol.* **16,** 334.
35. Potter, M. and Lieberman, R. (1970). *J. Exp. Med.* **132,** 737.
36. Harboe, M., Solheim, B.G., and Deverill, J. (1969). *J. Exp. Med.* **129,** 1217.
37. Gilman, A., Nisonoff, A., and Dray, S. (1964). *Immunochemistry* **1,** 109.
38. Oudin, J. and Bordenave, G. (1971). *Nature (London)* **231,** 86.
39. Braun, D.G. and Krause, R.M. (1968). *J. Exp. Med.* **128,** 969.
40. Eichmann, K. and Kindt, T.J. (1971). *J. Exp. Med.* **134,** 523.
40a. Kindt, T.J., Seide, R.K., Bokisch, V.A., and Krause, R.M. (1973). *J. Exp. Med.* **138,** 522.
40b. Braun, D.G. and Kelus, A.S. (1973). *J. Exp. Med.* **138,** 1248.
40c. Winfield, J.B., Pincus, J.E., and Mage, R.G. (1972). *J. Immunol.* **108,** 1278.
41. MacDonald, A.B. and Nisonoff, A. (1970). *J. Exp. Med.* **131,** 583.
42. Eichmann, K., Braun, D.G., Feizi, T., and Krause, R.M. (1970). *J. Exp. Med.* **131,** 1169.
43. Oudin, J. and Cazenave, P.A. (1971). *Proc. Nat. Acad. Sci. U.S.* **68,** 2616.
44. Cohn, M., Notani, G., and Rice, S.A. (1969). *Immunochemistry* **6,** 111.
45. Potter, M. and Leon, M.A. (1968). *Science* **162,** 369.
46. Lieberman, R. and Humphrey, W. (1971). *Proc. Nat. Acad. Sci. U.S.* **68,** 2510.
46a. Barstad, P., Rudikoff, S., Potter, M., Konigsberg, W., Cohn, M., and Hood, L., (1974). *Science* **183,** 962.
46b. Rudikoff, S., Mushinski, E.B., Potter, M., Glaudemans, C.P.J., and Jolley, M.E. (1973). *J. Exp. Med.* **138,** 1095.
47. Cosenza, H. and Köhler, H. (1972). *Science* **176,** 1027.

48. Cosenza, H. and Köhler, H. (1972). *Proc. Nat. Acad. Sci. U.S.* **69,** 2701.
49. Sher, A. and Cohn, M. (1972). *Eur. J. Immunol.* **2,** 319.
49a. Lieberman, R., Potter, M., Mushinski, E.B., Humphrey, W., Jr., and Rudikoff, S. (1974). *J. Exp. Med.* **139,** 983.
50. Kuettner, M.G., Wang, A.L., and Nisonoff, A. (1972). *J. Exp. Med.* **135,** 579.
51. Nisonoff, A. (1973). *In* "Genetic Control of Immune Responsiveness" (M. Landy and H.O. McDevitt, eds). Brook Lodge Symposium, May, 1972. p. 157. Academic Press, New York.
52. Eichmann, K. (1972). *Eur. J. Immunol.* **2,** 301.
53. Briles, D.E. and Krause, R.M. (1972). *J. Immunol.* **109,** 1311.
54. Blomberg, B., Geckeler, W., and Weigert, M.G. (1972). *Science* **177,** 178.
55. Carson, D. and Weigert, M. (1973). *Proc. Nat. Acad. Sci. U.S.* **70,** 235.
56. Weigert, M.G., Cesari, I.M., Yonkovich, S.J., and Cohn, M. (1970). *Nature (London)* **228,** 1045.
57. Appella, E. and Perham, R.N. (1967). *Cold Spring Harbor Symp. Quant. Biol.* **32,** 37.
58. Appella, E. and Perham, R.N. (1968). *J. Mol. Biol.* **33,** 963.
59. Pawlak, L.L. and Nisonoff, A. (1973). Unpublished data.
60. Pawlak, L.L. and Nisonoff, A. (1973). *J. Exp. Med.* **137,** 855.
60a. Pawlak, L.L., and Nisonoff, A. (1974). *Ann. Immunol. (Inst. Pasteur), Paris* **125 C,** 363.
60b. Eichmann, K. (1973). *J. Exp. Med.* **137,** 603.
60c. Imanishi, T. and Makela, O. (1973). *Eur. J. Immunol.* **3,** 329.
61. Pawlak, L.L., Hart, D.A., Nisonoff, A., Mushinski, E.B., and Potter, M. (1973). *Proc. 3rd Int. Convocation Immunol.,* p. 259. S. Karger, Basel.
62. Pawlak, L.L., Mushinski, E.B., Nisonoff, A., and Potter, M. (1973). *J. Exp. Med.* **137,** 22.
63. Bailey, D.W. (1971). *Transplantation* **11,** 325.
64. Edelman, G.M. and Gottlieb, P.D. (1970). *Proc. Nat. Acad. Sci. U.S.* **67,** 1192.
65. Eichmann, K. (1973). *J. Exp. Med.* **137,** 603.
65a. Eichmann, K., Tung, A.S., and Nisonoff, A. (1974). *Nature (London)* **250,** 509.
66. Roholt, O.A., Radzimski, G., and Pressman, D. (1965). *Science* **147,** 613.
67. MacDonald, A.B., Alescio, L., and Nisonoff, A. (1969). *Biochemistry* **8,** 3109.
68. Nisonoff, A., MacDonald, A.B., Hopper, J.E., and Daugharty, H. (1970). (In *Symp. Exp. Approaches to Homogeneous Antibody Populations, April 1969*) *Fed. Proc. Fed. Amer. Soc. Exp. Biol.* **29,** 72.
69. Spring-Stewart, S.B., Schroeder, K.W., and Nisonoff, A. (1971). *J. Exp. Med.* **134,** 765.
70. Spring-Stewart, S.B., and Nisonoff, A. (1973). *Contemp. Topics Mol. Immunol.* **2,** 99.
71. Jaton, J.C., Waterfield, M.D., Margolies, M.N., Bloch, K.J., and Haber, E. (1970). *Biochemistry* **10,** 1583.
72. Jaton, J.C., Waterfield, M.C., Margolies, M.N., and Haber, E. (1970). *Proc. Nat. Acad. Sci. U.S.* **66,** 959.
73. Oudin, J. and Michel, M. (1969). *J. Exp. Med.* **130,** 619.
74. Wang, A.C., Wang, I.Y.F., McCormick, J.N., and Fudenberg, H.H. (1969). *Immunochemistry* **6,** 451.
75. Pink, J.R.L., Wang, A.C., and Fudenberg, H.H. (1971). *Annu. Rev. Med.* **22,** 145.
76. Wang, A.C., Wilson, S.K., Hopper, J.E., Fudenberg, H.H., and Nisonoff, A. (1970). *Proc. Nat. Acad. Sci. U.S.* **66,** 337.
77. Wang, A.C., Gergely, J., and Fudenberg, H.H. (1973). *Biochemistry* **12,** 528.

78. Penn, G.M., Kunkel, H.G., and Grey, H.M. (1970). *Proc. Soc. Exp. Biol. Med.* **135**, 660.

79. Penn, G.M. (1972). Quoted in Natvig, J.B., and Kunkel, H.G. (1973). *Advan. Immunol.* **16**, 1.

79a. Seon, B.-K., Yagi, Y., and Pressman, D. (1973). *J. Immunol.* **110**, 345.

79b. Rudders, R.A., Yakulis, V.J., and Heller, P. (1973). *Amer. J. Med.* **55**, 215.

79c. Wolfenstein-Todel, C., Franklin, E.C., and Rudders, R.A. (1974). *J. Immunol.* **112**, 871.

80. Hilschmann, N., and Craig, L.C. (1965). *Proc. Nat. Acad. Sci. U.S.* **53**, 1403.

81. Dreyer, W.J. and Bennett, J.C. (1965). *Proc. Nat. Acad. Sci. U.S.* **54**, 864.

82. Milstein, C. (1967). *Nature (London)* **216**, 330.

83. Hood, L.E. and Ein, D. (1968). *Nature (London)* **220**, 764.

84. Brient, B. and Nisonoff, A. (1970). *J. Exp. Med.* **132**, 951.

85. Levin, A.S., Fudenberg, H.H., Hopper, J.E., Wilson, W.K., and Nisonoff, A. (1971). *Proc. Nat. Acad. Sci. U.S.* **68**, 169.

86. Nossal, G.J.V., Szenberg, A., Ada, G.L., and Austin, C.M. (1964). *J. Exp. Med.* **119**, 485.

87. Nossal, G.J.V., Warner, N.C., and Lewis, H. (1971). *Cell. Immunol.* **2**, 41.

88. Pernis, B., Forni, L., and Amante, L. (1971). *Ann. N.Y. Acad. Sci.* **190**, 420.

89. Kincaid, P.W., Lawton, A.R., Bockman, D.E., and Cooper, M.D. (1970). *Proc. Nat. Acad. Sci. U.S.* **67**, 1918.

90. Lawton, A.R., Asofsky, R., Hylton, M.B., and Cooper, M.D. (1972). *J. Exp. Med.* **135**, 277.

91. Pierce, C.W., Solliday, S.M., and Asofsky, R. (1972). *J. Exp. Med.* **135**, 675.

91a. Hopper, J.E. (1973). *Fed. Proc. Fed. Amer. Soc. Exp. Biol.* **32**, 989.

91b. Hopper, J.E., Noyes, C., Heinrickson, R.L., and Kingdon, H.S. (1973). *Clin. Res.* **21**, 581.

92. Tan, M. and Epstein, W. (1967). *J. Immunol.* **98**, 568.

93. Solomon, A. and McLaughlin, C.L. (1969). *J. Biol. Chem.* **244**, 3393.

94. Brient, B.W., Haimovich, J., and Nisonoff, A. (1971). *Proc. Nat. Acad. Sci. U.S.* **68**, 3136.

95. Sirisinha, S. and Eisen, H.N. (1971). *Proc. Nat. Acad. Sci. U.S.* **68**, 3130.

96. Sher, A. and Cohn, M. (1972). *J. Immunol.* **108**, 176.

96a. Spring-Stewart, S. and Nisonoff, A. (1973). *J. Immunol.* **110**, 679.

97. Hurez, D., Meshaka, G., Milhaesco, C., and Seligmann, M. (1968). *J. Immunol.* **100**, 69.

98. Seligmann, M., and Milhaesco, C. (1967). *In* "Third Nobel Symposium on Gamma Globulin" (J. Killander, ed.), p. 169. Interscience, New York.

99. Wilson, S.K., Hopper, J.E., and Nisonoff, A. (1971). Unpublished results.

100. Bordenave, G. (1971). *Ann. Inst. Pasteur, Paris* **120**, 292.

101. Sher, A., Lord, E., and Cohn, M. (1971). *J. Immunol.* **107**, 1226.

102. Wilson, S.K., Brient, B.W., and Nisonoff, A. (1971). *Ann. N.Y. Acad. Sci.* **190**, 362.

103. Hart, D.A., Wang, A-L., Pawlak, L.L., and Nisonoff, A. (1972). *J. Exp. Med.* **135**, 1293.

104. Hart, D.A., Pawlak, L.L., and Nisonoff, A. (1973). *Eur. J. Immunol.* **3**, 44.

104a. Pawlak, L.L., Hart, D.A., and Nisonoff, A. (1974). *Eur. J. Immunol.* **4**, 10.

105. Pawlak, L. L., Hart, D.A., and Nisonoff, A. (1973). *J. Exp. Med.* **137**, 1442.

106. Eichmann, K. (1974). *Eur. J. Immunol.* **4**, 296.

107. Ramseier, H. and Lindenmann, J. (1971). *J. Exp. Med.* **134**, 1083.

108. Binz, H. and Lindenmann, J. (1972). *J. Exp. Med.* **136**, 872.

108a. Ramseier, H. (1973). *Curr. Top. Microbiol. Immunol.* **60**, 31.

109. McKearn, T.J. (1974). *Science* **183,** 94.

109a. Lynch, R.G., Graff, R.J., Sirisinha, S., Simms, E.S., and Eisen, H.N. (1972). *Proc. Nat. Acad. Sci. U.S.* **69,** 1540.

110. Hannestad, K., Koa, M.S., and Eisen, H.N. (1972). *Proc. Nat. Acad. Sci. U.S.* **69,** 2295.

111. Yakulis, V., Bhoopalm, N., and Heller, P. (1972). *J. Immunol.* **108,** 1119.

112. Iverson, G.M. (1970). *Nature (London)* **227,** 273.

113. Janeway, C.A., Jr., and Paul, W.E. (1973). *Eur. J. Immunol.* **3,** 340.

114. Fraker, P.J., Cicurel, L., and Nisonoff, A. (1974). *J. Immunol.* **113,** 791.

115. Rodkey, L.S. (1974). *J. Exp. Med.* **139,** 712.

12

Theories of the Genetic Control of Diversity of Antibodies

I. INTRODUCTION

The basis of the variability of immunoglobulin structure has been alluded to in our discussions of amino acid sequences, allotypy, and idiotypy and is one of the most interesting problems in immunology. Whatever the ultimate answer, it is already evident that at least one aspect of the genetic mechanism is rarely encountered in biology; namely, the control of a single polypeptide chain by two genes. That additional unusual mechanisms are involved is predictable from the existence of a vast array of structurally related molecules with different antigen-binding specificities. There is no precedent for this among any other group of macromolecules. We will summarize here some of the current hypotheses and the relevant supporting arguments. Topics that will not be considered include cellular mechanisms in antibody biosynthesis and the properties of the immune response genes (1), which determine the capacity of an animal to respond to particular antigens.

At one time it was anticipated that the accumulation of sufficient data on amino acid sequences of V regions would elucidate the genetic basis of variability. Unfortunately, the data have by no means led to a consensus of opinion. A fundamental question concerns the number of V genes that are inherited in the germ line. At one extreme are those who believe that the experimental data support the inheritance of all V genes in the germ line. Another group of investigators holds that the number of inherited V genes is small and that the pool is diversified and magnified by somatic processes such as mutation or recombination. Although everyone in the field has thought about this question, a relatively small group of investigators has chosen to take sides, at least in print. Those who have proposed specific mechanisms have frequently done so with considerable ingenuity and have provided some of the most interesting reading material in theoretical immunology (e.g., 2–18). Each of the references cited has the additional merit of bringing together data in the literature relevant to the question of antibody diversity. A recent monograph by Smith (18) provides a thorough analysis of current theories.

It would not be practical to reproduce all the fine points of the arguments made by proponents of particular mechanisms. We shall try, however, to summarize some of the more cogent discussions. Before doing this we shall discuss RNA–DNA hybridization experiments, then briefly review other relevant data, much of which has been presented in detail in earlier chapters.

II. RNA–DNA HYBRIDIZATION

The measurement of RNA–DNA hybridization is a direct approach that may eventually establish the number of V genes in the germ line. (If the number of genes should prove to be small, a somatic mechanism for enlarging the pool would be necessary.) It is apparent from the range of antibody specificities that the number of different V genes expressed in a mature animal is very large. A minimum value would probably be several thousand and the actual number may be much higher. If the germ line theory is correct, all these genes would be present in every diploid cell. It is theoretically possible to estimate the number of genes by RNA–DNA hybridization. The approach being used is to isolate mRNA coding for the L or H chain from a mouse tumor producing large quantities of a myeloma protein (19–28a).[1] That such mRNA is active can be shown by its ability to mediate the production of the polypeptide chain in a cell-free system or in frog oocytes. By culturing the tumor cells in a radioactive medium or by trace-labeling with ^{125}I after isolation the mRNA can be obtained with a specific radioactivity high enough for hybridization experiments. Purification is facilitated by the fact that a large fraction of the mRNA in a typical mature plasma cell ($\sim 30\%$) is translated into immunoglobulin. A widely used method involves fractionation according to size; the length of the mRNA molecule varies with the size of the polypeptide chain it encodes. As a preliminary step, mRNA can be separated from ribosomal RNA by hybridizing the former to oligo(dT)-cellulose or to poly(U) (21,24); hybridization occurs

---

[1] This is only a partial list of investigations directed toward isolation of mRNA.

because a stretch of poly(A) is generally present on the 3' end of the mRNA strand, but not on rRNA. An important method, developed by Stevens and Williamson (27), exploits their discovery that mRNA for the H chain of a myeloma protein has affinity for that protein. (Details relating to the fine specificity have not yet been reported.) The mRNA is coprecipitated with the myeloma protein and antibody to the protein.

The mRNA for L chains has been reported to contain 850 (21), 1250 (26), or 1300 (28a) bases, rather than the 640 required to encode an L chain. Part of the difference is poly(A). In addition the polypeptide synthesized *in vitro* is actually larger than an L chain by at least 20 amino acids; a degradative process would be required to produce the L chain (19,21,24a,25,27a,27c).[2]

The percentage of DNA in the genome which is capable of hybridizing with radioactive mRNA can be estimated from the initial rate of hybridization in the presence of a large excess of DNA (28b). Possible sources of error include impurity of the mRNA, in particular the presence of unrelated RNA, capable of hybridization with irrelevant DNA on the strand containing the message. Also, in estimating the number of V genes, an important and unresolved question concerns the minimum degree of complementarity between the RNA and DNA that is required to permit the formation of stable hybrids. Coming from a plasma cell tumor, the mRNA for L chain is presumably homogeneous. The genes encoding V regions are necessarily heterogeneous. Assuming that the minimum complementary sequence needed for hybridization is 10–20 nucleotides, Delovitch and Baglioni estimated that the degree of amino acid sequence homology between L chains of the same V_κ subgroup is sufficient to permit hybridization of the mRNA for one L chain with the DNA encoding another L chain, but that hybridization involving different V_κ subgroups is less likely (22). A similar conclusion was reached by Leder *et al.* (28c) on the basis of known V_κ sequences and their experience in hybridizing globin mRNA with globin DNA from different animal species; they believe that stable hybrids would generally not form between mRNA for one V_κ subgroup and the V gene for another. Since the number of mouse V_κ subgroups is large (28d) the number of V genes may be grossly underestimated by this technique.

The data published so far are contradictory. Delovitch and Baglioni, who measured initial rates of hybridization to DNA of mRNA for mouse L chains, estimated that the number of V_κ plus C_κ genes is less than 40. Contrasting results were reported by Premkumar *et al.* (28), who utilized mRNA for mouse H chains, isolated as described above (27). The curve describing the rate of hybridization was found to be

---

[2] It is uncertain whether this occurs *in vivo*.

biphasic. The authors concluded that there are about 5000 genes which undergo rapid initial hybridization (because of the large number present). These were thought to be V_H genes. Another group of genes, which hybridize much more slowly, was believed to comprise C_H genes; an estimated total of about eight such genes was present. There is uncertainty in this interpretation because of the possible sources of error mentioned earlier, in particular the possible presence of additional stretches of RNA in the mRNA preparation, which might permit hybridization with DNA that does not code for immunoglobulin.

Subsequently, Honjo *et al.* (28a), using mRNA for a mouse κ chain, observed a reiteration frequency of only 30–50 DNA copies per genome. In contrast to the findings of Premkumar *et al.*, no highly reiterative genes were detected. The authors point out that the value they observed may be a minimum, since many V genes may have insufficient complementarity with the mRNA preparation to permit hybridization. They also note that at present the evidence that the 30 to 50 reiterated genes are indeed V genes is only inferential and that additional supporting data are needed.

When the mRNA was reverse-transcribed into DNA only half the message was copied (28a). The resulting DNA strand evidently included that portion which codes for the C_κ region since it cross-hybridized with mRNA coding for various κ chains. Using this material for hybridization the reiteration frequency for genes encoding C_κ was found to be three copies per haploid genome. This is consistent with genetic data which suggest the presence of a small number of C genes (Chapter 9, Section III,K).

In similar studies, Tonegawa *et al.* (28e) found that their mRNA preparation (specific for a mouse κ chain) hybridized with mouse DNA in a biphasic manner. About 20% appeared to hybridize with DNA sequences having a reiteration frequency of approximately 200 per genome. A major component, however, hybridized with sequences having a maximal reiteration frequency of less than 4. The authors were uncertain as to whether the 200 sequences represent V_κ genes, but favored the interpretation that they represented other types of DNA; i.e., they believe that their mRNA hybridized with fewer than four V_κ genes. On the assumption that hybridization would not occur with V_κ genes encoding nonhomologous V_κ subgroups the authors concluded that there is a very small number of germ line genes (perhaps only 1) for each subgroup.

It may be noted again that the presence of a small number of C genes and a larger number of V genes may necessitate a mechanism for uniting V and C pairs, since each V gene cannot exist in tandem with a C

gene in the germ line. The alternative, which seems less likely, is that joining occurs at the level of mRNA.

III. BASIC PREMISES RELEVANT TO THEORIES OF ANTIBODY DIVERSITY

In this section we will outline certain facts and concepts on which there is a general consensus of opinion and which provide a basis for various theories (to be discussed in the following section).

A. Clonal Selection

The clonal selection theory of Burnet (2) is now generally accepted. Small lymphocytes are known to have immunoglobulin receptors which are similar or identical to the antibodies that will later be synthesized by descendants of a cell. The receptors are believed to be produced initially without input of information from the antigen. The role of antigen is to combine with the receptors, thereby stimulating the differentiation and repeated cell division that results in the formation of a clone of cells, all producing the same antibody molecule. (The possibility of a switch within a cell, with respect to class of immunoglobulin produced, will be considered later.)

A selective rather than an instructive role for antigen was indicated by experiments that conclusively demonstrated that amino acid sequences control the three-dimensional conformation of the immunoglobulin molecule and its antigen-binding specificity. Thus, it was shown that an antibody molecule can regain its specificity after reduction of all disulfide bonds and complete unfolding in the presence of concentrated urea or guanidine (29,30). Upon refolding in the absence of antigen, followed by controlled reoxidation to reconstitute disulfide bonds, a substantial fraction of the original antibody activity was recovered; this indicates that the primary amino acid sequence controls specificity. (Similar experiments have been done with a number of enzymes.) More recent evidence, based on X-ray crystallography, indicates that many amino acids in the hypervariable regions of both the H and L chains make direct physical contact with the antigen when it combines with antibody (Chapter 5). These residues, which are widely spaced in the linear amino acid sequence, are brought into close juxtaposition during the folding process.

Another general premise of the clonal selection theory is that antibody molecules produced by a single cell are identical in structure, although it is possible that an occasional cell may produce more than one type of antibody molecule (31).

B. Two Genes, One Polypeptide

It appears that each polypeptide chain of an immunoglobulin is encoded by two genes controlling the V and C regions, respectively.[3] This property, which applies to very few proteins, was suggested by Dreyer and Bennett (5) when it became evident, from the amino acid sequence studies of Hilschmann and Craig (32), that a human κ chain comprises a variable and an invariant segment which are contiguous. Dreyer and Bennett proposed that there are multiple V_L genes and a single C_L gene (for each allotype), and suggested an insertion mechanism for connecting a member of the V_L gene pool with the C_L gene (Fig. 12.1).[4] Further support for the "two genes–one polypeptide" hypothesis is the association of different V region subgroups ($V_{\kappa I}$, $V_{\kappa II}$, etc.) with the same C_κ region (33). (It is generally agreed that each V_κ subgroup must be encoded by a different germ line gene.)

A related observation is the occurrence of the same V regions in association with different C regions (rather than the reverse). An example, first observed by Todd (Chapter 9) is the presence of the same allotypic markers of the *a* locus on H chains of different classes of rabbit immunoglobulins. The evidence is quite conclusive that the allotypic markers controlled by the *a* locus are on the V_H segment. Yet these markers are found in association with IgG, IgM, IgA, and with homocytotropic antibody (IgE). These findings are readily interpretable on the assumption that the *V* and *C* genes are separate entities and that a given *V* gene is capable of association with *C* genes controlling H chains of different classes. In addition, the same V_H subgroups, identified by sequence analysis, are found in association with the various heavy chain classes of immunoglobulin (Chapter 4).

Perhaps the strongest evidence supporting the concept of "two genes–one polypeptide chain" was the occurrence of two monoclonal proteins in the same patient (designated Til) with apparently identical V_H regions but different C_H regions (34). One protein was IgM and the other, IgG. Evidence for identity of the V_H regions of these proteins and

---

[3] Suggestions that separate genes may control the hinge region and individual C_H domains were discussed in relation to the proteins associated with heavy chain disease (Chapter 4, Section VII).

[4] Since all individuals possess λ chains with three or four minor variants of the basic sequence there actually must be at least three or four human C_λ genes.

RINGS OF NUCLEIC ACID
WITHIN CHROMOSOME

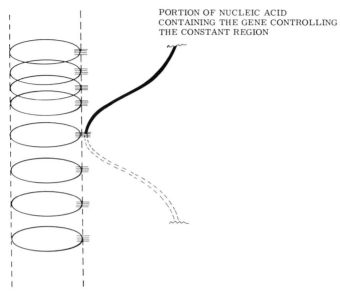

PORTION OF NUCLEIC ACID
CONTAINING THE GENE CONTROLLING
THE CONSTANT REGION

Fig. 12.1. Mechanism proposed by Dreyer and Bennett (5) to account for the existence of contiguous V and C regions in immunoglobulin polypeptide chains. Genetic material which codes for the constant portion of an L chain is inserted into that which codes for the variable region by a mechanism similar to the insertion of λ phage DNA into a bacterial chromosome. Current theories usually visualize the *V* genes as a linear array rather than as a series of rings, but there is no direct evidence on this point. Reprinted by permission of the authors.

of their L chains is discussed in Chapter 11, Section VIII. It is difficult to account for this observation on any basis other than the existence of separate *V* and *C* genes. Another early example of the presence of myeloma proteins of different classes, but with shared idiotype, was reported by Penn *et al.* (35), and a number of such cases have subsequently been documented (Chapter 11). In addition, Oudin and Michel have shown that IgM and IgG antibodies of the same specificity from an individual rabbit can share idiotype (36). Since idiotype must be a reflection of V region sequences, their observations on idiotype are consistent with the presence of the same V regions in association with C regions of different classes, and therefore with the hypothesis that there are separate *V* and *C* genes.

C. Switch in Class of Immunoglobulin Synthesized by a Cell; Translocation of Genes

To account for the data obtained with Til proteins it was proposed that a clone of malignant cells originally synthesized either Til IgG or IgM and that a switching mechanism occurred in one or more cells which repressed the gene controlling, say, C_μ and simultaneously derepressed the gene controlling C_γ. On the basis of these data and the shared idiotypic determinants in IgG and IgM discovered by Oudin and Michel, it was further proposed that a similar switching event occurs during *normal* immunoglobulin biosynthesis, i.e., that different cells of a single normal clone synthesize IgG and IgM (and perhaps other classes as well) and that the L chains and V_H regions of the molecules synthesized within that clone are identical (34). If, as seems probable (see below), the linkage of V and C regions takes place at the DNA level, this would require a relocation of the V gene from a position next to the gene encoding, say, C_μ to that encoding C_γ. This might occur by excision and reinsertion of the gene or by the formation of a loop, placing the V gene next to the appropriate C gene. A corollary of this proposal is that molecules of different classes made by the same clone of cells may have identical antigen-binding sites. The fact that the antigen-binding site is generally part of a major idiotypic determinant (37) lends additional weight to this hypothesis.

Although the nature of the switching, or translocation mechanism is obscure, it would appear that it involves only the expression of the C_H gene and does not affect the expression of the genes controlling the C_L, V_L, or V_H regions. The structural relationship between Til IgG and IgM and, hypothetically, between normal IgG and IgM from a single clone of cells is illustrated in Fig. 11.6.

D. Biological Evidence for a Genetic Switching Mechanism

A switch in biosynthesis, within a clone of cells, from one class of immunoglobulin to another class having the same antigen-binding specificity would be consistent with the "two genes-one polypeptide" hypothesis. Evidence for such a switch has been derived from experiments at the cellular level. Individual plasma cells from the bone marrow of patient Til were shown, with class-specific fluorescent antisera, to synthesize either IgG or IgM, but no individual cells producing both classes were identified (38). In a subsequent study it was found that 100% of plasma cells that were stained by fluorescent antiidiotypic antibodies directed to Til IgG were also stained by antiidiotypic antibodies prepared against Til IgM (39). Nearly all of the bone marrow plasma cells of the patient were stained by the fluorescent antiidiotypic reagents.

Early evidence for a switching mechanism was obtained by Nossal and co-workers (40). Single cell suspensions were made of lymphoid cells from rats that had been challenged with *Salmonella adelaide*. Antibody production by a single cell, isolated within a droplet, was monitored by measuring the capacity of the secreted antibody to immobilize *Salmonella*. If the antibody was inactivated by dilute mercaptoethanol, it was considered to be IgM; otherwise it was assumed to be IgG. Antibodies produced 2 or 3 days after immunization were IgM. At 4 days an appreciable number of single cells were making both IgG and IgM; at 14 days only IgG was synthesized. The secretion of both classes of immunoglobulin by a single cell 4 days after immunization was taken as evidence for a switching mechanism.

Pernis *et al.* (41) found, by fluorescence staining techniques, that an appreciable fraction of rabbit lymphoid cells (up to 15%) bear IgM on their surfaces but have IgG in their cytoplasm. In a heterozygous rabbit the surface IgM and internal IgG of a single cell are of the same allotype (*a* and *b* loci) (42). This supports the conclusion that the surface IgM is synthesized by the cell and is not absorbed from surrounding fluids. The authors concluded that their data are consistent with a switch, within a single cell, from the biosynthesis of IgM to IgG.

Evidence of another kind for a switch mechanism is derived from studies of suppression of immunoglobulin biosynthesis by the administration of anti-Ig antisera. For example, Kincade *et al.* treated 13-day chick embryos with goat anti-chicken IgM (43). When the chickens were subsequently bursectomized at hatching it was found that the biosynthesis of IgG, as well as IgM, was completely suppressed. Chickens not treated with anti-IgM, but bursectomized upon hatching, synthesize both IgG and IgM. The authors concluded that bursa cells synthesizing IgG arise exclusively from cells which had previously synthesized IgM, and which had IgM surface receptors through which the anti-IgM mediated its action. They further suggested that the switchover from IgM to IgG production does not normally occur in chicken peripheral tissues, as they could suppress IgM synthesis, without affecting IgG, in peripheral lymphoid cells.

Similar experiments have been carried out in other systems, both *in vivo* and *in vitro* (e.g., 44–46). Among the effects seen are suppression of IgG and IgA biosynthesis (as well as that of IgM) in the mouse by administration of anti-IgM and inhibition of a plaque-forming antibody response (both IgG and IgM) by incorporation of anti-IgM in culture medium. So far, suppression of IgM biosynthesis by anti-IgG has not been observed.

Such biological experiments do not in themselves provide evidence as to the structural relationship between the different classes of molecules. However, extrapolation of the data on dual myeloma proteins appearing in the same serum suggests that the various classes synthesized by a given cell line may share identical L chains and V_H regions.

We should note that some investigators are not satisfied that the existence of a switch mechanism, involving a change in class in immunoglobulin synthesized within a cell, has been completely established for normal cells; all of the evidence is indirect. We find it difficult, however, to conceive of an alternative mechanism, in the case of multiple myeloma, to account for the repeated occurrence of myeloma proteins of different classes but shared idiotype within the same individual.

E. Evidence for Joining of V and C Regions at the DNA Level

There are two types of evidence to indicate that fusion of V and C regions occurs at the level of DNA. First, there are data which suggest that V to C linkage does not occur between polypeptide chains. Second, there is support based on the occurrence of monoclonal proteins with unusual deletions, and on the *cis*-transcription of *V* and *C* genes, i.e., the utilization of *V* and *C* genes on the same chromosome in the production of an immunoglobulin polypeptide chain. These points are discussed below.

Evidence against joining of V and C regions at the polypeptide level has come from studies of the biosynthesis of both H and L chains (47,48). Although not definitive, the data are very suggestive. In principle, the experiments involve pulse-labeling of immunoglobulin-producing cells. The viable cells are exposed to short pulses (30 seconds to a few minutes) of tritiated leucine. The cells are chilled and lysed and the immunoglobulin is purified. The H or L chain is then cleaved into large fragments with cyanogen bromide or by an enzyme, and the gradient of radioactivity along the length of the chain is determined. For a chain synthesized as a single continuous unit the specific radioactivity of leucine should decrease from the C-to the N-terminus of the chain. In both sets of experiments the data fit this model fairly well but are not sufficiently precise for an unambiguous interpretation, owing in part to incomplete information on the amino acid sequences of the polypeptide chains, the leucine content of individual peptides, and the possible existence of intracellular pools, differing in size, of the chain segments.

The molecular size of mRNA capable of synthesizing L chains is also inconsistent with linkage at the polypeptide level (21,22,25,26,28a,

49), since the mRNA is large enough to encode the entire polypeptide chain; also a single homogeneous mRNA strand appears capable of mediating the synthesis of the entire polypeptide chain *in vitro*.

Perhaps the strongest evidence that a single message encodes both the V and C regions of an L chain is that of Brownlee *et al.*, who showed that a portion of the mRNA has a nucleotide sequence coding for the amino acid sequence which overlaps the V–C junction of the polypeptide (26).

Additional evidence for linkage of V and C regions at the DNA level is the existence of monoclonal H chains with large deletions. These are discussed in detail in Chapter 9, Section VII. In several instances the deletion involves a continuous stretch of amino acids comprising residues in both the V and C regions. While deletions of DNA are frequently observed, there are no known mechanisms for reproducibly deleting internal segments from mRNA or protein.[5]

Further support for the concept that V and C regions are not joined at the polypeptide level is derived from the studies of Mandy and Todd on allotypic markers present in individual rabbit γ chains (50). Utilizing antisera which recognize allotypic markers in both the V and C regions of the H chain (controlled by the *a* and *d* loci, respectively), they investigated the immunoglobulin of a rabbit whose parents were a^1d^{11}/a^1d^{11} and a^3d^{12}/a^3d^{12}, respectively; the rabbit was therefore of genotype a^1d^{11}/a^3d^{12}. The authors asked the question whether individual molecules have H chains only of the parental types (a1,d11 or a3, d12) or whether molecules of phenotypes a1,d12 and a3,d11 were also present. Nearly all the H chain population was found to be of one or the other parental type. This indicated that the sequence information for most H chains is derived from one chromosome. While not in itself conclusive, this experiment suggests that the fusion of V and C regions occurs in the genome, and is an intrachromosomal event. If joining of V and C polypeptides occurred, all combinations of allotypes might have been expected. Similar results were reported by Mage *et al.* (51), who used antisera specific for allotypic determinants on rabbit γ chains controlled by the *a* locus (V_H region) and the *e* locus (C_H region). Sensitive methods have, however, revealed the presence of a small percentage of polypeptide chains controlled by *V* and *C* genes on different chromosomes (Chapter 9).

---

[5] The deletion probably occurs after joining of *V* and *C* genes, since the joining mechanism must require recognition of the terminus of the *V* gene and the initial segment of the *C* gene. Also, a deletion in both the *V* and *C* genes before joining would require two separate genetic events and therefore is improbable.

F. Families of Genes

Genes controlling the immunoglobulins exist as three major groups or families. Members of each group are closely linked genetically to one another but not to genes comprising the other groups. They are probably present on separate autosomes. In the human, the families of genes are:

$$V_{\kappa Ia}, V_{\kappa Ib}, V_{\kappa II}, V_{\kappa IIIa}, V_{\kappa IIIb} \text{——} C_\kappa$$
$$V_{\lambda I}, V_{\lambda II}, V_{\lambda III}, V_{\lambda IV}, V_{\lambda 1} \text{——} C_{\lambda 1}, C_{\lambda 2}, C_{\lambda 3}, C_{\lambda 4}$$
$$V_{HI}, V_{HII}, V_{HIII} \text{——} C_{\gamma 1}, C_{\gamma 2}, C_{\gamma 3}, C_{\gamma 4}, C_\mu, C_{\alpha 1}, C_{\alpha 2}, C_\delta, C_\epsilon$$

There appears to be no restriction on the capacity of a V gene within a family to combine with any C gene belonging to the same family, but interactions between different families do not occur; e.g., no L chain has been detected which comprises a V_κ and a C_λ region. The most direct evidence for translocation, within a cell, of a V gene from one C gene to another, has so far been obtained for H chains; its occurrence in L chains is inferred on the basis of data already discussed.

The proportions of κ and λ chains vary, from 0 to 100%, among species (Chapter 7). The fact that κ chains are present in sharks and that λ chains are found in birds indicates that the $\kappa-\lambda$ divergence must have occurred at least 200×10^6 years ago.

G. Primordial Gene Encoding an Immunoglobulin Polypeptide Chain

Extensive studies of amino acid sequences have led to the suggestion that all immunoglobulins arose from a common ancestral gene about 330 nucleotides in length; i.e., large enough to encode a polypeptide chain of 110 residues. A common ancestry was suggested by Singer and Doolittle, who noted a similarity in the C-terminal segments of human H and L chains (52). Hill et al. observed a significant degree of homology ($\sim 25\%$) between a human C_κ and the rabbit $C_H 3$ sequence and also between the rabbit $C_H 2$ and rabbit $C_H 3$ domains (53). Many examples of such homologies, involving vertebrate species throughout the phylogenetic scale, have now accumulated (Chapter 7). The degree of homology between V_κ and C_κ or V_λ and C_λ is, however, marginal (about 15%), and the hinge region of the γ chain does not appear homologous to other segments of the chain. The genes coding for various classes and types of H and L chains, and the multiple C_H domains in a single H chain, are assumed to have arisen from the primordial gene by conventional genetic mechanisms of duplication and mutation.

H. Nature of the Amino Acid Substitutions in Variable Regions

Amino acid sequences have already been considered at some length. As a basis for discussion of theories of generation of diversity, we will briefly review here some of the patterns observed, using as an example the human V_κ region, which has been studied extensively. Milstein and Munro subdivide the types of substitutions observed in a V_κ subgroup into low-frequency variants, repeated variants, and hot spots (13). An example of a low-frequency variant is position 2 in human κ_{III} chains (terminology of L. Hood) where 17 of 18 proteins examined had an isoleucine residue and 1 had valine. An example of repeated variants is at position 10 in $V_{\kappa I}$ where 13 of 18 proteins had serine, 3 had threonine, and 2 phenylalanine. In the hot spots, or hypervariable positions, great variability is observed and no pattern has yet emerged. Among the low frequency and repeated variants a large proportion of the substitutions can be accounted for by a single base change in the nucleotide triplet encoding the amino acid residue.[6] In the hypervariable regions substitutions frequently require more than a single base change.

Most polypeptide chains belonging to the same V region subgroup have the same length, although exceptions occur (8,13).

I. Evidence for a Small Number of *C* Genes

The number of copies of genes for each C region (reiteration frequency) appears to be very limited. Evidence based on hybridization studies has already been discussed. Another type of evidence is the infrequency of crossovers. For example, no crossovers among genes controlling C_α and C_γ regions have been observed in mouse breeding colonies.[7] There have been only two reports of crossovers, involving V and C region genetic markers of rabbit H chains; crossovers in the region of the genome containing the various human C_H genes are also quite rare (Chapter 9), as are crossovers involving *V* and *C* genes in mice (Chapter 11). Strong evidence indicating that one or a very small number of genes controls a given human C_H region was the discovery of an individual whose serum contained a large proportion of IgG mole-

---

[6] When an amino acid is represented by more than one codon, the number of base changes is taken as the smallest value possible.

[7] A comparison of allotypes in wild and inbred mice suggests, however, that crossovers among genes controlling C_H regions of immunoglobulins may have occurred (although infrequently) in the natural population (Chapter 9).

cules with an H chain sequence characteristic of both IgG1 and IgG3 (Chapter 9, Section III). To explain this observation, Kunkel *et al.* (54) postulated that a mispairing of genes (unequal crossing-over) had occurred which resulted in the formation of a single gene encoding the C_H1 domain of IgG3 and the C_H2 and C_H3 domains of IgG1. A large fraction of the immunoglobulin of this individual consisted of such hybrid molecules. If there were multiple copies of each C_H gene, a single crossover event would be expected to affect only a small proportion of the immunoglobulin population. An individual possessing hybrid IgG2–IgG4 molecules has also been discovered (54a).

J. The Total Number of *V* Genes

Until the RNA–DNA hybridization experiments are clarified, one can only speculate as to the number of *V* genes in the germ line of an animal. The total number of different *V* genes would be greater than this value if somatic mutational processes take place; if so, the number might also be in a continual state of flux. It seems evident that the number of different *V* genes must be large to account for the enormous diversity of antibody populations with respect to specificity, affinity, and idiotype. The number of different antibodies, in the estimation of many observers, must be at least 10^5 and it may be orders of magnitude larger. As pointed out by Smith *et al.*, a total of 2×10^4 genes encoding H and L chains would occupy only 0.2% of the human haploid chromosome (8). A total of 10^4 V_H sequences and 10^4 V_L sequences could in theory give rise to 10^8 different antibody-combining sites. The potential number of genes that might be generated by somatic mutation is of course virtually unlimited.

An estimate of a *minimum* number of different V_L sequences can be made from the data of Quattrocchi *et al.*, who examined 52 monoclonal human κ chains and 50 λ chains by peptide mapping, and, when necessary by sequencing, and observed no identities (54b). From these results Smith *et al.* calculate that, at the 95% confidence level, there must be at least 400 different genes encoding human V_κ regions (8). (The data are of course not relevant to the question as to whether they are germ line genes.)

The number of *V* genes required would obviously be greatly reduced if a given H chain were capable of interacting with various L chains to form different, functional antibody molecules. We know that isolated H chains can recombine virtually indiscriminately with L chains, although preferential recombination with the autologous L chain is generally observed (Chapter 6). We have no information, however, as to what proportion of all possible H-L recombinants form useful molecules or whether the biosynthesis of an H chain of a particular structure within a cell places any restriction on the structure of the L chain that can be produced by the same cell; i.e., whether or not the biosynthesis of the two chains is completely independent.[8]

The number of V genes required could also be greatly reduced by the existence of antibody molecules of dual or multiple specificity. A few such examples are known. Thus, Schubert *et al.* observed that several mouse myeloma proteins, of 240 screened, showed activity against the Dnp group, as evidenced by precipitation with Dnp-protein conjugates, and also reacted with 5-acetyluracil or purine coupled to a protein carrier (55). These cross-reactions were surprising in view of the apparently unrelated structures of Dnp and the other two haptens. Eisen *et al.* found that mouse myeloma protein MOPC 315, which combines with ϵ-Dnp-L-lysine with an affinity of about $1 \times 10^7 \ M^{-1}$, also reacts with menadione, but with a K value about 15 times lower (56). Weaker cross-reactions ($K = 2-5 \times 10^4 \ M^{-1}$) were observed with 5-acetouracil caproate, caffeine, and riboflavin. These cross-reactions appear to involve the same active sites since the various compounds mentioned were capable of displacing labeled ϵ-Dnp-L-lysine from the myeloma protein.

Rosenstein *et al.* found that mouse myeloma protein 460, which reacts with both ϵ-Dnp-L-lysine and with 2-methyl-1,4-naphthaquinone 3-thioglycollate, can be modified chemically by various treatments so as to destroy one antibody activity but not the other (57). They postulated, therefore, that antibody-combining sites may be polyfunctional.[9] A more detailed discussion of their work, and further evidence for the polyfunctionality of the antibody combining site, is given in Chapter 10, Section XV. X-Ray crystallographic data indicate that the region of the active

---

[8] There is no evidence which proves that the biosynthesis of the two chains does not take place independently. It is of interest, however, that a large proportion of myeloma proteins of the IgG4 subclass are κ (58–60). This might be accounted for, without postulating biased synthesis, on the assumption that the C_κ and $C_{\gamma 4}$ regions interact with greater energy than C_λ and $C_{\gamma 4}$ and are therefore more likely to form a stable antibody molecule. A similar explanation might obtain for the preponderance of IgD myeloma proteins with λ chains. (The C_λ region of course interacts with the $C_H 1$ domain.)

[9] In searching for antibodies with dual or multiple specificity it is important to use myeloma proteins or homogeneous antibodies. The heterogeneity of normally induced antibody greatly reduces the possibility of demonstrating dual specificity; all antibodies in such a heterogeneous population react with the immunogen but only a small proportion might have specificity for any other individual antigen. This could account for the failure to identify multiple specificity in induced antibody populations.

site may indeed be large enough to accommodate unrelated small haptens in different segments of one site (Chapter 5).

Thus, evidence is accumulating that antibody molecules may be multispecific, and this concept is being widely discussed. Actually, it had been introduced on theoretical grounds in a remarkable paper published by Talmage in 1959 (60a).

Interesting data that may be relevant to this question were reported by Haimovich and du Pasquier, who worked with tadpoles, which possess a total of only 1 to 2×10^6 lymphocytes (61). They found that antibodies to the 2,4,6-trinitrophenyl or 2,4-dinitrophenyl group showed a degree of specificity comparable to those of animals possessing much larger numbers of lymphocytes. They estimate that the tadpole expresses at most 10^5 different antibody specificities at any moment. The authors suggest the possibility that a given cell or its progeny expresses different specificities at different times. (The rate of change would have to be substantial to account for the rapidity of the immune response in the tadpole.)

K. A Germ Line Gene for Each V Region Subgroup

There is general agreement among proponents of germ line and somatic theories that each V region subgroup must be encoded by at least one separate germ line gene. Molecules of each subgroup could otherwise appear in all individuals only through the same sets of parallel somatic mutations operating on a single gene; this seems highly improbable (6).

IV. THEORIES OF ANTIBODY DIVERSITY

The major theories describing mechanisms for the generation of antibody diversity, i.e., for V region variability, have themselves undergone evolution as more information on the structure and genetics of antibodies has become available. We will summarize several proposals in their current form and, in the next section, present arguments that have been made for and against these theories.

A. The Multigene Germ Line Theory

The multigene germ line theory, initially proposed by Szilard (3) and by Dreyer and Bennett (5) and espoused by Hood and Talmage (7), by Smith *et al.* (8,18), and by Garver and Hilschmann (16), proposes that a gene for each potential V region is represented in the germ line and that these multiple genes arose by normal processes of chemical evolution, i.e., by gene duplication followed by mutation and selection. The various V region families (V_κ, V_λ, V_H) need not have the same number of genes. Thus, the V region germ line genes are derived by the same mechanism that has been proposed for the generation of the various C region class and subclass genes. Mutations in V and C genes are selected during evolution on the basis of the capacity of the newly generated gene to encode a useful antibody polypeptide chain. According to the germ line theory the experience of one generation with respect to the efficacy of the various V genes is passed on to subsequent generations.

B. Somatic Mutation

Somatic mutation theories (2,3,10–15) postulate that the origin of diversity is a normal genetic event (mutation, deletion, insertion or recombination) which occurs in V genes at low frequency throughout the life of the individual. We will first consider mechanisms that do not involve recombination.

Proponents of somatic mutation believe that there is one or a very few stable germ line genes for each C region subclass and for each V region subgroup. Mutations may accumulate independently in single steps in each individual. The mutations of genes, proposed to occur over evolutionary time in the germ line theory, are postulated to take place within the lymphocytes of each individual of the species; i.e., each individual produces the necessary library of V region sequences *de novo*. In contrast to the germ line theory, in which selection acts at the level of the individual, the selective agent under somatic mutation acts upon cells. This agent is presumed to be exogenous antigen, which stimulates the expansion of clones of cells synthesizing L–H pairs that react effectively with that antigen. The probability of another mutation in the gene being expressed in the cell is then increased because of the expansion of the clone.

A question that arises in consideration of somatic mutation mechanisms is whether the hypervariable regions are true "hot spots" or whether mutations accumulate in these regions through some mechanism other than hypermutability. Some proponents of the theory prefer to assume that the rate of mutation is no greater in hypervariable regions than in the remainder of the V region, but that mutations of low frequency accumulate there because of antigenic selection, followed by expansion of the clone (e.g., 11,14); this mechanism would appear to be particularly wasteful of genetic material since many positions in the framework or nonhypervariable region are conserved and obviously cannot tolerate mutations.

C. Somatic Recombination

Hypotheses involving somatic recombination have been put forth by Smithies (62,62a) and by Gally and Edelman (15,63). The initial proposal of Gally and Edelman (63) has been modified somewhat, to permit recombination only between V genes belonging to the same subgroup (15). The data on sequences would argue strongly against recombination between members of different subgroups, since a comparison of κ chains has generally failed to reveal sequences containing the N-terminal region of one subgroup and the C-terminal region of another.

Gally and Edelman (15) proposed that there are clusters of V genes, encoding V_κ, V_λ, or V_H region subgroups. Each cluster evolved from a common precursor by gene duplication, unequal crossing-over and mutation. They suggest that a cluster might comprise 10–50 genes, a range much smaller than that required by the multigene germ line hypothesis but perhaps more than the minimum number needed if there is somatic mutation. During evolutionary time, mutations accumulate within the genes of each cluster, which are tandemly linked in the genome and are nonidentical. Somatic recombination occurs through the formation of an episome made up of portions of two adjacent V genes. The length of the episome is the same as that of a single V gene. The episome becomes circular, then migrates, and is inserted next to a C gene to form a single $V–C$ segment. During the insertion the circular episome is broken at a point next to the nucleotide triplet encoding the C-terminus of the V region. Variability is generated by using various portions of any two adjacent V genes. Cleavage, prior to reinsertion, must occur at the end of a triplet in order to avoid a frame shift. It should be noted that this translocation mechanism would also provide a means of implementing the switch in class of antibody that is proposed to occur within a single clone of cells.

D. Networks of Branched DNA

Smithies has proposed a model of the genome encoding immunoglobulin structure which deals with the problem of joining the same V region to different C regions and which allows for allotypic variation in the V_H region (as observed in rabbit immunoglobulins) (9). His model (Fig. 12.2) envisions an alternative configuration to the linear array of V_H regions postulated by the germ line theory. Smithies proposes that the DNA exists as a branched two-dimensional network. Thus, during transcription of the portion of the genome encoding the V_H region an RNA polymerase molecule would traverse a branched pathway rather

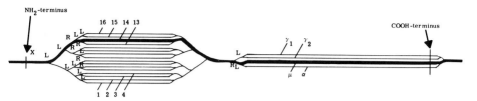

Fig. 12.2.   Illustration of the mechanism proposed by Smithies (9) for the generation of variability in V regions. The illustration shows a hypothetical locus for H chains with sixteen *V* genes (V_1 to V_{16}) and four *C* genes ($C_{\gamma 1}$, $C_{\gamma 2}$, C_{α}, C_{μ}). Each line represents a DNA double helix. Commitment to one of the possible proteins coded by the locus is determined by the random setting of its DNA forks in left (L) or right (R) configurations; X, represents a position at which allotypic variants could easily be found. The path of an RNA polymerase molecule is indicated by the heavy line; it would transcribe mRNA corresponding to V_{14}–C_{μ}. Note that the model provides for the sharing of the same V regions by different immunoglobulin classes and subclasses. Reprinted by permission of the author (9).

than the linear one characteristic of conventional transcription. At each branch point a randomly set switch would guide the polymerase into making a right or left turn. In the model shown in Fig. 12.2 the terminal segments of the gene are unbranched, thus providing invariant areas of the V_H polypeptide. A second branch point occurs along the chain where the C region (immunoglobulin class) to be synthesized is selected by a similar switch mechanism. Smithies also suggested a mechanism which would generate and replicate the network of branched DNA. For details the reader may consult reference 9.

E. *V* Genes Encoding Antibodies Directed to Histocompatibility Antigens

This is an interesting proposal, put forth by N. Jerne, that might explain the large concentration of antigen-sensitive cells directed against allogeneic histocompatibility antigens (12). The principal thesis is that the germ line *V* genes of an animal code for antibodies directed against histocompatibility antigens of the same species. Those lymphocytes in which mutations in *V* genes have not occurred are active against histocompatibility antigens. Lymphocytes synthesizing antibodies to self-constituents of the animal are destroyed or suppressed, unless their *V* genes have undergone mutations. These mutations result in the library of antibodies against foreign antigens. In the original proposal it was suggested that the mutations occur in the thymus. This would probably be modified now, insofar as humoral antibodies are concerned, since the latter are produced by B cells, which have not been processed by the thymus. Since the nature of the molecules conferring specificity to T cells is controversial, one cannot at this time decide whether Jerne's hypothesis is relevant to the diversity of specificities of those cells.

F. Partial Degradation of DNA with Subsequent Errors in Repair

As a mechanism of generating variability of sequence, Brenner and Milstein (64) postulated that the action of a cleavage enzyme and an exonuclease removes a portion of the DNA encoding an immunoglobulin polypeptide chain; this is followed by repair with error to generate a new gene. More specifically, they suggested that the initial cleavage occurs near the junction of the V and C genes, exposing a 3'-OH end. (This assumes that V and C genes are contiguous; to make this consistent with current thinking the deletion would have to occur after V–C joining.) An exonuclease then removes a portion of the V gene. The errors introduced during repair could be base-pairing mistakes or insertions and deletions. They suggest that the DNA strand repaired is not the one which is transcribed into RNA, and that the effect becomes manifest only after DNA replication and cell division. The initial cleavage was postulated to occur at the beginning of the C region, because the invariant nucleotide sequence would provide a consistent site of attack for the enzyme. The hypothesis therefore predicts that mutations should be more prevalent toward the C-terminal end of the V domain; this facet of the hypothesis has not been supported by data on amino acid sequences.

A modification of the hypothesis was put forth by Baltimore (65); it also involves cleavage and partial degradation of DNA, followed by errors in repair. Baltimore's hypothesis is based on the observation that the thymus of several species tested contains an enzyme, not found in most other tissues (66), which can add deoxyribonucleotides sequentially to a 3'-OH end in single- or double-stranded DNA. The nucleotide added does not have to be complementary to the second strand, and thus errors in repair might readily be introduced. After the addition of one or more nucleotides by this enzyme the DNA is repaired by the usual mechanism. It is further proposed that the sites of preferential initial cleavage by the endonuclease are adjacent to hypervariable regions. Since the enzyme is present in thymus cells, the proposal applies to the T cell recognition molecule, whose nature is uncertain. Baltimore states, however, that he has found a different replicative DNA polymerase in bursa (B) cells which also may make errors in repair (65). More recently, the presence of the transferase enzyme, first found in thymus, has also been reported in mouse plasmacytoma cells (66a), which are of B cell origin. (Its presence in B cells is still controversial.)

G. Episomal DNA Coding for Hypervariable Sequences

In 1970, T.T. Wu and E.A. Kabat compared the known amino acid sequences of a considerable number of mouse and human L chains and noted the existence of the hypervariable regions (67). The presence of hypervariable regions was subsequently established for H chains as well. To account for the hypervariability, Wu and Kabat suggested that these regions are encoded by short stretches of DNA which are inserted, like episomes, into the chromosomal DNA. This interesting hypothesis avoids the necessity of postulating the existence of "hot spots" in the DNA. Another possible explanation for the existence of hypervariable regions has already been discussed. It involves amplification of clones carrying mutations in those regions through interaction with antigen; additional mutations are then favored because of the large size of the clone.

V. STRENGTHS AND WEAKNESSES OF THE VARIOUS THEORIES

Nearly all arguments favoring one particular theory have been countered by alternative suggestions. We agree, however, with the proponents of somatic mutation that the localization of rabbit H chain allotypic markers to the V_H region provides very strong (although perhaps not decisive) evidence against the multigene germ line theory. This is one of the points to be discussed below.

A. Multigene Germ Line Theory

A relatively straightforward explanation for the diversity of V regions would of course be the inheritance of the relevant genes in the germ line. As already indicated, a few thousand V genes would not occupy a large proportion of a chromosome; and that there may indeed be a substantial number of V_κ genes in the germ line of the mouse is shown by the substantial number of V_κ subgroups already discovered (28c).

Hood and Talmage (7), Smith *et al.* (8), and Garver and Hilschmann (16) take the view that the germ line theory provides the simplest explanation for antibody diversity. In analyzing sequences within a human V_κ or V_λ subgroup, Hood and Talmage conclude that the nature of the variation is indistinguishable from that which occurs among the cytochromes c or hemoglobins of various species. (This comparison does not include the hypervariable regions of the immunoglobulins.) The similarities include the randomness of transversions (e.g., purine to pyrimidine) and transitions (e.g., purine to purine), and the tendency of G to mutate at a higher than normal frequency. They make the additional point that the substitutions which occur at a given position are very restricted; multiple substitutions might be expected to result from somatic mutation. (One might make the counterargument that only certain substitutions can be tolerated without disruption of the structure of the molecule.)

Another circumstance suggesting the presence of multiple germ line genes is the emergence of sub-subgroups as more proteins are sequenced; that is, linked substitutions along the chain in addition to those characterizing the subgroups. Each of these could well reflect an additional germ line gene.

Dayhoff (68), Hood and Talmage (7), and Smith *et al.* (8) have shown that it is possible to construct "phylogenetic trees" from V region sequences and that these closely resemble phylogenetic trees for sets of proteins (hemoglobins, etc.) that are related through evolution.

The method was first applied (to the cytochromes c of a wide variety of species, from *Neurospora* to man) by Fitch and Margoliash (69). The relatedness of two proteins of known sequence (mutation distance) is determined by the minimum number of nucleotide differences between the genes coding for the two polypeptides. A group of sequences (V_κ, for example), can be compared, and the mutation distance between every pair determined. A phylogenetic tree is constructed from these values in such a manner as to minimize total mutation distances among all proteins in the sample.

A simplified example is shown in Fig. 12.3. Proteins A and B are placed in the lower apex because they are most closely related. The length of the arm connecting B to the first apex (a hypothetical ancestor) is longer than that connecting A to the apex because B is more distally related to C. For details of construction of a tree using larger samples of proteins the reader is referred to reference 69. When the sample is large it becomes impractical to test all possible permutations in order to construct an optimal tree (containing a minimum total number of mutations) and a finite number of models is chosen for testing. In the case of the cytochromes c the tree generated entirely by computer analysis remarkably resembles the known pattern of evolution of species (69).

Mutation distances

	B	C
A	11	20
B		23

Resulting tree

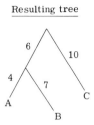

Fig. 12.3. Simplified illustration of the method of construction of a phylogenetic tree, according to Fitch and Margoliash (69).

A phylogenetic tree constructed by Hood and Talmage (7) from the first 20 N-terminal residues of 41 human κ and 23 λ proteins is shown in Fig. 12.4. Note that certain symbols, such as κI-III, represent hypothetical precursor molecules. (The actual structure of the precursor is predicted by the method.) The KL symbol in the figure is the hypothetical common precursor from which κ and λ chains are derived. The mutational distances shown on the tree would of course be much greater if the entire sequences were known and charted. More elaborate trees were subsequently constructed, on the basis of additional sequence data, by Smith *et al.*, who also present phylogenetic trees for mouse and human V_H regions (8).

In constructing a phylogenetic tree, the values for mutation distances are corrected for the statistical probability of back-mutations. For example, since the two mutations $x \rightarrow y \rightarrow x$, would not appear as a mutation at all, the number of mutations occurring during evolution appears, as a result of this effect, to be smaller than the actual value. A similar error can occur through a series of mutations such as the following:

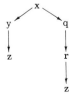

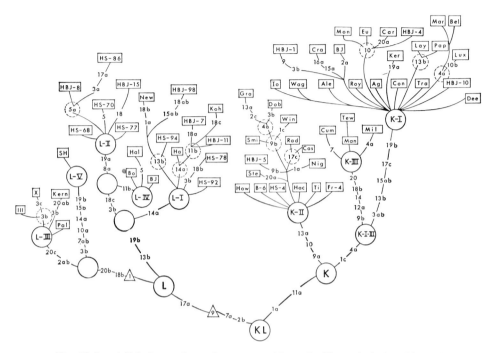

Fig. 12.4.   A "phylogenetic tree" constructed from the N-terminal 20 residues of 41 κ and 23 λ proteins by the method of Fitch and Margoliash (69), which reduces the number of mutations to a minimum. The 64 proteins are indicated by closed rectangles. Deletions are indicated by triangles and mutations by numbers. The letters a, b, or c indicate whether the first, second, or third nucleotide in the triplet is changed. Closed circles indicate L chain types of major V region subgroups. Dotted circles indicate subdivisions of the V region subgroups or highly improbable identical somatic mutations occurring in different individuals. Reprinted, by permission, from Hood and Talmage (7).

Complexities in constructing phylogenetic trees also arise when complete sequences are not known, or when two homologous proteins differ in length, necessitating arbitrary insertions or deletions for optimal alignment. These factors are taken into consideration in estimating values for mutation distances that appear on the tree.

On occasion the choice of a particular genealogy, used in constructing the tree, leads to insertion of a particular protein at a position less suitable than would be required by another genealogy, i.e., by a tree having a different structure. This is referred to as a "dislocation." Smith *et al.* state that somatic recombination among germ line genes (even those coding for a single subgroup) would tend to scramble genealogical relationships. They believe that the number of dislocations generated by somatic recombination would be much greater than the actual number observed.

1. WASTAGE OF GENETIC MATERIAL

A major objection raised against the germ line theory is that it is hard to conceive of an efficient system of evolution that would result in a useful library of V genes. If a very large array of genes has arisen as a result of repeated duplication and mutation, it is difficult to understand how genes that are ineffective, i.e., that encode a nonfunctional or useless polypeptide chain, can be eliminated by natural selection. (One can, of course, readily visualize preservation of useful genes.) The accumulation of useless genetic material in the germ line is perhaps more difficult to accept than its appearance in relatively short-lived lymphocytes, as required by somatic mutation.

2. PRESENCE OF ALLOTYPIC MARKERS IN THE V REGIONS OF RABBIT H CHAINS

One of the strongest arguments against the germ line theory is based on the presence of allotypic markers in rabbit V_H regions. It is well established that allotypic determinants controlled by the a locus, and by other loci, x and y, controlling a-negative molecules, are present on the Fd segment of rabbit H chains. It seems quite certain that these determinants are localized to V_H regions (Chapter 9). This poses a serious objection to the germ line theory. Suppose there were hundreds or thousands of genes encoding the V_H region of a given allotype. In a heterozygous a^1,a^2 rabbit one chromosome would carry a large number of a^1 genes and the other chromosome a comparable number of a^2 genes. During meiosis there would presumably be a high probability of a crossover leading to the formation of a chromosome carrying a^1 and a^2 genes. If this rabbit now were mated to an a^3,a^3 partner, some of the offspring would be phenotypically a1,a2,a3. With very rare exceptions (Chapter 9), no one has observed the presence of more than two allotypic markers controlled by the a locus in an individual rabbit, although thousands have been screened.[9a] This fact provides one of the strongest arguments against the multigene germ line theory. Proponents of the theory must postulate a special mechanism to prevent the occurrence of crossovers in a large, presumably linear array of genes. Smith *et al.* (8) present several possibilities to explain these data in the light of the germ line theory. One suggestion is that the a locus markers are actually not allelic but that each rabbit possesses multiple genes representing each of the three "allotypic" groups, which in actuality, are subgroups. What is inherited, according to his view, are two allelic regulatory genes,[10] which permit

---

[9a] This statement must be qualified because of recent data (see *Note added in proof,* p. 406). This weakens the argument against the germ line theory.

[10] One type of hypothetical regulatory gene would control the function of linking a V_H gene to a C_H gene, and would be specific for one V_H subgroup (8).

the expression of only one *V* gene on each chromosome. The absence of crossovers among the structural *a* locus genes would be explained on the basis that they are not allelic.

An alternative possibility (8) is that, by some special mechanism, interchromosomal crossing-over is prevented from occurring in this part of the rabbit genome. A third possibility is that three geographically isolated populations of rabbits evolved the three sets of genes independently, and that these are not true alleles and therefore do not cross over.

It should be noted that the existence of the *a* locus allotypes on V_H regions presents no major obstacle to the somatic mutation theory.

3. SPECIES-SPECIFIC AMINO ACID RESIDUES

Another focus of discussion, first considered by Doolittle (70), is the presence of amino acid residues at certain positions that are characteristic of a species. The term "species-specific" residue will be used to denote amino acid residues which are present at a given position in a V region (V_L or V_H) of one species but not another. In some instances a residue may be found in only one V region subgroup of a species but not at all in another species. Such a residue will still be referred to as "species-specific" despite its absence from some immunoglobulins of the species in which it is found. Capra *et al.* (71) prefer the term, "phylogenetically associated," to "species-specific" residue since closely related species often possess the same characteristic residue at a given position.

To illustrate this point, nearly all human λ chains investigated have proline at position 8, whereas glutamic acid or glutamine is present at the same position in mouse λ chains. Impressive examples of the existence of "species-specific" residues are to be found in the data of Capra *et al.* on V_{HIII} sequences, up to position 24, in various mammalian species (71). It was feasible to obtain these results with pooled, normal IgG fractions because of the remarkably small degree of heterogeneity of V_{HIII} sequences outside hypervariable regions and because nearly all proteins of the V_{HIII} subgroup possess an unblocked N-terminus.[11]

Capra *et al.* found that all mouse IgG molecules of the V_{HIII} subgroup have lysine at position 19 where each of 8 other species tested has arginine. Only the mouse and seal have lysine at position 3, where the other species examined have glutamine. In four of the species, glycine is present at position 10, whereas six other species have aspartic

---

[11] About two-thirds of the species investigated (all mammals) have unblocked H chains, comprising from 19 to 100% of the H chain population. Unblocked H chains were always homologous to human V_{HIII} in sequence.

acid at this position. Only the opposum (the only pouched mammal investigated) has isoleucine at position 2. Their data provide several other examples of distinct interspecies differences. Residues found in the normal V_{HIII} pool of a species were also present in V_{HIII} myeloma proteins of the same species.

As first pointed out by Doolittle, and supported by Capra *et al.*, such observations are difficult to reconcile with the multigene germ line theory (70,71). If the theory were correct it would seem necessary, during generation of a new species, that many *V* genes in a large array undergo the same mutations, in order to account for the existence of species-specific residues; this would require an unusual mechanism (see below). Capra *et al.* do not, however, argue against the possibility of limited duplication of *V* genes. (Duplication, followed by mutation of *C* genes is generally assumed to account for the existence of subclasses of IgG, whose patterns may differ markedly among even closely related species.)

In defense of the multigene theory, Smith *et al.* invoke either of two possible mechanisms, gene expansion or coevolution, to allow for the presence of species-specific residues in multigene systems (8). The gene expansion and contraction model postulates homologous but unequal crossing-over to expand or contract the number of related genes on a given chromosome. It assumes that, as a result of gene contraction, at some time during the evolution of a new species only a small number of genes of a given subgroup may be present. A mutation at a given position in one of the genes could be magnified by subsequent gene expansion so that most germ line genes would then carry that mutation, which would now encode a species-specific amino acid residue. Evolutionary selection pressures would favor retention of this gene, and its further expansion, if the mutation in question improved the viability of the newly emerging species. Smith *et al.* cite known examples of gene expansion and contraction to support their hypothesis.

As defined, gene expansion and contraction do not necessarily require large changes in the total amount of genetic material coding for V region sequences; one segment of the relevant portion of the genome might expand at the expense of another segment, leaving the total content of DNA encoding V regions about the same.

In the coevolution model multiple germ line genes evolve in parallel, with similar mutations occurring in many genes. Groups of genes that encode different V region subgroups follow different independent pathways. Species-specific residues would then arise as one line diverges from another. The mutations would not be entirely parallel since different genes in the same subgroup encode sequences that differ at various positions. Genetic mechanisms that would permit such spreading of favorable mutations are discussed by Callan (72) and by Gally and Edelman (15).

The existence of species-specific residues is, of course, less difficult to reconcile with somatic mutation than with the multigene theory. If there were, for example, only one germ line gene per V region subgroup, a single mutation at a given locus occurring within a species could result in the presence of a species-specific residue (although substitutions might occur through somatic mutation).

4. INHERITANCE OF THE CAPACITY TO SYNTHESIZE ANTIBODIES OF A GIVEN IDIOTYPIC SPECIFICITY

This phenomenon, discovered by Cohn *et al.* (73) and by Eichmann and Kindt (74), in their investigations of inbred mice and rabbit families, respectively, is discussed at some length in Chapter 11. A number of examples has been reported for inbred mice, where certain idiotypes appear regularly in association with the antibody of a particular specificity in some strains but not in others. These data strongly suggest that different outbred rabbits, or different mouse strains, differ with respect to their complement of germ line V genes. The data do not appear, however, to rule out somatic mutation processes. The cross-reactive idiotype might still appear by virtue of a small number of mutations of germ line genes (V_L and/or V_H), which would take place by a random process in most or all members of the strain. Also, even if cross-reactive idiotypes reflect germ line genes, this would not rule out somatic processes for the production of other idiotypes, which are not cross-reactive within a strain. Such noncross-reactive idiotypes are not uncommon (Chapter 11).

B. Somatic Mutation

Objections to the theory of multiple germ line genes, discussed in the previous section are, in a sense, arguments favoring its leading contenders, the somatic mutation and somatic recombination theories.

Somatic mutation is obviously conservative of genetic material in the germ line and is capable of generating a broad diversity of antibodies — perhaps much broader than that obtainable in a germ line. A major difficulty is that somatic mutation must involve considerable wastage of cells. Random mutations would inevitably lead to the production of a large proportion of antibody-like molecules which do not have a specificity useful to the host. It is also possible that many L and H chain pairs would not be capable of interacting with one another to form a stable molecule or a useful combining site. If, as seems likely, a precursor lymphocyte carries only one type of antibody receptor molecule, the wastefulness in terms of the cell population could be very great. Nevertheless, the lymphocyte population may be large enough to provide the necessary specificities, even if a large majority of the cells possess receptors that are never called into play.

Another difficulty arising from the somatic mutation theory concerns the conservation of allotypic determinants in rabbit V_H regions. Certain positions must be incapable of mutation to account for the presence of allotypic markers controlled by the a, x, or y loci on all or nearly all rabbit H chains.

Smith *et al.* (8) believe that patterns of amino acid sequences in L chains of human myeloma proteins are difficult to reconcile with somatic mutation of a small number of germ line genes. Consider myeloma proteins from different individuals with L chains of the $V_{\kappa I}$ subgroup. The "genealogy" of amino acid sequences indicate that all are derived from some common ancestral gene. The existing sequences indicate the presence of mutations (from an ancestral gene) which are common to some sequences but not to others. To illustrate this point:

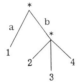

Sequences numbered 2, 3, and 4 (but not 1) have in common the mutations represented by branch b. This can readily be reconciled with mutations in a germ line; but since myeloma proteins arise separately in each individual it is difficult to understand how those individuals with sequences 2, 3, and 4 could share the mutations along branch b, i.e., how the same set of mutations could occur in each of the three individuals. This objection can be overcome by increasing the number of germ line genes for V region subgroups; i.e., by postulating different germ line genes for sequences denoted by asterisks in the illustration above. This becomes more difficult in dealing with an actual phylogenetic tree for $V_{\kappa I}$ sequences, where a number of branch points are encountered. The phylogenetic tree might also be reconciled with somatic mutation by postulating the existence of some type of somatic selection process which mimics normal protein evolution. These points are elaborated by Smith *et al.* (8) and by Smith (18).

Arguments based on the repeated occurrence in inbred mice of monoclonal proteins with similar or identical V regions are discussed in Section VI.

C. Somatic Recombination

Smith *et al.* (8) raise objections to the theory of somatic recombination. One is that they are unable to find evidence for crossovers within members of a subgroup, except near the C-terminus of V_κ. Second, as already indicated, they state that recombination would introduce severe dislocations, which are not observed, in phylogenetic trees. Finally they argue that if 10–50 recombining genes are present in each subgroup, the total number begins to approach that required by germ line models; the theory would therefore be subject to objections similar to those mounted against the germ line theory.

D. Episomes Coding for Hypervariable Regions

As discussed in Section IV,G the existence of episomes encoding hypervariable regions would account for the unusual pattern of amino acid substitutions seen in those regions (67). Where a large library of episomes would be stored in the cell and how they would be mobilized are difficult questions to answer on the basis of known genetic mechanisms.

Arguing for such a possibility is the demonstration by Kindt *et al.* (75) that different antistreptococcal antibody molecules, produced within the same rabbit, may share idiotype but differ with respect to V_H subgroup, as evidenced by the presence or absence of allotypic markers controlled by the *a* locus. Episomal insertions could account for these data. Additional support for this concept is the observation by Hopper (76) of shared idiotype in monoclonal proteins produced by the same individual; one protein is IgM(λ) and the other, IgG(κ).

VI. REPEATED OCCURRENCE OF MONOCLONAL PROTEINS WITH IDENTICAL V REGIONS

The data to be discussed here are relevant to current thinking on the subject of antibody diversity but do not in our estimation provide strong supporting evidence for or against germ line or somatic models.

Investigations of the structure of monoclonal proteins have revealed the repeated occurrence of polypeptide chains with identical structure. For example, several monoclonal λ chains, derived from individual BALB/c mice bearing plasma cell tumors, have been shown to possess identical amino acid sequences. These identical λ chains occurred in combination with H chains of different classes or as free Bence Jones proteins (77–79). In addition to eight identical λ chains, four others were found which differed in sequence in the V region by 1–3 amino acid residues (1–4 nucleotide interchanges in the DNA). All interchanges occurred in the hypervariable regions of the chain (near positions 30, 50 or 95) (78, 79).

Capra and Kunkel found that two patients with the benign disease, hypergammaglobulinemic purpura, had high titers of a monoclonal antiglobulin (IgG1, $V_{\kappa 1}$) (80,80a). The L chains of the proteins from two individuals had identical sequences through residue 40; at five of these positions each had an amino acid residue not encountered previously at that position in human κ chains. In addition their peptide maps were identical. This suggests that the remainder of the V regions may also prove to be identical. Striking similarities, although so far no identities, have been observed (81) among H or L chain sequences of certain human antiglobulins and cold agglutinins that exhibit cross-idiotypic specificity.

A number of examples of the sharing of idiotype by antibodies of the same specificity elicited in partially inbred rabbits or in inbred mice are discussed in Chapter 11. These results demonstrate the repeated occurrence of very similar or identical sequences in different animals of the same inbred family group or strain.

Proponents of the multigene germ line theory would argue that each shared sequence or idiotype reflects a separate germ line gene. To explain the limited number of variations in λ chains Smith *et al.* postulate that the mouse V_λ locus is small because its expansion began relatively recently (8). (In support of this concept is the fact that only about 3 to 5% of the L chains in the mouse are λ.) The exclusive occurrence of replacements in the hypervariable regions would be attributed to natural selection of such mutations, which alter the specificity of the antibody molecule so that different antigens in the environment can be recognized.

M. Cohn, who advocates somatic mutation, interprets the identical λ chain sequences as expressions of the same germ line gene, which he calls λ_0 (11). He postulates that the BALB/c mouse has a very small number of germ line genes controlling the V_λ region and that λ chains with different sequences arise through somatic mutation.[12] A lymphocyte synthesizing the variant will be stimulated if the receptor can recognize an antigen to which the animal is exposed. The relatively low frequency of occurrence of monoclonal mouse κ chains with identical sequences is attributed to the presence of a larger number of V_κ germ line genes.

The observation that identical myeloma proteins are very rare in humans was ascribed to the fact that, typically, a human is about 50 years old, whereas a mouse is less than 1 year old when afflicted with multiple myeloma (11). During the 50-year period a large number of structural variants might arise as a result of sequential mutations.

As suggested above, the repeated occurrence of certain idiotypes in inbred mice could reflect the presence of a germ line gene for each idiotype or, alternatively, could indicate that the relevant genes are related to germ line genes through a small number of mutations, which occur through a random somatic process in almost every mouse of that strain. If, in addition, the gene encodes a polypeptide chain of an immunoglobulin which reacts with an antigen that is prevalent in the animal species, clonal expansion would result in the regular appearance of the corresponding immunoglobulin molecule.

REFERENCES

1. McDevitt, H.O. and Benacerraf, B. (1969). *Advan. Immunol.* **11**, 31.
2. Burnet, M. (1959). "The Clonal Selection Theory of Acquired Immunity." University Press, Cambridge, England.
3. Lederberg, J. (1959). *Science* **129**, 1649.
4. Szilard, L. (1960). *Proc. Nat. Acad. Sci. U.S.* **46**, 293.
5. Dreyer, W.J. and Bennett, J.C. (1965). *Proc. Nat. Acad. Sci. U.S.* **54**, 864.
6. Hood, L., Gray, W.R., Sanders, B.G., and Dreyer, W.J. (1967). *Cold Spring Harbor Symp. Quant. Biol.* **32**, 133.
7. Hood, L.E. and Talmage, D.W. (1970). *Science* **168**, 325.
8. Smith, G.P., Hood, L., and Fitch, W.M. (1971). *Annu. Rev. Biochem.* **40**, 969.
9. Smithies, O. (1970). *Science* **169**, 882.
10. Lennox, E.S. and Cohn, M. (1967). *Annu. Rev. Biochem.* **36**, 365.
11. Cohn, M. (1971). *Ann. N.Y. Acad. Sci.* **190**, 529.
12. Jerne, N.K. (1971). *Eur. J. Immunol.* **1**, 1.
13. Milstein, C. and Munro, A.J. (1970). *Annu. Rev. Microbiol.* **24**, 335.
14. Milstein, C. and Pink, J.R.L. (1970). *Progr. Biophys. Mol. Biol.* **21**, 209.
15. Gally, J.A. and Edelman, G.M. (1972). *Annu. Rev. Genet.* **6**, 1.
16. Garver, F.A. and Hilschmann, N. (1971). *FEBS Lett.* **16**, 128.
17. Pink, R., Wang, A-C., and Fudenberg, H.H. (1971). *Annu. Rev. Med.* **22**, 145.

[12] The mouse myeloma protein, MOPC 315, differs considerably with respect to sequence in the C_λ region, indicating the presence of at least two C_λ genes (82).

18. Smith, G.P. (1973). "The Variation and Adaptive Expression of Antibodies." Harvard Univ. Press, Cambridge, Massachusetts.
19. Stavnezer, J. and Huang, R.C.C. (1971). *Nature New Biol.* **230**, 172.
20. Brownlee, G.G., Harrison, T.M., Mathews, M.B., and Milstein, C. (1972). *FEBS Lett.* **23**, 244.
21. Swan, D., Aviv, H., and Leder, P. (1972). *Proc. Nat. Acad. Sci. U.S.* **69**, 1967.
22. Delovitch, T.L. and Baglioni, C. (1973). *Proc. Nat. Acad. Sci. U.S.* **70**, 173.
23. Storb, U. (1972). *J. Immunol.* **108**, 755.
24. Stevens, R.H. and Williamson, A.R. (1972). *Nature (London)* **239**, 143.
24a. Milstein, C., Brownlee, G.G., Harrison, T.M., and Mathews, M.B. (1972). *Nature New Biol.* **239**, 117.
25. Mach, B., Faust, C., and Vassalli, P. (1973). *Proc. Nat. Acad. Sci. U.S.* **70**, 451.
26. Brownlee, G.G., Cartwright, E.M., Cowan, N.J., Jarvis, J.M., and Milstein, C. (1973). *Nature New Biol.* **244**, 236.
27. Stevens, R.H. and Williamson, A.R. (1973). *Proc. Nat. Acad. Sci. U.S.* **70**, 1127.
27a. Schechter, I. (1973). *Proc. Nat. Acad. Sci. U.S.* **70**, 2256.
27b. Smith, M., Stavnezer, J., Huang, R.C., Burdon, J.B., and Lane, C.D. (1973). *J. Mol. Biol.* **80**, 553.
27c. Tonegawa, S. and Baldi, I. (1973). *Biochem. Biophys. Res. Commun.* **51**, 81.
28. Premkumar, E., Shoyab, M., and Williamson, A.R. (1974). *Proc. Nat. Acad. Sci. U.S.*, **71**, 99.
28a. Honjo, T., Packman, S., Swan, D., Nau, M., and Leder, P. (1974). *Proc. Nat. Acad. Sci. U.S.* **71**, 3659.
28b. Britten, R.D. and Koyne, D.E. (1968). *Science* **161**, 529.
28c. Leder, P., Honjo, T., Packman, S., Swan, D., Nau, M., and Norman, B. (1974). *In* Proceedings ICN–UCLA Symposium on Molecular Biology (C.F. Fox, ed.). Academic Press, New York.
28d. Hood, L., McKean, D., Farnsworth, V., and Potter, M. (1973). *Biochemistry* **12**, 741.
28e. Tonegawa, S., Bernardini, A., Weimann, B.J., and Steinberg, C. (1974). *FEBS Lett.* **40**, 92.
29. Haber, E. (1964). *Proc. Nat. Acad. Sci. U.S.* **52**, 1009.
30. Whitney, P.L. and Tanford, C. (1965). *Proc. Nat. Acad. Sci. U.S.* **53**, 524.
31. Mäkelä, O. and Cross, A.M. (1970). *Progr. Allergy* **14**, 145.
32. Hilschmann, N. and Craig, L.C. (1965). *Proc. Nat. Acad. Sci. U.S.* **54**, 1403.
33. Hood, L.E. and Ein, D. (1968). *Nature (London)* **220**, 764.
34. Wang, A.C., Wilson, S.K., Hopper, J.E., Fudenberg, H.H., and Nisonoff, A. (1970). *Proc. Nat. Acad. Sci. U.S.* **66**, 337.
35. Penn, G.M., Kunkel, H.G., and Grey, H.M. (1970). *Proc. Soc. Exp. Biol. Med.* **135**, 660.
36. Oudin, J. and Michel, M. (1969). *J. Exp. Med.* **130**, 619.
37. Brient, B.W. and Nisonoff, A. (1970). *J. Exp. Med.* **132**, 951.
38. Wang, A-C., Wang, I.Y.F., McCormick, J.N., and Fudenberg, H.H. (1969). *Immunochemistry* **6**, 451.
39. Levin, A.S., Fudenberg, H.H., Hopper, J.E., Wilson, S.K., and Nisonoff, A. (1971). *Proc. Nat. Acad. Sci. U.S.* **68**, 169.
40. Nossal, G.J.V., Szenberg, A., Ada, G.L., and Austin, C.M. (1964). *J. Exp. Med.* **119**, 485.
41. Pernis, B., Forni, L., and Amante, L. (1971). *Ann. N.Y. Acad. Sci.* **190**, 420.
42. Pernis, B., Forni, L., and Amante, L. (1970). *J. Exp. Med.* **132**, 1001.

43. Kincade, P.W., Lawton, A.R., Bockman, D.E., and Cooper, M.D. (1970). *Proc. Nat. Acad. Sci. U.S.* **67,** 1918.
44. Lawton, A.R., Asofsky, R., Hylton, M.B., and Cooper, M.D. (1972). *J. Exp. Med.* **135,** 277.
45. Pierce, C.W., Solliday, S.M., and Asofsky, R. (1972). *J. Exp. Med.* **135,** 698.
46. Manning, D.D. and Jutilla, J.W. (1972). *J. Immunol.* **108,** 282.
47. Lennox, E.S., Knopf, P.M., Munro, A.J., and Parkhouse, R.H.E. (1967). *Cold Spring Harbor Symp. Quant. Biol.* **32,** 249.
48. Fleischman, J.B. (1967). *Biochemistry* **6,** 1311.
49. Scharff, M.D., Shapiro, A.L., and Ginsberg, B. (1967). *Cold Spring Harbor Symp. Quant. Biol.* **32,** 235.
50. Mandy, W.J. and Todd, C.W. (1970). *Biochem. Genet.* **4,** 59.
51. Mage, R.O., Young-Cooper, G.O., and Alexander, C. (1971). *Nature (London)* **230,** 63.
52. Singer, S.J. and Doolittle, R.F. (1966). *Science* **153,** 13.
53. Hill, R.L., Delaney, R., Fellows, R.E., and Lebovitz, H.E. (1966). *Proc. Nat. Acad. Sci. U.S.* **56,** 1765.
54. Kunkel, H.G., Natvig, J.B., and Joslin, F.G. (1969). *Proc. Nat. Acad. Sci. U.S.* **62,** 144.
54a. Natvig, J.B. and Kunkel, H.G. (1973). *Advan. Immunol.* **16,** 1.
54b. Quattrocchi, R., Cioli, D., and Baglioni, C. (1969). *J. Exp. Med.* **130,** 401.
55. Schubert, D., Jobe, A., and Cohn, M. (1968). *Nature (London)* **220,** 882.
56. Eisen, H.N., Michaelides, M.C., Underdown, B.J., Schulenberg, E.P., and Simms, E.S. (1970). *Fed. Proc. Fed. Amer. Soc. Exp. Biol.* **29,** 78.
57. Rosenstein, R.W., Musson, R.A., Armstrong, M.Y.K., Konigsberg, W.H., and Richards, R.R. (1972). *Proc. Nat. Acad. Sci. U.S.* **69,** 877.
58. Terry, W.D., Fahey, J.L., and Steinberg, A.G. (1965). *J. Exp. Med.* **122,** 1087.
59. Schur, P.H. (1972). *In* "Progress in Clinical Immunology" (R. Schwartz, ed.), Vol. I. Grune & Stratton, New York.
60. Skvaril, F., Morell, A., and Barandun, S. (1972). *Vox Sang.* **23,** 546.
60a. Talmage, D.W. (1959). *Science* **129,** 1643.
61. Haimovich, J. and du Pasquier, L. (1973). *Proc. Nat. Acad. Sci. U.S.* **70,** 1898.
62. Smithies, O. (1967). *Cold Spring Harbor Symp. Quant. Biol.* **32,** 161.
62a. Smithies, O. (1967). *Science* **157,** 267.
63. Gally, J.A. and Edelman, G.M. (1970). *Nature (London)* **227,** 341.
64. Brenner, S. and Milstein, C. (1966). *Nature (London)* **211,** 242.
65. Baltimore, D. (1974). *Nature (London)* **248,** 409.
66. Chang, L.M.S. and Bollum, F.J. (971). *J. Biol. Chem.* **246,** 909.
66a. Penit, C., Paraf, A., and Chapeville, F. (1974). *Nature (London)* **249,** 755.
67. Wu, T.T. and Kabat, E.A. (1970). *J. Exp. Med.* **132,** 211.
68. Dayhoff, M. (1969). "Atlas of Protein Sequence and Structure," p. 29. National Biomedical Research Foundation, Silver Spring, Maryland.
69. Fitch, W.M. and Margoliash, E. (1967). *Science* **155,** 279.
70. Doolittle, R.F. (1966). *Proc. Nat. Acad. Sci. U.S.* **58,** 1195.
71. Capra, J.D., Wasserman, R.L., and Kehoe, J.M. (1973). *J. Exp. Med.* **138,** 410.
72. Callan, H.G. (1967). *J. Cell. Sci.* **2,** 1.
73. Cohn, M., Notani, G., and Rice, S.A., (1969). *Immunochemistry* **6,** 111.
74. Eichmann, K. and Kindt, T.J. (1971). *J. Exp. Med.* **134,** 532.
75. Kindt, T.J., Klapper, D.G., and Waterfield, M.D. (1973). *J. Exp. Med.* **137,** 636.
76. Hopper, J.E. (1973). *Fed. Proc. Fed. Amer. Soc. Exp. Biol.* **32,** 989.

77. Appella, E. (1971). *Proc. Nat. Acad. Sci. U.S.* **68,** 590.
78. Weigert, M.G., Cesari, I.M., Yonkovich, S.J., and Cohn, M. (1970). *Nature (London)* **228,** 1045.
79. Cesari, I.M. and Weigert, M.G. (1973). *Proc. Nat. Acad. Sci. U.S.* **70,** 2112.
80. Capra, J.D. and Kunkel, H.G. (1970). *Proc. Nat. Acad. Sci. U.S.* **67,** 87.
80a. Capra, J.D., Kehoe, J.M., Winchester, R.J., and Kunkel, H.G. (1971). *Ann. N.Y. Acad. Sci.* **190,** 371.
81. Capra, J.D. and Kehoe, J.M. (1975). *Advan. Immunol.,* in press.
82. Schulenberg, E.P., Simms, E.S., Lynch, R.G., Bradshaw, R.A., and Eisen, H.N. (1971). *Proc. Nat. Acad. Sci. U.S.* **68,** 2623.

Index